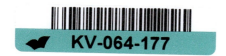

CANCER DRUG DISCOVERY AND DEVELOPMENT

SERIES EDITOR: Beverly A. Teicher, Genzyme Corporation
Framingham, MA, USA

For other titles published in this series, go to
www.springer.com/series/7625

Stem Cells and Cancer

Edited by

Rebecca G. Bagley, MS

Genzyme Corporation,
Framingham, MA, USA

Beverly A. Teicher, PhD

Genzyme Corporation,
Framingham, MA, USA

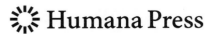 Humana Press

Editors
Rebecca G. Bagley
Genzyme Corporation
Framingham, MA
USA

Beverly A. Teicher
Genzyme Corporation
Framingham, MA
USA

ISBN: 978-1-60327-932-1   e-ISBN: 978-1-60327-933-8
DOI: 10.1007/978-1-60327-933-8
Springer Dordrecht Heidelberg London New York

Library of Congress Control Number: 2008944031

Printed on acid-free paper

Springer is part of Springer Science+Business Media (www.springer.com)

Preface

The recent surge in stem cell research has ignited a field of discovery into many human diseases including diabetes, neuropathologies, and cancer. Stem cell therapy is a promising approach to the treatment of many debilitating diseases to replace specific differentiated cells that have been lost or died. Although stem cells may provide therapeutic benefit under certain conditions, stem cells are often implicated in the initiation, progression, and therapeutic resistance of malignant disease.

This first edition of *Stem Cells and Cancer* is intended to give a current perspective on the role of stem cells in cancer and strategies for novel therapies directed toward tumor stem cells. Cancer stem cells remain a controversial topic and the criteria that define cancer stem cells are continuing to evolve. The current cancer stem cell hypothesis is presented in several chapters with distinctions made between the hierarchical and stochastic models of tumor cell development. "Stemness," self-renewal, pluripotency, clonality, and tumorigenicity are important concepts applied toward defining cancer stem cells. Signaling pathways such as Wnt, Sonic Hedgehog, Notch, and Bmi-1 that are involved in differentiation, proliferation, and survival are implicated in the malignant process. Additional chapters address the identification of cancer stem cell populations through the evaluation of molecular markers such as CD133, CD44, and CD24, for example, or by Hoechst dye exclusion to recognize "side populations." Mesenchymal and hematopoietic stem cells are described as well as mouse models that are employed to elucidate the properties and functionality of stem cells in cancer and the stem cell niche. This book encompasses a wide variety of human cancers that include but are not limited to leukemia, gliomas, breast, and prostate cancers. Resistance to conventional therapies, genetic vs. epigenetic changes that affect therapeutic response, and strategies to prevent disease recurrence are challenges that have been incorporated into this volume. *Stem Cells and Cancer* represents a compendium of cutting edge research by experts in the field and will be instrumental in the study of this intriguing line of investigation for many years to come.

Framingham, MA   *Rebecca G. Bagley*
Beverly A. Teicher

Contents

Contributors

ALISON L. ALLAN, PH.D. • *London Regional Cancer Program, London, ON, Canada Department of Anatomy and Cell Biology, University of Western Ontario, London, ON, Canada; Department of Oncology, University of Western Ontario, London, ON, Canada*

REBECCA G. BAGLEY, M.S. • *Genzyme Corporation, Framingham, MA, USA*

SURINDER K. BATRA, PH.D. • *Department of Biochemistry & Molecular Biology, Eppley Institute for Research in Cancer and Allied Diseases, University of Nebraska Medical Center, Omaha, NE, USA*

STEPHEN B. BAYLIN, MD • *Cancer Biology Division, The Sidney Kimmel Comprehensive Cancer Center, The Johns Hopkins University Medical Institutions, Baltimore, MD, USA*

JOHAN BENGZON, M.D., PH.D. • *Division of Neurosurgery, Rausing Laboratory, Department of Clinical Sciences, University Hospital, Lund, Sweden Lung Strategic Research Center for Stem Cell Biology and Cell Therapy, University Hospital, Lund, Sweden; Department of Pathology, Division of Neuropathology, University Hospital, Lund, Sweden*

KEITH L. BLACK, M.D. • *Department of Neurosurgery, Cedars-Sinai Medical Center, Los Angeles, CA, USA*

ANGELIKA M. BURGER, PH.D. • *Department of Pharmacology, Wayne State University, Karmanos Cancer Institute, Hudson-Webber Cancer Research Center, Detroit, MI, USA*

ANN F. CHAMBERS, PH.D. • *London Regional Cancer Program, London, ON, Canada; Department of Oncology, University of Western Ontario, London, ON, Canada; Department of Medical Biophysics, University of Western Ontario, London, ON, Canada*

LIANG CHENG, M.D. • *Department of Pathology and Urology, Indiana School of Medicine, Indianapolis, IN, USA; School of Medicine, Polytechnic University of the Marche Region, United Hospitals, Ancona, Italy; Department of Surgery, Cordoba University School of Medicine, Cordoba, Spain*

ALYSHA K. CROKER, B.Sc. • *London Regional Cancer Program, London, ON, Canada; Department of Anatomy and Cell Biology, University of Western Ontario, London, ON, Canada; Department of Oncology, University of Western*

*Ontario, London, ON, Canada; Department of Medical Biophysics,
University of Western Ontario, London, ON, Canada*

DARREL DAVIDSON, M.D., PH.D. • *Department of Pathology and Urology,
Indiana School of Medicine, Indianapolis, IN, USA*

ALBERT D. DONNENBERG, PH.D. • *Hillman Cancer Center, Research Pavillon,
Pittsburgh, PA, USA; Division of Hematology/Oncology, Department of Medicine,
University of Pittsburgh School of Medicine, Pittsburgh, PA, USA*

VERA S. DONNENBERG, PH.D. • *Hillman Cancer Center, Research Pavillon,
Pittsburgh, PA, USA; Department of Surgery, Heart, Lung, and Esophageal Surgery
Institute, University of Pittsburgh School of Medicine, Pittsburgh, PA, USA; Division
of Hematology/Oncology, Department of Medicine, University of Pittsburgh School
of Medicine, Pittsburgh, PA, USA*

JOSEPH DOSCH, B.S. • *University of Michigan Medical Center, Ann Arbor, MI, USA*

ELISABET ENGLUND, M.D., PH.D. • *Department of Pathology, Division of
Neuropathology, University Hospital, Lund, Sweden*

XIAOLONG FAN, M.D., PH.D. • *Division of Neurosurgery, Rausing Laboratory,
Department of Clinical Sciences, University Hospital, Lund, Sweden; Lung Strategic
Research Center for Stem Cell Biology and Cell Therapy, University Hospital, Lund,
Sweden*

KIMBERLY E. FOREMAN, PH.D. • *Breast Cancer Research Program, Cardinal
Bernardin Cancer Center, Loyola University Chicago, Maywood, IL, USA*

CHIARA GRISANZIO, M.D. • *Department of Pathology, Brigham and Women's
Hospital, Department of Medical Oncology, Harvard Medical School, Boston,
MA, USA*

BRETT M. HALL, PH.D. • *Integrated Biomedical Science Graduate Program,
The Ohio State University, Columbus, OH, USA; Center for Childhood Cancer,
The Research Institute at Nationwide Children's Hospital, Columbus, OH, USA*

NAOTSUGU HARAGUCHI, M.D., PH.D. • *Department of Gastroenterological Surgery,
Graduate School of Medicine, Osaka University, Osaka, Japan*

BIAO HE, PH.D. • *Department of Surgery, University of California San Francisco
Helen Diller Family Comprehensive Cancer Center, University of California San
Francisco, San Francisco, CA, USA*

XI HE, M.D. • *Stowers Institute for Medical Research, Kansas City, MO, USA*

MARY J.C. HENDRIX, PH.D. • *Children's Memorial Research Center, Chicago,
IL, USA*

SOFIA HONORIO, PH.D. • *Department of Carcinogenesis, Science Park Research
Division, University of Texas M.D. Anderson Cancer Center, Smithville, TX, USA;
Division of Nutritional Science, Department of Human Ecology, University of Texas
at Austin, Austin, TX, USA; Program in Molecular Carcinogenesis, Graduate School
of Biomedical Sciences, Houston, TX, USA*

JACLYN Y. HUNG, PH.D. • *Greehey Children's Cancer Research Institute, The University of Texas Health Science Center, San Antonio, TX, USA*

KEISUKKE IETA, M.D. • *Department of Surgery, Kyushu University, Medical Institute of Bioregulation, Beppu, Japan*

HIDESHI ISHII, M.D., PH.D. • *Department of Gastroenterological Surgery, Osaka University, Graduate School of Medicine, Osaka, Japan; Department of Surgery, Kyushu University, Medical Institute of Bioregulation, Beppu, Japan*

DAVID M. JABLONS, M.D. • *Department of Surgery, University of California San Francisco Cancer Centre, San Francisco, CA, USA*

STEFFEN KOSCHMIEDER, M.D. • *Department of Medicine, Hematology and Oncology, University of Munster, Munster, Germany*

CHEONG JUN LEE, M.D. • *University of Michigan Medical Center, Ann Arbor, MI, USA*

HANGWEN LI • *Department of Carcinogenesis, Science Park Research Division, University of Texas M.D. Anderson Cancer Center, Smithville, TX, USA; Division of Nutritional Science, Department of Human Ecology, University of Texas at Austin, Austin, TX, USA*

LINHENG LI, PH.D. • *Stowers Institute for Medical Research, Kansas City, MO, USA; Department of Pathology and Laboratory Medicine, University of Kansas Medical Center, Kansas City, KS, USA*

CHUN-PENG LIAO, PH.D. • *Department of Pathology, Department of Biochemistry and Molecular Biology, Keck School of Medicine, University of Southern California, Los Angeles, CA, USA*

GENTAO LIU, PH.D. • *Department of Neurosurgery, Cedars-Sinai Medical Center, Los Angeles, CA, USA; ImmunoCellular Therapeutics, Woodland Hills, CA, USA*

ANTONIO LOPEZ-BELTRA, M.D., PH.D. • *Department of Surgery, Cordoba University School of Medicine, Cordoba, Spain*

NAIRA V. MARGARYAN, D.V.M., PH.D. • *Children's Memorial Research Center, Chicago, IL, USA*

LUCIO MIELE, M.D., PH.D. • *Breast Cancer Research Program, Cardinal Bernardin Cancer Center, Loyola University Chicago, Maywood, IL, USA*

MURIELLE MIMEAULT, PH.D. • *Department of Biochemistry & Molecular Biology, Eppley Institute for Research in Cancer and Allied Diseases, University of Nebraska Medical Center, Omaha, NE, USA*

KOSHI MIMORI, M.D., PH.D. • *Department of Surgery, Kyushu University, Medical Institute of Bioregulation, Beppu, Japan*

RODOLFO MONITRONI, M.D. • *School of Medicine, Polytechnic University of the Marche Region, United Hospitals, Ancona, Italy*

MASAKI MORI, M.D., PH.D., F.A.C.S. • *Department of Gastroenterological Surgery, Graduate School of Medicine, Osaka University, Osaka, Japan; Department of Surgery, Kyushu University, Medical Institute of Bioregulation, Beppu, Japan*

MELIA G. NAFUS, B.S. • *Department of Biomedical Sciences, Cornell University, Ithaca, NY, USA*

ALEXANDER YU NIKITIN, M.D., PH.D. • *Department of Biomedical Sciences, Cornell University, Ithaca, NY, USA*

JOYCE E. OHM, PH.D. • *Cancer Biology Division, The Sidney Kimmel Comprehensive Cancer Center, The Johns Hopkins University Medical Institutions, Baltimore, MD, USA*

CLODIA OSIPO, PH.D. • *Breast Cancer Research Program, Cardinal Bernardin Cancer Center, Loyola University Chicago, Maywood, IL, USA*

BRYON E. PETERSEN, PH.D. • *Department of Pathology/Immunology & Medicine, University of Florida College of Medicine, Gainesville, FL, USA*

LYNNE-MARIE POSTOVIT, PH.D. • *Children's Memorial Research Center, Chicago, IL, USA; Schulich School of Medicine and Dentistry, University of Western Ontario, London, ON, Canada*

PAOLA RIZZO, PH.D. • *Breast Cancer Research Program, Cardinal Bernardin Cancer Center, Loyola University Chicago, Maywood, IL, USA*

JASON T. ROSS, B.S. • *Stowers Institute for Medical Research, Kansas City, MO, USA; Department of Pathology and Laboratory Medicine, University of Kansas Medical Center, Kansas City, KS, USA*

PRADIP ROY-BURMAN, PH.D. • *Department of Pathology, Department of Biochemistry and Molecular Biology, Keck School of Medicine, University of Southern California, Los Angeles, CA, USA*

LEIF G. SALFORD, M.D., PH.D. • *Division of Neurosurgery, Rausing Laboratory, Department of Clinical Sciences, University Hospital, Lund, Sweden*

DAVID H. SCOVILLE, B.S. • *Stowers Institute for Medical Research, Kansas City, MO, USA; Department of Pathology and Laboratory Medicine, University of Kansas Medical Center, Kansas City, KS, USA*

ELISABETH A. SEFTOR, B.S. • *Children's Memorial Research Center, Chicago, IL, USA*

RICHARD E.B. SEFTOR, PH.D. • *Children's Memorial Research Center, Chicago, IL, USA*

TOM SHUPE, PH.D. • *Department of Pathology/Immunology & Medicine, University of Florida College of Medicine, Gainesville, FL, USA*

SABINA SIGNORETTI, M.D. • *Department of Pathology, Brigham and Women's Hospital, Department of Medical Oncology, Harvard Medical School, Boston, MA, USA*

DIANE SIMEONE, M.D. • *University of Michigan Medical Center, Ann Arbor, MI, USA*

GILBERT H. SMITH, PhD • *Mammary Biology & Tumorigenesis Laboratory, Center for Cancer Research, National Cancer Institute, Bethesda, MD, USA*

LUIGI STRIZZI, M.D., PH.D. • *Children's Memorial Research Center, Chicago, IL, USA*

NICHOLAS J. SULLIVAN, B.S. • *Integrated Biomedical Science Graduate Program, The Ohio State University, Columbus, OH, USA; Center for Childhood Cancer, The Research Institute at Nationwide Children's Hospital, Columbus, OH, USA*

DEAN G. TANG, M.D., PH.D. • *Department of Carcinogenesis, Science Park Research Division, University of Texas M.D. Anderson Cancer Center, Smithville, TX, USA; Program in Molecular Carcinogenesis, Graduate School of Biomedical Sciences, Houston, TX, USA*

BEVERLY A. TEICHER, PH.D. • *Genzyme Corporation, Framingham, MA, USA*

DANIEL G. TENEN, M.D. • *Center for Life Sciences and Harvard Stem Cell Institute, Harvard Medical School, Boston, MA 02115, USA*

JASON L. TOWNSON, B.SC. • *London Regional Cancer Program, London, ON, Canada; Department of Medical Biophysics, University of Western Ontario, London, ON, Canada*

JUDITH A. VARNER, PH.D. • *Moores University of California San Diego Cancer Center, La Jolla, CA, USA*

ADAM YAGUI-BELTRAN, M.D. • *Department of Surgery, University of California San Francisco Helen Diller Family Comprehensive Cancer Center, University of California San Francisco, San Francisco, CA, USA; Department of Surgery, University of California San Francisco Cancer Centre, San Francisco, CA, USA*

JOHN S. YU, M.D. • *Department of Neurosurgery, Cedars-Sinai Medical Center, Los Angeles, CA, USA; ImmunoCellular Therapeutics, Woodland Hills, CA, USA*

SHAOBO ZHANG, M.D. • *Department of Pathology and Urology, Indiana School of Medicine, Indianapolis, IN, USA*

ZONGXIANG ZHOU, PH.D. • *Department of Biomedical Sciences, Cornell University, Ithaca, NY, USA*

I   INTRODUCTION TO CANCER STEM CELLS

1 The Cancer Stem Cell Hypothesis

Kimberly E. Foreman, Paola Rizzo,
Clodia Osipo, and Lucio Miele

ABSTRACT

The "cancer stem cell" hypothesis is receiving increasing interest and has become the object of considerable debate among cancer biologists and clinicians. This ongoing debate is focusing attention on the very definition of stemness and its significance in the context of a malignancy. From a therapeutic standpoint, the cancer stem cell hypothesis emphasizes the cellular heterogeneity in cancers, and the need to specifically target small cell populations that resemble tissue stem cells and are phenotypically different from the majority of cancer cells. Regardless of their origin, these cells divide slowly, have the ability to undergo asymmetric cell division and are highly resistant to conventional chemotherapeutics. These characteristics make them prime suspects as potential causes of disease recurrence and metastasis, which are the main causes of morbidity and mortality in oncology. This chapter provides an introduction to the cancer stem cell hypothesis, briefly summarizes the evidence supporting this theory and the aspects that remain controversial. Finally, we present a brief discussion of the possible therapeutic significance of cancer stem cells and the current efforts to target developmental pathways on which these cells depend.

Key Words: Cancer stem cells, Tumor-initiating cells, Stem cell niche, Targeted therapies

THE CANCER STEM CELL MODEL OF CARCINOGENESIS

For decades, the prevailing theory of cancer initiation and progression has been that cancers derive from the serial acquisition of genetic mutations by normal somatic cells. These mutations resulted in enhanced proliferation, inhibition of differentiation, and reduced capacity to undergo apoptosis. Each mutation would result in progressive "dedifferentiation" so that the tumor cells would continually lose their mature, tissue-specific attributes, and regress to a more primitive phenotype. As differentiated cells have limited life spans, it would be difficult for any given cell to acquire all the mutations necessary to become transformed, thus explaining the relatively uncommon occurrence of transformation. However, if initial mutations led to unrestrained proliferation, this would generate more cells that could potentially be affected by further oncogenic mutations. Once transformed, cancer cells would proliferate indefinitely and form a tumor where each viable tumor cell was in principle equally capable of forming a new tumor.

Recent findings suggest that this model may be overly simplistic. The "cancer stem cell hypothesis" has gained considerable interest in recent years *(1–3)*. This theory states that cells in a tumor are organized as a hierarchy similar to that of normal tissues, and are maintained by a small subset of

From: *Cancer Drug Discovery and Development: Stem Cells and Cancer,*
Edited by: R.G. Bagley and B.A. Teicher, DOI: 10.1007/978-1-60327-933-8_1,
© Humana Press, a part of Springer Science+Business Media, LLC 2009

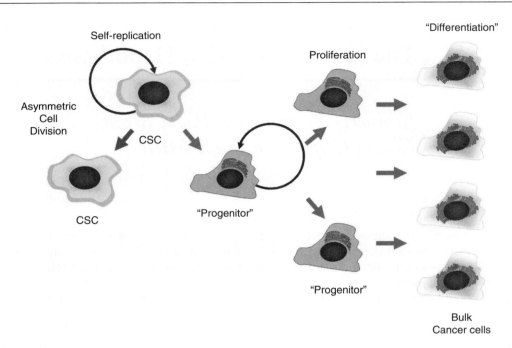

Fig. 1. The CSC hypothesis. CSCs are thought to maintain their numbers by slow self-replication, and produce other tumor cells by asymmetric cell division. In this process, cell division of a CSC generates a CSC and a transformed "progenitor-like" cell, which has limited self-renewal ability but are highly proliferative, similar to a transit-amplifying population in normal tissue. These progenitors give rise to more or less partially differentiated bulk tumor cells through a combination of proliferation and abortive differentiation.

tumor cells that are ultimately responsible for tumor formation and growth. These cells, defined as "cancer stem cells" (CSCs) or tumor initiating cells (TICs), possess several key properties of normal tissue stem cells including self-renewal (i.e., the ability of a cell to renew itself indefinitely in an undifferentiated state), unlimited proliferative potential, infrequent or slow replication, resistance to toxic xenobiotics, high DNA repair capacity, and the ability to give rise to daughter cells that differentiate. However, unlike highly regulated tissue stem cells, CSCs demonstrate dysregulated self-renewal/differentiation programs and produce daughter cells that arrest at various stages of differentiation. The daughter cells make up the bulk of the tumor and are characterized by rapid replication, limited proliferative potential, and the inability to form a new tumor. Only the CSC is able to initiate tumor formation as it is solely capable of self-renewal. A diagrammatic representation of the CSC hypothesis is shown in Fig. 1.

The strongest evidence for the CSC theory comes from studies in acute myelogenous leukemia (AML). Landmark studies by Dick and colleagues demonstrated that only rare cells in AML were able to initiate leukemia in murine models, and serial transplantation studies revealed these cells had a high self-renewal capacity *(4, 5)*. The cell responsible for tumor initiation was identified as having a CD34+CD38− phenotype, which was particularly interesting as bulk AML samples tend to be CD34−. Furthermore, CD34+CD38− is a phenotype characteristic of normal hematopoietic stem cells (HSC) indicating the putative CSCs may have a primitive phenotype. Bonnet et al. found that as few as 5×10^3 CD34+CD38− cells could engraft an immunocompromised mouse, while 100 times more CD34− or CD34+CD38+ cells from the same donor could not *(5)*. Importantly, the tumors derived from injection of the CD34+CD38− cells was heterogeneous and composed of a mixture of tumorigenic and nontumorigenic cells similar to the donor sample *(5)*. Since then, stem-like cells have been identified in a variety of human malignancies including other leukemias and solid tumors such as breast, colon, brain, head and neck, lung, pancreatic, nasopharyngeal cancers, and melanomas *(4–18)*. In many cases, a tumorigenic subset of cells could be reproducibly identified and isolated based on a distinct set of cell markers separating it from the nontumorigenic subset *(19)*. Attempts to isolate CSCs from other malignancies are underway in laboratories worldwide, and this list is likely to grow. Remarkably, even established cancer cell lines that have been grown in vitro for many years appear to contain CSC-like populations that can be isolated and are highly tumorigenic *(20, 21)*. The surface markers of CSCs from different tumor types are diverse, suggesting that their biological behaviors may be different as well.

One reason the CSC theory has generated such enthusiasm is that it may help explain long-standing problems in cancer biology. It is well-recognized that tumors are heterogeneous in terms of both functional heterogeneity and cellular composition. Functional heterogeneity refers to the observation that only a small portion of tumor cells can give rise to colonies in clonogenic assays in vitro or tumors in vivo. Under the traditional theory of tumor formation (also called the stochastic model), every tumor cell should be equally capable of forming a tumor. As tens to hundreds of thousands of tumor cells are needed to reproducibly initiate tumors in animal models, investigators concluded that the process was inefficient. However, with the CSC theory, the number of cells needed to form a tumor would simply be determined by the relative frequency of CSC in the tumor population. A sufficient number of CSCs must be present in the inoculum, since most cells in the line are proliferative but nontumorigenic. The phenotypic heterogeneity of tumors is also more easily explained by the CSC theory. Mutations in the CSC would be passed on to each daughter cell, and as the daughter cell differentiates, it may arrest at any one of numerous points prior to full maturation. In the stochastic model, the tumor cell would need to dedifferentiate to different degrees to form a phenotypically heterogeneous but genetically clonal population. Although the genomic instability associated with cancer clearly makes this possible, it is easier to envision an abortive version of the normal hierarchical differentiation program in a tissue as opposed to a random back-differentiation process affecting individual cells to different extents.

It has also been postulated that the CSC theory may explain why it is so difficult to treat cancer. If this model is correct, then directing cancer therapeutics at the bulk of rapidly replicating tumor cells is not likely to achieve tumor eradication, unless the CSCs are eliminated. This could explain the vexing problem faced by oncologists worldwide, who often can achieve complete clinical and pathological remissions of cancers with chemotherapy, only to see the cancers recur, often in metastatic and ultimately lethal forms. This clinical phenomenon implies that very small numbers of cells, sometimes undetectable even by sophisticated molecular diagnostic tools, are capable of causing tumor relapses. Standard chemotherapeutic strategies using mitotic poisons, DNA-damaging agents, antimetabolites, or even modern "targeted" agents such as growth factor receptor kinase inhibitors often are aimed at actively proliferating cells resulting in growth arrest and/or cell death. This strategy efficiently kills the daughter cells, but is much less effective against CSCs, which can remain quiescent for extended periods of time. Thus, tumors may shrink in response to traditional chemotherapy, even to the point where they are undetectable, yet CSCs often persist and eventually cause relapsed and metastatic disease *(2)*. Furthermore, when CSCs are exposed to and escape from chemotherapy-induced death, they may become more resistant to these insults and pass this on to their daughter cells. This may explain why recurrent cancers are often more resistant to treatment than primary disease. An additional characteristic of CSCs that makes them more difficult to eradicate than "bulk" cancer cells is their high level expression of ABC family transporters, which catalyze the ATP-dependent transport of toxic chemicals from the cell *(22)*. These molecules were originally identified as one of the main cause of multidrug resistance in cancers *(23)*. Evolutionarily, it is plausible that normal tissue stem cells would be particularly well protected against toxic insults, because of their fundamental role in tissue regeneration. Unfortunately, this property also makes the neoplastic counterparts of tissue stem cells highly resistant to many common chemotherapeutic drugs. Indeed, one of the most popular ways of isolating putative CSC population takes advantage of their ability to rapidly efflux DNA-binding fluorescent dyes such as Hoechst or 7-AAD, which is due to high level expression of ABC transporters. Cells that retain less dye appear as a "side population" (SP) in flow cytometry experiments. In several cases, SP cells have been shown to be enriched in putative CSCs (24–26).

WHERE DO CANCER STEM CELLS COME FROM?

While the CSC theory has offered possible new explanations for several key aspects of tumor biology, it has also raised new questions. Perhaps one of the most interesting, and yet difficult to answer, is what is the origin of the CSC? The answer to this question depends on our understanding of the stem cell differentiation process in normal tissues. If tissue stem cell differentiation is a "one way only" process, and partially differentiated cells cannot return to a "stem-like" program even when transformed, then the most obvious candidate precursor of the CSC is the tissue-specific stem cell that normally functions to replace dead and injured cells in tissues. Several points support this possibility. First, normal stem cells are already capable of indefinite self-renewal and generate more differentiated progenitors, most likely through asymmetric cell division. Even slightly more differentiated progenitor cells would have lost this ability and would have to reacquire self-renewal through mutations – a potentially complicated process. Second, tissue stem cells are long-lived and would be capable of accumulating the serial mutations necessary for transformation over the lifetime of the cell. Acquisition of multiple mutations would be more difficult for a short-lived cell. Finally, CSCs isolated from tumors tend to possess a primitive phenotype. As already mentioned, the putative CSC in AML has a CD34$^+$CD38$^-$ phenotype, which is the same as the HSC, while more differentiated cells (CD34$^+$CD38$^+$) could not initiate tumor formation (4, 5). Similarly, CSCs derived from various primary tumors or cultured cell lines routinely express other markers of normal tissue stem cells including CD133, nestin, c-kit, sox2, oct4, and musashi-1 (7, 8, 11, 27, 28). Clearly, it is simpler to conclude that CSCs derived from stem cells continue to express stem cell markers than to envision a more mature cell specifically regaining the ability to express these markers as a consequence of a random dedifferentiation event.

Nevertheless, formal proof that CSCs can only derive from normal tissue stem cells has yet to be obtained. At least theoretically, it is conceivable that the process of transformation puts a strong selective pressure on differentiated cells so that only cells that undergo the epigenetic changes necessary to restore "stemness" are capable of surviving transformation. In this model, reversion to a stem-like state is part of the transformation process. This is essentially a modified restatement of classical transformation models in which loss of differentiation results from a process of selection in a population of genomically unstable cells.

The feasibility of cloning organisms from somatic cell nuclei shows that under some circumstances the nucleus of a somatic cell can be reprogrammed all the way back to totipotency, generating a viable embryo and a complete organism. In fact, the recent demonstration that cells equivalent to human embryonic stem cells can be obtained from normal fibroblasts by transduction of specific factors supports the hypothesis that achieving stemness through dedifferentiation is possible, at least under some circumstances. Yu et al. recently showed that expression of oct4, sox2, nanog, and LIN28 in human dermal fibroblasts converts them into pluripotent cells with a phenotype virtually indistinguishable from embryonic stem cells (29). In another report, Takahashi et al. (30) showed that expression of Oct3/4, sox2, Klf4, and c-Myc can achieve the same result. The fact that the protooncogene c-Myc can be part of the reprogramming mix of genes supports the idea that under some conditions, the transformation process could reprogram a cell to a stem-like phenotype. It is important to note that these studies were conducted in fibroblasts and not epithelial cells. Can a similar process of reprogramming occur in common epithelial malignancies? A process of partial dedifferentiation has been known for years in epithelial cancers as epithelial-mesenchymal transition (EMT) *(31–34)*. This consists in loss of epithelial markers, such as tissue-specific cytokeratins, and adhesion molecules, such as E-cadherin, and acquisition of markers typical of mesenchymal cells, such as vimentin and N-cadherin. The process of EMT is thought to contribute to the ability of transformed epithelial cells to metastasize. In this model, cancer cells need to undergo EMT to migrate through the body, and once they seed distant metastatic sites, they can revert to a more or less "epithelial" phenotype through a process of mesenchymal-epithelial transition (MET). Several transcription factors such as Twist, Snail, or Slug and secretory proteins of the TGF-β family, including some bone morphogenetic proteins (BMPs), can induce the EMT program *(34)*. Vascular mimicry is thought to be a specialized form of EMT in which tumor cells can acquire an endothelial phenotype *(35, 36)*.

Thus, the question seems to be not whether or not differentiation plasticity is possible in epithelial cancer cells, but whether this process can go as far as generating a cell that has the functional characteristics of a stem cell. What a simple dedifferentiation model does not immediately explain is the hierarchical organization of cells in malignancies. If dedifferentiation is a secondary event that arises through selection and confers a selective advantage to less differentiated cells, why is there a hierarchical organization among neoplastic cells with a highly tumorigenic, dededifferentiated population capable of generating less tumorigenic, more differentiated cells? One possible explanation is that dedifferentiation is a highly improbable event, which produces a cell fate program that includes functional "stemness." Thus, only a few cells or even a single cell would have to undergo this process to generate a small population of CSCs. These then give rise to the rest of the cancer cell population through a process of hierarchical abortive differentiation that imperfectly recapitulates that of a normal tissue.

An intermediate possibility is that the CSC could originate not exclusively from tissue stem cells, but from a restricted number of cell populations including tissue stem cells and immature progenitor cells, which are immediately below tissue stem cells in the differentiation hierarchy and are capable of short-term self-replication. Experimental support for this hypothesis comes from several studies in leukemia where the introduction of oncogenic fusion gene products into hematopoietic progenitor cells resulted in AML in animal models. Cozzio et al. found that expression of the MLL-ENL fusion gene product in hematopoietic progenitor cells resulted in leukemia, albeit with less efficiency than when it was expressed in true hematopoietic stem cells *(37)*. Similar results were also found with the MOZ-TIF2 fusion gene product *(38)*. More recently, Somervaille and Cleary enforced MLL-AF9 expression in normal murine HSC and progenitor cells *(39)*. Using serial transplantation in mice, they discovered that the functional CSC expressed MAC-1 and Gr1, two markers associated with more mature cells *(39)*. Interestingly, the cells also expressed the stem cell marker c-kit, suggesting CSCs may express an unusual combination of cell markers *(39)*. Taken together, these studies clearly support the notion that AML may arise from either stem or progenitor cells in a mouse model; however, caution should be used in interpreting this data. Murine cells are generally easier to transform than human cells; hence, it is unclear if these findings are relevant to human disease *(40)*. A similar theory has been proposed for breast cancer *(41, 42)*. According to Dontu et al. *(41)*, the existence of ERα-negative breast cancers and ERα-positive breast cancers of variable biological aggressiveness may be explained by postulating that CSCs in these cancers originate from different cell populations. The most aggressive, undifferentiated ERα-negative cancers and poor-prognosis ERα-positive cancers would arise from the most primitive mammary stem cells, which are ERα-negative, while less aggressive ERα-positive cancers would arise from CSCs derived from intermediate progenitors that are ERα-positive. These can generate

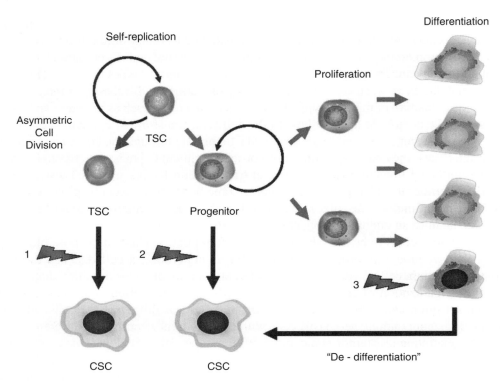

Fig. 2. Possible origins of CSCs. Three different but not mutually exclusive models are schematically presented. "Lightning" symbols indicate transforming mutations. CSCs may originate exclusively from the transformation of primitive tissue stem cells (TSC, model 1), or from the transformation of either TSC or progenitor cells (model 2). Alternatively, CSCs may originate from the transformation and dedifferentiation of more mature cells, which reacquire stem cell properties as a consequence of transforming mutations (model 3) (*see Color Plates*).

ERα-negative, rapidly proliferating "transit-amplifying" cells. This is a conceptually plausible model. However, experimentally it is difficult to distinguish it from a scenario in which all breast cancer arise from primitive, ERα-negative mammary stem cells, which lose their differentiation ability to variable degrees depending on the transforming mutations they undergo. Figure 2 represents three different, nonmutually exclusive models for the origin of CSCs.

OPEN QUESTIONS: LIMITATIONS OF THE EXPERIMENTAL EVIDENCE

An important issue that remains to be addressed is that almost all of the experimental evidence for the cancer stem cell model comes from studies in which human CSCs are transplanted into immunocompromised mice *(43, 44)*. Thus, a possible objection to the model is that selection protocols for CSCs could simply identify cells that are more adept at forming tumors in the xenogeneic microenvironment of an immunocompromised mouse. Given the limitations of current experimental models, this cannot be ruled out. However, if CSCs are essentially an artifact of xenograft models, it is not clear why human cancer cell lines of diverse tissue origins that have been grown in vitro for decades retain cell populations that exhibit stem-like characteristics very similar to CSCs isolated from primary tumors including increased expression of ABC transporters and asymmetric cell division, and are highly tumorigenic in mice. Specifically, it is not clear what selection pressure could explain the remarkable persistence of these CSC-like populations outside of the mouse microenvironment, if they are not necessary for continued in vitro propagation of the cell line. Strasser and colleagues have proposed that the reason so many human cancer cells are needed to initiate tumor formation is that the murine microenvironment is not appropriate for development of human cancers, and only a few cells are capable of overcoming this hostile environment *(43)*. These authors have taken the approach of genetically engineered mouse cells to develop lymphoma (primary Eμ-myc lymphomas), isolating subpopulations of the tumor cells based on the murine stem cell markers Sca-1 and AA4.1 (CD93), and examining tumor formation in syngeneic naïve, immunocompetent mice *(43)*. They report identify a small subpopulation (2–5%) of cells with stem-like characteristics, but found that Sca-1$^+$AA4.1^{hi} and Sca-1$^+$AA4.1^{lo} cells were equally capable of forming tumors *(43)*. These data have been interpreted as evidence against the universal validity of the cancer stem cell model. It should be pointed out that although xenograft models are certainly artificial, transgenic mouse models of carcinogenesis have important limitations of their own, and may or may not faithfully recapitulate human carcinogenesis. Typically, in these models a very potent oncogene is overexpressed in a target cell population, and the whole process of carcinogenesis and tumor progression is dramatically accelerated compared with human disease. Mouse cells are far more susceptible to transformation than human cells, and may be able to more easily reacquire functional "stemness." It is interesting to notice that the oncogene used in this particular experimental model, c-Myc, is also one of the stemness-inducing genes that can reprogram human fibroblasts to an embryonic stem cell-like phenotype. Thus, an alternate explanation for these data is that both Sca-1$^+$AA4.1^{hi} and Sca-1$^+$AA4.1^{lo} cells in this transgenic model have acquired functional "stemness" through a process of dedifferentiation, and can behave as CSCs. More sophisticated animal models will be required to gain further insights into this issue. These models should be based on human cells, but attempt to recapitulate as much as possible the human microenvironment. Such a humanized xenograft model has been generated for the mammary gland *(45)*, and should provide valuable information on putative breast cancer stem cells.

The controversy on the human relevance of CSC data obtained in xenograft models underscores the importance of tumor microenvironment in the biology of CSCs. Tumor-stroma interactions may indeed be critical in reprogramming cancer cell developmental pathways. Transforming growth factor (TGF)-β and bone morphogenetic proteins (BMPs) can be produced by tumor stroma, as can several other mediators of intercellular communication such as Wnt, Hedgehog, and Notch ligands. There is growing interest in studying the CSC "niche" as a potential therapeutic target. Normal stem cells are well known to require signals from their immediate environment, including stromal cells, microvascular endothelial cells, and extracellular matrix for their long-term survival and self-renewal. This specialized microenvironment is commonly referred to as the stem cell niche, and it is best understood in the hematopoietic system *(46)*. There is increasing evidence that CSCs also require microenvironmental signals from specialized niches *(47–49)* (Fig. 3). Autocrine and paracrine mediators secreted by the CSCs themselves or by other tumor cells may also play an important role, at least in some malignancies *(50, 51)*. How much autocrine or paracrine interactions contribute to the CSC niche is still unclear. However, at least under some circumstances CSCs can recreate a niche-like environment in the absence of other cell types. Putative breast cancer stem cells can form spheroids called "mammospheres" in suspension culture *(52, 53)*. Other putative CSCs can also form similar spheroids. Mammospheres contain few CSCs, and mostly consist of precursors and partially differentiated cells. Mammospheres can propagate in vitro and form secondary and tertiary mammospheres, which retain the original cellular composition. This implies that at least under some culture conditions, the CSCs themselves and their immediate progeny can form a functional niche that is capable of sustaining self-renewal, asymmetric cell division and partial differentiation.

Undoubtedly, much remains to be clarified and further studies are needed. These may well reveal that the origin of the functional CSC may vary based on the cell type involved and the specific nature of the oncogenic events leading to transformation.

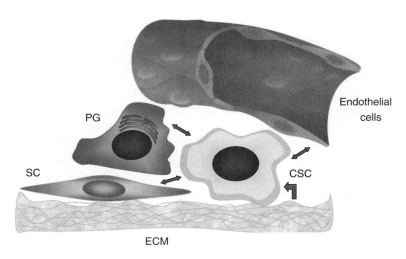

Fig. 3. The CSC "niche". In vivo, CSCs may require signals from their microenvironment to maintain their properties, as is the case for normal tissue stem cells. Microenvironmental signals may be received from endothelial cells, from various types of stromal cells (SC), such as fibroblasts, bone marrow stromal cells, or immunocytes infiltrating the tumor, from progenitor cells (PG) derived from the CSCs themselves, and/or from the extracellular matrix (ECM). It is likely that the cross-talk between CSCs and other cells is bidirectional. These signals may be therapeutically targeted to deprive CSCs of indispensable microenvironmental signals.

CLINICAL IMPLICATIONS: TARGETING CANCER STEM CELLS FOR THERAPY

Regardless of the origin of CSCs, perhaps the most important aspect of the cancer stem cell model is that it has drawn increasing attention to the hierarchical organization of malignancies. Cancers have been known for decades to be heterogeneous, but until recently the idea that the most abundant cancer cells derive from a much smaller and often elusive pool of stem-like cells was commonly accepted only in the field of leukemia. This model appears to apply to many solid tumors, and the list is growing by the day. Whatever their genesis, if human cancers do contain a small population of cells that proliferate slowly, are highly resistant to current chemotherapeutic regimens and could cause disease recurrence and metastasis, eradication of these cells may be necessary to achieve a long-lasting remission or cure. Thus, new therapies targeting the CSC must be developed if we hope to prevent or eliminate recurrent and metastatic disease. It has been proposed that identification of signaling pathways that are involved in self-renewal and are deregulated in CSCs may be an effective approach for novel target discovery *(2)*. Alternatively, the identification of proteins expressed preferentially by CSCs, such as CD96 in leukemia, could provide targets for antibody-based therapies or to modulate cell signaling and promote differentiation *(54)*. Yet another possibility is disrupting the interactions between CSCs and their niche *(48, 49)*. Several signaling pathways have been identified as playing critical roles in stem cell self-renewal including among others Notch, Wnt, and Hedgehog *(55)*. These pathways are evolutionarily ancient and have fundamental roles during development, when they control multiple cell fate decisions. They are primarily used for short-range intercellular communication utilizing secreted factors such as Hedgehog *(56)* or the Wnts *(57, 58)* or cell membrane-associated ligands such as Notch ligands Jagged and Delta *(59)*. Importantly, these pathways are involved in several of the phenomena we described above, from EMT *(60)* to CSC-niche communication *(46, 49, 51)*. Drugs that inhibit Notch signaling are in early clinical development and others are in the pipeline *(61)*, and Hedgehog inhibitors are not far behind. Interest in using Notch inhibitors to target CSCs is growing. In glioblastomas, elevated Notch expression has been associated with high nestin levels and is linked to a poor prognosis *(62, 63)*. Furthermore, Notch inhibition reduced the ability of brain CSCs to form tumors *(64)*. In breast cancer, Notch expression and activation has been associated with a poor prognosis, and studies indicate that Notch inhibitors can kill breast cancer cells in vitro *(65–67)*. As CSCs have been identified in primary breast cancers, there has been much interest in Notch signaling in breast CSCs *(6)*. Farnie et al. recently compared mammospheres derived from normal mammary tissue and human ductal carcinoma in situ (DCIS) and reported that activated Notch-1, Notch-4, and the downstream target Hes-1 were expressed in mammospheres from DCIS samples, but not those derived from normal breast tissue *(68)*. Notch inhibition with a γ-secretase inhibitor or a neutralizing Notch-4 antibody significantly reduced the ability of DCIS derived cells to form mammospheres *(68)*. These results suggest that Notch inhibition may be able to preferentially target breast CSCs, while sparing normal mammary stem cells. Laboratories around the world, including ours, are exploring the development of therapeutic regimens including Notch, Hedgehog, or Wnt inhibitors to target CSCs. Figure 4 shows a simplified representation of pathways that have been associated with CSC maintenance.

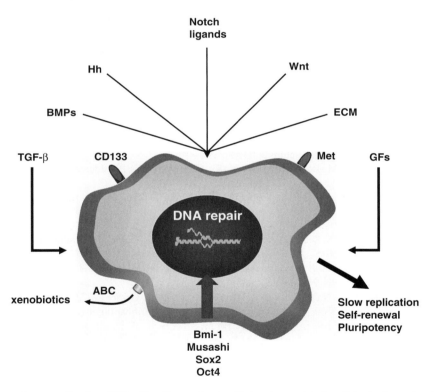

Fig. 4. Molecular pathways affecting CSCs. The figure shows a list, not meant to be all-inclusive, of pathways that have been shown to modulate the CSC phenotype. Extracellular signals delivered through the Hedgehog (Hh), Notch, Wnt pathways or through TGF-β and the related BMPs, or from ECM proteins and from growth factors such as hepatocyte growth factor (Met ligand) may all participate in regulating the maintenance, self-renewal, and differentiation of CSCs. Slow replication, ability to generate partially differentiated progenies (pluripotency) highly effective DNA repair, ability to eliminate xenobiotics through ABC family transporters (ABC), and expression of primitive membrane markers (CD133, Met) have been documented in many putative CSC populations isolated from tumors or cell lines. Transcription factors such as Bmi-1, Musashi, Sox2, Oct4, and others have been shown to be commonly expressed in putative CSCs and participate in controlling their phenotype.

CONCLUSIONS

The CSC hypothesis has sparked a tremendous increase in scientific interest in the hierarchical organization of cancer cells, the isolation of rare cellular subpopulations that may be responsible for treatment failures, and the role of microenvironmental niches in the maintenance of these populations. There are still many questions that remain unanswered, particularly surrounding the origin of CSC populations in human tumors and the interpretation of data generated by current experimental models. Yet, looking at cancers from the perspective offered by the CSC hypothesis may answer fundamental questions in tumor biology and open the way to paradigm shifts in our therapeutic approach to malignancies. Thus, it is reasonable to take the view that studying the mechanisms regulating the survival, self-renewal, and differentiation of normal and transformed stem cells could potentially lead to tremendous advances in the treatment of neoplastic diseases.

REFERENCES

1. Wicha MS, Liu S, Dontu G. Cancer stem cells: an old idea–a paradigm shift. Cancer Res 2006;66:1883–1890.
2. Song LL, Miele L. Cancer stem cells-an old idea that's new again: implications for the diagnosis and treatment of breast cancer. Expert Opin Biol Ther 2007;7:431–438.
3. Pardal R, Clarke MF, Morrison SJ. Applying the principles of stem-cell biology to cancer. Nat Rev Cancer 2003;3:895–902.
4. Lapidot T, Sirard C, Vormoor J, Murdoch B, Hoang T, Caceres-Cortes J, Minden M, Paterson B, Caligiuri MA, Dick JE. A cell initiating human acute myeloid leukaemia after transplantation into SCID mice. Nature 1994;367:645–648.
5. Bonnet D, Dick JE. Human acute myeloid leukemia is organized as a hierarchy that originates from a primitive hematopoietic cell. Nat Med 1997;3:730–737.
6. Al Hajj M, Wicha MS, Benito-Hernandez A, Morrison SJ, Clarke MF. Prospective identification of tumorigenic breast cancer cells. Proc Natl Acad Sci USA 2003;100:3983–3988.
7. Singh SK, Hawkins C, Clarke ID, Squire JA, Bayani J, Hide T, Henkelman RM, Cusimano MD, Dirks PB. Identification of human brain tumour initiating cells. Nature 2004;432:396–401.
8. Singh SK, Clarke ID, Terasaki M, Bonn VE, Hawkins C, Squire J, Dirks PB. Identification of a cancer stem cell in human brain tumors. Cancer Res 2003;63:5821–5828.
9. Prince ME, Sivanandan R, Kaczorowski A, Wolf GT, Kaplan MJ, Dalerba P, Weissman IL, Clarke MF, Ailles LE. Identification of a subpopulation of cells with cancer stem cell properties in head and neck squamous cell carcinoma. Proc Natl Acad Sci USA 2007;104:973–978.
10. O'Brien CA, Pollett A, Gallinger S, Dick JE. A human colon cancer cell capable of initiating tumour growth in immuno-deficient mice. Nature 2007;445:106–110.
11. Ricci-Vitiani L, Lombardi DG, Pilozzi E, Biffoni M, Todaro M, Peschle C, De Maria R. Identification and expansion of human colon-cancer-initiating cells. Nature 2007;445:111–115.
12. Schatton T, Murphy GF, Frank NY, Yamaura K, Waaga-Gasser AM, Gasser M, Zhan Q, Jordan S, Duncan LM, Weishaupt C, Fuhlbrigge RC, Kupper TS, Sayegh MH, Frank MH. Identification of cells initiating human melanomas. Nature 2008;451:345–349.
13. Seigel GM, Hackam AS, Ganguly A, Mandell LM, Gonzalez-Fernandez F. Human embryonic and neuronal stem cell markers in retinoblastoma. Mol Vis 2007;13:823–832.
14. Ho MM, Ng AV, Lam S, Hung JY. Side population in human lung cancer cell lines and tumors is enriched with stem-like cancer cells. Cancer Res 2007;67:4827–4833.
15. Zen Y, Fujii T, Yoshikawa S, Takamura H, Tani T, Ohta T, Nakanuma Y. Histological and culture studies with respect to ABCG2 expression support the existence of a cancer cell hierarchy in human hepatocellular carcinoma. Am J Pathol 2007;170:1750–1762.
16. Wang J, Guo LP, Chen LZ, Zeng YX, Lu SH. Identification of cancer stem cell-like side population cells in human nasopharyngeal carcinoma cell line. Cancer Res 2007;67:3716–3724.
17. Olempska M, Eisenach PA, Ammerpohl O, Ungefroren H, Fandrich F, Kalthoff H. Detection of tumor stem cell markers in pancreatic carcinoma cell lines. Hepatobiliary Pancreat Dis Int 2007;6:92–97.
18. Haraguchi N, Inoue H, Tanaka F, Mimori K, Utsunomiya T, Sasaki A, Mori M. Cancer stem cells in human gastrointestinal cancers. Hum Cell 2006;19:24–29.

19. Dalerba P, Dylla SJ, Park IK, Liu R, Wang X, Cho RW, Hoey T, Gurney A, Huang EH, Simeone DM, Shelton AA, Parmiani G, Castelli C, Clarke MF. Phenotypic characterization of human colorectal cancer stem cells. Proc Natl Acad Sci USA 2007;104:10158–10163.
20. Kondo T. Stem cell-like cancer cells in cancer cell lines. Cancer Biomark 2007;3:245–250.
21. Setoguchi T, Taga T, Kondo T. Cancer stem cells persist in many cancer cell lines. Cell Cycle 2004;3:414–415.
22. Lou H, Dean M. Targeted therapy for cancer stem cells: the patched pathway and ABC transporters. Oncogene 2007;26:1357–1360.
23. Donnenberg VS, Donnenberg AD. Multiple drug resistance in cancer revisited: the cancer stem cell hypothesis. J Clin Pharmacol 2005;45:872–877.
24. Hadnagy A, Gaboury L, Beaulieu R, Balicki D. SP analysis may be used to identify cancer stem cell populations. Exp Cell Res 2006;312:3701–3710.
25. Hirschmann-Jax C, Foster AE, Wulf GG, Nuchtern JG, Jax TW, Gobel U, Goodell MA, Brenner MK. A distinct "side population" of cells with high drug efflux capacity in human tumor cells. Proc Natl Acad Sci USA 2004;101:14228–14233.
26. Hirschmann-Jax C, Foster AE, Wulf GG, Goodell MA, Brenner MK. A distinct "side population" of cells in human tumor cells: implications for tumor biology and therapy. Cell Cycle 2005;4:203–205.
27. Collins AT, Berry PA, Hyde C, Stower MJ, Maitland NJ. Prospective identification of tumorigenic prostate cancer stem cells. Cancer Res 2005;65:10946–10951.
28. Hemmati HD, Nakano I, Lazareff JA, Masterman-Smith M, Geschwind DH, Bronner-Fraser M, Kornblum HI. Cancerous stem cells can arise from pediatric brain tumors. Proc Natl Acad Sci USA 2003;100:15178–15183.
29. Yu J, Vodyanik MA, Smuga-Otto K, Antosiewicz-Bourget J, Frane JL, Tian S, Nie J, Jonsdottir GA, Ruotti V, Stewart R, Slukvin II, Thomson JA. Induced pluripotent stem cell lines derived from human somatic cells. Science 2007;318:1917–1920.
30. Takahashi K, Tanabe K, Ohnuki M, Narita M, Ichisaka T, Tomoda K, Yamanaka S. Induction of pluripotent stem cells from adult human fibroblasts by defined factors. Cell 2007;131:861–872.
31. Hugo H, Ackland ML, Blick T, Lawrence MG, Clements JA, Williams ED, Thompson EW. Epithelial-mesenchymal and mesenchymal–epithelial transitions in carcinoma progression. J Cell Physiol 2007;213:374–383.
32. Peinado H, Olmeda D, Cano A. Snail, Zeb and bHLH factors in tumour progression: an alliance against the epithelial phenotype? Nat Rev Cancer 2007;7:415–428.
33. Gupta PB, Mani S, Yang J, Hartwell K, Weinberg RA. The evolving portrait of cancer metastasis. Cold Spring Harb Symp Quant Biol 2005;70:291–297.
34. Yang J, Mani SA, Weinberg RA. Exploring a new twist on tumor metastasis. Cancer Res 2006;66:4549–4552.
35. Hendrix MJ, Seftor RE, Seftor EA, Gruman LM, Lee LM, Nickoloff BJ, Miele L, Sheriff DD, Schatteman GC. Transendothelial function of human metastatic melanoma cells: role of the microenvironment in cell-fate determination. Cancer Res 2002;62:665–668.
36. Hess AR, Margaryan NV, Seftor EA, Hendrix MJ. Deciphering the signaling events that promote melanoma tumor cell vasculogenic mimicry and their link to embryonic vasculogenesis: role of the Eph receptors. Dev Dyn 2007;236:3283–3296.
37. Cozzio A, Passegue E, Ayton PM, Karsunky H, Cleary ML, Weissman IL. Similar MLL-associated leukemias arising from self-renewing stem cells and short-lived myeloid progenitors. Genes Dev 2003;17:3029–3035.
38. Huntly BJ, Shigematsu H, Deguchi K, Lee BH, Mizuno S, Duclos N, Rowan R, Amaral S, Curley D, Williams IR, Akashi K, Gilliland DG. MOZ-TIF2, but not BCR-ABL, confers properties of leukemic stem cells to committed murine hematopoietic progenitors. Cancer Cell 2004;6:587–596.
39. Somervaille TC, Cleary ML. Identification and characterization of leukemia stem cells in murine MLL-AF9 acute myeloid leukemia. Cancer Cell 2006;10:257–268.
40. Rangarajan A, Weinberg RA. Opinion: Comparative biology of mouse versus human cells: modelling human cancer in mice. Nat Rev Cancer 2003;3:952–959.
41. Dontu G, El Ashry D, Wicha MS. Breast cancer, stem/progenitor cells and the estrogen receptor. Trends Endocrinol Metab 2004;15:193–197.
42. Kalirai H, Clarke RB. Human breast epithelial stem cells and their regulation. J Pathol 2006;208:7–16.
43. Kelly PN, Dakic A, Adams JM, Nutt SL, Strasser A. Tumor growth need not be driven by rare cancer stem cells. Science 2007;317:337.
44. Hill RP. Identifying cancer stem cells in solid tumors: case not proven. Cancer Res 2006;66:1891–1895.
45. Kuperwasser C, Chavarria T, Wu M, Magrane G, Gray JW, Carey L, Richardson A, Weinberg RA. Reconstruction of functionally normal and malignant human breast tissues in mice. Proc Natl Acad Sci USA 2004;101:4966–4971.
46. Scadden DT. The stem cell niche in health and leukemic disease. Best Pract Res Clin Haematol 2007;20:19–27.
47. Gilbertson RJ, Rich JN. Making a tumour's bed: glioblastoma stem cells and the vascular niche. Nat Rev Cancer 2007;7:733–736.

48. Baguley BC. Tumor stem cell niches: a new functional framework for the action of anticancer drugs. Recent Patents Anticancer Drug Discov 2006;1:121–127.

49. Yang ZJ, Wechsler-Reya RJ. Hit 'em where they live: targeting the cancer stem cell niche. Cancer Cell 2007;11:3–5.

50. Hoelzinger DB, Demuth T, Berens ME. Autocrine factors that sustain glioma invasion and paracrine biology in the brain microenvironment. J Natl Cancer Inst 2007;99:1583–1593.

51. Fodde R, Brabletz T. Wnt/beta-catenin signaling in cancer stemness and malignant behavior. Curr Opin Cell Biol 2007;19:150–158.

52. Dontu G, Wicha MS. Survival of mammary stem cells in suspension culture: implications for stem cell biology and neoplasia. J Mammary Gland Biol Neoplasia 2005;10:75–86.

53. Liu S, Dontu G, Wicha MS. Mammary stem cells, self-renewal pathways, and carcinogenesis. Breast Cancer Res 2005;7:86–95.

54. Hosen N, Park CY, Tatsumi N, Oji Y, Sugiyama H, Gramatzki M, Krensky AM, Weissman IL. CD96 is a leukemic stem cell-specific marker in human acute myeloid leukemia. Proc Natl Acad Sci USA 2007;104:11008–11013.

55. Katoh M. Networking of WNT, FGF, Notch, BMP, and Hedgehog signaling pathways during carcinogenesis. Stem Cell Rev 2007;3:30–38.

56. Tung DC, Chao KS. Targeting hedgehog in cancer stem cells: how a paradigm shift can improve treatment response. Future Oncol 2007;3:569–574.

57. Cho RW, Wang X, Diehn M, Shedden K, Chen GY, Sherlock G, Gurney A, Lewicki J, Clarke MF. Isolation and molecular characterization of cancer stem cells in MMTV-Wnt-1 murine breast tumors. Stem Cells 2008;26:364–371.

58. Korkaya H, Wicha MS. Selective targeting of cancer stem cells: a new concept in cancer therapeutics. BioDrugs 2007;21:299–310.

59. Dontu G, Jackson KW, McNicholas E, Kawamura MJ, Abdallah WM, Wicha MS. Role of Notch signaling in cell-fate determination of human mammary stem/progenitor cells. Breast Cancer Res 2004;6:R605–R615.

60. Bailey JM, Singh PK, Hollingsworth MA. Cancer metastasis facilitated by developmental pathways: Sonic hedgehog, Notch, and bone morphogenic proteins. J Cell Biochem 2007;102:829–839.

61. Rizzo P, Osipo C, Foreman KE, Miele L. Rational targeting of Notch signaling in cancer. Oncogene 2008;27:5124–31.

62. Shih AH, Holland EC. Notch signaling enhances nestin expression in gliomas. Neoplasia 2006;8:1072–1082.

63. Phillips HS, Kharbanda S, Chen R, Forrest WF, Soriano RH, Wu TD, Misra A, Nigro JM, Colman H, Soroceanu L, Williams PM, Modrusan Z, Feuerstein BG, Aldape K. Molecular subclasses of high-grade glioma predict prognosis, delineate a pattern of disease progression, and resemble stages in neurogenesis. Cancer Cell 2006;9:157–173.

64. Fan X, Matsui W, Khaki L, Stearns D, Chun J, Li YM, Eberhart CG. Notch pathway inhibition depletes stem-like cells and blocks engraftment in embryonal brain tumors. Cancer Res 2006;66:7445–7452.

65. Reedijk M, Odorcic S, Chang L, Zhang H, Miller N, McCready DR, Lockwood G, Egan SE. High-level coexpression of JAG1 and NOTCH1 is observed in human breast cancer and is associated with poor overall survival. Cancer Res 2005;65:8530–8537.

66. Dickson BC, Mulligan AM, Zhang H, Lockwood G, O'Malley FP, Egan SE, Reedijk M. High-level JAG1 mRNA and protein predict poor outcome in breast cancer. Mod Pathol 2007;20:685–693.

67. Zang S, Ji C, Qu X, Dong X, Ma D, Ye J, Ma R, Dai J, Guo D. A study on Notch signaling in human breast cancer. Neoplasma 2007;54:304–310.

68. Farnie G, Clarke RB, Spence K, Pinnock N, Brennan K, Anderson NG, Bundred NJ. Novel cell culture technique for primary ductal carcinoma in situ: role of Notch and epidermal growth factor receptor signaling pathways. J Natl Cancer Inst 2007;99:616–627.

2

Tumor Stem Cells and Malignant Cells, One and the Same

Beverly A. Teicher

ABSTRACT

Cancer is a proliferative, invasive, and metastatic disease often caused by repeated tissue insults resulting in accumulation of genetic abnormalities that rarely produce malignant cells. The survival of mouse L1210 leukemia was determined for inoculations of 1 cell up to 10^6 cells. The survival times varied in a log-linear manner with the inoculum cell number from 19 days with 1 cell to 7 days with 10^6 cells implanted. In preclinical tumor models or in patients, tumor nodules of 10^8–10^9 cells are advanced cancer. Malignant cells frequently secrete growth modulatory substances that regulate their growth and alter growth of normal cells. Whether the metastatic malignant cell is the same or significantly different from the primary lesion malignant cell remains a topic of active investigation. Reaching a detectable lesion takes 10 years. Genetic instability produces variants in the primary tumor and metastases that are more heterogeneous than the early disease. The argument that cancer arises only from the tissue stem cell populations and that cancer stem cells comprise perhaps 1 in 100,000 or 1 in 10,000 cells within the tumor leads to the notion that agents that selectively kill cancer stem cells will not decrease the tumor mass. The cells that initiate, sustain, and populate cancers are malignant cells. Cancer stem cell notion is useful if it leads to important research questions and to better therapeutics.

Key Words: Colony forming units, Malignant cells, Genetic instability, Metastasis, L1210 leukemia

INTRODUCTION

Cancer is a proliferative, invasive, and metastatic disease that is frequently caused by repeated insults to a tissue resulting in accumulation of genetic abnormalities that, by rare chance, produce a malignant cell. Cancer cells are genetically aberrant and instable. Some cancers begin as a single clone (and a few remain clonal) and other arise from a field of repeatedly damaged cells. The search for an understanding of cancer and for the key as to how to control and ablate malignant disease often returns to the remarkable processes of normal tissue/embryo development and normal tissue repair. The "well-behaved" proliferative and self-limiting biology of wound repair, gut lining replacement, liver regeneration, skin renewal, and bone marrow generation of hematopoietic cells has taught us that cell proliferation and differentiation are a constant process in complex organisms and are well-controlled under normal circumstances.

The concept of a stem cell was put forth by Till and McCulloch to describe the ability of a single mouse bone marrow cell to produce a colony of cells in the mouse spleen and later to describe the

From: *Cancer Drug Discovery and Development: Stem Cells and Cancer,*
Edited by: R.G. Bagley and B.A. Teicher, DOI: 10.1007/978-1-60327-933-8_2,
© Humana Press, a part of Springer Science+Business Media, LLC 2009

ability of similar single bone marrow cells to give to colonies of varied types in cell culture (1, 2). A colony-forming unit (CFU) is an individual cell that is able to clone itself into a colony of identical cells. A CFU is a measure of viable bacterial numbers or a measure of viable mammalian malignant cells in a culture. In reconstituting the immune system of lethally irradiated mice, bone marrow cells from syngeneic donors are intravenously injected into the recipient animals and colonies form in the spleen. Each colony is the progeny of a pluripotent stem cell; therefore, the number of colonies is a measure of the number of stem cells. These findings led to the notion that cancer can arise from multiply insulted cells that by rare chance have aberrantly turned on genes that normally are expressed only by normal tissue "stem" cells. Thus, cancer cells have aberrantly reverted to a dedifferentiated proliferative state. These malignant cells are trying to build a tissue but they are abnormal and lethal. Indeed, an area of therapeutic investigation has a goal to discover agents that can terminally differentiate malignant cells to a quiescent nonproliferative state.

EARLY OBSERVATIONS

An interesting aspect of the current cancer stem cell debate regards the number of human tumor cells required to initiate the growth of a subcutaneous nodule in immunodeficient mice. A very large number of variables would need to be optimized to achieve reliable data from such observations. A historical perspective looking at syngeneic mouse tumors may help. The L1210 and P388 mouse leukemias were developed in 1948 and 1955, respectively (3–5). L1210 and P388 leukemias were both chemically induced in a DBA/2 mouse by painting the skin with methylcholanthrene. The leukemias have been propagated in DBA/2 mice by implanting intraperitoneally 0.1 mL of a diluted ascetic fluid containing either 10^5 L1210 cells or 10^6 P388 cells. These mouse leukemias were the first tumors used for large-scale drug discovery screening programs by the national drug development program instituted in 1954 by Congress, which directed the National Cancer Institute to start a program. The Cancer Chemotherapy National Service Center (CCNSC) screen consisted of three mouse tumors: L1201 leukemia, SA-180 sarcoma, and mammary adenocarcinoma 755 (6). Over the years, the primary screen varied from the original three tumors to L1210 plus two arbitrarily selected tumors to L1210 plus Walker 256 carcinosarcoma to L1210 plus P388 leukemia to L1210 plus B16 melanoma or Lewis lung carcinoma. In 1976, a change occurred in the NCI primary screen. The new screen included a panel of colon, breast, and lung tumor models (mouse and human); however, compounds were initially screened in P388 leukemia (7).

Skipper and Schabel and colleagues explored the growth characteristics of the L1210 and P388 leukemias in mice (8, 9). The testing was conducted in a hybrid of DBA/2 hosts. Tumor cell implant sites were intraperitoneal injection, subcutaneous implant, intravenous injection, and intracranial injection. For L1210 leukemia with an inoculum of 10^5 cells, the mean days of survival and tumor cell doubling times for these implant sites were 8.8, 9.9, 6.4, and 7.0 days and 0.34, 0.46, 0.45, and 0.37 days, respectively (Fig. 1). The mean survival times of mice implanted with L1210 cells by these various routes was determined for inoculations of 1 cell up to 10^6 cells. The survival times varied in a log-linear manner with the inoculum cell number. Thus, when the mice were implanted with 1 L1210 cell by intraperitoneal injection, they survived 19 days and when the mice were implanted with 10^6 L1210 cells intraperitoneally, they survived 7 days (Fig. 1). Similar studies were conducted with P388 leukemia. For P388 leukemia (10^6 cells), the mean days of survival and the tumor doubling times for the same implant sites were 10.3, 13.0, 8.0, and 8.0 days and 0.44, 0.52, 0.68, and 0.63 days, respectively. From these studies, it must be concluded that every L1210 and P388 cell is a cancer stem cell.

Skipper and Schabel applied similar analyses to solid tumors especially the mouse Ridgway osteogenic sarcoma (10). In preclinical tumor models or in patients, tumor nodules of 10^8–10^9 cells are

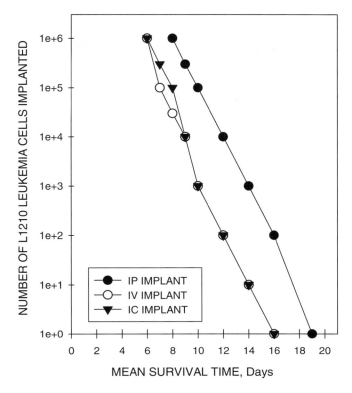

Fig. 1. Mean survival times of mice inoculated with various numbers of murine L1210 leukemia cells injected intraperitoneally, intravenously, or intracranially. These data form the basis for the in vivo bioassay method for determining the number of L1210 cells surviving after treatment of L1210 tumor-bearing mice with therapy. From these survival curves, it was determined that from: (1) intraperitoneal inoculation of L1210 cell-generation time = 0.55 days; the lethal number of L1210 cells = 1.5×10^9; (2) intravenous inoculation the L1210 cell-generation time = 0.43 days; and (3) intracranial inoculation the L1210 cell-generation time = 0.46 days (8,9).

advanced cancer (Fig. 2) (10, 11). One source of variability in the response of drug-sensitive tumor cells to a drug is the heterogeneity of the blood supply such that the drug does not reach the tumor cells distal from the blood supply in sufficient concentration to be lethal. Thus, the pharmacokinetics and concentration of a drug required to kill tumor cells distal from vasculature should be documented. In addition, the physiologic heterogeneity of tumor masses as a source of varied treatment response, Skipper and Schabel considered the heterogeneity of tumor stem cells, defined as cells capable of unlimited proliferative thrust, caused by the inherent genetic instability of malignant cells to be a source of variable treatment response. Skipper and Schabel considered various types of tumor stem cells that might account for fluctuation in response to chemotherapy in similarly treated individuals bearing a specific cancer, and classifications of cancers by chemotherapeutic effect. Fluctuating ratios of treatment responsive to treatment resistant stem cells, as predicted by the mutation theory, could account for one patient responding to a drug and the next not responding. Differences in tumor growth fraction and differences in tumor distribution into pharmacologic sanctuaries could also strongly influence a patient's response to therapy. Treatment resistant stem cells are primarily responsible for the failure of the best available chemotherapy to cure responsive, refractory, and very refractory experimental neoplasms. These data examined suggest that differences in the resistant to responsive stem cell ratios in different types of cancer may account for their being classified as responsive, refractory, or very refractory (12).

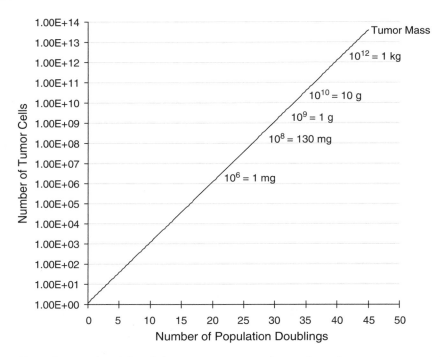

Fig. 2. Tumor cell numbers and weight of the tumor mass are shown. In patients, tumors are advanced at first presentation or at recurrence after initial noncurative therapy *(10,11)*.

TUMOR CELL HETEROGENEITY

Experience with the heterogeneous response of well-controlled preclinical tumor models grown in inbred strain of mice led investigators in the mid-1980s to believe that the assumption that there should be a common pattern of cellular heterogeneity for histologically identical types of cancer was not warranted *(13)*. Although malignant disease may develop from a single transformed cell, even in tumors where the single cell has diversified to heterogeneous cell phenotypes, evidence of a clonal origin still exists *(14)*. Although Foulds concluded that tumor evolution (progression) is characterized by permanent, irreversible changes, we recognize today that cell remain very plastic and adaptable and can often modulate their biology to changes in the microenvironment *(15)*. During molecular progression of tumors, neoplastic cells accumulate increasing genetic alterations that are generated by mutational events, genetic instability *(16, 17)*. Tumor cell genetic instability ensures that malignant disease contains heterogeneous, phenotypically diverse tumor subpopulations *(14)*. Tumor cell diversification mechanisms may be similar or identical to normal development during embryonic and postembryonic diversification and development. Tumor cell subpopulations can influence the properties of other subpopulations in the tumor including proliferation, sensitivity to drugs, immunogenicity, and metastatic potential *(14, 18–20)*.

Understanding the biology of malignant cells (cancer stem cells) that allows them to escape the constraints that normally regulate cell growth and differentiate is critical. Malignant cells frequently secrete growth modulatory substances that regulate their own growth (autocrine) and/or alter the growth of normal cells (paracrine) in the vicinity of the malignancy (Fig. 3) *(21)*. A malignant tumor whose growth depends upon the release of autocrine and paracrine growth factors may be vulnerable to treatment with specific receptor antagonists or growth factor neutralizing antibodies.

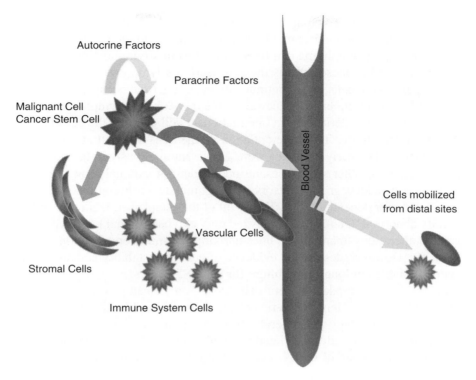

Fig. 3. Malignant cells can have abscopal effects on the host through secretion of paracrine factors and can produced autocrine factors that can sustain proliferation of the malignancy.

HEMATOPOIESIS AS A MODEL

Analogies for the development of malignancy have been sought in the processes of normal aging and in the differentiation of cells in the hematopoietic system *(22, 23)*. The incidence of many cancers increase with age because of increased probability of DNA changes that may allow occurrence of a malignant cell and because some of the alterations associated with normal aging increase the susceptibility of cells to carcinogenic events. In normal aging, there is a decrease in DNA repair capacity and a decline in cellular immune reactivity that could contribute to permitting malignant growth *(22)*. Normal hematopoiesis, the formation of the many cell types in blood, is a process of development, self-renewal through mitosis, and differentiation of hematopoietic stem cells, the source cell of all blood cell lineages *(24)*. Because most blood cells have relatively short lifespans, hematopoietic stem cells continuously replicate themselves through self-renewal to prevent depletion of the stem cell pool while simultaneously differentiating into multiple lineages of the varied blood cell types. The fate choice of hematopoietic cells to either self-renew or differentiate is controlled by intrinsic mechanisms and extrinsic signals from the environment or the stem cell niche *(25)*. In adults, the hematopoietic stem cell number is relatively constant under normal conditions. Bone marrow hematopoietic stem cells appear quiescent; however, the majority divide regularly as shown by their slow constant incorporation of radio-labeled nucleotides *(26, 27)*. There are two proposed mechanisms by which asymmetric cell division may be achieved called divisional asymmetry and environmental asymmetry. In divisional asymmetry, specific cell fate determinants in the genome, RNA, and proteins are distributed unequally during cell division. After cell division, only one daughter cell receives the determinants, thus retaining the hematopoietic stem cell fate while the other daughter differentiates.

In environmental asymmetry, one hematopoietic stem cell niche and retains the stem cell identity, while the other enters a different environment favoring its differentiation *(24)*.

The first human leukemia-lymphoma cell lines were Burkitt's lymphoma lines developed in 1963 *(28)*. The most widely used of these lines is the Raji Burkitt's lymphoma *(29)*. The term "cell line" indicates that the population of cells grew continuously in culture (to this day); therefore, the cells were "immortal" or capable of continuous self-renewal. Some the leukemia-lymphoma cell lines were presumed to be monoclonal that is derived from one malignant cell and that the current multiclonal lines emerged during extended culture. The differentiation of the cells arrested at a discrete stage during maturation of the lineage. The early cell lines were grown autonomously in basic nutrient media supplemented with fetal calf (or other serum) serum independent of external growth factors, although, in some cases, exogenously added growth factors could stimulate proliferation. Later cell lines were selected to be growth factor dependent *(30)*. Nearly all of the established leukemia and lymphoma cell lines are genetically abnormal. Of 429 lines analyzed only two had normal karyotypes *(31)*. In addition to gross cytogenetic alterations, many of the lines harbor point mutations deletions and amplifications of specific genes *(32)*. However, despite the evidence of genetic instability and abnormality, these cell lines have remained "stable" in long-term culture for nearly 50 years.

An interesting case is the impact of stem cell "dose" on hematopoietic recovery in autologous blood stem cell recipients *(23)*. Hematopoietic cells collected from blood and reinfused into patients following high-dose chemotherapy are generally termed "stem cells," even though the population of cells contains true stem cells and differentiated progenitor cells *(33, 34)*. Mobilized blood stem cell quantity, identified by expression of CD34, may be the strongest predictor of days to hematopoietic recovery (i.e., platelets and neutrophils) in autologous blood stem cell recipients *(35)*. The majority of patients will recover if a stem cell dose of $\geq 5 \times 10^6$/kg stem cells are infused, which corresponds to 3.5×10^8 cells *(36)*. Bone marrow engraftment is the result of early undifferentiated stem and progenitor cell self-renewal and differentiation. The rate of engraftment is dependent, in part, on the number and type of stem cells infused. Using a genetically engineered model cell to represent human leukemia stem cells, Hope et al. tracked these human leukemia stem cells in SCID mice and found that the leukemia stem cells were not functionally homogeneous *(37)*. Like normal hematopoietic stem cells, some human leukemia stem cells divided rarely and underwent self-renewal rather than commitment after cell division and others demonstrated heterogeneity in self-renewal potential.

METASTASIS

The detection of circulating tumor cells in the blood and lymph system and micrometastases has been investigated through multiple eras of cancer research because of the potential importance of these cells to prognosis and therapeutic approaches *(38)*. The first publication of circulating tumor cells was in 1869 when Ashworth reported cancer cells in the blood of a patient at autopsy *(39)*. In the decade 1955–1965, 5,000 cancer patients were tested for circulating tumor cells using 20 different cytological methods; however, it was finally realized that the tests used were not sufficiently discriminatory *(40)*. When immunohistochemical detection methods were developed and more recently with the development of PCR techniques, interest in documenting a connection between circulating tumor cell numbers and stage of disease and in detecting occult metastases renewed *(41–43)*. Although the accuracy of methods for detecting tumor cells in circulation has markedly improved over the years, the application of these data to determination of the most appropriate treatment regimen for individual patients has yet to occur. It is not clear whether circulating tumor cells are enriched for cancer "stem cells," malignant cells that can initiate metastasis or whether circulating tumor cells reflect the quality of the primary lesion vasculature or other properties of the malignant disease *(44, 45)*. There is no doubt that malignant cells must be plastic and adaptive to altering environments and stress. The capacity

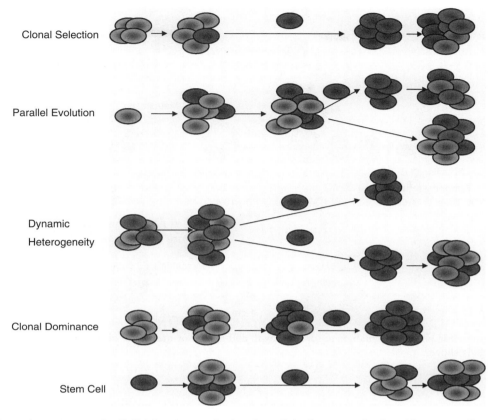

Clonal Selection

Parallel Evolution

Dynamic
Heterogeneity

Clonal Dominance

Stem Cell

Fig. 4. The various patterns of cell division that can lead to the cellular heterogeneity found in most malignant disease.

of some malignant cells to make epithelial to mesenchymal transition and then return to an epithelial phenotype is an example of the plasticity of malignant cells *(44)*. During wound healing processes normal cells can undergo these changes as well.

Metastasis is a critical characteristic of malignant disease *(45)* (Fig. 4). The placement of a cancer stem cell in the metastatic process and understanding whether the metastatic malignant cell is the same or significantly different from the malignant cell of the primary lesion remains a topic of active investigation. The clonal selection hypothesis is that cell populations with metastatic capacity are subpopulations within the primary lesion. The parallel evolution model theorizes that metastasis occurs early in malignant disease and evolves along a different path than the primary lesion. The dynamic heterogeneity hypothesis indicates that metastatic variants arise within the primary tumor, and these variants spread and evolve further at secondary sites. The notion of clonal dominance is that more virulent metastatic subclones occur within the primary tumor and outgrow the original malignant cells and eventually dominate the primary lesion and metastases. The stem cell model indicates that only cancer stem cells and not the majority population of the tumor have the capacity to metastasize and establish distant lesions *(46–48)*.

Gatenby and Gillies proposed a model for the somatic evolution of invasive cancer as overcoming a series of barriers to proliferation *(49)*. Tumor development and the genotypic and phenotypic heterogeneity of cancer cell populations is described using an equivalence principle such that multiple alterations in the cell may allow to successfully adapt to and overcome a critical barrier moving toward malignancy. During tumor initiation, progression and metastasis, approximately 30 generation

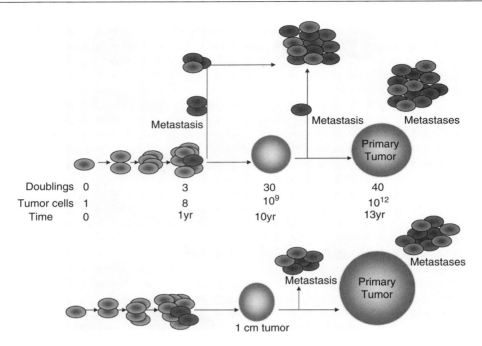

Fig. 5. Two possible patterns of malignant tumor growth and spread of metastatic disease over time and malignant cell doublings is shown.

times or about 10 years are required for a single malignant cell to produce a palpable mass of about 1 cm³ composed of about 10^9 tumor cells *(45)* (Fig. 5). Over the course of these 10 years to reach a clinically detectable lesion, genetic instability produces variants in the primary tumor and metastases that are more heterogeneous than the early disease. A lethal tumor burden of 10^{12} tumor cells could be expected after 10 cell doublings or 3 years from detection of the disease without treatment.

CARCINOGENESIS

Chemical carcinogen-induced rat mammary tumors provided an in vivo model for the early cancer stem cell hypothesis *(50)*. In the rat mammary gland, epithelial stem cells insulted by a chemical targeting DNA can give rise to more-rapidly proliferating benign stem cells, which retain some response to normal growth-controlling factors. These altered but benign stem cells can also differentiate to a degree. The genetic instability of these cells results in the generation of malignant cells in subsequent generations with loss of response to growth-controlling factors, decreased capacity for differentiation and escape from immune surveillance. The cells which then compose the malignant disease have departed in critical ways from the normal epithelial stem cells of origin and continue to suffer from genetic instability and to evolve.

Colony formation is a demonstration of self-renewal capacity. It was noted early that colony-forming human epidermal cells were heterogeneous in capacity for sustained growth and that the potential for continued growth from a single cell could be predicted from the phenotype of the colony produced *(51)*. Three types of colonies were described: (1) holocolonies characterized as large with a smooth perimeter containing mainly small cells that may be considered the most undifferentiated population; (2) paracolonies characterized as being small with a highly irregular perimeter containing cells that are large and flattened and appear terminally differentiated; and (3) merocolonies characterized by medium to large size and a wrinkled perimeter with heterogeneous cells. In the case of normal cells, the transitions from holoclone (stem-like) to meroclone to paraclone (terminally differentiated) are thought to be unidirectional and result in progressively restricted growth potential. However, malignant cells have increased plasticity and may dedifferentiate toward holoclone states or abnormally differentiate forming giant multinucleated cells that no longer proliferate. Locke et al. studied seven well-established human cancer cell lines from varied histology and found that cell lines generated from carcinomas produced cell culture colony patterns similar to those produced by the stem and amplifying cells of normal epithelia as described earlier *(52)*. The cancer cell lines appeared to maintain a subpopulation of "stem cells" during passage of the line. The heterogeneity of the colonies produced from the cancer cell lines indicates that the stem cell property of asymmetrical division persists in cancer cell lines but is shifted toward stem cell self-renewal. Thus, malignant cells attempt to recapitulate the behavior of normal tissue cells; however, their behavior is aberrant and detrimental. Malignant cells are damaged cells that have dedifferentiated, returned to the behavior of embryonic cells rather than dying or being recognized as abnormal by the immune system.

The skin epidermis is a normal tissue that is continuously confronted with physiochemical traumas from the environment *(53)*. The skin undergoes continual rejuvenation through homeostasis and is primed to undergo wound repair in response to injury. The epidermis has tissue "stem cells," which both self-perpetuate and give rise to the differentiating cells that constitute the tissue. The TGFβ pathway is involved in the control of proliferation of many cells. The loss of response to TGFβ proliferation control is a necessary step in malignant transformation *(54–56)*. In the absence of TGFβ, proliferation control, squamous cell carcinomas spontaneously develop in mice *(57)*. These tumors have many of the characteristics of invasive squamous cell carcinomas.

Although some may argue that the embryological, stem-like properties of tumors and tumor cell lines indicate that the malignant cell originates only from tissue stem cells, this argument seems unnecessary to explain the dedifferentiated properties of the malignant cell *(58)*. The argument that cancer arises only from the stem cell populations of tumor that comprise perhaps 1 in 100,000 or 1 in 10,000 cells within the tumor leads to the notion that treatment agents that selectively kill the cancer stem cell will not result in decrease in the tumor mass. Classic studies and recent studies show that with some tumor cell lines inoculation of mice with few cells from 1 to 10 can produce tumors that are lethal to the host *(59)*. Most transplantable tumor models are carried out with the implant for 10^5–10^7 tumor cells primarily due to the impatience of the experimentalist, who would like to see a palpable nodule in 1 or 2 weeks and not in several months or years. Generally, if a tumor nodule is not palpable in 2 or 3 weeks, the tumor is considered a no take. The timeline for these studies is that of the experimentalist not reflective of the nature of cell proliferation. Although it appears that only a minute proportion of human tumor cells can grow readily and rapidly in mice, syngeneic tumor models indicate that inoculums of many fewer cells that divide quite rapidly in the murine host yield lethal malignant disease in a short time *(60)*.

CONCLUSIONS

In most incarnations, the cancer stem cell is very similar to a normal tissue stem cell. The cancer stem hypothesis has been advanced to describe how a cancer originates, how it is sustained, and what makes it drug resistant. Among the properties of tissue stem cells in the adult are the relative quiescence manifested by infrequent cell divisions, resistance to drugs/toxins mediated by ABC transporters, active DNA repair pathways and resistance to apoptosis. The cancer stem cell has been defined as a cell involved in malignant disease process that possess the capacity to self-renew and give rise to the heterogeneous lineages of cancer cells that comprise the tumor. Whether the malignant cells with long term self-renewal capacity that sustain the cancer arose from tissue stem cells that acquired mutations leading to a differentiation block and malignancy or whether more differentiated cells acquired mutations that dedifferentiated them and resulted in a malignant cell capable of self-renewal has not been determined. Thus, the use of the term "stem cell" may not be accurate. The cells that initiate, sustain, and populate cancers are malignant cells *(61, 62)*. The notion of the cancer stem cell is useful, if it leads important research questions being addressed and to better therapeutics being developed. The self-renewal, pluripotency, and drug resistance of malignant cells is a product of their abnormality and genetic instability.

REFERENCES

1. Till JE, McCulloch EA. Early repair processes in marrow cells irradiated and proliferating in vivo. Radiat Res 1963; 18: 96–105.
2. McCulloch EA, Till JE. Perspectives on the properties of stem cells. Nature Med 2005; 11: 10276–8.
3. Law LW, Dunn TB, Boyle PJ, Miller JH. Observations on the effect of a folic acid antagonist on transplantable lymphoid leukemias in mice. J Natl Cancer Inst 1949; 10: 179–92.
4. Dawe CJ, Potter M. Morphologic and bioloigc progression of a lymphoid neoplasm of the mouse in vivo and in vitro. Amer J Pathol 1957; 33: 603.
5. Waud WR. Murine L1210 and P388 leukemias. In: Anticancer Drug Development Guide: Preclinical Screening, Clinical Trials and Approval. BA Teicher Ed. Humana Press Inc, Totowa, NJ 1997; pp59–74.
6. Goldin A, Serpick AA, Mantel NA. A commentary, experimental screening procedures and clinical predictability value. Cancer Chemother Rep 1966; 50: 173–218.
7. Goldin A, Vendetti JM, Muggia FM, Rozencweig M, DeVita VT. New animal models in cancer chemotherapy. In: Fox BW (ed.) Advances in Medical Oncology, Research and Education, Vol 5. Basis for Cancer Therapy I. New York: Pergamon. 1979; 113–22.
8. Skipper HE, Schabel FM, Wilcox WS, Laster WR, Trader MW, Thompson SA. Experimental evaluation of potential anticancer agents. XVIII. Effects of therapy on viability and rate of proliferation of leukemia cells in various anatomic sites. Cancer Chemother Reps 1965; 47: 41–65.
9. Schabel FM Jr, Griswold DP Jr, Laster WR Jr, Corbett TH, Lloyd HH. Quantitative evaluation of anticancer agent activity in experimental animals. Pharmacol Ther (A) 1977; 1: 411–435.
10. Schabel FM Jr, Griswold DP Jr, Corbett TH, Laster WR Jr. Increasing the therapeutic response rates to anticancer drugs by applying the basic principles of pharmacology. Cancer 1984; 54(6 suppl): 1160–7.
11. De Vita VT Jr, Young RC, Canellos GP. Combination versus single agent chemostherapy: a review of the basis for selection of drug treatment of cancer. Cancer 1975; 35: 98–110.
12. Skipper HE, Schabel FM Jr. Tumor stem cell heterogeneity: implications with respect to classification of cancers by chemotherapeutic effect. Cancer Treat Reps 1984; 68: 43–61.
13. Martin DS, Balis ME, Fisher B, Frei E, Freireich EJ, Heppner GH, Holland JF, Houghton JA, Houghton PJ, Johnson RK, Mittelman A, Rustum Y, Sawyer RC, Schmid FA, Stolfi RL, Young CW. Role of murine tumor models in cancer treatment research. Cancer Res 1986; 46: 2189–92.
14. Nicolson GL. Tumor cell instability, diversification and progression to the metastatic phenotype: from oncogene to oncofetal expression. Cancer Res 1987; 47: 1473–87.
15. Foulds L. Neoplastic Development. New York: Academic Press, 1975.
16. Nowell PC. The clonal evolution of tumor cell populations. Science 1976; 194: 23–8.
17. Nowell PC. Mechanisms of tumor progression. Cancer Res 1986; 46: 2203–7.
18. Heppner GH, Miller BE, Miller FR. Tumor subpopulation interactions in neoplasms. Biochim Biophys Acta 1984; 695: 215–26.
19. Miller FR. Intratumor immunologic heterogeneity. Cancer Metastasis Rev 1982; 1: 319–34.
20. Miller FR. Tumor subpopulations intereactions in metastasis. Invasion Metastasis 1983; 3: 234–42.
21. Walsh JH, Karnes WE, Cuttitta F, Walker A. Autocrine growth factors and solid tumor malignancy. West J Med 1991; 155: 152–63.
22. Ebbesen P. Cancer and normal ageing. Mech Ageing Develop 1984; 25: 269–83.
23. Pecora AL. Impact of stem cell dose on hematopoietic recovery in autologous blood stem cell recipients. Bone Marrow Transplant 1999; 23 (suppl 2): S7–S12.
24. Huang X, Cho S, Spangrude GJ. Hematopoietic stem cells: generation and self-renewal. Cell Death Differentiation 2007; 14: 1851–9.

25. Moore KA, Lemischka IR. Stem cells and their niches. Science 2006; 311: 1880–5.

26. Bradford GB, Williams B, Rossi R, Bertoncello I. Quierscence, cycling and turnover in the primitive hematopoietic stem cell compartment. Exp Hematol 1997; 25: 445–53.

27. Cheshier SH, Morrison SJ, Liao X, Weissman IL. In vivo proliferation and cell cycle kinetics of long-term self-renewing hematopoietic stem cells. Proc Natl Acad Sci USA 1999; 96: 3120–5.

28. Drexler HG, Matsuo Y, MacLeod AF. Continuous hematopoietic cell lines as model systems for leukemia-lymphoma research. Leukemia Res 2000; 24: 881–911.

29. Pulvertaft RJV. Cytology of Burkitt's tumor (African lymphoma). Lancet 1964; i: 238–40.

30. Drexler HG, Zaborski M, Quentmeier H. Cytokine response profiles of human myeloid factor-dependent human leukemia cell lines. Leukemia 1997; 11: 701–8.

31. Dexler HG (editor). The Leukemia-lymphoma Cll Lines Factsbook. San Diego, CA: Academic Press, 2000.

32. Drexler HG, Fombonne S, Matsuo Y, Hu ZB, Hamaguchi H, Uphoff CC .P53 alterations in human leukemia-lymphoma cell lines: in vitro artifact or prerequisite for cell immortalization ? Leukemia 2000; 14: 198–206.

33. Krause DS, Fackler MJ, Civin CI, Stratford May W. CD34: structure, biology and clinical utility. Blood 1996; 87: 1–13.

34. Berardi AC, Wang A, Levine JD, Lopez P, Scadden DT. Functional isolation and characterization of human hematopoietic stem cells. Science 1995: 267: 104–8.

35. Furness SGB, McNagny K. Beyond mere markers: functions for CD34 family of sialomucins in hematopoiesis. Immunol Res 2006; 34: 13–32.

36. Pecora AL, Preti RA, Gleim GW, Jennis A, Zahos K, Cantwell S, Doria L, Isaacs R, Gillio AP, Michelis MA, Brochstein JA. CD34+CD33– cells influence days to engraftment and transfusion requirements in autologous blood stem cell recipients. J Clin Oncol 1998; 16: 2093–104.

37. Hope KJ, Jin L, Dick JE. Acute myeloid leukemia originates from a hierarchy of leukemia stem cell classes that differ in self-renewal capacity. Nature Immunol 2004; 5: 738–43.

38. Ghossein RA, Bhattacharya S, Rosai J. Molecular detection of micrometastases and circulating tumor cells in solid tumors. Clin Cancer Res 1999; 5: 1950–60.

39. Ashworth TR. A case of cancer in which cells similar to those in the tumors were seen in the blood after death. Australian Med J 1869; 14: 146.

40. Christopherson W. Cancer cells in the peripheral blood: a second look. Acta Cytol 1965; 9: 169–74.

41. Moss TJ, Sanders DG. Detection of neuroblastoma cells in blood. J Clin Oncol 1990; 8: 736–40.

42. Pelkey TJ, Frierson HF, Bruns DE. Molecular and immunological detection of circulating tumor cells and micrometaseses from solid tumors. Clin Chem 1996; 42: 1369–81.

43. Campana D, Pui CH. Detection of minimal residual disease in acute leukemias: methodological advances and clinical significance. Blood 1995; 85: 1416–34.

44. Scheel C, Onder T, Karnoub A, Weinberg RA. Adaptation versus selection: the origins of metastatic behavior. Cancer Res 2007; 67: 11476–80.

45. Talmadge JE. Clonal selection of metastasis within the life history of a tumor. Cancer Res 2007; 67: 11471–5.

46. Gray JW. Evidence emerges for early metstasis and parallel evolution of primary and meststatic tumors. Cancer Cell 2003; 4: 4–6.

47. Schmidt-Kittler O, Ragg T, Daskalakis A, Granzow M, Ahr A, Blankenstein TJ, Kaufmann M, Diebold J, Arnholdt H, Mullor P, Bischoff J, Harich D, Schlimok G, Riethmuller G, Eils R, Klein CA. From latent disseminated cells to overt metastasis: genetic analysis of systemic breast cancer progression. Proc Natl Acad Sci USA 2003; 100: 7737–42.

48. Weigelt B, Glas AM, Wessels LF, Witteveen AT, Peterse JL, Van't Veer LJ. Gene expression profiles of primary breast tumors maintained in distant metastases. Proc Natl Acad Sci USA 2003; 100: 15901–5.

49. Gatenby RA, Gillies RJ. A microenvironmental model of carcinogenesis. Nature 2008; 8: 56–61.

50. Rudland PS. Stem cells and the development of mammary cancers in experimental rats and in humans. Cancer Mestastasis Rev 1987; 6: 55–83.

51. Barrandon Y, Green H. Three clonal types of keratinocyte with different capacities for multiplication. Proc Natl Acad Sci USA 1987; 84: 2302–6.

52. Locke M, Heywood M, Fawell S, Mackenzie IC. Retention of intrinsic stem cell hierarchies in carcinoma-derived cell lines. Cancer Res 2005; 65: 8944–50.

53. Fuchs E. Skin stem cells: rising to the surface. J Cell Biol 2008; 180: 273–84.

54. Teicher BA. Malignant cells, directors of the malignant process: role of transforming growth factor-beta. Cancer Metastasis Rev 20: 133–143, 2001.

55. Pinkas J, Teicher BA. TGF-b in cancer and as a therapeutic target. Biochem Pharmacol 72: 523–529, 2006.

56. Teicher BA. Transforming growth factor-b and the immune response to malignant disease. Clin Cancer Res 2007; 13: 6247–51.

57. Guasch G, Schober M, Pasolli HA, Conn EB, Polak L, Fuchs E. Loss of TGFb signaling destabilizes homeostasis and promotes squamous cell carcinomas in stratified epithelia. Cancer Cell 2007; 12: 313–27.

58. Wicha MS, Liu S, Dontu G. Cancer stem cells: an old idea – a paradigm shift. Cancer Res 2006; 66: 1883–90.

59. Kelly PN, Dakic A, Adams JM, Nutt SL, Strasser A. Tumor growth need not be driven by rare cancer stem cells. Science 2007; 317: 337.

60. Adams JM, Kelly PN, Dakic A, Nutt SL, Strasser A. Response to comment on: "Tumor growth need not be driven by rare cancer stem cells". Science 2007; 318: 1722d.

61. Hill RP, Perris R, "Destemming" cancer stem cells. J Natl Cancer Inst 2007; 99: 1435–40.

62. Hill RP. Identifying cancer stem cells in solid tumors: case not proven. Cancer Res 2006; 66: 1891–6.

II   THE STEM CELL NICHE

3

Mesenchymal Stem Cells in Tumor Stroma

Nicholas J. Sullivan and Brett M. Hall

ABSTRACT

Mesenchymal stem cells (MSC) are defined, minimally, as cells that display a fibroblastic morphology in cell culture, exhibit a robust self-renewal capacity, and retain the ability to undergo trilineage differentiation into adipocytes, chondrocytes, and osteoblasts. MSC can be isolated from diverse tissues but are most commonly isolated from red bone marrow. Accumulating evidence suggests that bone marrow MSC can be mobilized into the periphery to serve as regenerative stem cells at sites of injury and inflammation. Although the *in vivo* biology of MSC is poorly understood, several studies have demonstrated that MSC can be selectively recruited into tumors. Following engraftment within tumor stroma, MSC proliferate and acquire an activated phenotype similar tumor-associated fibroblasts (TAF). Tumor-homing properties of MSC have lead to their utility as therapeutic cell-based antitumor protein delivery vehicles. However, with a greater appreciation for the influential role that the tumor microenvironment can serve during tumor initiation, promotion, and progression, MSC may enhance tumor progression following acquisition of TAF-like characteristics. A more comprehensive delineation of the biological role of MSC within tumor stroma will improve our understanding pf tumor-stroma interactions and facilitate future development of MSC-based clinical therapies.

Key Words: Mesenchymal stem cell (MSC), Tumor microenvironment, Tumor-associated fibroblast (TAF), Stromagenesis, Myofibroblast, Desmoplasia, Tumor stroma

INTRODUCTION

Carcinomas are solid tumors that arise from malignant epithelial cells and represent the most common type of cancer in humans. However, it is becoming increasingly clear that malignant cells are supported by nonepithelial tumor stroma that shape a given tumor microenvironment. Tumor stroma can be generally divided into four main components: *(1)* tumor vasculature, *(2)* inflammatory immune cells, *(3)* extracellular matrix (ECM)/soluble growth factors, and *(4)* tumor-associated fibroblasts (TAF) (Fig. 1). Bidirectional paracrine communications between connective tissue fibroblasts and epithelial cells are vital for normal tissue homeostasis, and a comparable but progressive intimacy continues throughout tumor development. Although mesenchymal cell fibroblasts (herein referred to as fibroblasts) can enhance tumor growth and metastasis by means of promoting angiogenesis *(1)*, epithelial–mesenchymal transition *(2)*, and progressive genetic instability *(3, 4)*, there is also evidence that healthy tumor microenvironments can act in a dominant manner to inhibit tumor growth *(5)*.

From: *Cancer Drug Discovery and Development: Stem Cells and Cancer,*
Edited by: R.G. Bagley and B.A. Teicher, DOI: 10.1007/978-1-60327-933-8_3,
© Humana Press, a part of Springer Science+Business Media, LLC 2009

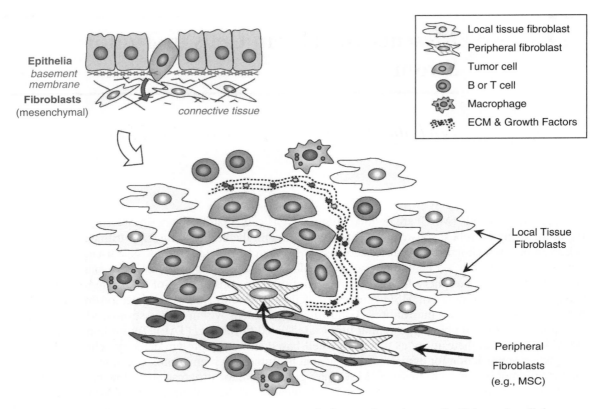

Fig. 1. Similar to an organ, solid tumor masses are composed of a complex mixture of cellular and acellular components, which together comprise the tumor microenvironment. Following loss of basement membrane integrity, tumor cells invade into the underlying connective tissue and interact directly with local mesenchymal fibroblasts. Subsequent tumor and fibroblast cell expansion promotes recruitment of immune cells, peripheral mesenchymal fibroblasts, and *de novo* production and remodeling of extracellular matrix (ECM) (*see Color Plates*).

These studies suggest that acquisition of genetic or biologic alterations may be a prerequisite for fibroblasts to enhance tumor progression *(3, 5–7)*. Although the model for progressive genetic lesions within tumor cells and tumor stroma is compelling, recent evidence suggests that clonal somatic mutations are rare within human TAF *(8)*.

TAF originate from local and, to a lesser degree, peripheral fibroblasts (Fig. 1). Tissue-specific fibroblasts demonstrate heterogeneous phenotypes *(9)*, which can confound the biological impact of fibroblasts in a given tumor microenvironment. In addition, molecular characterization of fibroblasts both in culture and *in vivo* can be highly variable *(10–12)*. For example, normal fibroblasts express common mesenchymal markers such as vimentin or fibroblast-specific protein 1 (FSP1), and upon activation, α-smooth-muscle-actin and fibroblast-activation protein (FAP) are expressed *(13)*. Further exacerbating their molecular variability is that fibroblasts can coexpress various mesenchymal cell markers, and a definitive hierarchal phenotype for fibroblasts is currently undefined. One of the primary biologic functions of fibroblasts *in vivo* is to maintain the integrity of connective tissue. Hence, fibroblasts produce multiple growth factors and ECM proteins including types I, III, IV, and V collagen, laminin, and fibronectin. Additionally, fibroblasts remodel ECM through production of a series of matrix metalloproteinases (MMPs) and tissue inhibitor of metalloproteinases (TIMPs). Fibroblasts are also critical players in normal wound healing, where they acquire an "activated" phenotype resulting in increased proliferation and production of ECM constituents and growth factors *(13, 14)*.

MESENCHYMAL STEM CELLS

The *in vivo* ontogeny and subsequent biology of bone marrow-derived mesenchymal stem cells (MSC) is poorly understood, and therefore, the phenotypic definition of MSC remains controversial *(11)*. Consequently, MSC are most commonly studied *in vitro*, and their tissue culture characteristics can differ dramatically between laboratories, perhaps due to different isolation methods and culture conditions. Nevertheless, the minimal definition of human MSC (hMSC) or murine MSC is mesenchymal cells that display a fibroblastic morphology in cell culture, exhibit a robust self-renewal capacity *(15)*, and retain the capacity to undergo trilineage differentiation into adipocytes, chondrocytes, and osteoblasts *(16, 17)*. Common sources of adult human MSC include bone marrow, compact bone, peripheral blood, and adipose tissue, and the majority of MSC populations can be isolated and expanded in plastic tissue culture plates. Although they express common mesenchymal markers, no exclusive MSC-specific marker is known, thus exemplifying their heterogeneous nature. Nevertheless, MSC are known to express CD73, CD90, CD105 (endoglin), and CD106 (VCAM-1). In contrast, MSC lack all hematopoietic and endothelial lineage markers and are generally CD34 negative *(11, 16, 18)*. Murine MSC display a similar phenotype, which can vary slightly across inbred strains *(17)*.

Although *in vitro* analysis has facilitated the characterization of MSC, the physiological role of MSC in tissue maintenance and repair has recently become more appreciated. Local resident multipotent MSC are well-recognized for their roles in normal tissue maintenance as well as response to injury, but a regenerative resident stem cell population in terminally differentiated tissues such as the CNS and heart appears to be absent or severely reduced. Thus, it has been postulated that bone marrow-derived cells, including MSC, are essential for support of normal adult tissue homeostasis as well as wound healing *(19)*. However, further *in vivo* data are needed to fully define the participation of MSC during normal non-hematopoietic tissue maintenance and regeneration *(11)*.

TUMOR STROMAGENESIS

Although Stephen Paget's "Seed and Soil" Hypothesis was postulated in 1889 to describe permissive metastatic microenvironments in breast cancer patients *(20)*, the role of tumor stroma during tumor progression has only recently gained widespread acceptance. Normal fibroblastic stroma preserves epithelial cell quiescence and effectively inhibits epithelial cell transformation and consequent tumorigenesis as demonstrated in normal breast epithelium *(21)* and other reports of stromal dominance over neoplastic cells *(5, 22)*. However, damaged stroma (by age, injury or inflammation, genetic mutation, or cancer cell influence) can provide a more supportive microenvironment for expanded tumor growth *(3, 23–27)*.

Beacham and Cukierman recently introduced a progressive model for tumor stromagenesis that highlights a reversible "primed" stroma during tumor initiation and an irreversible "activated" stroma (also defined as reactive stroma) during later stage tumorigenesis. While primed tumor stroma initially responds to carcinoma cell invasion much like they would to inflammatory stimuli, they subsequently promote tumorigenesis. This response was reversible and primed tumor stroma was able to return to a quiescent state without tumor progression. Activated stroma, in contrast, represents an irreversible phase of tumor stromagenesis and generally correlates with a desmoplastic reaction *(14)*. Subsequent dysregulated fibrotic responses are marked by overt expansion of fibroblasts within the tumor stroma and overproduction of ECM proteins and growth factors.

TUMOR-ASSOCIATED FIBROBLASTS

Normal epithelium interacts with the underlying stromal compartment through a basement membrane composed mainly of collagen IV and laminin. However, during tumorigenesis, this homeostatic setting gives rise to noninvasive, premalignant, dysplastic, and hyperplastic epithelial cells (i.e., carcinoma *in situ* (CIS)). Upon progression to carcinoma, the previously uncompromised basement membrane is degraded and malignant epithelial cells invade into the underlying reactive stroma *(28)*. Invasive carcinoma cells are then free to directly interact with activated fibroblasts, commonly referred to as TAF *(29, 30)*, carcinoma-associated fibroblasts (CAF) *(1)*, or reactive stroma *(31)*. Haddow *(1972)* and Dvorak *(1986)* were the first to describe tumors as "wounds that do not heal" *(32, 33)*, but in contrast to wound healing, TAF remain in a chronic state of activation and ultimately support tumor progression. Reactive stroma is found in most if not all solid tumors and is often a prognostic indicator of poor clinical outcomes *(5, 34–36)*.

Upon acquiring an activated phenotype, TAF resemble smooth muscle cells and are often referred to as myofibroblasts *(28)*. They retain a fibroblastic spindle-shaped morphology, but unlike their normal counterparts, express extensive and highly organized α-smooth-muscle-actin stress fibers. Although TAF exhibit an increase in both proliferation and motility, they are concurrently capable of enhancing the growth and invasiveness of carcinoma cells as well as normal epithelial cells. For example, Barcellos-Hoff *et al.* demonstrated that an increased incidence of mammary carcinoma following transplantation of nontransformed mammary epithelial cells into irradiated mammary gland stroma was, in part, due to up-regulated paracrine mediators *(23)*. TAF provide carcinoma cells with an extensive variety of promitogenic factors such as transforming growth factor-β (TGF-β), basic fibroblast growth factor (bFGF), epidermal growth factor (EGF), insulin-like growth factor (IGF), interleukin-6 (IL-6), and hepatocyte growth factor (HGF), many of which can also be derived from carcinoma cells. TAF can also enhance tumor angiogenesis through production of stromal-cell derived factor-1 (SDF-1/CXCL-12) and vascular endothelial growth factor (VEGF) *(37)*. Finally, the disorganized appearance and dynamic remodeling of the tumor microenvironment is, in part, due to TAF over-expression of MMP and ECM proteins.

THERAPEUTIC POTENTIAL OF MESENCHYMAL STEM CELLS

Rationale for the therapeutic exploitation of MSC has been validated by the extensive characterization of two primary MSC properties: (1) MSC are capable of homing to sites of inflammation such as tumors *(38, 39)* and (2) MSC are poorly immunogenic *(40–42)*. Although poorly understood, the capacity of MSC to home or perhaps be recruited to sites of inflammation holds clinical implications, particularly for delivery of antitumor agents. An extensive body of experimental evidence suggests that they are recruited to the tumor microenvironment where they contribute as TAF. For example, we and others have shown that bone marrow-derived MSC and cancer cell lines display robust intercellular interactions *in vitro* and *in vivo* *(39, 43–49)*, and several studies have demonstrated a selective recruitment and engraftment of intravenously delivered hMSC to the tumor site in melanoma, breast, and brain tumor xenograft models *(39, 44, 45, 50)*. Furthermore, primary hMSC acquire a phenotype of activated fibroblasts following 3D collagen coculture with colon carcinoma cells or TGF-β1 *(51)*. Finally, an elegant study by Ishii *et al.* demonstrated that non-lymphoid bone marrow-derived cells contribute to both tumor-associated vasculature and TAF in a syngeneic mouse model *(52)*.

Poor immunogenicity, the second therapeutic property of MSC, complements their capacity to home to and persist within tumor microenvironments. Although much of the experimental evidence to date has been obtained from cell culture studies, strong evidence supports that bone marrow-derived MSC escape recognition by alloreactive peripheral blood mononuclear cells both *in vitro* and *in vivo* *(41, 53–56)*. Although the immunosuppressive properties of MSC remain inadequately defined, it reinforces their potential clinical utility as cellular antitumor delivery vehicles. For example, there would be a reduced need for autologous or MHC-matched MSC, and allogeneic MSC could be genetically engineered to express a soluble antitumor agent of choice (e.g., IFN-β) *(39)*.

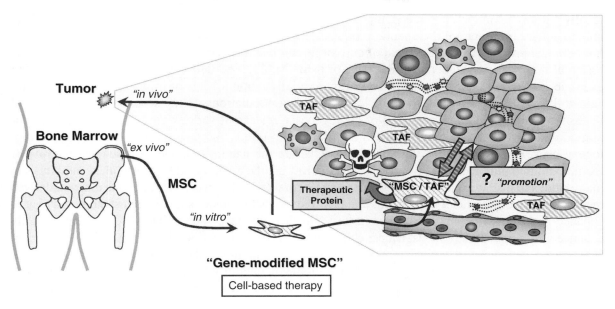

Fig. 2. A "Trojan Horse" anticancer therapy. Bone marrow MSC are isolated from bone marrow and expanded in tissue culture. MSC, *in vitro*, are gene-modified to produce a given antitumor protein and are then reintroduced back into the cancer patient. Given the strong affinity for tumors, MSC selectively engraft and expand within the tumor microenvironment and produce locally concentrated levels of select antitumor proteins (*see Color Plates*).

A THERAPEUTIC "DOUBLE-EDGED SWORD"

MSC-based cellular therapies are based on the "Trojan Horse" principle, in that, gene-modified MSC tend to preferentially engraft within expanding tumors. Once embedded within tumor stroma, MSC become activated, expand, and elevate their metabolic activity. As a consequence, secretion of the predetermined antitumor protein can reach locally elevated concentrations and prevent tumor growth (Fig. 2) *(43)*. However, under some circumstances, MSC may actually promote tumor progression. For example, MSC can enhance tumor growth rates through production of paracrine interleukin-6 (IL-6) *(57, 58)*, and MSC display immunosuppressive effects that can interfere with antitumor immune surveillance *(55, 56)*. These data illustrate the need to better understand biologic consequences of MSC-tumor interactions before MSC-based therapies can truly be successful in the clinical setting. Should injection of gene-modified MSC integrate within tumor stroma and enhance tumor growth rates, survival, or metastasis, the clinical consequences of the MSC therapies would predictably lead to disease progression and highly unfavorable clinical outcomes.

CONCLUSIONS

MSC represent a relatively well-defined *ex vivo* cell population with complex and poorly understood biology *in vivo (11, 18)*. MSC can be readily isolated from multiple tissues, yet red bone marrow remains the most commonly cited source in both humans and mice *(16, 17)*. The first indication that hMSC had a natural affinity for tumors was reported by Studeny *et al.* in 2002 *(39)*. In this and a subsequent study, Studeny *et al.* demonstrated that hMSC, administered intravenously, were able to integrate and persist within tumor stroma of preestablished human melanoma and breast cancer xenografts *(39, 44)*. They also demonstrated that MSC could deliver therapeutic doses of IFN-β locally within the tumor, and indeed, these studies were the first to show that gene-modified MSC are able to deliver intratumoral therapeutic proteins. The use of cell-based delivery systems such as MSC hold clinical promise and a great deal of current research is focused in this area. Conversely, it is also essential that we better understand the risks of using MSC-based delivery in the clinical setting. For example, we do not understand why MSC preferentially home to sites of injury or tumors. It is presumed that MSC are recruited to assist local fibroblast populations during wound repair (e.g., ECM deposition and remodeling, induction of angiogenesis, release of various growth factors, and immunomodulation), and it is likely that MSC are drawn into tumor microenvironments under similar biological cues. However, a lingering question is what are the natural biological consequences of MSC recruitment into tumor stroma? Bone and bone marrow are the common sites of secondary metastasis in many adult and pediatric cancers, and given that MSC are derived from a prevalent bone marrow-derived mesenchymal fibroblast cell population, it is possible that MSC, under some circumstances, may act to enhance tumor growth, survival, and metastasis. In fact, we have shown that MSC can significantly enhance a subpopulation of breast cancer cell growth rates in vitro and in vivo (57, 58). Taken together, MSC-based anticancer therapies represent an exciting and novel therapeutic approach for cancer patients, but a better understanding of how MSC home to, engraft within, and ultimately impact tumor behavior will be essential before we can realize the full potential of MSC-based delivery systems.

REFERENCES

1. Orimo A, Gupta PB, Sgroi DC, et al. Stromal fibroblasts present in invasive human breast carcinomas promote tumor growth and angiogenesis through elevated SDF-1/CXCL12 secretion. Cell 2005;121(3):335–48.
2. Radisky DC, Levy DD, Littlepage LE, et al. Rac1b and reactive oxygen species mediate MMP-3-induced EMT and genomic instability. Nature 2005;436(7047):123–7.
3. Kurose K, Hoshaw-Woodard S, Adeyinka A, Lemeshow S, Watson PH, Eng C. Genetic model of multi-step breast carcinogenesis involving the epithelium and stroma: clues to tumour-microenvironment interactions. Hum Mol Genet 2001;10(18):1907–13.
4. Moinfar F, Man YG, Arnould L, Bratthauer GL, Ratschek M, Tavassoli FA. Concurrent and independent genetic alterations in the stromal and epithelial cells of mammary carcinoma: implications for tumorigenesis. Cancer research 2000;60(9):2562–6.
5. Kenny PA, Bissell MJ. Tumor reversion: correction of malignant behavior by microenvironmental cues. Int J Cancer 2003;107(5):688–95.
6. Hill R, Song Y, Cardiff RD, Van Dyke T. Selective evolution of stromal mesenchyme with p53 loss in response to epithelial tumorigenesis. Cell 2005;123(6):1001–11.
7. McCullough KD, Coleman WB, Ricketts SL, Wilson JW, Smith GJ, Grisham JW. Plasticity of the neoplastic phenotype *in vivo* is regulated by epigenetic factors. Proc Natl Acad Sci USA 1998;95(26):15333–8.
8. Qiu W, Hu M, Sridhar A, et al. No evidence of clonal somatic genetic alterations in cancer-associated fibroblasts from human breast and ovarian carcinomas. Nature genetics 2008;40:650–5.
9. Rinn JL, Bondre C, Gladstone HB, Brown PO, Chang HY. Anatomic demarcation by positional variation in fibroblast gene expression programs. PLoS genetics 2006;2(7):e119.
10. Cukierman E, Pankov R, Stevens DR, Yamada KM. Taking cell-matrix adhesions to the third dimension. Science 2001;294(5547):1708–12.
11. Javazon E H, Beggs K J, Flake A W. Mesenchymal stem cells: paradoxes of passaging. Exp Hematol 2004;32(5):414–25.
12. Kenny PA, Lee GY, Myers CA, Neve RM, Semeiks JR, Spellman PT, Lorenz K, Lee EH, Barcellos-Hoff MH, Peterson OW, Gray JW, Bissell MJ. The morphologies of breast cancer cell lines in three-dimensional assays correlate with their profiles of gene expression. Mol Oncol 2007;1:84–96.
13. Kalluri R, Zeisberg M. Fibroblasts in cancer. Nat Rev Cancer 2006;6(5):392–401.
14. Beacham DA, Cukierman E. Stromagenesis: the changing face of fibroblastic microenvironments during tumor progression. Semin Cancer Biol 2005;15(5):329–41.
15. Colter DC, Class R, DiGirolamo CM, Prockop DJ. Rapid expansion of recycling stem cells in cultures of plastic-adherent cells from human bone marrow. Proc Natl Acad Sci USA 2000;97(7):3213–8.
16. Pittenger MF, Mackay AM, Beck SC, et al. Multilineage potential of adult human mesenchymal stem cells. Science 1999;284(5411):143–7.
17. Peister A, Mellad JA, Larson BL, Hall BM, Gibson LF, Prockop DJ. Adult stem cells from bone marrow (MSCs) isolated from different strains of inbred mice vary in surface epitopes, rates of proliferation, and differentiation potential. Blood 2004;103(5):1662–8.

18. Dominici M, Le Blanc K, Mueller I, et al. Minimal criteria for defining multipotent mesenchymal stromal cells. The International Society for Cellular Therapy position statement. Cytotherapy 2006;8(4):315–7.

19. Phinney DG, Prockop DJ. Concise review: mesenchymal stem/multipotent stromal cells: the state of transdifferentiation and modes of tissue repair–current views. Stem cells (Dayton, Ohio) 2007;25(11):2896–902.

20. Paget S. The distribution of secondary growths in cancer of the breast. Lancet 1889;1:571–3.

21. Kuperwasser C, Chavarria T, Wu M, et al. Reconstruction of functionally normal and malignant human breast tissues in mice. Proc Natl Acad Sci USA 2004;101(14):4966–71.

22. Maffini MV, Soto AM, Calabro JM, Ucci AA, Sonnenschein C. The stroma as a crucial target in rat mammary gland carcinogenesis. J Cell Sci 2004;117(Pt 8):1495–502.

23. Barcellos-Hoff MH, Ravani SA. Irradiated mammary gland stroma promotes the expression of tumorigenic potential by unirradiated epithelial cells. Cancer Res 2000;60(5):1254–60.

24. Bissell MJ, Labarge MA. Context, tissue plasticity, and cancer: are tumor stem cells also regulated by the microenvironment? Cancer cell 2005;7(1):17–23.

25. Kurose K, Gilley K, Matsumoto S, Watson PH, Zhou XP, Eng C. Frequent somatic mutations in PTEN and TP53 are mutually exclusive in the stroma of breast carcinomas. Nat Genet 2002;32(3):355–7.

26. Sternlicht MD, Lochter A, Sympson CJ, et al. The stromal proteinase MMP3/stromelysin-1 promotes mammary carcinogenesis. Cell 1999;98(2):137–46.

27. Tlsty TD, Hein PW. Know thy neighbor: stromal cells can contribute oncogenic signals. Curr Opin Genet Dev 2001;11(1):54–9.

28. Mueller MM, Fusenig NE. Friends or foes – bipolar effects of the tumour stroma in cancer. Nat Rev Cancer 2004;4(11):839–49.

29. Kunz-Schughart LA, Knuechel R. Tumor-associated fibroblasts (part II): functional impact on tumor tissue. Histol Histopathol 2002;17(2):623–37.

30. Kunz-Schughart LA, Knuechel R. Tumor-associated fibroblasts (part I): Active stromal participants in tumor development and progression? Histol Histopathol 2002;17(2):599–621.

31. Rowley DR. What might a stromal response mean to prostate cancer progression?Cancer Metastasis Rev 1998;17(4):411–9.

32. Dvorak HF. Tumors: wounds that do not heal. Similarities between tumor stroma generation and wound healing. N Engl J Med 1986;315(26):1650–9.

33. Haddow A. Molecular repair, wound healing, and carcinogenesis: tumor production a possible overhealing? Adv Cancer Res 1972;16:181–234.

34. De Wever O, Mareel M. Role of tissue stroma in cancer cell invasion. J Pathol 2003;200(4):429–47.

35. Hasebe T, Mukai K, Tsuda H, Ochiai A. New prognostic histological parameter of invasive ductal carcinoma of the breast: clinicopathological significance of fibrotic focus. Pathol Int 2000;50(4):263–72.

36. Kurosumi M, Tabei T, Inoue K, et al. Prognostic significance of scoring system based on histological heterogeneity of invasive ductal carcinoma for node-negative breast cancer patients. Oncol Rep 2003;10(4):833–7.

37. Karnoub AE, Dash AB, Vo AP, et al. Mesenchymal stem cells within tumour stroma promote breast cancer metastasis. Nature 2007;449(7162):557–63.

38. Ortiz LA, Gambelli F, McBride C, et al. Mesenchymal stem cell engraftment in lung is enhanced in response to bleomycin exposure and ameliorates its fibrotic effects. Proc Natl Acad Sci USA 2003;100(14):8407–11.

39. Studeny M, Marini FC, Champlin RE, Zompetta C, Fidler IJ, Andreeff M. Bone marrow-derived mesenchymal stem cells as vehicles for interferon-beta delivery into tumors. Cancer Res 2002;62(13):3603–8.

40. Uccelli A, Moretta L, Pistoia V. Immunoregulatory function of mesenchymal stem cells. Eur J Immunol 2006;36(10):2566–73.

41. Tse WT, Pendleton JD, Beyer WM, Egalka MC, Guinan EC. Suppression of allogeneic T-cell proliferation by human marrow stromal cells: implications in transplantation. Transplantation 2003;75(3):389–97.

42. Le Blanc K, Ringden O. Immunobiology of human mesenchymal stem cells and future use in hematopoietic stem cell transplantation. Biol Blood Marrow Transplant 2005;11(5):321–34.

43. Hall B, Andreeff M, Marini F. The participation of mesenchymal stem cells in tumor stroma formation and their application as targeted-gene delivery vehicles. Handb Exp Pharmacol 2007(180):263–83.

44. Studeny M, Marini FC, Dembinski JL, et al. Mesenchymal stem cells: potential precursors for tumor stroma and targeted-delivery vehicles for anticancer agents. J Natl Cancer Inst 2004;96(21):1593–603.

45. Nakamizo A, Marini F, Amano T, et al. Human bone marrow-derived mesenchymal stem cells in the treatment of gliomas. Cancer Res 2005;65(8):3307–18.

46. Zhu W, Xu W, Jiang R, et al. Mesenchymal stem cells derived from bone marrow favor tumor cell growth in vivo. Exp Mol Pathol 2006;80(3):267–74.

47. Houghton J, Stoicov C, Nomura S, et al. Gastric cancer originating from bone marrow-derived cells. Science 2004;306(5701):1568–71.

48. Prindull G, Zipori D. Environmental guidance of normal and tumor cell plasticity: epithelial mesenchymal transitions as a paradigm. Blood 2004;103(8):2892–9.

49. Hombauer H, Minguell JJ. Selective interactions between epithelial tumour cells and bone marrow mesenchymal stem cells. Br J Cancer 2000;82(7):1290–6.

50. Hall B, Dembinski J, Sasser AK, Studeny M, Andreeff M, Marini F. Mesenchymal stem cells in cancer: tumor-associated fibroblasts and cell-based delivery vehicles. Int J Hematol 2007;86(1):8–16.

51. Emura M, Ochiai A, Horino M, Arndt W, Kamino K, Hirohashi S. Development of myofibroblasts from human bone marrow mesenchymal stem cells cocultured with human colon carcinoma cells and TGF beta 1. In Vitro Cell Dev Biol Anim 2000;36(2):77–80.

52. Ishii G, Sangai T, Oda T, et al. Bone-marrow-derived myofibroblasts contribute to the cancer-induced stromal reaction. Biochem Biophys Res Commun 2003;309(1):232–40.

53. Di Nicola M, Carlo-Stella C, Magni M, et al. Human bone marrow stromal cells suppress T-lymphocyte proliferation induced by cellular or nonspecific mitogenic stimuli. Blood 2002;99(10):3838–43.

54. Bartholomew A, Sturgeon C, Siatskas M, et al. Mesenchymal stem cells suppress lymphocyte proliferation in vitro and prolong skin graft survival in vivo. Exp Hematol 2002;30(1):42–8.

55. Aggarwal S, Pittenger MF. Human mesenchymal stem cells modulate allogeneic immune cell responses. Blood 2005;105(4):1815–22.

56. Djouad F, Plence P, Bony C, et al. Immunosuppressive effect of mesenchymal stem cells favors tumor growth in allogeneic animals. Blood 2003;102(10):3837–44.

57. Sasser AK, Mundy BL, Smith KM, et al. Human bone marrow stromal cells enhance breast cancer cell growth rates in a cell line-dependent manner when evaluated in 3D tumor environments. Cancer Lett 2007;254(2):255–64.

58. Sasser AK, Sullivan NJ, Studebaker AW, Hendey LF, Axel AE, Hall BM. Interleukin-6 is a potent growth factor for ER-alpha-positive human breast cancer. Faseb J 2007;21(13):3763–70.

III Molecular Pathways and Gene Expression

4

Wnt Signaling in Cancer: From Embryogenesis to Stem Cell Self-Renewal

Adam Yagui-Beltrán, Biao He, and David M Jablons

ABSTRACT

Over the years, the role of the Wingless-int (Wnt) signaling pathway during embryogenesis has been the focus of many researchers, its role being fundamental for physiological organogenesis. More recently, during adulthood, the Wnt signaling pathway has been found to be involved in the regulation of a myriad of cellular processes, including cellular motility, proliferation, differentiation, survival, and apoptosis. It is therefore unsurprising that when this pathway becomes aberrant through anomalous regulation that cancer ensues. Indeed, this developmental pathway has been involved in cancers of the blood, thyroid, breast, lung, prostate, and colon. Key is the role that Wnt signaling plays in the regulation of stem cell fates, all within tightly regulated "niches." Careful dissection of the various mechanisms controlling this pathway and the subsequent understanding of their functional significance during tissue homeostasis; how it affects stem cells and how it may contribute to carcinogenesis will result in new molecular-based disease markers and novel therapeutic agents to specifically target these diseases.

Key Words: Wnt, Hedgehog, Notch, Cancer, Embryogenesis, Organogenesis, Tissue homeostasis, Extracellular matrix, Niche, Stem cell, Novel cell substitution therapies, Cancer stem cell

EMBRYOGENESIS AND ITS REQUIREMENTS

The formation of a multicellular organism requires the occurrence of the following elements that need to be perfectly coordinated in time and space: cells need to be able to proliferate; they also need to follow different yet specific fates of cellular differentiation to ultimately ensemble and organize into functioning organs. Indeed cell fate specification and the combination of complex gene regulatory networks (GRNs) are paramount for the processes of embryo and organogenesis *(1)*. GRNs will determine through the provision of a diverse array of patterns of gene expression the phenotype of individual cells. Intrinsic elements such as transcription factors released by cells in a timely manner provide the coordinates that delineate their individual fate. Extrinsic factors will play a role in influencing cells as groups in their transition through various states of differentiation. The "Signal Transduction" machinery integrating intrinsic and extrinsic factors is the ultimate denominator that provides the fate coordinates of specific cell populations. It is therefore imperative to understand the interplay between the

From: *Cancer Drug Discovery and Development: Stem Cells and Cancer,*
Edited by: R.G. Bagley and B.A. Teicher, DOI: 10.1007/978-1-60327-933-8_4,
© Humana Press, a part of Springer Science+Business Media, LLC 2009

various intrinsic and extrinsic factors in GRNs in order to elucidate the mechanisms governing cell fate assignment. The Cybernetics and Information Theory, reviewed by Rodbell *(2)*, proposed the existence of a signal, a transducer, and an effector, as well as a process of amplification happening during the transduction operation. This model has allowed a useful platform for the study and evaluation of signaling molecules in various organisms for the last few decades. Lack of knowledge on the quantitative aspects of signal transduction in biological processes led to the question of noise within the model, an issue that is known to be crucially important in the original "Information Theory." It is only recently that the concept of "noise," as being the subtle variations in the transduction pathway that will ultimately determine the outcome of the transduction process as a whole, is being considered in biological signal transduction models. Elegant experiments performed in single-cell organisms indicate that noise is an important element in the overall functionality of transcriptional networks and that they play a role in embryogenesis *(3–5)*. Consideration of this matter will lead to more precise perspectives on the way transcriptional networks operate during the development of an organism. It is widely accepted, through cumulative data from various research groups, over the last couple of decades, that there are six main signaling transduction pathways in the cell *(6)*: Wnt (Wingless/Int1), Hedgehog (Hh), Notch, Receptor Tyrosine Kinase (RTK), Steroid Hormone Receptor, and Bone Morphogenic Proteins (BMP). In combination, they represent the basic machinery for the determination of cell fate during development. They are thought to act in parallel, to ultimately enhance specific genes that result in cell type-specific combinations of transcription factors responsible for cellular states and behavior *(6, 7)*. This view is generally accepted as it has been proven in the photoreceptor cellular fate determination in the *Drosophila* model *(8, 9)* and in the eight-cell embryo of *C. elegans* during the specification of blastomeres *(10–12)*. The combined activity of transcription factors in these examples is precisely defined through specific temporospatial coordinates of GRNs. Nevertheless, there is increasing evidence that points toward more subtle interactions between elements of the signaling pathways governing cell fate, and it logically follows that a careful dissection of those interactions will help us understand better what actually happens during embryogenesis, organogenesis, tissue homeostasis, and repair *(13–16)*. This knowledge will be fundamental to the understanding of the consequences ensuing when these signaling pathways go haywire causing a mélange of alterations to stem cell cycling ultimately resulting in cancer. We will now focus our attention on the Wnt signaling cascade and describe some of its cross-regulatory interrelationships with some of the other signaling pathways responsible for cell-fate specification, to then examine the concept of homeostatic and "cancer" stem cells and their intimate orchestrating relationships with their microenvironment and with the Wnt pathway.

WNT SIGNAL TRANSDUCTION

This signaling pathway was named after the *wingless* gene, the Drosophila homologous gene of the first mammalian Wnt gene characterized, *int-1 (17)*. Wnt genes are responsible for encoding secreted cysteine-rich glycoproteins that bind with a myriad of receptors to then trigger changes in gene expression modifying cell behavior, cell adhesion, and cell polarity. In mammals, Wnt proteins comprise a family of 19 highly conserved signaling molecules and Wnt signaling has been described in at least three pathways *(18)*. The best studied and characterized Wnt pathway is the canonical signaling cascade (Fig. 1), in which Wnt ligands bind to two distinct families of cell surface receptors, the Frizzled (Fz) receptor family and the LDL receptor-related protein (LRP) family, and activate target genes through the stabilization of beta-catenin in the nucleus *(19)*. The noncanonical pathway is comprised of the Wnt/Ca2+ cascade where Wnt proteins signal through the activation of calmodulin kinase II and protein kinase C, this leads to an increase in intracellular Ca2+. Wnt can also signal noncanonically through Jun N-terminal kinase (JNK) (known as the planar cell polarity pathway), controlling cytoskeletal rearrangements and cell polarity *(20)*. The large repertoire of Wnt ligands,

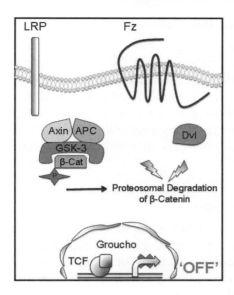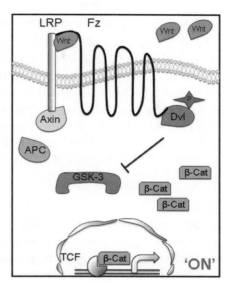

Fig. 1. The canonical Wnt transduction pathway. Proteosomal degradation of beta-catenin via its phosphorylation occurs in the absence of Wnt ligands. Downstream Wnt target genes are maintained repressed (OFF). Degradation of active beta-catenin is reduced upon binding of Wnts. Accumulation and translocation of beta-catenin into the nucleus leads to binding to T cell factors and activation of target genes (ON). *APC* Adenomatous polyposis coli; *Dvl* Dishevelled; *GSK* Glycogen synthase kinase; *TCF* T cell factor.

receptors, Wnt activators, and antagonists and their complex interactions elicit a wide variety of cellular responses, making the Wnt signaling pathway essential for embryogenesis, organogenesis, postnatal development, tissue repair, and homeostasis. There is increasing understanding that these functions occur through the effects of the pathway on rare pluripotent stem cells and it is not surprising that aberrations in this pathway may lead to many types of human cancer.

The Canonical Wnt Pathway

The canonical Wnt pathway is activated consequent to binding of Wnt ligands to their Frizzled (Fz) receptors and low-density lipoprotein receptor-related proteins-5/6 (LRP-5/6) coreceptors. Subsequent activation of the cytoplasmic phosphoprotein, Disheveled (Dvl) inhibits a cytoplasmic complex made of Glycogen Synthase Kinase 3 (GSK-3), Axin, Adenomatous Polyposis Coli (APC) to then inhibit the phosphorylation.

Polyposis Coli (APC) then inhibit the phosphorylation of beta-catenin by GSK-3*(21)*. The release and stabilization of hypophosphorylated beta-catenin leads to its cytoplasmic accumulation and subsequent translocation, with the help of BCL9, to the nucleus *(22–24)*. There, it interacts with DNA-bound T cell factor (TCF)/lymphoid enhancer protein (LEF) family members to activate transcription of target genes. In the absence of the Wnt signal, the TCF/DNA-binding proteins form a complex with Groucho and act as repressors of Wnt target genes *(25)*, the complex mediates proteosomal degradation of beta-catenin via its phosphorylation *(21, 26)*. Groucho can interact with histone deacetylases making the DNA refractory to transcriptional activation *(27)*. As beta-catenin penetrates the nucleus, it competes with Groucho for binding to TCF/LEF, recruits Pygopus, and converts the TCF repressor complex into a transcriptional activator complex (Fig. 1). Numerous target genes, such as c-Myc, cyclin D1, MMP7, and WISP have been identified and characterized. A comprehensive list of Wnt target genes may be found on the Internet at http://www.stanford.edu/~rnusse/wntwindow.html.

The Noncanonical Wnt Pathway

Apart from the Wnt/Ca2+ cascade where Wnt proteins signal through the activation of Calmodulin Kinase II and Protein Kinase C, leading to increased intracellular Ca2+, the noncanonical Wnt pathway can also influence cell polarity through the Jun N-terminal Kinase (JNK) signaling cascade *(20)*. Interestingly, Wnt has also been described to atypically signal via the Receptor Tyrosine Kinase (RTK) pathway *(28)* and a newly discovered cascade involving the Cyclic Adenosine Monophosphate (cAMP) pathway activating Protein Kinase A downstream of specific Wnts ultimately playing a role in myogenesis. A crucial element in the latter process is the phosphorylation and subsequent activation of the cAMP response element-binding (CREB) *(29)*.

Wnt Ligands

Wnt proteins are highly conserved, secreted glycoproteins of approximately 40 kDa in size. They characteristically have a high number of conserved cysteine residues. In humans, 19 Wnt proteins have been identified to date, and they are produced by a variety of different cellular types *(30)*. Essential for the functionality of Wnt proteins is the process of cysteine palmitoylation; moreover cells that secrete Wnt proteins require Porcupine (Porc), which is homologous to some of the acyltransferases in the endoplasmic reticulum. The studies suggest that Porc could be the enzyme responsible for cysteine palmitoylation of the Wnt proteins *(31–33)*. Research in *Drosophila* has shown that the seven-transmembrane proteins Wntless (WIs) and Evenness interrupted (Evi) are crucial for the adequate secretion of Wnts. WIs/Evi are primordially localized to the Golgi apparatus, and studies in which WIs/Evi were suppressed, Wnt-producing cells retained their Wnt proteins. Extracellular heparan sulfate proteoglycans (HSPGs) also seem to be involved in the transportation and stabilization of Wnt proteins *(34–36)*.

Wnt Receptors and Antagonists

Wnt signaling transduction starts when Wnt proteins interact with the members of two distinct and specific families of cell surface receptors, the Frizzled (Fz) protein family and the LRP family of cell surface receptors. Wnt ligands bind to Fz proteins through an extracellular N-terminal cysteine-rich domain (CRD). Most Wnt proteins have a promiscuous relationship with multiple Fz receptor proteins. There are ten Fz proteins that have been identified to date. Their molecular structure is comparable to that of the seven-transmembrane G protein-coupled receptors suggesting that Fz proteins may utilize heterotrimeric G proteins to transmit Wnt signals *(37, 38)*. Expression of cell surface receptors LRP5 or LRP6 (single-pass transmembrane molecules of the LRP family of receptors) is required in conjunction with Fz to adequately relay Wnt signaling. Studies validating a trimeric complex formation between Wnt molecules, Fz, and LRP5/6 are still ongoing *(39)*. Derailed and Ror2, two tyrosine kinase receptors have been demonstrated to bind to Wnts. Derailed couples to Wnt via its extracellular WIF (Wnt inhibitory factor) domain, and Ror2 does it via a Wnt CRD motif. More studies to understand the signaling mechanisms downstream of these alternative Wnt receptors are obviously required *(40, 41)*. Secreted inhibitory proteins can sequester Wnt ligands from their receptors. The secreted Frizzled-related proteins (SFRPs) and the Wnt inhibitory factor-1 (WIF-1) are good examples of these inhibitory proteins. In humans, the SFRP family comprises five members, each one of them containing a CRD domain. SFRPs may act as agonists and antagonists of Wnt, highlighting their complex biological nature *(42–44)*. WIF-1 contains a unique, evolutionarily conserved WIF domain and five epidermal growth factor (EGF)-like repeats and it is not homologous in sequence with SFRPs. The Dickkopf (Dkk) family of extracellular Wnt inhibitors antagonizes Wnt signaling relay by the inactivation of LRP5/6, and Dkk representing a third class of Wnt inhibitors *(45)*.

CROSS-TALK BETWEEN WNT AND OTHER SIGNAL TRANSDUCTION PATHWAYS DURING EMBRYOGENESIS AND CANCER

Even though this chapter specifically pertains to the Wnt signaling pathway and its involvement in development, cell renewal, and carcinogenesis, it is mandatory to briefly explore how Wnt interacts with some of the other key developmental pathways in order to gain some sort of perspective on its functionality during physiology and pathology. Other pathways will be explored in detail in specific cellular contexts elsewhere in the book.

Notch Signal Transduction

Notch belongs to a family of single-transmembrane-domain receptors that have an extracellular domain consisting of EGF-like repeats and an intracellular domain with a seven Ankyrin (ANK) repeats *(46–49)*. The intracellular domain of Notch (NICD) behaves as a membrane-bound transcription factor that is freed by an interaction between Notch and its ligands, Delta and Serrate *(50)*. NICD once free is able to translocate into the nucleus of the cell, to then interact with CSL (CBF in vertebrates, Suppressor of Hairless *[Su(H)]* in *Drosophila*, and LAG-1 in *C. elegans*), to subsequently drive the transcription of target genes. Recent studies from various research groups indicate that the cleavage of NICD seems to require endocytic trafficking or the localization of Notch to a specific endocytic compartment, adding complexity to this system *(51–57)*.

INTERFACE BETWEEN WNT AND NOTCH

Evidence regarding the interplay between Wingless and Notch was first discovered in the context of wing patterning and development in *Drosophila(58, 59)*. In this organism, Wnt and Notch reiteratively drive the development and patterning of the wing *(60, 61)*. Initially they synergize in the early formation of the wing primordium *(58, 62)*. At a later stage Notch signal transduction promotes *wingless* expression at the future wing margin *(63, 64)*. On the other hand, Wingless after its increased expression, promotes the transcription and expression of Notch ligands, Serrate and Delta on either side of its expression domain, inducing a positive-feedback loop that patterns the wing margin through the continuous expression of Wingless and Notch *(62, 65, 66)*. The severe sensitivity observed in developing *Drosophila* wing margin to the dosage of *Wingless* and *Notch* may explain some of the interactions observed between these two proteins in this particular organism. Loss of one *Notch* allele produces a wing phenotype, so it is not particularly surprising that considering its close association with *Wingless*, alterations in the dosage of the latter has dramatic effects on wing formation. Taken together, these results make the haploid-insufficient phenotype of *Notch* a sensitive assay to identify and characterize the proteins that interact genetically with Notch *(58, 67–70)*. Therefore, the mutual enhancement of mutations in *Wingless* and *Notch* has a simple explanation in the GRNs that drive wing organogenesis. Close and mutual interactions between *Notch* and *Wingless* (where Wnt signal transduction promotes the expression of Notch) have also been observed in vertebrates, during somitogenesis and muscle formation *(71, 72)*, during the formation of skin precursors *(73)*, and during the patterning of rhombomeres *(74)*. This pattern of regulatory relationship between two or more network elements of distinctive developmental pathways in differing physiological and embryogenic contexts makes it act similarly to the mode of action of a network motif *(75)*.

Although the model of "modular transcription networks" as described is of paramount importance, it is not sufficient to fully explain how Wnt and Notch signaling interrelate as illustrated through studies of the mutant *Notch* alleles *Abruptex (Ax)* and *Microchaete defective (Mcd)* in *Drosophila(13, 58, 76, 77)*. These mutants encode proteins that behave as gain-of-function Notch receptors, that allow Su(H)-independent Notch activity in the peripheral nervous system (PNS) during the prepatterning stage of development. However, during lateral inhibition and wing patterning, they provide

Su(H)-dependent activity *(13, 77–79)*. Moreover, *Ax* and *Mcd* can synergize with loss-of-function of *Wingless* and their phenotype can be partially recovered by gain-of-function Wingless signal transduction *(58)*. The results of these studies may suggest that Wingless and Notch can also interact in an antagonistic mode. It could be argued that this way of interaction may be due to the existence of targets that are differentially repressed by one pathway and antagonized by the other. This explanation though, can be problematic because frequently both modes of regulation act simultaneously on the same target gene. This gives rise to the possibility of there being a level of interaction that bypasses the transcriptional network. This is supported by epistasis analyses performed on PNS and muscle precursor specification in *Drosophila(6, 80–82)*. These experiments are based on the model described so far, that Wingless transduction presets a prepattern by forming equivalence groups through positional information. Notch on the other hand, acts on these groups to limit their neural potential to as few as one or two cells, via lateral inhibition. In the absence of Wingless, there is a subsequent lack of prepattern. When there is no prepattern PNS specification, Notch is not able to perform its duty. In a double mutant for *Notch* and *Wingless*, the lack of Wingless should be dominant over the absence of Notch, explaining that more clearly: when there is no prepattern, there is no need for lateral inhibition. Equally, the phenotypic characteristics of a *Notch, Wingless* double mutant ought to be identical to that of *Wingless* mutant *Drosophila* embryos alone. Interestingly, what was seen during specification of muscle founders in these organisms did not quite corroborate the expected phenotypes just highlighted, and indicated that a certain component of the *Wingless* mutant phenotype is because of *Notch*. Brennan et al. and Carmena et al. observed that loss of Wingless transduction in the fly embryos resulted in loss of precursors and that *Notch* mutants demonstrated more precursors, however and interestingly, double mutant *Notch/Wingless* embryos were found to have some precursors, suggesting that loss of *Notch* may be responsible for rescuing the loss of *Wingless* function *(82, 83)*. This phenomenon has also been seen in the specification of precursors of the *Drosophila* adult nervous system *(79, 84, 85)*. The activity of a transcriptional response element, exclusively Wingless dependent, in the embryonic visceral mesoderm *Ubx* gene demonstrated that the enhancer effects of Notch were exclusively targeting Wingless, independent of Su(H), and not due to some other peripheral pathway *(13, 69, 86)*. One could attempt to explain these results through complex GRNs with undiscovered regulatory elements, however, the easiest explanation is that in addition to the Wnt/Notch modular network, Notch is able to regulate Wnt transduction, via a constrained functional interaction between some of their specific elements *(87)*. The detailed genetic analyses described above and that led to the discovery of further mechanisms of interaction between Wnt and Notch signaling are logistically not possible in vertebrates. Despite these experimental limitations, there is evidence that also in vertebrates, there are developmental circumstances in which Wnt signaling is associated with high Notch signaling and vice versa, demonstrating clear antagonism. In other circumstances, such as during somitogenesis, where the central pattern generator of development is the Notch-driven spatiotemporal cycles of gene expression, it has been possible to identify the regulatory motif in which Delta expression is under the control of Wnt signaling transduction *(71, 72, 88, 89)*. When the results of these studies are considered together, one may conclude that the Wnt and Notch signaling pathways play an interactive role in common GRNs. Their interaction reflects an intimate functional relationship between both pathways and furthermore, a mechanistic interlocking of some of their component elements in a way that makes them part of the same information-processing network *(87)*.

Hedgehog Signal Transduction

The Hh signaling pathway is involved in embryonic patterning as well as stem cell proliferation, homeostasis, growth, and cancer. The *Hh* gene was initially identified as a secreted signaling protein required for specification of positional identity in the *Drosophila* embryonic segment *(90–94)*. In *Drosophila*, Hh is also involved in patterning of imaginal disc-derived adult structures such as the appendages, the eye, and the abdominal cuticle. In mammals there are three *Hh* genes: *Sonic, Indian*, and *Desert hedgehog* *(Shh, Ihh*, and *Dhh)*. They play essential roles in the patterning of many organs during embryogenesis, and it has been shown that aberrant Hh signaling is responsible for many developmental malformations *(90–94)*. The intramolecular cleavage and lipid modification reaction catalyzed by the carboxyl-terminal portion of the Hh protein precursor is the initiator of this signaling transduction cascade. The resultant amino-terminal peptide, esterified on its C-terminus to a cholesterol molecule (HhNp) is responsible for most known signaling actions of the Hh protein. In mammals, ShhNp proteins undergo further palmitoylation at its N-terminus and this additional step is dependent on prior addition of a cholesterol group, believed to exaggerate the activity of the protein in certain cellular contexts *(95, 96)*. Contrasting to other signaling pathways, intracellular Hh signaling occurs by sequential repressive interactions. Two transmembrane proteins, the tumor-suppressor Patched (Ptch) and the proto-oncogene Smoothened (Smo) are responsible for regulating Hh transduction initiation and transduction *(91, 92, 94)*. Ptch is a 12-span transmembrane protein. Smo belongs to the seven-transmembrane receptor family showing close similarity to the Fz receptor family in the Wnt signal transduction pathway. In the quiescent state of the Hh pathway the activity of Smo is suppressed by Ptch. Upon stimulation by Hh, Smo becomes activated after release of its inhibition, resulting in the signaling transcriptional cascade. There is enough scientific evidence to demonstrate an interaction between Hh and Ptch and between Ptch and Smo, resulting in the proposal of a heteromeric receptor model for this pathway. In this model, Hh binds to Ptch within the Ptch/Smo complex, releasing the activity of Smo without the disintegration of Ptch and Smo. Dissimilar in vivo localization of Ptch and Smo despite physiological relationships between Hh and Ptch, indicate that alternative models to explain this signal transduction pathway ought to be considered *(94, 97, 98)*. How activation of Smo relates to some of the cytoplasmic components of the Hh pathway, including the serine/threonine protein kinase Fused (Fu), Suppressor of Fused (Su(fu)), the kinesin-like protein Costal-2 (Cos-2), and the transcription factor Cubitus interruptus (Ci; Gli in mammals) is still not entirely clear *(91, 92, 97, 99, 100)*. In *Drosophila*, these molecules interact and aggregate to form a microtubule-anchored cytoplasmic complex mainly, it seems, through the action of Cos2. In the absence of Hh, protein kinase A phosphorylates Ci (Ci155), which is then cleaved into an N-terminal transcriptional repressor (Ci75) *(100)*. Stimulation via Hh leads to disintegration of the cytoplasmic complex from the microtubules, followed by nuclear translocation of the full-length Ci transcriptional activator, which in turn leads to transcriptional activation of Hh target genes *(101, 102)*, including *Ptch*, which feedbacks in an inhibitory manner *(103)*. In mammals several but not all homologs to the *Drosophila* Hh cytoplasmic proteins have been identified, many of which have multiple isoforms. The inhibitory transcriptional function of Ci in mammals seems to occur through Gli-3, while Gli-1 and Gli-2 behave as activators of the pathway. However, a lot remains unknown in the mammalian Hh pathway and its complexities.

INTERFACE BETWEEN WNT AND HEDGEHOG

Wnt and Hh signal transduction processes are fundamentally crucial for the physiological development of diverse epithelial tissues such as hair follicles, the teeth, and the gastrointestinal tract *(26, 104, 105)*. Ectopic activation or abnormally elevated expression of these signaling molecules may lead to cancer, whereas their inhibition may be responsible for developmental abnormalities in a variety of tissues *(106, 107)*. Evidence regarding the interplay between Wnt and Hh has been reported in embryonic organ morphogenesis and although both pathways have been described to occur in the context of epithelial-mesenchymal interactions, the specific mechanisms governing their mutual regulatory mechanisms remain to be relatively under explored *(108–113)*. In cancer, however, there is an increasing body of evidence linking the Wnt signaling pathway with Hedgehog. A study by Van den Brink et al. in 2004 described Ihh to be a negative regulator of the Wnt pathway during colonic epithelial cell differentiation *(114)*. Gli-1 has been shown to inhibit the proliferation of colorectal cancer cells via the suppression of Wnt *(115)*. Furthermore, another recent study found Gli-1 to suppress Wnt through SFRP-1, an antagonist of Wnt and a transcriptional target of Hh signaling *(115)*. Clearly, as the complexity of the Hh signaling pathway is dissected, newer insights into how this embryonic pathway cross-talks with Wnt and its components will arise, which in turn will elucidate those relationships that are crucial to cell-fate definition and how their deregulation may lead to neoplasia.

WNT, NICHES, STEM CELLS, AND THEIR FATES

Over the last few years, stem cells have acquired significant protagonism as priceless research tools for scientists and as a potential resource for novel cell substitution therapies for a variety of benign and malignant diseases. Crucial to stem cells and their function is their microenvironment and as such they cannot be evaluated in isolation. Therefore, before we explore the concept of "cancer stem cells" and their link to the Wnt signaling pathway, we must tackle the issue of niches and microenvironments in stem cell biology. The field of somatic stem cell biology has been around for over half a century and mouse embryonic stem cells have been utilized for a long time too. One of most important revolutions in the field was the isolation in 1998 of human embryonic stem cells (hESCs) by Thomson et al. Controversial and speculative reports on somatic stem cell plasticity fueled the revolution and served as one of the basis of regenerative medicine. The realization of the therapeutic potential of stem cells is unsurprising. However, in order to achieve tangible novel therapies, a careful understanding of the molecular mechanisms controlling stem cell fates and their niches is mandatory. In biology, the concept of niche in a solely architectural sense is insufficient. A biological niche ought to have, like in ecology, a sustaining function. The simple geography of stem cells is not enough to define a niche. The niche must have both anatomical and functional dimensions, allowing its dwelling stem cells to self-renew and repopulate. Indeed, somatic stem cells have restricted function outside their niche. A good example is the hematopoietic stem cell, which has the ability to regenerate successfully the entire blood and the immune system. These cells are able to circulate the body with limited or no function outside specific anatomical locations. Precise cues from particular sites signal these stem cells to survive, and to fluctuate in numbers and fates according to appropriate relevant physiological situations. When stem cells are exposed to physiological challenges, the niche is able to provide them with the adequate modulatory signals to guarantee satisfactory responses. It is this rich dynamism that makes the concept of "stem cell niche" rather attractive and important to diseases where stem cells play a role, be it in degenerative or malformative diseases, or in cancer. If we can understand how the niche functionally modulates stem cells, the quest to find novel therapies for all these diseases will be made easier. We will now highlight some of the progress that has been made on specific key issues intrinsically relating to stem cells and to their niche to try and understand what makes stem cells self-renew as opposed to differentiate to then analyze the role of Wnt in this fascinating processes.

The Extracellular Matrix

Early work in *Drosophila* and *C. elegans* led to the discovery that germ stem cells are localized at the distal end of a tapered structure, and that they seem to be dependent on interactions with somatic cells at the end of that structure that help them maintain their "stemness" *(116–118)*. These studies showed that the niche is composed of heterologous cell populations, and it led to the identification in mammals of osteoblasts in the bone marrow compartment, and the endothelium in the brain *(119–122)*. Currently, there is controversy, on whether there is the need for other cell types, apart from the stem cell, for the adequate functionality of the niche and this has been highlighted by two studies in *Drosophila*. These studies showed that the posterior mid-gut populations of cells are able to yield daughter enterocytes and enteroendocrine cells. These stem cells do not need direct contact with a heterologous cell type. Interestingly, they were found to have Armadillo (a beta-catenin paralogue) specifically localized at the interface between the stem cell and its descendent enteroblast. These stem cells localize to the basement membrane that separates them from surrounding muscle cells. A plausible explanation is that it is this basement membrane that provides a specific microenvironment within the continuum of the intestine. A microenvironment, which is composed of extracellular matrix and other noncellular components together are able to regulate the cells within that niche without the necessity of heterologous cells. There are also mammalian examples demonstrating that the extracellular matrix exerts a regulatory function on stem cells. In the skin, β-1 integrins have been found to be differentially expressed on primitive cells and to engage in constrained localization of a stem-cell population via presumed crosstalk with matrix glycoprotein ligands *(123, 124)*. In the nervous system, lack of Tenascin C changes neural stem cell number and function in the subventricular zone *(125)*. In the blood system, deletion of Tenascin C affects primitive cell populations, suggesting its involvement in the various hematopoietic stem (HS)-cell niches *(126)*. Another good example is Osteopontin (OPN), a matrix protein that is also involved in cell-mediated immunity and metastasis. OPN has been recently shown to play an important function in the regulation of hematopoietic stem-cell niches. OPN production fluctuates significantly with osteoblast activation, and animals deficient in OPN show an increased number of HS-cells. OPN was shown to limit the number of stem cells under homeostatic conditions or with stimulation, behaving as some sort of constrain regulating these blood stem cells. It is evident from these examples that many extracellular matrix components offer localizing niches that may in turn provide stimulatory and or inhibitory effects on the stem-cell population.

Paracrine Wnt Actions and the Niche

The physicality of a specific niche is important – it is an active process with defined characteristics. Equally important are the signals governing the physical organization of the niche. These signals and how they work are not fully understood. Experiments in mice have shown that ephrins and their RTK receptors are prominent mediators of structural boundaries and that they are involved in the organization of intestinal epithelial cells. When these molecules are aberrantly expressed, abnormal organization of the crypt and intestinal villus occurs, affecting the stem cells thereby located. The change in tissue topography and orientation of primitive and differentiating cells results in abnormal growth. Wnt proteins as well as their antagonists contribute at different levels in the niche, in a paracrine manner, to impair differentiation and to promote proliferation. A careful dissection of the specific Wnt molecular events responsible for the architectural organization of the niche and the stem cells contained within it is important, in order to understand how their aberrant regulation leads to cancer initiation and progression *(127)*.

So far, we have highlighted the importance of the niche for the adequate survival and maintenance of stem cell population. These cells together with matrix glycoproteins and the three-dimensional spaces that they create are the ultrastructure of the stem cell niche. Secreted proteins (by Wnt and other developmental pathways) offer a paracrine level of control that influences the stem cells, how they behave and what fate they follow. We will now explore how the Wnt pathway, essential during embryogenesis, influences stem cells in the context of tissue maintenance and then in cancer.

WNT IN STEM CELL HOMEOSTASIS AND REGENERATION

We have explored how the Wnt signaling pathway plays a crucial role during embryogenesis and organogenesis: examples include morphogenesis of the gastrointestinal tract, mammary gland, cardiovascular system, and bone marrow *(128–130)*. Interesting, recent data by Morrisey et al. demonstrated the importance of Wnt in the regulation of epithelial and mesenchymal lung development during gestation *(131)* and the specific importance of Wnt-2, Wnt-5a, Wnt-7b in lung maturation was elegantly elucidated through mouse knockout studies *(132–135)*. In addition to its involvement in orchestrating many of the processes governing embryogenesis, Wnt, unsurprisingly, is also involved in tissue homeostasis and regeneration. A good example for this role of Wnt in tissue repair is that of muscle regeneration: a study published in 2003, which emanated from the observation that injecting adult skeletal CD45+ stem cells into the circulation led to muscle restoration, resulted in the question of whether CD45+ stem cells, resident in muscle possessed a role in physiological regeneration *(136)*. The study found that CD45+ stem cells isolated from regenerating muscle were able to successfully produce functioning myoblasts, as opposed to nonmyogenic CD45+ stem cells isolated from injured muscle. Injection of sFRP2 and sFRP3, two Wnt antagonists, into regenerating muscle, resulted in a decrease in the myogenic CD45+ stem cell population, highlighting the potential role of Wnt in various degenerative neuromuscular pathologies *(136)*. There are many other examples that accentuate the involvement of the Wnt transduction pathway in the regeneration of the bile duct, the kidney, and the liver subsequent to trauma *(137–140)*. Furthermore, a crucial role of Wnt is its involvement in the maintenance of stem and progenitor cells in various tissues, including the blood, gut, prostate, nervous system, and the skin *(128, 129, 136, 141–144)*. A relatively new study in mice has shown that ectopic Wnt transduction enhances the stem cell activity of mammary glands in vivo *(140)*. The group found that Wnt effectors are able to promote the accumulation of mouse mammary progenitor cells (measured by Hoeschst dye exclusion) both in vivo and in vitro. Furthermore, they proposed that Wnt-induced progenitor amplification is a likely culprit factor in tumor initiation. Corroborating this work, they demonstrated that mammary glands from mice resistant to tumors, showed fewer progenitor side populations; when these animals were crossed to mice overexpressing Wnt, the progenitor populations were reduced, and subsequently all downstream tumorigenic events *(140)*. This leads to now move on to explore in more thorough detail some of the aspects of stem cells in the context of neoplasia.

STEM CELLS AND CANCER

Tumor tissue architecture may display many features of normal structures, with a cellular hierarchy that controls the balance between cell renewal and cell death. We have seen how interactions between cancer and stromal cells rely on deregulated physiological feedback mechanisms that in normal circumstances control tissue homeostasis *(145–148)*. Normal stem cells must have three characteristics; the ability to self-renew to allow maintenance of a population of undifferentiated stem cell pool throughout life; a strict regulation of stem-cell number; and they must have the capacity to undergo a wide range of differentiation processes in order to clonally repopulate functional cells within a tissue *(149)* (Fig. 2). Stem cells have been shown to differ in their intrinsic ability to self-renew and differentiate into defined cell types *(150)*. The concept of "cancer stem cell" describes a cancer cell that has the power to self-renew resulting in another cancerous stem cell as well as a cell that will give rise to the phenotypically diverse cancer cell populations *(151–153)*. These latter cells are thought to represent the bulk-tumor proliferative cell pool, that respond to chemoradiotherapy, however leaving the cancer stem cell population unaffected, resulting in the eventual repopulation of the tumor and cancer recurrence *(153)*. A proposed model for carcinogenesis as a result of a persistent state of injury repair proposes that accumulation of oncogenic events during this state may "lock" activated otherwise homeostatic stem cells in a permanent Wnt driven position that ultimately leads to cancer stem cells *(154)* (Fig. 3).

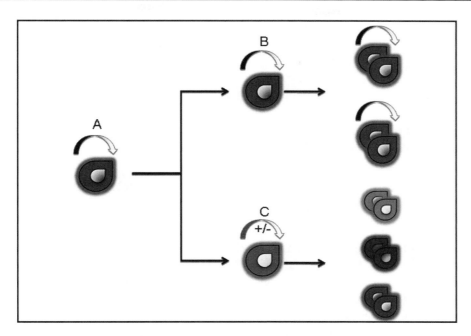

Fig. 2. Stem cell fate: to self-renew or to differentiate? Diagram A represents a powerful stem cell (SC) with self-renewal abilities, represented by the *black arrow*. These pluripotent SCs can result in more stem cells; B and/or SCs that have chosen the fate to differentiate, shown in C (orange, purple, and blue cells). The "*plus and minus (+/−) sign*" means that these cells although closely related to SCs, have limited self-renewal functions, and represent the progenitor cell population.

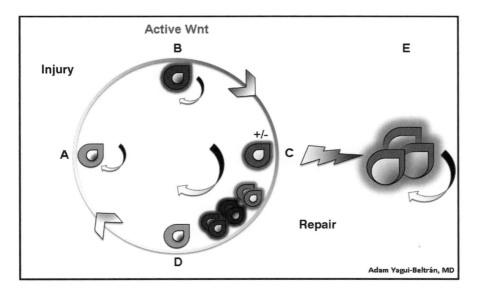

Fig. 3. Tissue homeostasis and carcinogenesis through stem cell cycling. Quiescent stem cell (SC) with inactive Wnt: (A) Upon tissue trauma, Wnt transduction leads to activation of homeostatic SCs: (B) These cells produce more pluripotent SCs as well as progenitor cells with limited proliferative power: (C) that produce specialized differentiated cells (shown in orange, purple, and blue) in order to regenerate the tissue. Upon repair, SCs cycle into a quiescent state: (D and A). Accumulation of oncogenic events may "lock" activated SCs in a permanent Wnt driven state leading to cancer stem cells: (E) [adapted from Beachy et al. *(154)*].

Cancer stem cells were initially discovered in hematological cancers, where only a small subpopulation of cancer cells was able, upon transplantation, to extensively proliferate and aggressively repopulate *(155–158)*. In the cancer stem-cell model, disruption of genes responsible for the regulation of stem-cell renewal is predictably important. There is considerable evidence demonstrating that only a subset of cells in a particular cancer displays characteristics of self-renewal. It is proposed that the microenvironment or the niche, as explained above, provides the necessary signals needed for the stem cells to continue escaping the constrains that normally restrict their capacity to self-renew and allows them, upon exit from their niche to undergo differentiation (Figs. 2 and 3).

CONCLUSIONS: WNT: FROM EMBRYOGENESIS TO STEM CELL FATE AND CANCER

An extraordinary amount of data from various research groups have demonstrated, corroborated, and reinforced the role of the Wnt signaling pathway throughout development and later in tissue homeostasis and cancer in adulthood (Table 1). Because of the large number of genes in the Wnt signaling pathway and their extensive functions in differing physiological and pathological contexts, a significant percentage of developmental decisions during the life on a human may be governed by a Wnt signal. Hence, it is not quite unexpected that anomalies in the orchestration of Wnt may result in various pathological processes, including neoplasia, as it has been shown in many types of human cancer (Table 1). Certainly we are steadily accumulating data that is allowing us to dissect in detail the Wnt signaling pathway, a complex yet strictly regulated transduction apparatus with numerous roles. Ironically, the precise mechanisms of the individual, precise events during Wnt transduction processes still need to be resolved. Examples of this include but are not limited to understanding the mechanisms of Wnt secretion and presentation to cells; how Wnt binds to the Fz/LRP complex and signals to Dvl; the mechanisms by which proteins within the beta-catenin degradation complex are regulated and how positive and negative Wnt regulators are integrated in the nucleus to initiate the transcriptional machinery to execute the events that will lead to downstream cellular physiological or pathological events. At the start of the chapter, we explored the concept of "cell fate specification" (Fig. 1), and its driving force, a combination of complex gene regulatory networks or GRNs *(1)*. This notion provides a useful framework in which biochemical signals can be located and explored. We explored the concept of noise as an intrinsic element within a biological system, and recent studies mostly in yeast and prokaryotes, postulate that noise is part of the framework of gene expression *(167–170)*. Two components of "noise" within this system were highlighted: intrinsic noise, defined as that associated with the biochemistry of the transcriptional machinery of any individual cell, and extrinsic noise that is due to cell-to-cell variation in transcriptional regulatory components. Hayward et al. proposed a third type of noise, with importance during the embryogenesis of multicellular organisms, a noise resultant from single genes that have to function cooperatively *(171)*. In this respect, the Wnt signaling pathway plays a fundamentally crucial role in controlling this noise; and it operates during cell fate assignments in development and stem cell regulation (Figs. 1–3). When this mechanism becomes anomalous and fails, deregulation results, potentially leading to malformations - during early life or cancer in adulthood. This functional "modularity" of Wnt in controlling such important cellular processes is further enriched and consequently complicated by its interaction with other developmental signaling pathways such as Hedgehog and Notch. Understanding the complex cross talk between Wnt and these other pathways, is undoubtedly important, and will improve our understanding of their mechanisms of action during stem cell-fate decision, renewal, and malignant conversion. We know that the Wnt pathway is strongly associated with cell fate and self-renewal, with that in mind, and with the many novel available research tools such as purified Wnt ligands, stimulatory

Table 1
Examples of Wnt signaling involvement in human neoplasia

Tumor	Author	Notes
Multiple myeloma	Derksen et al. *(159)*	Stimulation of growth by Wnt ligands. Dominant negative TCF-4 inhibits growth
Lymphoblastic leukemia	Chung et al. *(160)*	Overexpression of dominant negative beta-catenin or dominant TCF inhibits proliferation
Adenocarcinoma of the colon	Suzuki et al. *(161)*	Restoration of SFRP in colorectal cancer cells limits WNT signaling
Pleural mesothelioma	Lee et al. *(162)*	Restoration by transfection of the SFRP gene construct into cell lines lacking SFRP expression results in apoptosis and growth suppression
Adenocarcinoma of the lung	You et al. *(163)*	Inhibition of Wnt-2-mediated signaling induces apoptosis through inactivation of Survinin
Osteosarcoma	Hoang et al. *(164, 165)*	Expression of Dkk3 and LRP5 inhibits cancer cell growth in vitro
Oral squamous cell carcinoma	Sogabe et al. *(166)*	Ectopic expression of SFRPs inhibits cancer cell proliferation in vitro

of inhibitory small molecules, and RNAis, we will be able to tackle the challenging task of translating knowledge about the Wnt machinery into significant, pharmacologically relevant strategies to intervene in the diseases that its anomalous function causes *(32, 172–175)*. Additionally and paramount to the functionality of Wnt and its role in stem cell fate and renewal are their microenvironment or niches. We have explored these earlier, and we have learned that they are fundamental for survival of the stem cells that they host. Tumor initiation and progression is increasingly being linked to the microenvironment, and therefore a better understanding of how it is regulated affecting proliferation and self-renewal of homeostatic and cancer stem cells is a growing field in both science and medicine. In conclusion, we can argue that by integrating all these aspects relating to Wnt during normal processes of stem cell self-renewal, differentiation, and cancer, we are moving forward in our quest to find a wide array of novel therapies not only for cancer but also for many other diseases.

ACKNOWLEDGMENT

The work is supported by the Kazan Foundation and the NIH/NCI R011R01CA093708-01A3 Grant. We would like to express our enormous gratitude for the thorough, meticulous and careful constructive reading and feedback of our manuscript by our dear colleague Dr. Geneviève Clément from the Thoracic Oncology Laboratory, Department of Surgery at the University of California San Francisco.

REFERENCES

1. Davidson, E.H. and D.H. Erwin, *Gene regulatory networks and the evolution of animal body plans*. Science, 2006. 311(5762): pp. 796–800.
2. Rodbell, M., Nobel lecture. Signal transduction: evolution of an idea. Biosci Rep, 1995. 15(3): pp. 117–33.

3. Suel, G.M., et al., An excitable gene regulatory circuit induces transient cellular differentiation. Nature, 2006. 440(7083): pp. 545–50.

4. Suel, G.M., et al., Tunability and noise dependence in differentiation dynamics. Science, 2007. 315(5819): pp. 1716–9.

5. Maamar, H., A. Raj, and D. Dubnau, Noise in gene expression determines cell fate in Bacillus subtilis. Science, 2007. 317(5837): pp. 526–9.

6. Martinez Arias, A. and A. Stewart, Molecular Principles of Animal Development, 2002, New York, NY: Oxford University Press.

7. Barolo, S. and J.W. Posakony, Three habits of highly effective signaling pathways: principles of transcriptional control by developmental cell signaling. Genes Dev, 2002. 16(10): pp. 1167–81.

8. Silver, S.J. and I. Rebay, Signaling circuitries in development: insights from the retinal determination gene network. Development, 2005. 132(1): pp. 3–13.

9. Voas, M.G. and I. Rebay, Signal integration during development: insights from the Drosophila eye. Dev Dyn, 2004. 229(1): pp. 162–75.

10. Rose, L.S. and K.J. Kemphues, Early patterning of the C. elegans embryo. Annu Rev Genet, 1998. 32: pp. 521–45.

11. Newman-Smith, E.D. and J.H. Rothman, The maternal-to-zygotic transition in embryonic patterning of Caenorhabditis elegans. Curr Opin Genet Dev, 1998. 8(4): pp. 472–80.

12. Platzer, U. and H.P. Meinzer, Genetic networks in the early development of Caenorhabditis elegans. Int Rev Cytol, 2004. 234: pp. 47–100.

13. Brennan, K., et al., The abruptex mutations of notch disrupt the establishment of proneural clusters in Drosophila. Dev Biol, 1999. 216(1): pp. 230–42.

14. Carmena, A., S. Speicher, and M. Baylies, The PDZ protein Canoe/AF-6 links Ras-MAPK, Notch and Wingless/Wnt signaling pathways by directly interacting with Ras, Notch and Dishevelled. PLoS ONE, 2006. 1: p. e66.

15. Strutt, D., et al., Asymmetric localization of frizzled and the determination of notch-dependent cell fate in the Drosophila eye. Curr Biol, 2002. 12(10): pp. 813–24.

16. Tomlinson, A. and G. Struhl, Delta/Notch and Boss/Sevenless signals act combinatorially to specify the Drosophila R7 photoreceptor. Mol Cell, 2001. 7(3): pp. 487–95.

17. Rijsewijk, F., et al., The Drosophila homolog of the mouse mammary oncogene int-1 is identical to the segment polarity gene wingless. Cell, 1987. 50(4): pp. 649–57.

18. Widelitz, R., Wnt signaling through canonical and non-canonical pathways: recent progress. Growth Factors, 2005. 23(2): pp. 111–6.

19. Akiyama, T., Wnt/beta-catenin signaling. Cytokine Growth Factor Rev, 2000. 11(4): pp. 273–82.

20. Veeman, M.T., J.D. Axelrod, and R.T. Moon, A second canon. Functions and mechanisms of beta-catenin-independent Wnt signaling. Dev Cell, 2003. 5(3): pp. 367–77.

21. Nusse, R., Cell biology: relays at the membrane. Nature, 2005. 438(7069): pp. 747–9.

22. Kramps, T., et al., Wnt/wingless signaling requires BCL9/legless-mediated recruitment of pygopus to the nuclear beta-catenin-TCF complex. Cell, 2002. 109(1): pp. 47–60.

23. Krieghoff, E., J. Behrens, and B. Mayr, Nucleo-cytoplasmic distribution of beta-catenin is regulated by retention. J Cell Sci, 2006. 119(Pt 7): pp. 1453–63.

24. Sampietro, J., et al., Crystal structure of a beta-catenin/BCL9/Tcf4 complex. Mol Cell, 2006. 24(2): pp. 293–300.

25. Cavallo, R.A., et al., Drosophila Tcf and Groucho interact to repress Wingless signalling activity. Nature, 1998. 395(6702): pp. 604–8.

26. Logan, C.Y. and R. Nusse, The Wnt signaling pathway in development and disease. Annu Rev Cell Dev Biol, 2004. 20: pp. 781–810.

27. Chen, G., et al., A functional interaction between the histone deacetylase Rpd3 and the corepressor groucho in Drosophila development. Genes Dev, 1999. 13(17): pp. 2218–30.

28. Oishi, I., et al., The receptor tyrosine kinase Ror2 is involved in non-canonical Wnt5a/JNK signalling pathway. Genes Cells, 2003. 8(7): pp. 645–54.

29. Chen, A.E., D.D. Ginty, and C.M. Fan, Protein kinase A signalling via CREB controls myogenesis induced by Wnt proteins. Nature, 2005. 433(7023): pp. 317–22.

30. Miller, J.R., The Wnts. Genome Biol, 2002. 3(1): p. REVIEWS3001.

31. Hofmann, K., A superfamily of membrane-bound O-acyltransferases with implications for Wnt signaling. Trends Biochem Sci, 2000. 25(3): pp. 111–2.

32. Willert, K., et al., Wnt proteins are lipid-modified and can act as stem cell growth factors. Nature, 2003. 423(6938): pp. 448–52.

33. Zhai, L., D. Chaturvedi, and S. Cumberledge, Drosophila wnt-1 undergoes a hydrophobic modification and is targeted to lipid rafts, a process that requires porcupine. J Biol Chem, 2004. 279(32): pp. 33220–7.

34. Banziger, C., et al., Wntless, a conserved membrane protein dedicated to the secretion of Wnt proteins from signaling cells. Cell, 2006. 125(3): pp. 509–22.

35. Bartscherer, K., et al., Secretion of Wnt ligands requires Evi, a conserved transmembrane protein. Cell, 2006. 125(3): pp. 523–33.

36. Lin, X., Functions of heparan sulfate proteoglycans in cell signaling during development. Development, 2004. 131(24): pp. 6009–21.

37. Bhanot, P., et al., A new member of the frizzled family from Drosophila functions as a Wingless receptor. Nature, 1996. 382(6588): pp. 225–30.

38. Liu, T., et al., G protein signaling from activated rat frizzled-1 to the beta-catenin-Lef-Tcf pathway. Science, 2001. 292(5522): pp. 1718–22.

39. Tamai, K., et al., LDL-receptor-related proteins in Wnt signal transduction. Nature, 2000. 407(6803): pp. 530–5.

40. Lu, W., et al., Mammalian Ryk is a Wnt coreceptor required for stimulation of neurite outgrowth. Cell, 2004. 119(1): pp. 97–108.

41. Mikels, A.J. and R. Nusse, Purified Wnt5a protein activates or inhibits beta-catenin-TCF signaling depending on receptor context. PLoS Biol, 2006. 4(4): pp. e115.

42. Hsieh, J.C., et al., A new secreted protein that binds to Wnt proteins and inhibits their activities. Nature, 1999. 398(6726): pp. 431–6.

43. Jones, S.E. and C. Jomary, Secreted frizzled-related proteins: searching for relationships and patterns. Bioessays, 2002. 24(9): pp. 811–20.

44. Uren, A., et al., Secreted frizzled-related protein-1 binds directly to Wingless and is a biphasic modulator of Wnt signaling. J Biol Chem, 2000. 275(6): pp. 4374–82.

45. Fedi, P., et al., Isolation and biochemical characterization of the human Dkk-1 homologue, a novel inhibitor of mammalian Wnt signaling. J Biol Chem, 1999. 274(27): pp. 19465–72.

46. Ehebauer, M.T., et al., High-resolution crystal structure of the human Notch 1 ankyrin domain. Biochem J, 2005. 392(Pt 1): pp. 13–20.

47. Nam, Y., et al., Structural requirements for assembly of the CSL.intracellular Notch1.Mastermind-like 1 transcriptional activation complex. J Biol Chem, 2003. 278(23): pp. 21232–9.

48. Nam, Y., et al., Structural basis for cooperativity in recruitment of MAML coactivators to Notch transcription complexes. Cell, 2006. 124(5): pp. 973–83.

49. Zweifel, M.E., et al., Structure and stability of the ankyrin domain of the Drosophila Notch receptor. Protein Sci, 2003. 12(11): pp. 2622–32.

50. Kopan, R., Notch: a membrane-bound transcription factor. J Cell Sci, 2002. 115(Pt 6): pp. 1095–7.

51. Bray, S.J., Notch signalling: a simple pathway becomes complex. Nat Rev Mol Cell Biol, 2006. 7(9): pp. 678–89.

52. Ehebauer, M., P. Hayward, and A.M. Arias, Notch, a universal arbiter of cell fate decisions. Science, 2006. 314(5804): pp. 1414–5.

53. Le Borgne, R., Regulation of Notch signalling by endocytosis and endosomal sorting. Curr Opin Cell Biol, 2006. 18(2): pp. 213–22.

54. Jaekel, R. and T. Klein, The Drosophila Notch inhibitor and tumor suppressor gene lethal (2) giant discs encodes a conserved regulator of endosomal trafficking. Dev Cell, 2006. 11(5): pp. 655–69.

55. Moberg, K.H., et al., Mutations in erupted, the Drosophila ortholog of mammalian tumor susceptibility gene 101, elicit non-cell-autonomous overgrowth. Dev Cell, 2005. 9(5): pp. 699–710.

56. Thompson, B.J., et al., Tumor suppressor properties of the ESCRT-II complex component Vps25 in Drosophila. Dev Cell, 2005. 9(5): pp. 711–20.

57. Vaccari, T. and D. Bilder, The Drosophila tumor suppressor vps25 prevents nonautonomous overproliferation by regulating notch trafficking. Dev Cell, 2005. 9(5): pp. 687–98.

58. Couso, J.P. and A. Martinez Arias, Notch is required for wingless signaling in the epidermis of Drosophila. Cell, 1994. 79(2): pp. 259–72.

59. Hing, H.K., X. Sun, and S. Artavanis-Tsakonas, Modulation of wingless signaling by Notch in Drosophila. Mech Dev, 1994. 47(3): pp. 261–8.

60. Klein, T. and A.M. Arias, The vestigial gene product provides a molecular context for the interpretation of signals during the development of the wing in Drosophila. Development, 1999. 126(5): pp. 913–25.

61. Zecca, M. and G. Struhl, Recruitment of cells into the Drosophila wing primordium by a feed-forward circuit of vestigial autoregulation. Development, 2007. 134(16): pp. 3001–10.

62. Klein, T. and A.M. Arias, Interactions among Delta, Serrate and Fringe modulate Notch activity during Drosophila wing development. Development, 1998. 125(15): pp. 2951–62.

63. Diaz-Benjumea, F.J. and S.M. Cohen, Serrate signals through Notch to establish a Wingless-dependent organizer at the dorsal/ventral compartment boundary of the Drosophila wing. Development, 1995. 121(12): pp. 4215–25.

64. Neumann, C.J. and S.M. Cohen, A hierarchy of cross-regulation involving Notch, wingless, vestigial and cut organizes the dorsal/ventral axis of the Drosophila wing. Development, 1996. 122(11): pp. 3477–85.

65. Micchelli, C.A., E.J. Rulifson, and S.S. Blair, The function and regulation of cut expression on the wing margin of Drosophila: Notch, Wingless and a dominant negative role for Delta and Serrate. Development, 1997. 124(8): pp. 1485–95.

66. de Celis, J.F. and S. Bray, Feed-back mechanisms affecting Notch activation at the dorsoventral boundary in the Drosophila wing. Development, 1997. 124(17): pp. 3241–51.

67. Mahoney, M.B., et al., Presenilin-based genetic screens in Drosophila melanogaster identify novel notch pathway modifiers. Genetics, 2006. 172(4): pp. 2309–24.

68. Go, M.J. and S. Artavanis-Tsakonas, A genetic screen for novel components of the notch signaling pathway during Drosophila bristle development. Genetics, 1998. 150(1): pp. 211–20.

69. Langdon, T., et al., Notch receptor encodes two structurally separable functions in Drosophila: a genetic analysis. Dev Dyn, 2006. 235(4): pp. 998–1013.

70. Verheyen, E.M., et al., Analysis of dominant enhancers and suppressors of activated Notch in Drosophila. Genetics, 1996. 144(3): pp. 1127–41.

71. Aulehla, A., et al., Wnt3a plays a major role in the segmentation clock controlling somitogenesis. Dev Cell, 2003. 4(3): pp. 395–406.

72. Aulehla, A. and B.G. Herrmann, Segmentation in vertebrates: clock and gradient finally joined. Genes Dev, 2004. 18(17): pp. 2060–7.

73. Estrach, S., et al., Jagged 1 is a beta-catenin target gene required for ectopic hair follicle formation in adult epidermis. Development, 2006. 133(22): pp. 4427–38.

74. Cheng, Y.C., et al., Notch activation regulates the segregation and differentiation of rhombomere boundary cells in the zebrafish hindbrain. Dev Cell, 2004. 6(4): pp. 539–50.

75. Alon, U., An Introduction to Systems Biology: Design Principles of Biological Circuits, 2006, Boca Raton, FL: Chapman & Hall.

76. Arias, A.M., New alleles of Notch draw a blueprint for multifunctionality. Trends Genet, 2002. 18(4): pp. 168–70.

77. Heitzler, P. and P. Simpson, Altered epidermal growth factor-like sequences provide evidence for a role of Notch as a receptor in cell fate decisions. Development, 1993. 117(3): pp. 1113–23.

78. de Celis, J.F. and S.J. Bray, The Abruptex domain of Notch regulates negative interactions between Notch, its ligands and Fringe. Development, 2000. 127(6): pp. 1291–302.

79. Ramain, P., et al., Novel Notch alleles reveal a Deltex-dependent pathway repressing neural fate. Curr Biol, 2001. 11(22): pp. 1729–38.

80. Brennan, K., et al., Wingless modulates the effects of dominant negative notch molecules in the developing wing of Drosophila. Dev Biol, 1999. 216(1): pp. 210–29.

81. Suzuki, D. and Griffiths, A., An Introduction to Genetic Analysis, 1976, New York, NY: W. H. Freeman.

82. Brennan, K., M. Baylies, and A.M. Arias, Repression by Notch is required before Wingless signalling during muscle progenitor cell development in Drosophila. Curr Biol, 1999. 9(13): pp. 707–10.

83. Carmena, A., et al., Combinatorial signaling codes for the progressive determination of cell fates in the Drosophila embryonic mesoderm. Genes Dev, 1998. 12(24): pp. 3910–22.

84. Brennan, K., et al., A functional analysis of Notch mutations in Drosophila. Genetics, 1997. 147(1): pp. 177–88.

85. Heitzler, P. and P. Simpson, The choice of cell fate in the epidermis of Drosophila. Cell, 1991. 64(6): pp. 1083–92.

86. Lawrence, N., et al., Notch signaling targets the Wingless responsiveness of a Ubx visceral mesoderm enhancer in Drosophila. Curr Biol, 2001. 11(6): pp. 375–85.

87. Hayward, P., T. Kalmar, and A.M. Arias, Wnt/Notch signalling and information processing during development. Development, 2008. 135(3): pp. 411–24.

88. Galceran, J., et al., LEF1-mediated regulation of Delta-like1 links Wnt and Notch signaling in somitogenesis. Genes Dev, 2004. 18(22): pp. 2718–23.

89. Pourquie, O., The segmentation clock: converting embryonic time into spatial pattern. Science, 2003. 301(5631): pp. 328–30.

90. McMahon, A.P., More surprises in the Hedgehog signaling pathway. Cell, 2000. 100(2): pp. 185–8.

91. Ingham, P.W., Transducing Hedgehog: the story so far. EMBO J, 1998. 17(13): pp. 3505–11.

92. Goodrich, L.V. and M.P. Scott, Hedgehog and patched in neural development and disease. Neuron, 1998. 21(6): pp. 1243–57.

93. Lee, J.J., et al., Secretion and localized transcription suggest a role in positional signaling for products of the segmentation gene hedgehog. Cell, 1992. 71(1): pp. 33–50.

94. Kalderon, D., Transducing the hedgehog signal. Cell, 2000. 103(3): pp. 371–4.
95. Porter, J.A., K.E. Young, and P.A. Beachy, Cholesterol modification of hedgehog signaling proteins in animal development. Science, 1996. 274(5285): pp. 255–9.
96. Pepinsky, R.B., et al., Identification of a palmitic acid-modified form of human Sonic hedgehog. J Biol Chem, 1998. 273(22): pp. 14037–45.
97. Denef, N., et al., Hedgehog induces opposite changes in turnover and subcellular localization of patched and smoothened. Cell, 2000. 102(4): pp. 521–31.
98. Stone, D.M., et al., The tumour-suppressor gene patched encodes a candidate receptor for Sonic hedgehog. Nature, 1996. 384(6605): pp. 129–34.
99. Taipale, J., et al., Effects of oncogenic mutations in Smoothened and Patched can be reversed by cyclopamine. Nature, 2000. 406(6799): pp. 1005–9.
100. Aza-Blanc, P., et al., Proteolysis that is inhibited by hedgehog targets Cubitus interruptus protein to the nucleus and converts it to a repressor. Cell, 1997. 89(7): pp. 1043–53.
101. Robbins, D.J., et al., Hedgehog elicits signal transduction by means of a large complex containing the kinesin-related protein costal2. Cell, 1997. 90(2): pp. 225–34.
102. Chen, C.H., et al., Nuclear trafficking of Cubitus interruptus in the transcriptional regulation of Hedgehog target gene expression. Cell, 1999. 98(3): pp. 305–16.
103. Freeman, M., Feedback control of intercellular signalling in development. Nature, 2000. 408(6810): pp. 313–9.
104. Hooper, J.E. and M.P. Scott, Communicating with Hedgehogs. Nat Rev Mol Cell Biol, 2005. 6(4): pp. 306–17.
105. Gregorieff, A. and H. Clevers, Wnt signaling in the intestinal epithelium: from endoderm to cancer. Genes Dev, 2005. 19(8): pp. 877–90.
106. Taipale, J. and P.A. Beachy, The Hedgehog and Wnt signalling pathways in cancer. Nature, 2001. 411(6835): pp. 349–54.
107. McMahon, A.P., P.W. Ingham, and C.J. Tabin, Developmental roles and clinical significance of hedgehog signaling. Curr Top Dev Biol, 2003. 53: pp. 1–114.
108. Noramly, S., A. Freeman, and B.A. Morgan, Beta-catenin signaling can initiate feather bud development. Development, 1999. 126(16): pp. 3509–21.
109. Bitgood, M.J. and A.P. McMahon, Hedgehog and Bmp genes are coexpressed at many diverse sites of cell-cell interaction in the mouse embryo. Dev Biol, 1995. 172(1): pp. 126–38.
110. Reddy, S., et al., Characterization of Wnt gene expression in developing and postnatal hair follicles and identification of Wnt5a as a target of Sonic hedgehog in hair follicle morphogenesis. Mech Dev, 2001. 107(1–2): pp. 69–82.
111. Heemskerk, J. and S. DiNardo, Drosophila hedgehog acts as a morphogen in cellular patterning. Cell, 1994. 76(3): pp. 449–60.
112. Silva-Vargas, V., et al., Beta-catenin and hedgehog signal strength can specify number and location of hair follicles in adult epidermis without recruitment of bulge stem cells. Dev Cell, 2005. 9(1): pp. 121–31.
113. Iwatsuki, K., et al., Wnt signaling interacts with Shh to regulate taste papilla development. Proc Natl Acad Sci USA, 2007. 104(7): pp. 2253–8.
114. van den Brink, G.R., et al., Indian Hedgehog is an antagonist of Wnt signaling in colonic epithelial cell differentiation. Nat Genet, 2004. 36(3): pp. 277–82.
115. Akiyoshi, T., et al., Gli1, downregulated in colorectal cancers, inhibits proliferation of colon cancer cells involving Wnt signalling activation. Gut, 2006. 55(7): pp. 991–9.
116. Crittenden, S.L., et al., A conserved RNA-binding protein controls germline stem cells in Caenorhabditis elegans. Nature, 2002. 417(6889): pp. 660–3.
117. Xie, T. and A.C. Spradling, A niche maintaining germ line stem cells in the Drosophila ovary. Science, 2000. 290(5490): pp. 328–30.
118. Kiger, A.A., H. White-Cooper, and M.T. Fuller, Somatic support cells restrict germline stem cell self-renewal and promote differentiation. Nature, 2000. 407(6805): pp. 750–4.
119. Palmer, T.D., A.R. Willhoite, and F.H. Gage, Vascular niche for adult hippocampal neurogenesis. J Comp Neurol, 2000. 425(4): pp. 479–94.
120. Calvi, L.M., et al., Osteoblastic cells regulate the haematopoietic stem cell niche. Nature, 2003. 425(6960): pp. 841–6.
121. Zhang, J., et al., Identification of the haematopoietic stem cell niche and control of the niche size. Nature, 2003. 425(6960): pp. 836–41.
122. Kiel, M.J., et al., SLAM family receptors distinguish hematopoietic stem and progenitor cells and reveal endothelial niches for stem cells. Cell, 2005. 121(7): pp. 1109–21.
123. Jones, P.H. and F.M. Watt, Separation of human epidermal stem cells from transit amplifying cells on the basis of differences in integrin function and expression. Cell, 1993. 73(4): pp. 713–24.

124. Jensen, U.B., S. Lowell, and F.M. Watt, The spatial relationship between stem cells and their progeny in the basal layer of human epidermis: a new view based on whole-mount labelling and lineage analysis. Development, 1999. 126(11): pp. 2409–18.

125. Garcion, E., et al., Generation of an environmental niche for neural stem cell development by the extracellular matrix molecule tenascin C. Development, 2004. 131(14): pp. 3423–32.

126. Ohta, M., et al., Suppression of hematopoietic activity in tenascin-C-deficient mice. Blood, 1998. 91(11): pp. 4074–83.

127. Batlle, E., et al., Beta-catenin and TCF mediate cell positioning in the intestinal epithelium by controlling the expression of EphB/ephrinB. Cell, 2002. 111(2): pp. 251–63.

128. Reya, T., et al., A role for Wnt signalling in self-renewal of haematopoietic stem cells. Nature, 2003. 423(6938): pp. 409–14.

129. Korinek, V., et al., Depletion of epithelial stem-cell compartments in the small intestine of mice lacking Tcf-4. Nat Genet, 1998. 19(4): pp. 379–83.

130. Brennan, K.R. and A.M. Brown, Wnt proteins in mammary development and cancer. J Mammary Gland Biol Neoplasia, 2004. 9(2): pp. 119–31.

131. Weidenfeld, J., Wnt signaling and pulmonary fibrosis. Am J Pathol, 2003. 162(5): pp. 1393–7.

132. Weidenfeld, J., et al., The WNT7b promoter is regulated by TTF-1, GATA6, and Foxa2 in lung epithelium. J Biol Chem, 2002. 277(23): pp. 21061–70.

133. Li, C., et al., Wnt5a participates in distal lung morphogenesis. Dev Biol, 2002. 248(1): pp. 68–81.

134. Shu, W., et al., Wnt7b regulates mesenchymal proliferation and vascular development in the lung. Development, 2002. 129(20): pp. 4831–42.

135. Yamaguchi, T.P., et al., A Wnt5a pathway underlies outgrowth of multiple structures in the vertebrate embryo. Development, 1999. 126(6): pp. 1211–23.

136. Polesskaya, A., P. Seale, and M.A. Rudnicki, Wnt signaling induces the myogenic specification of resident CD45+ adult stem cells during muscle regeneration. Cell, 2003. 113(7): pp. 841–52.

137. Shackel, N.A., et al., Identification of novel molecules and pathogenic pathways in primary biliary cirrhosis: cDNA array analysis of intrahepatic differential gene expression. Gut, 2001. 49(4): pp. 565–76.

138. Surendran, K. and T.C. Simon, CNP gene expression is activated by Wnt signaling and correlates with Wnt4 expression during renal injury. Am J Physiol Renal Physiol, 2003. 284(4): pp. F653–62.

139. Monga, S.P., et al., Changes in WNT/beta-catenin pathway during regulated growth in rat liver regeneration. Hepatology, 2001. 33(5): pp. 1098–109.

140. Liu, B.Y., et al., The transforming activity of Wnt effectors correlates with their ability to induce the accumulation of mammary progenitor cells. Proc Natl Acad Sci USA, 2004. 101(12): pp. 4158–63.

141. Bhardwaj, G., et al., Sonic hedgehog induces the proliferation of primitive human hematopoietic cells via BMP regulation. Nat Immunol, 2001. 2(2): pp. 172–80.

142. Owens, D.M. and F.M. Watt, Contribution of stem cells and differentiated cells to epidermal tumours. Nat Rev Cancer, 2003. 3(6): pp. 444–51.

143. Pinto, D., et al., Canonical Wnt signals are essential for homeostasis of the intestinal epithelium. Genes Dev, 2003. 17(14): pp. 1709–13.

144. Perez-Losada, J. and A. Balmain, Stem-cell hierarchy in skin cancer. Nat Rev Cancer, 2003. 3(6): pp. 434–43.

145. Szabowski, A., et al., c-Jun and JunB antagonistically control cytokine-regulated mesenchymal-epidermal interaction in skin. Cell, 2000. 103(5): pp. 745–55.

146. Donjacour, A.A. and G.R. Cunha, Stromal regulation of epithelial function. Cancer Treat Res, 1991. 53: pp. 335–64.

147. Sternlicht, M.D., et al., The stromal proteinase MMP3/stromelysin-1 promotes mammary carcinogenesis. Cell, 1999. 98(2): pp. 137–46.

148. Muller, A., et al., Involvement of chemokine receptors in breast cancer metastasis. Nature, 2001. 410(6824): pp. 50–6.

149. Al-Hajj, M., et al., Therapeutic implications of cancer stem cells. Curr Opin Genet Dev, 2004. 14(1): pp. 43–7.

150. Bixby, S., et al., Cell-intrinsic differences between stem cells from different regions of the peripheral nervous system regulate the generation of neural diversity. Neuron, 2002. 35(4): pp. 643–56.

151. Wicha, M.S., S. Liu, and G. Dontu, Cancer stem cells: an old idea – a paradigm shift. Cancer Res, 2006. 66(4): pp. 1883–90; discussion 1895–6.

152. Sell, S., Stem cell origin of cancer and differentiation therapy. Crit Rev Oncol Hematol, 2004. 51(1): pp. 1–28.

153. Houghton, J., et al., Stem cells and cancer. Semin Cancer Biol, 2007. 17(3): pp. 191–203.

154. Beachy, P.A., S.S. Karhadkar, and D.M. Berman, Tissue repair and stem cell renewal in carcinogenesis. Nature, 2004. 432(7015): pp. 324–31.

155. Park, C.H., D.E. Bergsagel, and E.A. McCulloch, Mouse myeloma tumor stem cells: a primary cell culture assay. J Natl Cancer Inst, 1971. 46(2): pp. 411–22.
156. Bruce, W.R. and H. Van Der Gaag, A quantitative assay for the number of murine lymphoma cells capable of proliferation in vivo. Nature, 1963. 199: pp. 79–80.
157. Wodinsky, I. and C.J. Kensler, Growth of L1210 leukemia cells. Nature, 1966. 210(5039): pp. 962.
158. Bergsagel, D.E. and F.A. Valeriote, Growth characteristics of a mouse plasma cell tumor. Cancer Res, 1968. 28(11): pp. 2187–96.
159. Derksen, P.W., et al., Illegitimate WNT signaling promotes proliferation of multiple myeloma cells. Proc Natl Acad Sci USA, 2004. 101(16): pp. 6122–7.
160. Chung, E.J., et al., Regulation of leukemic cell adhesion, proliferation, and survival by beta-catenin. Blood, 2002. 100(3): pp. 982–90.
161. Suzuki, H., et al., Epigenetic inactivation of SFRP genes allows constitutive WNT signaling in colorectal cancer. Nat Genet, 2004. 36(4): pp. 417–22.
162. Lee, A.Y., et al., Expression of the secreted frizzled-related protein gene family is downregulated in human mesothelioma. Oncogene, 2004. 23(39): pp. 6672–6.
163. You, L., et al., Inhibition of Wnt-2-mediated signaling induces programmed cell death in non-small-cell lung cancer cells. Oncogene, 2004. 23(36): pp. 6170–4.
164. Hoang, B.H., et al., Expression of LDL receptor-related protein 5 (LRP5) as a novel marker for disease progression in high-grade osteosarcoma. Int J Cancer, 2004. 109(1): pp. 106–11.
165. Hoang, B.H., et al., Dickkopf 3 inhibits invasion and motility of Saos-2 osteosarcoma cells by modulating the Wnt-beta-catenin pathway. Cancer Res, 2004. 64(8): pp. 2734–9.
166. Sogabe, Y., et al., Epigenetic inactivation of SFRP genes in oral squamous cell carcinoma. Int J Oncol, 2008. 32(6): pp. 1253–61.
167. Kaern, M., et al., Stochasticity in gene expression: from theories to phenotypes. Nat Rev Genet, 2005. 6(6): pp. 451–64.
168. Elowitz, M.B., et al., Stochastic gene expression in a single cell. Science, 2002. 297(5584): pp. 1183–6.
169. Gregor, T., et al., Probing the limits to positional information. Cell, 2007. 130(1): pp. 153–64.
170. Raser, J.M. and E.K. O'Shea, Control of stochasticity in eukaryotic gene expression. Science, 2004. 304(5678): pp. 1811–4.
171. Arias, A.M. and P. Hayward, Filtering transcriptional noise during development: concepts and mechanisms. Nat Rev Genet, 2006. 7(1): pp. 34–44.
172. Boutros, M., et al., Genome-wide RNAi analysis of growth and viability in Drosophila cells. Science, 2004. 303(5659): pp. 832–5.
173. Lepourcelet, M., et al., Small-molecule antagonists of the oncogenic Tcf/beta-catenin protein complex. Cancer Cell, 2004. 5(1): pp. 91–102.
174. Meijer, L., et al., GSK-3-selective inhibitors derived from Tyrian purple indirubins. Chem Biol, 2003. 10(12): pp. 1255–66.
175. Lum, L., et al., Identification of hedgehog pathway components by RNAi in Drosophila cultured cells. Science, 2003. 299(5615): pp. 2039–45.

5

PTEN in Hematopoietic and Intestinal Stem Cells and Cancer

Jason T. Ross, David H. Scoville, Xi He, and Linheng Li

ABSTRACT

In this chapter, we discuss the roles of the tumor suppressor PTEN in regulating stem cells of the hematopoietic and intestinal systems as well as its contributions to carcinogenesis in these tissues. Stem cells in continually renewing tissues must balance the necessity to maintain their respective tissue with the requirement to preserve the stem cell pool throughout adult life. Hematopoietic stem cells (HSCs) are tasked with sustaining the various cell types of the blood while intestinal stem cells must continually regenerate the gut epithelium. PTEN, a dual-specificity phosphatase able to target proteins and lipids, is the sole antagonist of the PI3K/AKT signaling pathway. PI3K/AKT signaling is often activated by growth factors and typically results in the stimulation of cellular outcomes such as proliferation, inhibition of apoptosis, and migration. Functional studies of PTEN loss in animal models have indicated a role for PTEN as a protective agent for stem cells that promote quiescence, as PTEN-deficient animals exhibit overproliferative stem and progenitor cells and are prone to proliferative disorders and cancer development. However, from these and other studies including accumulated clinical evidence, it is not likely that PTEN acts alone to stimulate malignant transformation. Indeed, HSCs in PTEN-deficient animals become exhausted and unable to sustain a healthy hematopoietic system. Rather, PTEN appears to function as a restrictive factor that prevents unregulated proliferation, which leaves stem and progenitor cells susceptible to additional mutations/deregulation, such as in Wnt/β-catenin signaling, that results in overt cancer. Additional study into PTEN/PI3K/AKT signaling should provide further insight into self-renewal mechanisms of adult stem cells that may aid in distinguishing normal stem cells from their cancer-initiating counterparts.

Key Words: Stem cells, Hematopoiesis, Intestine, Cancer, PTEN

INTRODUCTION

The PI3K/AKT pathway plays important roles in cell survival, proliferation, migration, and differentiation in a variety of tissues and cell types. As many of these cellular processes can become hijacked in cancers, many components of this pathway are considered proto-oncogenes, and PTEN, the sole antagonist of PI3K *in vivo*, is considered a major tumor suppressor *(1–3)*. In this chapter, we will begin by providing an overview of the biochemistry of the PI3K/AKT signaling pathway.

From: *Cancer Drug Discovery and Development: Stem Cells and Cancer,*
Edited by: R.G. Bagley and B.A. Teicher, DOI: 10.1007/978-1-60327-933-8_5,
© Humana Press, a part of Springer Science+Business Media, LLC 2009

We will discuss known functions of PTEN in normal stem cells in both the hematopoietic and intestinal systems. Finally, we will address the roles of PTEN and PI3K/AKT signaling in contributing to tumorigenesis in these tissues.

THE PTEN/PI3K/AKT SIGNALING PATHWAY

Central to this pathway is phosphatidylinositol-3-kinase (PI3K), which can phosphorylate both protein and lipid substrates and functions as a dimer of regulatory and catalytic subunits. We will focus on the class Ia PI3Ks as they are the best studied and most relevant in terms of tumor formation. PI3K is normally held in the cytoplasm in an inactive state. Once a ligand (usually a growth factor) binds to its respective receptor tyrosine kinase (RTK) (usually a growth factor receptor) at the plasma membrane, the RTK becomes fully activated by autophosphorylation and subsequently transduces signals downstream through multiple effectors, one of which is PI3K. RTKs can activate PI3K through one of the several mechanisms involving release of autoinhibition of PI3K and a shift in its localization from the cytoplasm to the plasma membrane, bringing PI3K in close proximity to phosphatidylinositol-(4,5)-bisphosphate (PIP_2), its primary lipid substrate.

Activated PI3K catalyzes the conversion of PIP_2 to phosphatidylinositol-(3,4,5)-triphosphate (PIP_3). PIP_3 molecules allow for recruitment of phosphatidylinositol-dependent kinase 1 (PDK-1) and protein kinase B (PKB or more commonly AKT) to the plasma membrane where PDK-1 phosphorylates and promotes activation of AKT. Phosphatase and tensin homolog (PTEN) is the lone antagonist of PI3K/AKT signaling *in vivo*. As a lipid and protein phosphatase, PTEN catalyzes the opposing reaction of PI3K, converting PIP_3 into PIP_2 and blocking the activation of AKT by preventing its localization to the membrane *(1, 2)* (Fig. 1).

As the main effector of activated PI3K, the Ser/Thr kinase AKT has many cellular substrates that it can both activate and inhibit via phosphorylation to mediate outcomes that ultimately promote cellular survival and proliferation. Specifically, AKT prevents glycogen synthase kinase 3 beta (GSK3β) from phosphorylating and contributing to the degradation of CyclinD1 and c-MYC, allowing for these factors to foster cell cycle progression. In addition to blocking the degradation of CyclinD1, AKT can act to increase its levels within the cell. AKT does this as well as act to decrease levels of cell cycle inhibitors such as p27[KIP1] by affecting the activity of Forkhead box transcription factors (FOXOs). Furthermore, AKT can inactivate p27[KIP1] directly. As well as driving progression through the cell cycle, AKT also leads to increases in protein translation via indirect activation of mammalian target of rapamycin (mTOR) *(1, 2)*. Additionally AKT phosphorylates proapoptotic factors BAD (which inhibits Bcl-2) and Caspase 9 to block their promotion of apoptosis. AKT phosphorylates the FOXOs and inhibits their induction of expression of apoptotic-promoting genes such as BIM, as seen in Fig. 1. Also, AKT can indirectly promote the export of p53 out of the nucleus via Mdm2, thereby preventing p53's well-known roles in cell cycle arrest and apoptosis *(1, 2)*.

It is not surprising that components driving and/or mediating PI3K/AKT signaling are considered proto-oncogenes, and PTEN is well characterized as a potent tumor suppressor, since this pathway directly regulates processes of growth and survival. In fact, mutations in components of the PTEN/PI3K/AKT pathway have been found in a variety of cancers including gliobastomas, breast, endometrial and ovarian cancers, hepatocellular and renal cell carcinomas, as well as cancers of the hematopoietic and gastrointestinal systems *(1, 4)*. Furthermore, greater than 40% of human colorectal carcinomas have been found to possess mutations resulting in deregulation of this pathway. Similar mutations have also been characterized in various kinds of leukemia and lymphoma. A common target of genetic mutation in many of these human neoplasms appears to be PTEN as it is often deleted or unable to properly function *(5, 6)*. Recently, new insight into the roles of PTEN/PI3K/AKT signaling in the maintenance of

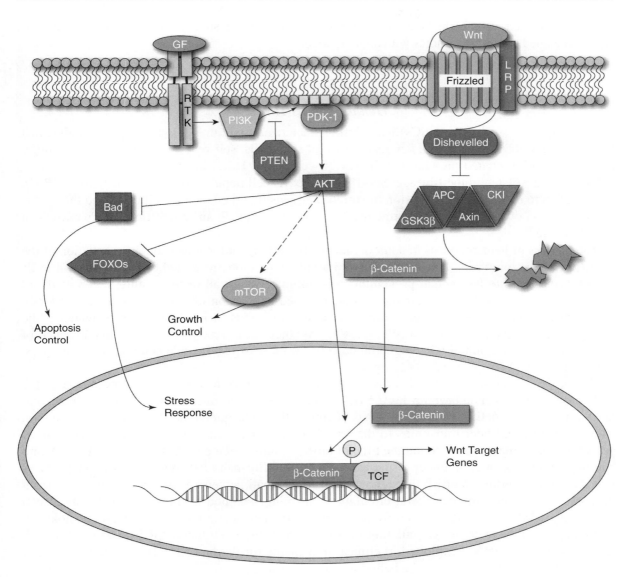

Fig. 1. Pertinent signaling pathways discussed in this chapter. On the *left*, the PI3K/AKT pathway is depicted. Binding of a growth factor (GF) to its respective receptor tyrosine kinase (RTK) at the cell surface results in activation of PI3K. Upon activation, PI3K phosphorylates certain phospholipids allowing for recruitment of phosphatidylinositol-dependent kinase-1 (PDK-1) and AKT followed by activation of AKT by PDK-1. Once active, AKT acts on multiple molecular targets; several that are mentioned in this chapter are shown. AKT inhibits proapoptotic factors such as BAD, and the Forkhead box transcription factors (FOXOs). AKT can also upregulate the activity of mammalian target of rapamycin (mTOR), which leads to increased protein translation and subsequent cell growth. The sole inhibitor of PI3K/AKT signaling is phosphatase and tensin homolog (PTEN), which reverses the reaction catalyzed by PI3K. On the *right*, the canonical Wnt pathway is depicted. Binding of Wnt ligand to the Frizzled cell surface receptor recruits lipoprotein-related protein (LRP) coreceptor for full activation of the signaling complex. Activated Frizzled inhibits degradation of β-catenin by a destruction complex that includes adenomatous polyposis coli (APC), Axin, casein kinase I, and glycogen synthase kinase 3β. This allows β-catenin to accumulate and translocate into the nucleus to bind to LEF/TCF transcription factors and drive the expression of Wnt-responsive genes. Recent studies indicate AKT phosphorylation may enhance β-catenin activity.

tissue-specific stem cells in the hematopoietic system and in the intestine, as well as in carcinogenesis, has been gained via in vivo studies with animal models.

PTEN, HSCS, AND CANCER

Hematopoiesis/HSCs

Hematopoietic stem cells (HSCs) were first characterized more than 40 years ago by studies that led to a proposal for defining the key features of all stem cells: self-renewal capacity and the ability to generate differentiated progeny *(7)*. It was 20 years until HSCs in the mouse were definitively identified and isolated in the Lineage⁻ Sca-1⁺ c-kit⁺ (LSK) cell population of the bone marrow (BM), which refers to their lack of expression of various antigens found on mature cell types and their positive expression of two cell-surface proteins, Sca-1 and c-kit; *(8, 9)* since that time HSCs have been widely studied.

The process of hematopoiesis in adult organisms is ongoing and involves the differentiation of the most primitive, long-term HSCs (LT-HSCs) initially into more restricted, short-term stem cells (ST-HSCs), then into less potent progenitors, and ultimately into all of the mature, committed cell types of the blood, at least in part through coordinated expression of cell-specific genes *(10–12)*. These phenotypically different cells carry out various functions of the blood, one of which is the transport of oxygen via red blood cells (RBCs). Another is the establishment and maintenance of innate and acquired immunity via white blood cells (WBCs), which include neutrophils, monocytes, macrophages, and lymphocytes *(11)* (Fig. 2a).

Hematopoiesis arises in a transient fashion as blood is first formed by yolk-sac mesoderm in the early mouse embryo at embryonic day 7.5 (E7.5); this is termed primitive hematopoiesis. Somewhat later at E9.5 to 10, definitive hematopoiesis begins in the aorta-gonad mesonephros (AGM) region and/or placenta and later transitions to the fetal liver after E11, and continues for the duration of prenatal development *(13)*. Around the time of birth, definitive hematopoiesis shifts to the BM, and continues there for the remainder of the animal's normal lifespan *(10)*. While the vast majority of HSCs are found within the BM, throughout adult life a small percentage of HSCs will egress from the marrow and enter the peripheral circulation. Seemingly related to this is the well-established finding that HSCs can be mobilized from the BM to the peripheral blood by certain chemokines, including granulocyte colony-stimulating factor (G-CSF), stem cell factor (SCF), and Flt-3 ligand. Indeed, such methods are exploited in clinical transplants for therapy *(14)*. HSC mobilization can also result from compromises to the hematopoietic system such as massive blood loss or myelosuppression (sub-lethal irradiation or chemotherapy), and a major homing site of mobilized cells during mobilization is the spleen, where extramedullary hematopoiesis can occur *(15)*. Research into HSC mobilization/homing has emphasized the importance of the HSC niche, the identification of which was a milestone in the field.

Ray Schofield first proposed the hypothesis that a physically limited microenvironment (niche) exists *in vivo*, where stem cells normally reside and stably maintain self-renewal potential. After cell division, one daughter cell remains in the niche (self-renewal) and the other is forced out of the niche, where it loses its capacity to self-renew and commits to differentiation *(16)*. Evidence supporting this hypothesis came from *in vitro* studies of HSC-supporting stromal cell lines and *in vivo* identification of germline stem cell-supporting niche cells in the *Drosophila* ovary and testis *(17–24)*. More recent studies put forth evidence proposing what came to be known as the HSC endosteal niche, the key player of which is a subpopulation of bone-lining, osteoblast cells that express N-cadherin and function as niche cells *(25–28)*. This concept was recently augmented to include the vascular niche as additional studies found that HSCs can also closely associate with endothelial cells of the vasculature in the BM and spleen,

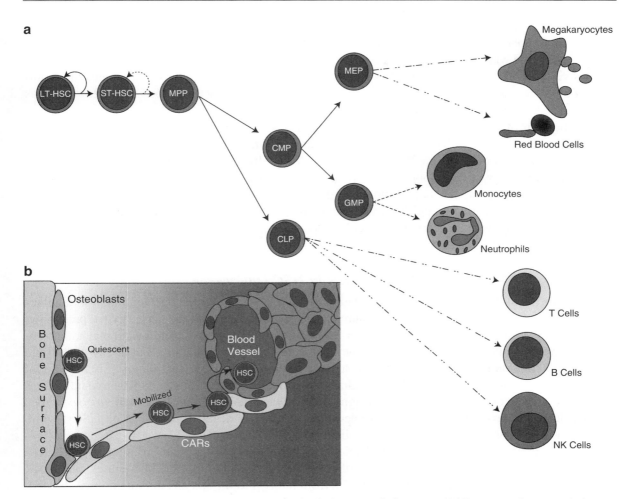

Fig. 2. Pictorial representation of lineage development in the hematopoietic system. (**a**) Long-term hematopoietic stem cells (LT-HSC) give rise to short-term hematopoietic stem cells (ST-HSC), and while both cell types share the potential for multilineage differentiation, ST-HSCs are much more restricted in their ability to self-renew as compared to LT-HSCs. Multipotent progenitors (MPP) that lack self-renewal capacity will give rise to common lymphoid progenitors (CLP) and common myeloid progenitors (CMP). CLPs will ultimately give rise to T- and B-lymphocytes as well as natural killer (NK) cells. CMPs differentiate into granulocyte-macrophage progenitors (GMP) and megakaryocyte-erythroid progenitors (MEP), which will give rise to neutrophils and monocytes/macrophages and megakaryocytes and erythrocytes, respectively. (**b**) Depiction of potential HSC/niche physical interactions. HSCs have been found to associate with osteoblasts lining the surface of bone and vascular endothelial cells. Additional work has shown HSCs closely associate with CXCL12-abundant reticulocytes (CARs), which may form networks to facilitate trafficking of HSCs into and out of the bone marrow, such as during mobilization.

indicating that these cells can also act as niche for HSCs *(29–31)*. Studies into these two niches suggest they have complementary roles in regulating HSCs. The endosteal niche maintains HSC quiescence to preserve the stem cell pool, while the vascular niche likely functions to promote HSC proliferation, differentiation, and mobilization to meet the continual demands of hematopoiesis *(32)*. Yet these are not the only niches identified within BM. Studies have identified a population of stromal cells, termed CXCL12-abundant reticular (CAR) cells, that are located both adjacent to the endosteum and perivascularly. Given roles of CXCL12-CXCR4 signaling in HSC maintenance, CAR cells appear to be an important component of the HSC niche *in vivo (33, 34)* (Fig. 2b). Additionally, studies have elucidated a role for osteoclasts in contributing to microenvironmental regulation of HSC behavior primarily by degradation of endosteal components promoting mobilization of hematopoietic progenitors in response to stress *(35)*. And while not involved in direct physical attachment to HSCs, neurons of the sympathetic nervous system (SNS) have been found to be involved in regulating HSC microenvironment and mobilization by affecting bone metabolism and expression of the chemotactic factor CXCL12, which has known roles directing trafficking of HSCs *(36)*.

Identification of the stem cell niche in this system has highlighted the various roles of external signals that regulate HSCs. These include cytokines and growth factors and well-studied developmental signaling pathways such as the Wnt, Notch, and BMP pathways. An extensive amount of research over the years has shown the importance of these various signals in regulating activities of HSCs that include self-renewal, proliferation, migration, and differentiation. In this section, we will focus on the PI3K/AKT signaling pathway and its major antagonist, PTEN, and discuss how this pathway both regulates normal HSCs and contributes to leukemogenesis.

The Role of PTEN in HSC Quiescence

Stem cells in adult tissues must delicately balance the need for continually generating new daughter cells to replenish those lost in the normal maintenance of that tissue with the necessity for preserving the stem cell pool over the life of the organism. To attain this balance, it is widely held that adult stem cells are predominantly quiescent, entering the cell cycle very infrequently so that at any given time only a small fraction of the stem cell pool is actively dividing while the vast majority is held under cell cycle arrest. This balance is partly maintained by the interplay of positive and negative influences on the state of stem cells, including various signaling pathways such as Wnt and Notch. *In vivo* studies into the functional loss of PTEN have revealed it to be a major negative influence on HSCs, while PI3K/AKT signaling is an opposing, positive influence.

Genetic deletion of PTEN in the BM of mice initially results in increased proliferation of HSCs. This overstimulation is evidenced by a shift of HSCs from the G0 to G1/S/G2/M phases of the cell cycle. Linked to this is the mobilization of HSCs from the BM to the spleens in mutant mice. Indeed, the transient expansion of HSCs does not occur in the BM, but rather within the spleen. This excessive proliferation coupled with the dissociation from the restrictive endosteal niche ultimately exhausts the stem cell pool causing its long-term decline and impaired ability to sustain reconstitution of a depleted hematopoietic system. PTEN mutant mice develop myeloproliferative disorder (MPD), and acute leukemia formation develops in mice transplanted with PTEN-deficient HSCs. The observation that PTEN mutant mice display both a depletion of normal HSCs and increased leukemia formation led to the hypothesis of a cancer stem cell (CSC) *(37–39)* population forming in these animals. Treatment with rapamycin, a drug that inhibits the activity of mTOR, prevented development of hematopoietic malignancy in PTEN-deficient animals and inhibited generation/maintenance of potential CSCs *(40, 41)*. Overall it appears that PTEN is an important factor in restricting overproliferation of HSCs and may act alone, or more likely, in concert with other cellular components to distinguish between CSCs and normal stem cells. In fact, recent work supports this latter possibility. Studies into PTEN deficiency in HSCs mediated by an alternative method of PTEN gene deletion have produced new insight. While mutant mice developed MPD that progressed to acute leukemia in a similar fashion to previous studies, when this PTEN-deficient mouse model was combined with a reduction in β-catenin expression, the incidence of leukemia was significantly decreased and its progression was substantially delayed *(42)*. These results indicate that β-catenin activity may be subject in part to PTEN/PI3K/AKT regulation and that PTEN/mTOR signaling, while important, might not account for all of the PTEN mutant phenotype.

The Role of PTEN in Leukemia

The PTEN tumor suppressor gene was cloned to a region on human chromosome 10 in 1997, and that same year genetic mutations in PTEN were first linked to human conditions such as Cowden disease and several human cancers including those of the breast, prostate, endometrium, brain, and skin *(43–51)*. A year later, studies showed that a small percentage of malignant lymphomas involve mutations in the PTEN gene *(6)*. Inactivating mutations of this tumor suppressor are not the only mechanism for its involvement in cancer development. Studies have shown numerous human leukemias and lymphomas display decreased expression of PTEN both at the mRNA and protein level, as well as at the increased levels of phosphorylated AKT (indicative of PI3K activity) *(52, 53)*.

Indeed, the role for PTEN as a potent tumor suppressor was confirmed in the studies of PTEN deletion in the BM of mice. Accompanying defects in the HSC compartment, mice lacking PTEN develop MPD that progresses to acute myeloid leukemia (AML) and acute lymphoid leukemia (ALL), following a similar disease course as that seen in human patients *(40, 41)*. Supporting this tumor suppressor role, forced expression of PTEN in ALL cells causes a reduction in their proliferation and slows their passage through the cell cycle in a AKT-dependent manner *(54, 55)*. Furthermore, forced expression of PTEN in other PTEN-null ALL cell lines, in addition to these effects on cell growth, has also demonstrated its importance in promoting p53-mediated apoptosis. Mdm2, a primary regulator of p53 whose subcellular localization is controlled by AKT, is in turn regulated by PTEN. As expected, in PTEN-null ALL cells, Mdm2 is localized in the nucleus and actively represses p53, functioning in an antiapoptotic manner. Forced expression of PTEN in these cells results in repression of Mdm2, both by antagonizing PI3K/AKT signaling, thereby resulting in the relocalization of Mdm2 to the cytoplasm, as well as by direct binding of PTEN to p53, diminishing the effect of Mdm2 *(56)*.

PTEN, ISCS, AND CANCER

Intestinal Development/ISCs

Extensive research into the intestine has resulted in this organ being one of the best defined in terms of development and cancer formation, but interestingly the location of intestinal stem cells (ISCs) has remained controversial for many years. To briefly summarize the formation of the small intestine, during gastrulation endoderm is specified to a stratified cuboidal epithelium until midgestation in most vertebrates *(57)*. During mid-to-late gestation, signals from mesenchyme induce the adjacent epithelium to evaginate and form finger-like projections into the intestinal lumen called villi. The intervening regions between villi consist of undifferentiated, proliferative cells that shortly after birth invaginate to form clefts in the submucosa called crypts; these crypts continue to develop during the first few weeks of postnatal development in rodents *(58, 59)*. While the molecular mechanism controlling this morphogenesis remains to be elucidated, a wealth of evidence suggests signaling pathways such as Wnt, Hedgehog, and BMP play crucial roles *(60–66)*.

In the adult small intestine, the single layer of columnar epithelium is comprised of the well-organized, repetitive villi and crypts formed during development. The villi are populated by terminally differentiated cells including enterocytes, goblet cells, and enteroendocrine cells (which function in absorption and secretion, respectively), and the crypts house the intestinal stem and progenitors along with a mature, secretory cell type called Paneth cells *(67–71)* (Fig. 3).

ISCs, much like HSCs, are defined by their ability to generate more stem cells (self-renewal) and their capacity for multilineage differentiation. Initial evidence for the existence of ISCs came from studies of mutant mouse strains that indicated a monoclonal nature for crypts, that is, a single crypt was generated from a single ISC *(72–74)*. While it has been known for some time that ISCs reside in crypts, as mentioned their exact position within the crypt–villus axis has remained unresolved. Early

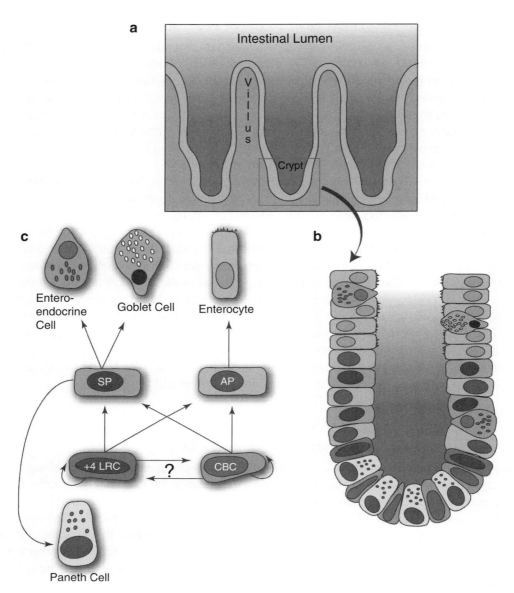

Fig. 3. Diagram of small intestinal architecture. (**a**) Pictorial representation of the crypt-villus axis in the small intestinal epithelium. Invaginations into the gut submucosa called crypts harbor the stem and progenitor cells of this tissue. As cells differentiate, they migrate up into finger-like projections into the gut lumen called villi. (**b**) An enlarged view of an intestinal crypt. (**c**) A diagram of lineage development in the intestine. Putative intestinal stem cells – label retaining cells at the +4 position (+4 LRC) and crypt-based columnar cells (CBCs) are able to give rise to secretory progenitor (SP) and absorptive progenitor (AP) cells. Enteroendocrine and Goblet cells as well as enterocytes migrate up into the villus, while Paneth cells migrate to the crypt base. The relationship between +4 LRCs and CBCs and their potential to give rise to each other remain undetermined *(see Color Plates)*.

studies indicated that ISCs existed at the base of the crypt intermingled with Paneth cells; these putative ISCs were termed crypt-based columnar (CBC) cells because of their location and morphology *(70, 74, 75)*. Due to the research of stem cells in other adult tissues that indicated them to be quiescent or extremely slow cycling, the technique of long-term label retention was employed in the intestine. These later experiments identified a quiescent cell that localized to a position that was (on average)

4 cells up (+4 position) from the crypt base and above Paneth cells and was termed the +4 label retaining cell (LRC) due to its position and quiescent nature *(26, 76–79)*. More recent work has supported the presence of putative ISCs at both of these positions, continuing the debate over ISC location. One elegant study that centered around lineage tracing experiments of Lgr5-expressing cells at the crypt base supports CBCs as ISCs, while experiments demonstrating colocalization of molecules with +4 LRCs such as Musashi-1, phosphorylated-PTEN, phosphorylated-AKT, sFRP5, and Wip1 phosphatase support the +4 LRC as the ISC *(64, 80–85)*. It is certainly possible that continued research in this field will conclusively prove one or the other of these potential ISCs to be the bona fide stem cell of the intestine, or it may well be that these disparate studies are revealing a scenario in the intestine not unlike that recently identified in the hematopoietic system.

A recent study into the expression of the niche factor N-cadherin in HSCs revealed a heretofore unrealized heterogeneity in the LT-HSC population, with microarray and functional assays indicating that there are in actuality two populations of these long-term stem cells: those that are most quiescent and held in reserve, and those that are more metabolically active and primed to receive stimulatory signals to proliferate, differentiate, and mobilize. Indeed, it appears that the so-called "reserved" HSCs can give rise to "primed" HSCs as needed, and vice versa. This dynamic may also exist in the intestine, with the +4 LRC representing a "reserved" pool of stem cells that cycle very infrequently, and the more active CBCs playing the role of "primed" stem cells that meet the demands of this continually regenerating tissue. In times of stress or damage, as one of these ISCs is lost it might be replaced by the other *(86)* (Fig. 3).

Although definitive localization of ISCs within intestinal crypts remains elusive, a great deal of insight has been gained into the biology of these cells, primarily from genetic and molecular immunohistochemical studies that have indicated the importance of several developmental signaling pathways in regulating ISCs. Adhering to our focus on PTEN in this chapter, we will look at the role of this PI3K antagonist in ISCs and intestinal carcinogenesis.

The Role of PTEN in ISC function

Recently, insight into the role of PTEN in the regulation of ISCs has been gained by functional studies similar to those conducted in the hematopoietic system *(40, 41)*. Widespread deletion of PTEN in adult mice leads to generation of hamartomatous intestinal polyps, a specific type of polyp with both epithelial and stromal involvement. Investigation into this disease process revealed that, much like in HSCs, PTEN acts as a negative regulator of the cell cycle in stem and progenitor (ISC/p) cells within intestinal crypts. When PTEN is deleted in these cells, they shift from a largely quiescent/slow-cycling population to a more active/proliferative state. Additionally, within PTEN mutant intestine, the number of ISC/p cells increases and they become aberrantly localized, a feature similar to the mobilization of HSCs. These aberrant ISC/p cells were found at the initiation sites of both crypt fission and crypt budding, processes that, while common during early intestinal development, are, with the exception of during injury repair, quite rare in the adult and indicative of polyposis formation *(84, 87–89)*. Importantly, the proliferation of ISC/p cells was not the only factor leading to polyposis development. As mentioned, hamartomatous polyps have both the epithelial and stromal components. Indeed, these mutant mice also lose PTEN expression within intestinal stroma, resulting in overgrowth and mislocalization of stromal cells in close proximity to aberrant ISC/p cells. This deregulated stroma may provide stimulatory signals that contribute to polyp formation *(84)*.

This functional evidence indicates that these deregulated ISC/p cells may have undergone a phenotypic switch from normal stem cells to CSCs. Although not a specific CSC marker, nuclear localized β-catenin, considered critical in the process of stem cell activation, was observed within these cells, supporting their identity as stem cells. β-catenin is the primary effector of the Wnt signaling pathway. In the absence of Wnt ligand, β-catenin is targeted for degradation by a destruction complex that includes adenomatous polyposis coli (APC), Axin, casein kinase I, and glycogen synthase kinase 3β. Activation of the Wnt receptor complex that includes Frizzled and the coreceptor lipoprotein-related protein (LRP) results in the repression of the destruction complex via Disheveled, allowing β-catenin to accumulate and translocate into the nucleus to bind to LEF/TCF transcription factors and drive the expression of Wnt-responsive genes *(86)* (Fig. 1).

Indeed, while cells possessing nuclear localized β-catenin have been identified at the putative ISC position and costained with other ISC markers, they are relatively rare in normal, adult intestine. In the characterization of PTEN mutant mice, multiple cells with nuclear β-catenin were seen in intestinal polyps and particularly at sites of crypt fission and budding *(64, 84, 90)*. Moreover, investigation into the mechanism of tumor formation in PTEN mutant mice revealed new insight into the molecular link between β-catenin nuclear activity and PTEN/PI3K/AKT signaling. A novel AKT phosphorylation site was identified on β-catenin at Ser552, and distribution of β-catenin phosphorylated on Ser552 was restricted to the nucleus *(84, 91, 92)*. It is likely that while PTEN mutation removes the sole negative regulator of PI3K/AKT signaling, this pathway's activity is still controlled by input signals and may require further dysregulation of upstream signaling including insulin growth factor (IGF), fibroblast growth factor (FGF), and epidermal growth factor (EGF) pathways and/or Wnt signaling for carcinogenesis to occur.

The Role of PTEN in Intestinal Polyposis and Colorectal Cancer

As stated earlier, mutations in PTEN occur in a variety of human cancers, and those of the gastrointestinal tract are no exception. In fact over 40% of human colorectal carcinomas involve mutations of the PI3K/AKT pathway, a large number of which result in reduced or absent PTEN function *(5)*. Also Cowden disease, a rare autosomal dominant disorder in humans characterized by development of multiple hamartomatous lesions including intestinal polyps, results from genetic mutation of PTEN *(93)*. Indeed, the conditional PTEN knockout mouse model discussed above exhibits this disorder *(84)*. Additionally, another human genetic disorder Bannayan-Riley-Ruvalcaba Syndrome also presents with multiple hamartomas in various tissues, including the gastrointestinal tract, and has been linked to mutations in PTEN *(94)*.

Yet mutation of PTEN alone is not the only deregulation of this pathway that can contribute to cancer formation. Amplifications of genomic regions containing the AKT and PI3K catalytic domain (PI3KCA) genes, as well as the mutations in the regulatory subunit of PI3K, are well characterized in colon tumors. Specifically, mutations in PI3KCA have been found in 32% of colorectal cancers. Additionally, genetic screens of colorectal carcinomas have found other pathway components such as PDK-1 to be mutated in these neoplasms *(95)*.

CONCLUDING REMARKS

In this chapter, we have discussed the need for tissue-specific stem cells to balance the replenishment of lost cells with the maintenance of the stem cell pool throughout the life of an organism. Furthermore, we have discussed the recent findings of two pools of stem cells with different states – reserved vs. primed – in the hematopoietic system and the possibility of such a dichotomy within the intestine. Recent *in vivo* studies investigating functional loss of PTEN in two different adult tissues have revealed PTEN as an important factor in preserving the balance between long-term maintenance and routine tissue replenishment. In both the hematopoietic system and the intestine, deletion of PTEN resulted in overproliferation of stem cells and ultimately carcinogenesis. Indeed, the status of PI3K/

AKT pathway components as oncogenes and PTEN as a tumor suppressor is well established. However, the studies discussed herein suggest a role for PTEN beyond simply that of restraint of PI3K/AKT signaling. It is possible that PTEN is one of the factors that contribute to the delineation of reserved/primed stem cells. As the sole antagonist to the stimulatory PI3K/AKT pathway, it may function in restraining reserved stem cells and promoting their recalcitrance to stimuli. Likewise downregulation of PTEN's expression and/or activity in primed stem cells may contribute to their responsiveness to such positive signals.

Additionally, it may well be that mutation and loss of PTEN, while leading to excessive proliferation of stem cells and their progeny, does not directly result in overt cancer. It is likely that additional deregulation of other pathways, such as Wnt/β-catenin signaling, contributes to conversion of a normal stem/progenitor cell to a CSC identity that mediates malignant transformation (Fig. 4). Additional study into PTEN/PI3K/AKT signaling and its differential phenotypic outcomes in normal and cancer stem cells should provide insight into self-renewal mechanisms in these two stem cell populations and may lead to identification of potential therapeutic targets for eliminating CSCs without adversely affecting normal tissue stem cells.

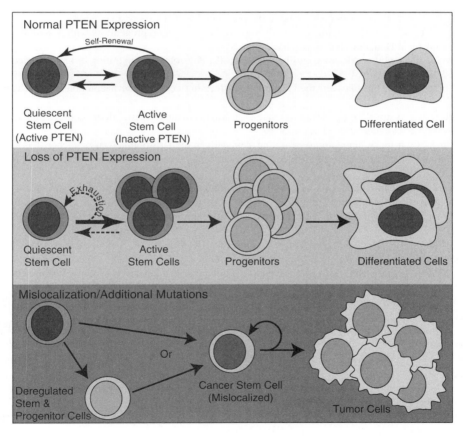

Fig. 4. Model of role of PTEN in stem cell behavior and tumor formation. Stem cells possessing functional PTEN undergo self-renewing divisions and generate daughter progenitor cells that transiently proliferate prior to differentiation to mature cell types (*upper panel*). Loss of PTEN results in overproliferation of stem cells leading to their exhaustion and development of proliferative disorders involving progeny (*middle panel*). Mislocalization of stem/progenitor cells may contribute to accumulation of additional mutations, resulting in deregulation of other signaling pathways leading to transformation of normal cells to cancer stem cells that will give rise to bulk tumor cells and overt cancer formation (*lower panel*).

REFERENCES

1. Vivanco I, Sawyers CL. The phosphatidylinositol 3-Kinase AKT pathway in human cancer. Nat Rev Cancer 2006;2(7):489–501.
2. Cully M, You H, Levine AJ, Mak TW. Beyond PTEN mutations: the PI3K pathway as an integrator of multiple inputs during tumorigenesis. Nat Rev Cancer 2006;6(3):184–92.
3. Stiles B, Groszer M, Wang S, Jiao J, Wu H. PTENless means more. Dev Biol 2004;273(2):175–84.
4. Mutter GL. Pten, a protean tumor suppressor. Am J Pathol 2001;158(6):1895–8.
5. Parsons DW, Wang TL, Samuels Y, et al. Colorectal cancer: mutations in a signalling pathway. Nature 2005;436:792.
6. Sakai A, Thieblemont C, Wellmann A, Jaffe ES, Raffeld M. PTEN gene alterations in lymphoid neoplasms. Blood 1998;92(9):3410–5.
7. Till JE, McCulloch EA, Siminovitch L. A stochastic model of stem cell proliferation, based on the growth of spleen colony-forming cells. Proc Natl Acad Sci USA 1964;51:29–36.
8. Spangrude GJ, Heimfeld S, Weissman IL. Purification and characterization of mouse hematopoietic stem cells. Science 1988;241:58–62.
9. Ikuta K, Weissman IL. Evidence that hematopoietic stem cells express mouse c-kit but do not depend on steel factor for their generation. Proc Natl Acad Sci USA 1992;89:1502–6.
10. Shivdasani RA, Orkin SH. The transcriptional control of hematopoiesis. Blood 1996;87:4025–39.
11. Cantor AB, Orkin SH. Hematopoietic development: a balancing act. Curr Opin Genet Dev 2001;11:513–9.
12. Shizuru JA, Negrin RS, Weissman IL. Hematopoietic stem and progenitor cells: clinical and preclinical regeneration of the hematolymphoid system. Annu Rev Med 2005;56:509–38.
13. Li L. Finding the hematopoietic stem cell niche in the placenta. Dev Cell 2005;8(3):297–8.
14. Thomas J, Liu F, Link DC. Mechanisms of mobilization of hematopoietic progenitors with granulocyte colony-stimulating factor. Curr Opin Hematol 2002;9:183–9.
15. Wright DE, Wagers AJ, Gulati AP, Johnson FL, Weissman IL. Physiological migration of hematopoietic stem and progenitor cells. Science 2001;294:1933–6.
16. Schofield R. The relationship between the spleen colony-forming cell and the haemopoietic stem cell. Blood Cells 1978;4:7–25.
17. Lin H, Spradling AC. A novel group of pumilio mutations affects the asymmetric division of germline stem cells in the Drosophila ovary. Development 1997;124:2463–76.
18. Xie T, Spradling AC. A niche maintaining germ line stem cells in the Drosophila ovary. Science 2000;290:328–30.
19. Tulina N, Matunis E. Control of stem cell self-renewal in Drosophila spermatogenesis by JAK-STAT signaling. Science 2001;294:2546–9.
20. Kiger AA, Jones DL, Schulz C, Rogers MB, Fuller MT. Stem cell self-renewal specified by JAK-STAT activation in response to a support cell cue. Science 2001;294:2542–5.
21. Moore KA, Ema H, Lemischka IR. In vitro maintenance of highly purified, transplantable hematopoietic stem cells. Blood 1997;89:4337–47.
22. Hackney JA, Charbord P, Brunk BP, Stoeckert CJ, Lemischka IR, Moore KA. A molecular profile of a hematopoietic stem cell niche. Proc Natl Acad Sci USA 2002;99:13061–6.
23. Wineman J, Moore K, Lemischka I, Muller-Sieburg C. Functional heterogeneity of the hematopoietic microenvironment: rare stromal elements maintain long-term repopulating stem cells. Blood 1996;87:4082–90.
24. Wineman JP, Nishikawa S, Muller-Sieburg CE. Maintenance of high levels of pluripotent hematopoietic stem cells in vitro: effect of stromal cells and c-kit. Blood 1993;81:365–72.
25. Calvi LM, Adams GB, Weibrecht KW, et al. Osteoblastic cells regulate the haematopoietic stem cell niche. Nature 2003;425:841–6.
26. Zhang J, Niu C, Ye L, et al. Identification of the haematopoietic stem cell niche and control of the niche size. Nature 2003;425:836–41.
27. Arai F, Hirao A, Ohmura M, et al. Tie2/angiopoietin-1 signaling regulates hematopoietic stem cell quiescence in the bone marrow niche. Cell 2004;118:149–61.
28. Hosokawa K, Arai F, Yoshihara H, et al. Function of oxidative stress in the regulation of hematopoietic stem cell-niche interaction. Biochem Biophys Res Commun 2007;363(3):578–83.
29. Kopp HG, Avecilla ST, Hooper AT, Rafii S. The bone marrow vascular niche: home of HSC differentiation and mobilization. Physiology (Bethesda) 2005;20:349–56.
30. Kiel MJ, Yilmaz OH, Iwashita T, Terhorst C, Morrison SJ. SLAM family receptors distinguish hematopoietic stem and progenitor cells and reveal endothelial niches for stem cells. Cell 2005;121:1109–21.
31. Kopp HG, Avecilla ST, Hooper AT, et al. Tie2 activation contributes to hemangiogenic regeneration after myelosuppression. Blood 2005;106(2):505–13.

32. Yin T, Li L. The stem cell niches in bone. J Clin Invest 2006;116(5):1195–201.

33. Ara T, Tokoyoda K, Sugiyama T, Egawa T, Kawabata K, Nagasawa T. Long-term hematopoietic stem cells require stromal cell-derived factor-1 for colonizing bone marrow during ontogeny. Immunity 2003;19(2):257–67.

34. Sugiyama T, Kohara H, Noda M, Nagasawa T. Maintenance of the hematopoietic stem cell pool by CXCL12-CXCR4 chemokine signaling in bone marrow stromal cell niches. Immunity 2006;25(6):977–88.

35. Kollet O, Dar A, Shivtiel S, et al. Osteoclasts degrade endosteal components and promote mobilization of hematopoietic progenitor cells. Nat Med 2006;12(6):657–64.

36. Katayama Y, Battista M, Kao WM, et al. Signals from the sympathetic nervous system regulate hematopoietic stem cell egress from bone marrow. Cell 2006;124(2):407–21.

37. Al-Hajj M, Becker MW, Wicha M, Weissman I, Clarke MF. Therapeutic implications of cancer stem cells. Curr Opin Genet Dev 2004;14(1):43–7.

38. Reya T, Morrison SJ, Clarke MF, Weissman IL. Stem cells, cancer, and cancer stem cells. Nature 2001;414 (6859):105–11.

39. Clarke MF, Fuller M. Stem cells and cancer: two faces of eve. Cell 2006;124(6):1111–5.

40. Yilmaz OH, Valdez R, Theisen BK, et al. Pten dependence distinguishes haematopoietic stem cells from leukaemia-initiating cells. Nature 2006;441(7092):475–82.

41. Zhang J, Grindley JC, Yin T, et al. PTEN maintains haematopoietic stem cells and acts in lineage choice and leukaemia prevention. Nature 2006;441:518–22.

42. Guo W, Lasky JL, Chang CJ, et al. Multi-genetic events collaboratively contribute to Pten-null leukaemia stem-cell formation. Nature 2008;453:529–33.

43. Liaw D, Marsh DJ, Li J, et al. Germline mutations of the PTEN gene in Cowden disease, an inherited breast and thyroid cancer syndrome. Nat Genet 1997;16(1):64–7.

44. Rhei E, Kang L, Bogomolniy F, Federici MG, Borgen PI, Boyd J. Mutation analysis of the putative tumor suppressor gene PTEN/MMAC1 in primary breast carcinomas. Cancer research 1997;57(17):3657–9.

45. Cairns P, Okami K, Halachmi S, et al. Frequent inactivation of PTEN/MMAC1 in primary prostate cancer. Cancer Res 1997;57(22):4997–5000.

46. Kong D, Suzuki A, Zou TT, et al. PTEN1 is frequently mutated in primary endometrial carcinomas. Nature Genet 1997;17(2):143–4.

47. Risinger JI, Hayes AK, Berchuck A, Barrett JC. PTEN/MMAC1 mutations in endometrial cancers. Cancer Res 1997;57(21):4736–8.

48. Tashiro H, Blazes MS, Wu R, et al. Mutations in PTEN are frequent in endometrial carcinoma but rare in other common gynecological malignancies. Cancer Res 1997;57(18):3935–40.

49. Rasheed BK, Stenzel TT, McLendon RE, et al. PTEN gene mutations are seen in high-grade but not in low-grade gliomas. Cancer Res 1997;57(19):4187–90.

50. Wang SI, Puc J, Li J, et al. Somatic mutations of PTEN in glioblastoma multiforme. Cancer Res 1997;57(19):4183–6.

51. Guldberg P, thor Straten P, Birck A, Ahrenkiel V, Kirkin AF, Zeuthen J. Disruption of the MMAC1/PTEN gene by deletion or mutation is a frequent event in malignant melanoma. Cancer Res 1997;57(17):3660–3.

52. Abbott RT, Tripp S, Perkins SL, Elenitoba-Johnson KS, Lim MS. Analysis of the PI-3-Kinase-PTEN-AKT pathway in human lymphoma and leukemia using a cell line microarray. Mod Pathol 2003;16(6):607–12.

53. Yang J, Liu J, Zheng J, et al. A reappraisal by quantitative flow cytometry analysis of PTEN expression in acute leukemia. Leukemia 2007;21(9):2072–4.

54. Xu Z, Stokoe D, Kane LP, Weiss A. The inducible expression of the tumor suppressor gene PTEN promotes apoptosis and decreases cell size by inhibiting the PI3K/Akt pathway in Jurkat T cells. Cell Growth Differ 2002;13(7):285–96.

55. Seminario MC, Precht P, Wersto RP, Gorospe M, Wange RL. PTEN expression in PTEN-null leukaemic T cell lines leads to reduced proliferation via slowed cell cycle progression. Oncogene 2003;22(50):8195–204.

56. Zhou M, Gu L, Findley HW, Jiang R, Woods WG. PTEN reverses MDM2-mediated chemotherapy resistance by interacting with p53 in acute lymphoblastic leukemia cells. Cancer Res 2003;63(19):6357–62.

57. de Santa Barbara P, van den Brink GR, Roberts DJ. Development and differentiation of the intestinal epithelium. Cell Mol Life Sci 2003;60(7):1322–32.

58. Calvert R, Pothier P. Migration of fetal intestinal intervillous cells in neonatal mice. Anat Rec 1990;227(2):199–206.

59. Schmidt GH, Winton DJ, Ponder BA. Development of the pattern of cell renewal in the crypt-villus unit of chimaeric mouse small intestine. Development 1988;103:785–90.

60. Korinek V, Barker N, Moerer P, et al. Depletion of epithelial stem-cell compartments in the small intestine of mice lacking Tcf-4. Nature Genet 1998;19:379–83.

61. Kim BM, Mao J, Taketo MM, Shivdasani RA. Phases of canonical Wnt signaling during the development of mouse intestinal epithelium. Gastroenterology 2007;133(2):529–38.

62. Madison BB, Braunstein K, Kuizon E, Portman K, Qiao XT, Gumucio DL. Epithelial hedgehog signals pattern the intestinal crypt-villus axis. Development 2005;132:279–89.

63. Bitgood MJ, McMahon AP. Hedgehog and Bmp genes are coexpressed at many diverse sites of cell-cell interaction in the mouse embryo. Dev Biol 1995;172(1):126–38.

64. He XC, Zhang J, Tong WG, et al. BMP signaling inhibits intestinal stem cell self-renewal through suppression of Wnt-beta-catenin signaling. Nature Genet 2004;36:1117–21.

65. Haramis AP, Begthel H, van den Born M, et al. De novo crypt formation and juvenile polyposis on BMP inhibition in mouse intestine. Science 2004;303:1684–6.

66. Batts LE, Polk DB, Dubois RN, Kulessa H. Bmp signaling is required for intestinal growth and morphogenesis. Dev Dyn 2006;235(6):1563–70.

67. Cheng H. Origin, differentiation and renewal of the four main epithelial cell types in the mouse small intestine. IV. Paneth cells. Am J Anat 1974;141(4):521–35.

68. Cheng H. Origin, differentiation and renewal of the four main epithelial cell types in the mouse small intestine. II. Mucous cells. Am J Anat 1974;141(4):481–501.

69. Cheng H, Leblond CP. Origin, differentiation and renewal of the four main epithelial cell types in the mouse small intestine. V. Unitarian Theory of the origin of the four epithelial cell types. Am J Anat 1974;141(4):537–61.

70. Cheng H, Leblond CP. Origin, differentiation and renewal of the four main epithelial cell types in the mouse small intestine. I. Columnar cell. Am J Anat 1974;141(4):461–79.

71. Cheng H, Leblond CP. Origin, differentiation and renewal of the four main epithelial cell types in the mouse small intestine. III. Entero-endocrine cells. Am J Anat 1974;141(4):503–19.

72. Hermiston ML, Green RP, Gordon JI. Chimeric-transgenic mice represent a powerful tool for studying how the proliferation and differentiation programs of intestinal epithelial cell lineages are regulated. Proc Natl Acad Sci USA 1993;90:8866–70.

73. Roth KA, Hermiston ML, Gordon JI. Use of transgenic mice to infer the biological properties of small intestinal stem cells and to examine the lineage relationships of their descendants. Proc Natl Acad Sci USA 1991;88:9407–11.

74. Bjerknes M, Cheng H. Clonal analysis of mouse intestinal epithelial progenitors. Gastroenterology 1999;116:7–14.

75. Bjerknes M, Cheng H. The stem-cell zone of the small intestinal epithelium. IV. Effects of resecting 30% of the small intestine. Am J Anat 1981;160(1):93–103.

76. Cheshier SH, Morrison SJ, Liao X, Weissman IL. In vivo proliferation and cell cycle kinetics of long-term self-renewing hematopoietic stem cells. Proc Natl Acad Sci USA 1999;96(6):3120–5.

77. Cotsarelis G, Sun TT, Lavker RM. Label-retaining cells reside in the bulge area of pilosebaceous unit: implications for follicular stem cells, hair cycle, and skin carcinogenesis. Cell 1990;61(7):1329–37.

78. Marshman E, Booth C, Potten CS. The intestinal epithelial stem cell. Bioessays 2002;24(1):91–8.

79. Potten CS, Owen G, Booth D. Intestinal stem cells protect their genome by selective segregation of template DNA strands. J Cell Sci 2002;115:2381–8.

80. Barker N et al., Barker N, van Es JH, Kuipers J, et al. Identification of stem cells in small intestine and colon by marker gene Lgr5. Nature 2007.

81. Imai T, Tokunaga A, Yoshida T, et al. The neural RNA-binding protein Musashi1 translationally regulates mammalian numb gene expression by interacting with its mRNA. Mol Cell Biol 2001;21(12):3888–900.

82. Gregorieff A, Pinto D, Begthel H, Destree O, Kielman M, Clevers H. Expression pattern of Wnt signaling components in the adult intestine. Gastroenterology 2005;129:626–38.

83. Tumbar T, Guasch G, Greco V, et al. Defining the epithelial stem cell niche in skin. Science 2004;303:359–63.

84. He XC, Yin T, Grindley JC, et al. PTEN-deficient intestinal stem cells initiate intestinal polyposis. Nature Genet 2007;39(2):189–98.

85. Demidov ON, Timofeev O, Lwin HNY, Kek C, Appella E, Bulavin DV. Wip1 phosphatase regulates p53-dependent apoptosis of stem cells and tumorigenesis in the mouse intestine. Cell Stem Cell 2007;1(2):180–90.

86. Scoville DH, Sato T, He XC, Li L. Current view: intestinal stem cells and signaling. Gastroenterology 2008;134(3):849–64.

87. Brittan M, Wright NA. Gastrointestinal stem cells. J Pathol 2002;197:492–509.

88. Potten CS, Booth C, Tudor GL, et al. Identification of a putative intestinal stem cell and early lineage marker; musashi-1. Differentiation 2003;71:28–41.

89. Asai R, Okano H, Yasugi S. Correlation between Musashi-1 and c-hairy-1 expression and cell proliferation activity in the developing intestine and stomach of both chicken and mouse. Dev Growth Differ 2005;47(8):501–10.

90. Lowry WE, Blanpain C, Nowak JA, Guasch G, Lewis L, Fuchs E. Defining the impact of beta-catenin/Tcf transactivation on epithelial stem cells. Genes Dev 2005;19(13):1596–611.

91. Tian Q, Feetham MC, Tao WA, et al. Proteomic analysis identifies that 14-3-3zeta interacts with beta-catenin and facilitates its activation by Akt. Proc Natl Acad Sci USA 2004;101:15370–5.
92. Taurin S, Sandbo N, Qin Y, Browning D, Dulin NO. Phosphorylation of beta-catenin by cyclic AMP-dependent protein kinase. J Biol Chem 2006;281(15):9971–6.
93. Liaw D, Marsh DJ, Li J, et al. Germline mutations of the PTEN gene in Cowden disease, an inherited breast and thyroid cancer syndrome. Nature Genet 1997;16:64–7.
94. Marsh DJ, Kum JB, Lunetta KL, et al. PTEN mutation spectrum and genotype-phenotype correlations in Bannayan-Riley-Ruvalcaba syndrome suggest a single entity with Cowden syndrome. Hum Mol Genet 1999;8(8):1461–72.
95. Samuels Y, Ericson K. Oncogenic PI3K and its role in cancer. Curr Opin Oncol 2006;18(1):77–82.

6

Transcription Factors in Cancer Stem Cells of the Hematopoietic Lineage

Steffen Koschmieder and Daniel. G Tenen

ABSTRACT

Hematopoietic transcription factors play a crucial role in the proliferation and commitment of hematopoietic stem cells (HSCs) and during the differentiation into their mature progeny. Genetic evidence suggests that perturbance of the function of critical transcription factors can result in increased HSC self-renewal, deregulated proliferation, and a block in differentiation, ultimately leading to acute leukemia. The leukemia-initiating cells have been isolated to near homogeneity, and gene expression arrays of these cells have revealed both similarities and disparities between leukemic stem and progenitor cells and their normal counterparts. Most striking was the finding that the leukemia-initiating cells found in AML can resemble HSCs or committed progenitor cells. These studies have also shown that disruption of the function of single transcription factors can induce acute leukemia in mice. Moreover, dysfunction of these factors has been described in human leukemias, and their functional restoration may lead to the eradication of malignant stem cells.

Key Words: Hematopoietic stem cells, Leukemic stem cells, Tumor stem cells, Acute myeloid leukemia, PU.1, CCAAT enhancer binding protein alpha

LEUKEMIC STEM CELLS

The term "tumor stem cells" has been used as early as 1959 by Manzini to explain the fact that patients relapse after initial remission of their malignant tumor *(1)*. The term "leukemic pluripotent stem cells" was coined by E. A. McCulloch in 1983 *(2)* since leukemia-associated chromosomal aberrations (i.e., G6PDH isoforms or immunoglobulin rearrangements) were present in more than one lineage suggesting that they occurred in an immature cell that gave rise to the various lineages involved *(3, 4)*. Since a stem cell is characterized by its ability to both self-renew and differentiate into mature progenitor cells of various lineages, any experimental system must address these capabilities when assessing tumor stem cells. The first convincing evidence for the presence of tumor stem cells was provided by Bonnet and Dick in 1997 who clearly demonstrated that the leukemia-initiating cells resided in a rare population of CD34+CD38neg cells *(5)*. The CD34+CD38neg population but not the bulk CD34+CD38+ population was able to initiate acute myeloid leukemia- (AML-) like disease upon transplantation into NOD/SCID mice, and the authors showed that these cells possessed the ability to both self-renew and differentiate into CD34+CD38+ cells in the recipient mice *(5)*.

From: *Cancer Drug Discovery and Development: Stem Cells and Cancer,*
Edited by: R.G. Bagley and B.A. Teicher, DOI: 10.1007/978-1-60327-933-8_6,
© Humana Press, a part of Springer Science + Business Media, LLC 2009

It should be noted that using the term "stem cell" (i.e., cancer stem cell, tumor stem cell, or leukemic stem cell) for malignancy-initiating or -maintaining cells may suggest that these malignant cells are similar to their normal counterparts. However, there are several reasons why the term "stem cell" may not reflect the biology of malignancy: first, the biology of cells that cause or maintain tumors has not been rigorously defined to date for most tumors (i.e., their ability to initiate and/or maintain tumors in vivo is not known). Second, they comprise a heterogeneous population of cells. Third, many differences have already been described between normal and so-called malignant stem cells. And finally, the frequency and biology of these cells varies from one tumor entity to the other, prohibiting a generalization of the term tumor stem cells. However, until more information is gathered about the nature of tumor-initiating and tumor-maintaining cells and since the hematopoietic system may indeed be a good example for a close relation between normal and malignant stem cells, we will adopt the term "leukemic stem cells" in the present review when discussing leukemia-initiating cells.

ROLE OF TRANSCRIPTION FACTORS IN NORMAL HEMATOPOIESIS

Hematopoietic development and maintenance of the hematopoietic cell system in the adult organism depends on a tightly regulated interplay between external factors (i.e., growth factors) and cell-intrinsic factors, such as transcription factors. The cells maintaining active human hematopoiesis migrate during embryonic development from the yolk sac to a region in the dorsal aorta (AGM region), then to liver and spleen, until reaching the final destination within the bone marrow. During these phases, hematopoietic stem and progenitor cells proliferate and differentiate, giving rise to their mature progeny. In the adult, the bone marrow is the major site of hematopoietic cell production except for cells of the T cell lineage which are produced in the thymus. Hematopoietic transcription factors play a major role in the governing of all of the above-mentioned processes, and targeted disruption of the genes encoding these factors in mice has elucidated the unique functions of each of these factors, including AML1 (6), CCAAT/enhancer-binding protein alpha (CEBPA) (7), PU.1 (8), GATA-1 (9), and SCL (10, 11). Through their DNA binding and transactivating properties, these transcription factors regulate the expression of an array of hematopoietic genes such as growth factor receptor genes, thus enhancing or limiting the commitment of cells toward a certain hematopoietic lineage.

A hierarchy of hematopoietic transcription factors exists where certain factors act earlier during development and others come into play at later stages. SCL acts during the speciation of the earliest hematopoietic cell elements before the separation of hematopoietic and endothelial precursors, and abrogation of SCL in knockout mice leads to embryonic lethality via anemia and complete lack of both yolk sac hematopoiesis and angiogenesis (10, 11). AML1 knockout mice display complete absence of definitive hematopoiesis but not of blood vessel development (6), suggesting that AML1 primarily acts on cells which are already committed to the hematopoietic lineage. Moreover, there are SCL binding motifs in the AML1 gene promoter, and SCL knockout mice display strong downregulation of AML1 expression (12), placing AML1 downstream of SCL during development. PU.1 expression is regulated by AML1 (13), and disruption of the PU.1 gene results in hematopoietic stem cell (HSC) defects that disrupt their differentiation into B cells and myeloid cells (8). Finally, the CEBP transcription factor family of genes regulates the commitment and maturation of myeloid cells without affecting the other cell lineages. Interestingly, even the CEBP members work through a hierarchy: while in the absence of CEBPA, no mature granulocytes are produced (7), granulocytes do form in the absence of the downstream factor, CEBP epsilon (CEBPE), but they show severe functional defects, mainly through altered production of secondary granule proteins (14, 15). This list is a (simplified) example for the close interaction between hematopoietic transcription factors, and many other factors have been shown to play important roles to warrant proper development and maintenance of the hematopoietic system in the vertebrate organism.

EFFECTS OF TRANSCRIPTION FACTORS IN NORMAL HEMATOPOIETIC STEM CELLS

The function of HSCs is subject to stringent regulation by hematopoietic transcription factors. However, several reports have indicated that requirements for individual factors may be different between HSCs in the developing embryo and the adult organism. While SCL and AML1, as well as members of the Hox family, have been demonstrated to be indispensable for the specification of fetal liver HSC *(6, 10, 11)*, SCL and AML1 appear less critical for the maintenance of HSC in the adult organism *(16, 17)*. Conversely, the Polycomb gene Bmi-1 was shown to be redundant in fetal liver HSCs but proved to be essential for HSC self-renewal in the adult organism *(18, 19)*.

In addition, transcription factors, which primarily act as lineage-restricted transcription factors, such as CEBPA and PU.1, have been described to also act on the HSC level. CEBPA knockout mice display a differentiation block at the CMP/GMP transition *(20)*, which results in a complete lack of granulocytes *(7)*. However, CEBPA knockout mice also show increased HSC self-renewal and competitive repopulation activity as compared to wild-type cells, and this was associated with increased expression of Bmi-1 *(20)*. These results suggest that CEBPA, which is expressed at low levels in HSCs, suppresses HSC self-renewal during normal hematopoiesis.

PU.1 expression is also low in HSCs and increases significantly during monocytic differentiation *(21)*. Since PU.1 knockout mice die perinatally, conditional PU.1 knockout mice were generated. These mice display reduced HSC maintenance after PU.1 had been excised *(22)*, leading to regeneration of the bone marrow by wild-type HSCs (PU.1 excision was not complete). PU.1-deficient HSCs also failed to generate myeloid and lymphoid progenitors and harbored a maturation arrest at the GMP stage of differentiation *(22)*. Conditional knockout mice showed that neither CEBPA nor PU.1 was required in more mature myeloid or lymphoid cells, once the HSC to CLP or CMP/GMP stages were bypassed *(22)*. These findings even further underscore the hierarchical organization of the hematopoietic system and show that fine tuning of both the timing and concentration of the expression of each transcription factor are crucial for their proper function.

ROLE OF TRANSCRIPTION FACTORS IN HUMAN LEUKEMIA

AML can be regarded as a model disease for tumor stem cell biology *(5)*. After significant therapeutic progress has been made in the eradication of AML blasts with up to 80% of all patients achieving complete morphologic remission, the major problem of AML treatment now lies in the high relapse rate, resulting in poor long-term disease-free survival. Cytogenetic analysis has shown that leukemia in most cases recurs from malignant cell clones that are initially present in the bone marrow of the patients. Thus, current concepts aim at defining and eradicating the leukemia-initiating and -maintaining malignant stem cell populations to reduce the incidence of relapses.

The most frequent molecular aberrations found in AML are chromosomal translocations involving transcription factor genes, such as AML1-ETO (t8;21), CBFB-SMMHC (inv16), and PML-RARA (t15;17). However, closer study of the cytogenetically normal AML cases revealed abnormalities in the expression and/or function of hematopoietic transcription factors. In depth analysis of these factors was performed using transgenic mice, and these experiments clearly demonstrated that perturbations of single transcription factors can result in aberrant differentiation of HSCs and can ultimately lead to overt acute leukemia. Examples include PU.1 and CEBPA as well as translocation products such as MOZ-TIF2 and MLL-AF9. The following sections will briefly describe the phenotypes obtained by manipulation of these transcription factor circuits.

PU.1 DEREGULATION TRANSFORMS HEMATOPOIETIC STEM CELLS

PU.1 is expressed at low levels in hematopoietic stem and progenitor cells, and its expression increases during B cell differentiation and during myeloid differentiation toward granulocyte-macrophage progenitor cells (GMPs) and macrophages. PU.1 knockout mice die soon after birth, displaying a lack of B-lymphoid and mature myeloid cells *(8)*. Conditional PU.1 knockout mice display a defect of HSC repopulating activity and perturbed maturation of CMPs and CLPs *(22)*.

To better understand the regulation of this important transcription factor gene, transgenic mice were generated using the PU.1 promoter to drive GFP expression. However, these mice did not express GFP suggesting that additional gene-regulatory elements are required for proper PU.1 expression. Therefore, P1 artificial chromosome (PAC-) transgenic mice were established carrying a 91-kb DNA fragment surrounding the PU.1 gene *(23)*. Expression of the reporter gene (Thy1.1) in these mice mimicked the expression of PU.1 and its cell-specific expression pattern. DNAse hypersensitive site analysis was performed to identify genomic regions critical for PU.1 gene regulation, and this analysis revealed, among other sites, a 3.5-kb region located 14 kb upstream of the PU.1 transcriptional start site. This site showed DNAse hypersensitivity in myeloid cells but not in T cells, reflecting high PU.1 expression in myeloid but no expression in T cells *(23)*. When this 3.5-kb element was added to the promoter and transgenic mice were produced, these mice expressed PU.1 in a similar fashion as wild-type mice *(24)*. These results confirm that PU.1 expression is regulated via both the promoter and a distal upstream regulatory element (termed "URE") recapitulating the in vivo regulation of the PU.1 gene.

Interestingly, targeted disruption of this 3.5-kb URE in mice produced intriguing results *(25)*: these knockout mice did not show complete abrogation of PU.1 expression, but PU.1 expression was rather downregulated to approximately 20% of control levels (PU.1 hypomorphic mice). These mice showed decreased B cell and macrophage numbers while the number of granulocytic cells was unaltered. However, in addition, PU.1 hypomorphic mice developed AML-like disease with 100% penetrance. Preleukemic myeloid progenitor cells were increased in numbers and displayed an abnormal surface immunophenotype. Moreover, these cells showed disrupted M-CSF and GM-CSF receptor expression but retained G-CSF signaling. Cytogenetic analysis of the leukemic blasts revealed frequent cytogenetic abnormalities with a high proportion of chromosome 15 trisomies. The murine c-myc gene is located on chromosome 15, and it is intriguing to speculate that c-myc overexpression ultimately transformed these PU.1 hypomorphic preleukemic cells to become leukemic stem cells. The leukemia was transferable upon transplantation of leukemic cells into NOD/SCID mice *(25)*. To answer the question which cell population confers the leukemia, FACS-sorted HSCs from leukemic PU.1 hypomorphic mice were transplanted into NOD-SCID recipients. The recipient mice developed AML-like disease after 9–12 weeks, suggesting that leukemic stem cells resided in the HSC compartment in PU.1 knockdown-induced AML *(26)*. In an attempt to identify early transforming events, HSCs from preleukemic mice were FACS-sorted and subjected to microarray expression analysis. This analysis revealed strong downregulation of two related transcription factors, c-jun and JunB, and, interestingly, together with PU.1, these factors were downregulated in a major proportion of human AML cases. In order to study the functional relevance of these aberrations, each of these genes was reintroduced into PU.1 hypomorphic cells. Intriguingly, retroviral restoration of PU.1 and c-jun expression was able to rescue myeloid differentiation of murine AML blasts. Moreover, lentiviral restoration of junB (but not c-jun) of preleukemic murine HSCs antagonized malignant cell growth and abrogated development of leukemia in transplanted NOD-SCID mice. These results clearly demonstrate that disruption of a single critical transcription factor (PU.1) can render HSCs susceptible to acquire additional transforming events and become true leukemic stem cells. Furthermore, these results suggest that a certain degree of reduction, rather than a complete loss, of a lineage-indispensable transcription factor can induce AML.

In addition to AML-like disease, a proportion of PU.1 hypomorphic mice developed aggressive T cell lymphomas (27). When mice were analyzed before the onset of T cell lymphomas, early T cell progenitors were increased in numbers and were found to harbor increased levels of PU.1, while the differentiation into more mature T cell precursors was inhibited. In contrast to this PU.1 overexpression in T cell progenitors, lymphoma cells harbored low PU.1 levels, and enforced retroviral PU.1 expression in these lymphoma cells reduced their growth (27). These data suggest that PU.1 downregulation is crucial for proper T cell development but is dispensable for T cell lymphomagenesis. The lymphomas were transplantable into NOD/SCID mice. Genome-wide screening for aberrant methylation patterns of these malignant cells revealed methylation of tumor suppressor genes such as Id4 in the lymphomas, and overexpression of Id4 in the T cell lymphoma cells inhibited their growth in vivo (27). Together, these results show that downmodulation of PU.1 may be a critical initial step to render T cell progenitors susceptible for malignant transformation into tumor stem cells. Complete transformation does not rely on PU.1 overexpression but rather involves methylation of critical tumor suppressor genes.

In humans, mutations of the PU.1 gene have been described in 7% of patients with AML (28). These mutations largely result in decreased synergistic activity of PU.1 with interacting proteins such as c-jun or AML1 on target promoters. Other studies found either no PU.1 mutations or a lower frequency of these mutations in AML, but the reason for this discrepancy is not known at present. However, PU.1 expression and/or function is decreased by several oncogenic proteins involved in AML pathogenesis, such as FLT3-ITD (29), and PML-RARA (30). In addition to PU.1 gene mutations, a polymorphism in the human counterpart of the PU.1 URE which was discussed above was found more frequently in patients with complex-karyotype AML (31). This polymorphism resulted in decreased binding of the chromatin remodeling protein SATB1 to the PU.1 URE and suppressed PU.1 expression in human leukemic HSCs and GMPs (31). Together, these data imply PU.1 as a major regulator of hematopoietic differentiation and as an important tumor suppressor in leukemic stem cells.

CEBPA

CCAAT enhancer binding protein alpha (CEBPA) belongs to the leucine zipper family of transcription factors and interacts with other members of this family (i.e., CEBPB, CEBPE) to form heterodimers and transactivate its target genes, such as the G-CSF receptor promoter. CEBPA was shown to be essential for proper granulocytic development (7). Since one of the hallmarks of human AML is a block in granulocytic differentiation, alterations of CEBPA expression and/or function were studied. Indeed, CEBPA gene mutations were found in AML (32), particularly in the large subgroup of cytogenetically normal AML cases, and these results have been confirmed by others (33–42). Seven percent of all patients with AML and 15% of cytogenetically normal AML cases harbored somatic CEBPA mutations. In addition, several cases of familial AML were described and found to harbor germline CEBPA mutations (39, 43). Interestingly, in the majority of cases, biallelic so-called C- and N-terminal mutations were found in the same patient, with the C-terminal mutation completely disrupting DNA binding and the N-terminal mutation abolishing the translation of the full-length p42 isoform but retaining the p30 isoform of the protein (32). p30 is generated from an internal AUG codon on the

CEBPA mRNA and was subsequently shown to inhibit the function of p42. Thus, CEBPA mutant cases display a strong reduction in active CEBPA protein in the AML blasts.

Whether CEBPA mutations or lack of the p42 CEBPA protein isoform are sufficient to transform HSCs and cause AML is not entirely clear at present. However, recently, p30 knockin mice have been generated to address these questions *(44)*.

Heterozygous CEBPA$^{p30/p42}$ mice develop normally without any evidence of hematopoietic defects or leukemia. Conversely, CEBPA$^{p30/p30}$ homozygous knockin mice show significant phenotypic alterations: the Mendelian ratio of this genotype is lower than expected due to significant perinatal lethality which was most likely caused by perinatal hypoglycemia, similar to what has been described for CEBPA$^{-/-}$ mice *(45)*. However, differently from CEBPA$^{-/-}$ mice, a fraction of CEBPA$^{p30/p30}$ mice survived (4/89 mice). These mice developed lethal AML-like disease between 9 and 14 months with anemia and an increase of myeloid blasts (Mac-1$^+$Gr-1^{lo} by FACS) in the bone marrow as well as myeloid infiltration of the spleen and the liver. Interestingly, hematopoietic abnormalities were already detectable at 2 months of age and progressed over 6–14 months, ultimately resulting in overt leukemia. These phases included neutropenia in young mice (<2 months), granulocyte hyperproliferation (2–6 months), and increase of c-kit$^+$ granulocytic precursor cells (>6 months). FACS analysis of the bone marrow showed that normal HSC, CMP, GMP, and MEP populations were strongly suppressed and replaced by the leukemic population. The leukemic cells showed increased BrdU labeling suggestive of increased cycling. Further analysis of these cells in vitro revealed that they possessed increased self-renewal capacity in serial replating clonogenic assays and that they continued to produce Mac-1$^+$c-kit$^+$ cells in long-term cultures. Similarly to CEBPA mutant AML cases, karyotypic abnormalities were not observed in the leukemic cells.

The disease proved to be transplantable, and recipient mice died of leukemia 9–18 weeks post-transplant. In order to identify the leukemia-initiating cell population, either FACS-purified HSC or progenitors (CMP, GMP, MEP), or Mac-1$^+$c-kit$^+$ committed progenitors or Mac-1$^+$c-kit$^{lo/-}$ mature myeloid cells were transplanted (2,000 cells each) into irradiated recipients, using 250,000 cells as wild-type competitors. Intriguingly, engraftment of CEBPA$^{p30/p30}$ cells was only detected when committed progenitors were used as donor cells and was restricted to the myeloid lineage, while engraftment of CEBPA$^{p30/p42}$ cells was restricted to HSC donor cells conferring multilineage engraftment. Mice receiving CEBPA$^{p30/p30}$ cells developed AML, and this leukemia was again transplantable into secondary recipients, using Mac-1$^+$c-kit$^+$ cells as a source. Interestingly, gene expression profiling of the leukemic cells revealed similarities between this mouse model and a retroviral mouse model of MLL-AF9-induced AML-like disease, with a significant fraction of the upregulated genes being involved in cellular self-renewal programs. These results clearly define phenotypically committed progenitor cells that have aberrantly acquired self-renewal capacities as the leukemia-initiating population in this model, and the authors go on to speculate that the type of leukaemia-initiating cell (progenitor-like vs. HSC-like such as shown for the PU.1 hypomorphic mouse model discussed above) may determine the long-term prognosis of the leukemia.

In addition to CEBPA gene mutations, other mechanisms leading to disruption of CEBPA expression or function have been described in AML and other acute leukemias: CEBPA was shown to be aberrantly overexpressed in B-Precursor-ALL and function as an oncogene in these cells *(46, 47)*. In addition, CEBPA expression was found to be suppressed in AML either by promoter methylation or by transcriptional repression. Gene silencing of the CEBPA gene promoter by hypermethylation was found in approximately 30% of AML patients *(48)*. In other cases, granulocytic differentiation was disrupted by suppression of CEBPA transcription by the oncogenic fusion protein AML1-ETO resulting from a t(8;21) chromosomal translocation *(32)*. A third mechanism of CEBPA alteration was found to involve inhibition of proper CEBPA protein translation by increased RNA binding proteins and was described in AML *(49, 50)* and CML blast crisis *(51)*.

The above-mentioned results illustrate the numerous mechanisms of how AML cells may acquire a block of CEBPA-induced cell cycle arrest and differentiation. Similar mechanisms have been found in other malignancies including several solid tumors, such as lung cancer *(52, 53)* and hepatocellular carcinoma *(54, 55)*. However, leukemia-initiating cell populations have not yet been defined for most of these diseases.

OTHER TRANSCRIPTION FACTORS

Several other transcription factors have been implicated in the transformation of hematopoietic cells, leading to AML-like disease in the mouse. Several of these models have been interrogated for the presence and nature of leukemic stem cells.

The model of leukemias arising from self-renewing committed progenitors has been substantiated by several retroviral mouse models. Mice transplanted with MLL-ENL transduced bone marrow were found to develop AML-like disease *(56)*, and the authors showed that transduction of HSCs or committed progenitor cells (GMPs) was equally efficient to generate the leukemia, demonstrating self-renewal capacities in leukemic committed progenitors. Similar results have been obtained using MLL-AF9 *(57)* and MOZ-TIF2 *(58)*, while the BCR-ABL oncogene was able to transform HSCs but not progenitors *(58)*. Biphenotypic acute leukemia in addition to AML and ALL was described in mice transplanted with MLL-GAS7 transduced bone marrow cells *(59)*, and the leukemia-initiating cells were found to co-express myeloid (Mac-1) and lymphoid (B220) markers. Biphenotypic leukemia-initiating cells can also lead to pure myeloid leukemias, as shown in mice transplanted with CALM-AF10 transduced bone marrow *(60)*. These mice develop AML-like disease. However, only HSCs aberrantly expressing the lymphoid marker B220 were capable of efficiently transferring the leukemia. Intriguingly, these cells were found to have undergone immunoglobulin rearrangements, suggesting that they were derived from transformed committed B cells or B cell precursors *(60)*. In line with these results, the lymphoid transcription factor Pax5 was found to be strongly downregulated in the leukemia-initiating cells, and Pax5 knockout cells have been described earlier to possess myeloid differentiation potential *(61)*.

Other transcription factors involved in transforming HSCs or committed progenitors to generate acute leukemia include junB *(62)*, SALL4 *(63)*, ß-catenin *(64, 65)*, c-myc *(66)*, and many others.

In summary, these data show that hematopoietic transcription factors play a major role in the maintenance, self-renewal, and differentiation of HSCs. In addition, in vivo studies have defined critical mechanisms for transformation of HSCs or progenitors to become leukemia-initiating cells, and the understanding of these mechanisms has helped elucidate mechanisms of stem cell transformation in other cancers.

REFERENCES

1. Makino S. The role of tumor stem-cells in regrowth of the tumor following drastic applications. Acta Unio Int Contra Cancrum 1959;15(Suppl 1):196–8.
2. McCulloch EA. Stem cells in normal and leukemic hemopoiesis (Henry Stratton Lecture, 1982). Blood 1983;62(1):1–13.
3. Fialkow PJ, Gartler SM, Yoshida A. Clonal origin of chronic myelocytic leukemia in man. Proc Natl Acad Sci USA 1967;58(4):1468–71.
4. Arnold A, Cossman J, Bakhshi A, Jaffe ES, Waldmann TA, Korsmeyer SJ. Immunoglobulin-gene rearrangements as unique clonal markers in human lymphoid neoplasms. N Engl J Med 1983;309(26):1593–9.
5. Bonnet D, Dick JE. Human acute myeloid leukemia is organized as a hierarchy that originates from a primitive hematopoietic cell. Nat Med 1997;3(7):730–7.
6. Okuda T, van Deursen J, Hiebert SW, Grosveld G, Downing JR. AML1, the target of multiple chromosomal translocations in human leukemia, is essential for normal fetal liver hematopoiesis. Cell 1996;84(2):321–30.
7. Zhang DE, Zhang P, Wang ND, Hetherington CJ, Darlington GJ, Tenen DG. Absence of granulocyte colony-stimulating factor signaling and neutrophil development in CCAAT enhancer binding protein alpha-deficient mice. Proc Natl Acad Sci USA 1997;94(2):569–74.

8. Scott EW, Simon MC, Anastasi J, Singh H. Requirement of transcription factor PU.1 in the development of multiple hematopoietic lineages. Science 1994;265(5178):1573–7.

9. Pevny L, Simon MC, Robertson E, et al. Erythroid differentiation in chimaeric mice blocked by a targeted mutation in the gene for transcription factor GATA-1. Nature 1991;349(6306):257–60.

10. Robb L, Lyons I, Li R, et al. Absence of yolk sac hematopoiesis from mice with a targeted disruption of the scl gene. Proc Natl Acad Sci USA 1995;92(15):7075–9.

11. Shivdasani RA, Mayer EL, Orkin SH. Absence of blood formation in mice lacking the T-cell leukaemia oncoprotein tal-1/SCL. Nature 1995;373(6513):432–4.

12. Landry JR, Kinston S, Knezevic K, et al. Runx genes are direct targets of Scl/Tal1 in the yolk sac and fetal liver. Blood 2008;111(6):3005–14.

13. Huang G, Zhang P, Hirai H, et al. PU.1 is a major downstream target of AML1 (RUNX1) in adult mouse hematopoiesis. Nat Genet 2008;40(1):51–60.

14. Yamanaka R, Kim GD, Radomska HS, et al. CCAAT/enhancer binding protein epsilon is preferentially up-regulated during granulocytic differentiation and its functional versatility is determined by alternative use of promoters and differential splicing. Proc Natl Acad Sci USA 1997;94(12):6462–7.

15. Lekstrom-Himes J, Xanthopoulos KG. CCAAT/enhancer binding protein epsilon is critical for effective neutrophil-mediated response to inflammatory challenge. Blood 1999;93(9):3096–105.

16. Mikkola HK, Klintman J, Yang H, et al. Haematopoietic stem cells retain long-term repopulating activity and multipotency in the absence of stem-cell leukaemia SCL/tal-1 gene. Nature 2003;421(6922):547–51.

17. Ichikawa M, Asai T, Saito T, et al. AML-1 is required for megakaryocytic maturation and lymphocytic differentiation, but not for maintenance of hematopoietic stem cells in adult hematopoiesis. Nat Med 2004;10(3):299–304.

18. Lessard J, Sauvageau G. Bmi-1 determines the proliferative capacity of normal and leukaemic stem cells. Nature 2003;423(6937):255–60.

19. Park IK, Qian D, Kiel M, et al. Bmi-1 is required for maintenance of adult self-renewing haematopoietic stem cells. Nature 2003;423(6937):302–5.

20. Zhang P, Iwasaki-Arai J, Iwasaki H, et al. Enhancement of hematopoietic stem cell repopulating capacity and self-renewal in the absence of the transcription factor C/EBP alpha. Immunity 2004;21(6):853–63.

21. Akashi K, Traver D, Miyamoto T, Weissman IL. A clonogenic common myeloid progenitor that gives rise to all myeloid lineages. Nature 2000;404(6774):193–7.

22. Iwasaki H, Somoza C, Shigematsu H, et al. Distinctive and indispensable roles of PU.1 in maintenance of hematopoietic stem cells and their differentiation. Blood 2005;106(5):1590–600.

23. Li Y, Okuno Y, Zhang P, et al. Regulation of the PU.1 gene by distal elements. Blood 2001;98(10):2958–65.

24. Okuno Y, Huang G, Rosenbauer F, et al. Potential autoregulation of transcription factor PU.1 by an upstream regulatory element. Mol Cell Biol 2005;25(7):2832–45.

25. Rosenbauer F, Wagner K, Kutok JL, et al. Acute myeloid leukemia induced by graded reduction of a lineage-specific transcription factor, PU.1. Nat Genet 2004;36(6):624–30.

26. Steidl U, Rosenbauer F, Verhaak RG, et al. Essential role of Jun family transcription factors in PU.1 knockdown-induced leukemic stem cells. Nat Genet 2006;38(11):1269–77.

27. Rosenbauer F, Owens BM, Yu L, et al. Lymphoid cell growth and transformation are suppressed by a key regulatory element of the gene encoding PU.1. Nat Genet 2006;38(1):27–37.

28. Mueller BU, Pabst T, Osato M, et al. Heterozygous PU.1 mutations are associated with acute myeloid leukemia. Blood 2003;101(5):2074.

29. Zheng R, Friedman AD, Levis M, Li L, Weir EG, Small D. Internal tandem duplication mutation of FLT3 blocks myeloid differentiation through suppression of C/EBPalpha expression. Blood 2004;103(5):1883–90.

30. Mueller BU, Pabst T, Fos J, et al. ATRA resolves the differentiation block in t(15;17) acute myeloid leukemia by restoring PU.1 expression. Blood 2006;107(8):3330–8.

31. Steidl U, Steidl C, Ebralidze A, et al. A distal single nucleotide polymorphism alters long-range regulation of the PU.1 gene in acute myeloid leukemia. J Clin Invest 2007;117(9):2611–20.

32. Pabst T, Mueller BU, Zhang P, et al. Dominant-negative mutations of CEBPA, encoding CCAAT/enhancer binding protein-alpha (C/EBPalpha), in acute myeloid leukemia. Nat Genet 2001;27(3):263–70.

33. Preudhomme C, Sagot C, Boissel N, et al. Favorable prognostic significance of CEBPA mutations in patients with de novo acute myeloid leukemia: a study from the Acute Leukemia French Association (ALFA). Blood 2002;100(8):2717–23.

34. Gombart AF, Hofmann WK, Kawano S, et al. Mutations in the gene encoding the transcription factor CCAAT/enhancer binding protein alpha in myelodysplastic syndromes and acute myeloid leukemias. Blood 2002;99(4):1332–40.

35. Snaddon J, Smith ML, Neat M, et al. Mutations of CEBPA in acute myeloid leukemia FAB types M1 and M2. Genes Chromosomes Cancer 2003;37(1):72–8.

36. Barjesteh van Waalwijk van Doorn-Khosrovani S, Erpelinck C, Meijer J, et al. Biallelic mutations in the CEBPA gene and low CEBPA expression levels as prognostic markers in intermediate-risk AML. Hematol J 2003;4(1):31–40.

37. Frohling S, Schlenk RF, Stolze I, et al. CEBPA mutations in younger adults with acute myeloid leukemia and normal cytogenetics: prognostic relevance and analysis of cooperating mutations. J Clin Oncol 2004;22(4):624–33.

38. Frohling S, Schlenk RF, Krauter J, et al. Acute myeloid leukemia with deletion 9q within a noncomplex karyotype is associated with CEBPA loss-of-function mutations. Genes Chromosomes Cancer 2005;42(4):427–32.

39. Smith ML, Cavenagh JD, Lister TA, Fitzgibbon J. Mutation of CEBPA in familial acute myeloid leukemia. N Engl J Med 2004;351(23):2403–7.
40. Bienz M, Ludwig M, Leibundgut EO, et al. Risk assessment in patients with acute myeloid leukemia and a normal karyotype. Clin Cancer Res 2005;11(4):1416–24.
41. Shih LY, Huang CF, Lin TL, et al. Heterogeneous patterns of CEBPalpha mutation status in the progression of myelodysplastic syndrome and chronic myelomonocytic leukemia to acute myelogenous leukemia. Clin Cancer Res 2005;11(5):1821–6.
42. Lin LI, Chen CY, Lin DT, et al. Characterization of CEBPA mutations in acute myeloid leukemia: most patients with CEBPA mutations have biallelic mutations and show a distinct immunophenotype of the leukemic cells. Clin Cancer Res 2005;11(4):1372–9.
43. Sellick GS, Spendlove HE, Catovsky D, Pritchard-Jones K, Houlston RS. Further evidence that germline CEBPA mutations cause dominant inheritance of acute myeloid leukaemia. Leukemia 2005;19(7):1276–8.
44. Kirstetter P, Schuster MB, Bereshchenko O, Moore S, Dvinge H, Kurz E, Theilgaard-Mönch K, Månsson R, Pedersen TA, Pabst T, Schrock E, Porse BT, Jacobsen SE, Bertone P, Tenen DG, Nerlov C. Modeling of C/EBPalpha mutant acute myeloid leukemia reveals a common expression signature of committed myeloid leukemia-initiating cells. Cancer Cell 2008;13(4): 299–310.
45. Wang ND, Finegold MJ, Bradley A, et al. Impaired energy homeostasis in C/EBPalpha knockout mice. Science 1995;269(5227):1108–12.
46. Chapiro E, Russell L, Radford-Weiss I, et al. Overexpression of CEBPA resulting from the translocation t(14;19)(q32;q13) of human precursor B acute lymphoblastic leukemia. Blood 2006;108(10):3560–3.
47. Akasaka T, Balasas T, Russell LJ, et al. Five members of the CEBP transcription factor family are targeted by recurrent IGH translocations in B-cell precursor acute lymphoblastic leukemia (BCP-ALL). Blood 2007;109(8):3451–61.
48. Lin TC, Lee CY, Tien HF, Hu CY, Tang JL, Lin LI. Tumor Suppressor activity of CCAAT/enhancer binding protein Alpha is epigenetically down-regulated in acute myeloid leukemia. Blood 2007;110(11):2113A.
49. Helbling D, Mueller BU, Timchenko NA, et al. The leukemic fusion gene AML1-MDS1-EVI1 suppresses CEBPA in acute myeloid leukemia by activation of Calreticulin. Proc Natl Acad Sci USA 2004;101(36):13312–7.
50. Helbling D, Mueller BU, Timchenko NA, et al. CBFB-SMMHC is correlated with increased calreticulin expression and suppresses the granulocytic differentiation factor CEBPA in AML with inv(16). Blood 2005;106(4):1369–75.
51. Perrotti D, Cesi V, Trotta R, et al. BCR-ABL suppresses C/EBPalpha expression through inhibitory action of hnRNP E2. Nat Genet 2002;30(1):48–58.
52. Halmos B, Huettner CS, Kocher O, Ferenczi K, Karp DD, Tenen DG. Down-regulation and antiproliferative role of C/EBPalpha in lung cancer. Cancer Res 2002;62(2):528–34.
53. Costa DB, Li S, Kocher O, et al. Immunohistochemical analysis of C/EBPalpha in non-small cell lung cancer reveals frequent down-regulation in stage II and IIIA tumors: a correlative study of E3590. Lung Cancer 2007;56(1):97–103.
54. Birkenmeier EH, Gwynn B, Howard S, et al. Tissue-specific expression, developmental regulation, and genetic mapping of the gene encoding CCAAT/enhancer binding protein. Genes Dev 1989;3(8):1146–56.
55. Tan EH, Hooi SC, Laban M, et al. CCAAT/enhancer binding protein alpha knock-in mice exhibit early liver glycogen storage and reduced susceptibility to hepatocellular carcinoma. Cancer Res 2005;65(22):10330–7.
56. Cozzio A, Passegue E, Ayton PM, Karsunky H, Cleary ML, Weissman IL. Similar MLL-associated leukemias arising from self-renewing stem cells and short-lived myeloid progenitors. Genes Dev 2003;17(24):3029–35.
57. Krivtsov AV, Twomey D, Feng Z, et al. Transformation from committed progenitor to leukaemia stem cell initiated by MLL-AF9. Nature 2006;442(7104):818–22.
58. Huntly BJ, Shigematsu H, Deguchi K, et al. MOZ-TIF2, but not BCR-ABL, confers properties of leukemic stem cells to committed murine hematopoietic progenitors. Cancer Cell 2004;6(6):587–96.
59. So CW, Karsunky H, Passegue E, Cozzio A, Weissman IL, Cleary ML. MLL-GAS7 transforms multipotent hematopoietic progenitors and induces mixed lineage leukemias in mice. Cancer Cell 2003;3(2):161–71.
60. Deshpande AJ, Cusan M, Rawat VP, et al. Acute myeloid leukemia is propagated by a leukemic stem cell with lymphoid characteristics in a mouse model of CALM/AF10-positive leukemia. Cancer Cell 2006;10(5):363–74.
61. Nutt SL, Heavey B, Rolink AG, Busslinger M. Commitment to the B-lymphoid lineage depends on the transcription factor Pax5. Nature 1999;401(6753):556–62.
62. Passegue E, Wagner EF, Weissman IL. JunB deficiency leads to a myeloproliferative disorder arising from hematopoietic stem cells. Cell 2004;119(3):431–43.
63. Ma Y, Cui W, Yang J, et al. SALL4, a novel oncogene, is constitutively expressed in human acute myeloid leukemia (AML) and induces AML in transgenic mice. Blood 2006;108(8):2726–35.
64. Jamieson CH, Ailles LE, Dylla SJ, et al. Granulocyte-macrophage progenitors as candidate leukemic stem cells in blast-crisis CML. N Engl J Med 2004;351(7):657–67.
65. Zhao C, Blum J, Chen A, et al. Loss of beta-catenin impairs the renewal of normal and CML stem cells in vivo. Cancer Cell 2007;12(6):528–41.
66. Felsher DW, Bishop JM. Reversible tumorigenesis by MYC in hematopoietic lineages. Mol Cell 1999;4(2):199–207.

7

Stem Cell Chromatin Patterns and DNA Hypermethylation

Joyce E. Ohm and Stephen B. Baylin

ABSTRACT

Normal development requires carefully orchestrated cellular remodeling on both a global and gene-specific/tissue-specific level. Heritable changes in gene expression that occur independently of alterations in the primary DNA sequence are deemed "epigenetic," and are largely characterized by a tightly regulated program of active and repressive histone modifications. In this chapter, we will discuss the histone modifications that help modulate gene expression during development, as well as the normal stem/progenitor cell epigenetic remodeling proteins, including polycomb group (PcG) proteins, which control these modifications. Intriguingly, the methylation of CpG dinucleotides in DNA also plays a critical role during both normal and malignant epigenetic reprogramming. DNA methylation is a critical mediator of both X-chromosome inactivation and paternal and maternal imprinting, the variable regulation of tissue/cell specific activation of genes required for successful differentiation of alternate cell lineages, and the permanent silencing of genes required for stem/progenitor cell maintenance and pluripotency. Aberrant DNA methylation is a key component of the malignant epigenetic programs that are pervasive in all types of cancer and are thought to contribute to tumor initiation and progression. The clustering of silenced genes within single cell pathways and the remarkable frequency with which epigenetically silenced genes are being identified within any given cancer type begs the question of whether gene silencing is a series of random events resulting in an enhanced survival of a premalignant clone, or whether silencing is the result of a directed, instructive program for silencing initiation reflective of the cells of origin for tumors. We hypothesize that a combination of both chromatin and DNA regulatory networks controlling stem cell epigenetics may go awry in cells that give rise to tumors and during tumor progression. In this regard, the current chapter stresses the hypothesis that the malignant epigenetic program is linked, at least for silencing of some cancer genes, to the epigenetic control of stem/precursor cell gene expression patterns.

Key Words: Stem cells, Epigenetics, Chromatin, DNA methylation, Polycomb, Cancer

THE EPIGENETIC TOOL BOX

Epigenetics is the study of heritable changes in gene expression that occur independently of alterations in the primary DNA sequence. Gene expression changes occurring during development are, by their nature, epigenetic. Assuming that within an individual the genetic code is faithfully replicated and remains uniform from cell to cell, then epigenetics is left to orchestrate the activation and inactivation, or lack of activation, of genes required for successful development of alternate cell lineages during

From: *Cancer Drug Discovery and Development: Stem Cells and Cancer,*
Edited by: R.G. Bagley and B.A. Teicher, DOI: 10.1007/978-1-60327-933-8_7,
© Humana Press, a part of Springer Science + Business Media, LLC 2009

development. The precision required for the generation, from a single fertilized egg, of upwards of ten trillion cells in a human body, which are capable of representing all of the various biology and functional components of differentiated organs, requires a masterfully coordinated, multifaceted program.

An understanding of the complexity of epigenetic regulation and the role these networks play in normal stem/progenitor cell differentiation must begin with an understanding of the tools that a cell uses to control the chromatin structure and how DNA is packaged for function - this packaging constitutes the groundwork of epigenetics. Within a cell, DNA is packaged into chromatin by wrapping 147 bp of DNA around nucleosome complexes. These complexes are composed of four different histone proteins: H2A, H2B, H3, and H4 (Fig. 1a), each arranged in pairs to form a histone octamer. The DNA that surrounds this complex is called the nucleosome, and is the fundamental unit of chromatin and plays a key role in gene expression *(1, 2)*. Chromatin can be divided into two main subtypes: euchromatin is generally considered to be permissive for gene transcription and is characterized by nucleosomes, which are more variably spaced and linearly arranged. Heterochromatin, in contrast, is restricted for the access of transcription factors by its densely packed nucleosome spacing along the DNA. The result is generally transcriptional repression and gene silencing *(1, 2)* (Fig. 1).

The structure of chromatin and the associated gene transcription is controlled by covalent modifications to the tails of the histone proteins resulting in what has been termed as "histone code" that regulates chromatin-DNA interactions. The histone code is much more complex than originally proposed *(3, 4)*, and to date, at least eight different classes of histone modifications have been characterized, reviewed in *(5)*. These include acetylation, lysine and arginine methylation, phosphorylation, ubiquitylation, sumoylation, ADP ribosylation, deimination, and proline isomerization. For the purpose of this chapter,

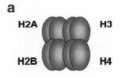

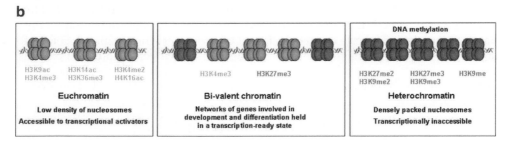

Fig. 1. Chromatin structure and histone modifications. (**a**) The nucleosome is composed of four different histone proteins: H2A, H2B, H3, and H4 (Fig. 1a), each arranged in pairs to form a histone octamer. DNA is packaged into chromatin by wrapping 147 bp of DNA around the nuclosome resulting in the fundamental unit of chromatin. (**b**) Euchromatin (*left panel*) is associated with actively transcribed genes. H3 is preferentially modified with active chromatin marks, and histones bearing these active marks (*green ovals*) are widely dispersed providing an open chromatin setting favorable for active transcription. Conversely, heterochromatin (*right panel*) is characteristic of silent gene promoter, and is associated with histones arranged in a more compacted nucleosomal configuration typical for transcriptionally repressed promoters. On these histones (*red ovals*), H3 is preferentially modified with several repressive methylation marks, and in some cases, the addition of DNA methylation. Networks of genes involved in development and differentiation are sometimes held in a transcription-ready state in stem cells called bivalent chromatin (*center panel*). In this intermediate state, the histones contain the transcriptional activating mark H3K4me3 and the repressive modification H3K27me3 (*see Color Plates*).

we will focus upon a subset of these modifications that have been closely linked to the activation or repression of genes. Key marks for active transcription include the acetylation of H3 lysine 9 and 14 (H3K9ac, H3K14ac) and H4K16 (H4K16ac), the di and trimethylation of H3 Lysine 4 (H3K4me2, H3K4me3), and the trimethylation of H3 lysine 36 (H3K36me3). In contrast, heterochromatin displays an enrichment of di-and tri-methylated H3 lysine 27 (H3K27me2, H3K27me3), and mono, di, and trimethylation of H3 lysine 9 (H3K9me, H3K9me2, H3K9me3), which are all chromatin modifications linked to transcriptional repression (Fig. 1). Many of the enzymes responsible for these histone modifications have also been identified. The known acetyltransferases, deacetylases, lysine methyltransferases, and lysine demethylases for these modifications have been recently reviewed in detail *(5, 6)*.

Another important epigenetic modification that is closely associated with gene silencing is DNA methylation. There are four known DNA methyltransferases in mammals: DNMT1, DNMT3a, DNMT3b, and DNMT3L *(7–9)*. These methyltransferases directly modify the CpG dinucleotides in DNA via the addition of methyl groups to cytosine. DNMT1 is generally considered to be a maintenance methyltransferase that is required for faithfully copying the epigenetic modifications to the daughter strands of DNA with each cell replication, while DNMT3a and DNMT3b are though to play a role in de novo methylation of DNA. The expression of the DNMT3L isoform is largely confined to embryonic cells, and its mechanisms of action and DNA targets are less well understood. DNA methylation is considered to be a more permanent, heritable mark relative to histone modifications. Although distinct experimental evidence exists to suggest that active and direct DNA demethylation can take place *(10–12)*, and the transient wave of global demethylation that occurs during embryonic development is well recognized, the specific mechanisms outside of base excision corrections by DNA glycosylases *(11)* are still not known, and no known, independently confirmed, DNA demethylases have been directly identified. The activation and inactivation of lineage specific genes required for different tissues and organs, as well as the permanent inactivation of pluripotency-associated genes in terminally differentiated cells, uses a complex combination of active and repressive histone and DNA modifications (Fig. 2), and many more of which are likely to be discovered. Aberrant DNA methylation is a hallmark of most cancers, and these heritable repressive modifications can be observed in even the earliest premalignant and hyperplastic lesions, accumulate throughout tumor progression, and contribute significantly to the biology of cancer *(13–16)*. As a result, we and others have hypothesized that errors in the carefully orchestrated network of histone and DNA epigenetic modifications required for normal development and differentiation from stem/progenitor cells may play a key role in tumor initiation and progression.

EPIGENETIC CHANGES DURING NORMAL DEVELOPMENT

Extensive chromatin remodeling occurs on a global level during development (Fig. 2). ES cells have a remarkably open, active, transcriptionally permissive chromatin structure, much of which is lost with lineage commitment *(17)*. As embryonic stem (ES) cells differentiate, they lose pluripotency. Structural chromatin proteins become more stably associated with chromatin in differentiated cells, reviewed in *(17)*, and there is also an increase in regions of condensed heterochromatin and an increase in the global levels of the accompanying repressive histone modifications associated with differentiation *(17, 18)*. The extent that adult tissue-specific stem/progenitor cells retain this global permissive chromatin status is likely tied to the extent with which they retain pluripotency. Enrichment of individual histone modifications also varies on a global level during different stages of development. For example, the methylation of H3K4 is enhanced globally in the post-blastocyst phase as developmental and tissue specific genes are activated *(18)*. The enhanced condensation of chromatin

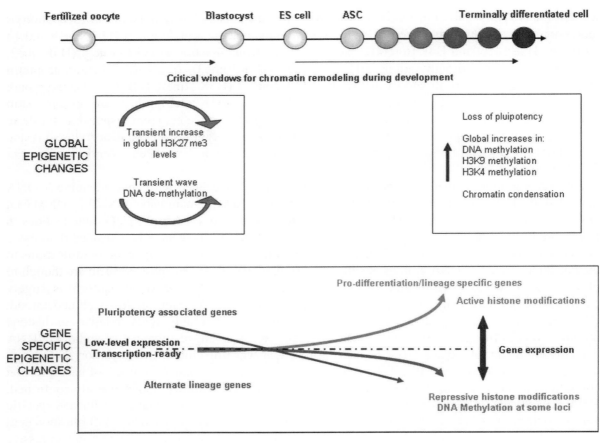

Fig. 2. Global and gene specific epigenetic changes during development. Histone modifications and DNA methylation are modulated on a global level during development during several critical windows for chromatin remodeling. In the pre-blastocyst phase, the key long-term gene transcription repression mark, H3K27me3, mediated by the Polycomb group (PcG) of transcriptional repressors, and DNA methylation undergo inversely correlated waves of enrichrichment. With terminal differentiation in normal cells, we see a loss of pluripotency, chromatin condensation, and global increases in DNA methylation and H3K4 and H3K9 methylation compared with ES cells. A model (*lower panel*) of normal activation and gene silencing of different groups of developmental genes on a local, gene specific level demonstrates that in stem and progenitor cells, important developmental and lineage specific genes are held in a bivalent, transcription-ready, low expression state (*dotted black line*). With differentiation, and in a specific lineage, some prodifferentiation and lineage specific genes must be activated (*green solid line*), while those genes required for alternate lineages (*red solid line*) must be permanently silenced. The divergent expression status of these two groups of genes is controlled at least in part by the enrichment of active and repressive histone modifications at their promoters. Pluripotency-associated genes (*blue solid line*) must be permanently silenced in terminally differentiated cells, and this is accomplished by the combination of enrichment for repressive chromatin modifications and for at least some genes, DNA methylation. The complex remodeling of these different classes of genes results in a critical window for chromatin remodeling, which may leave genes vulnerable to inappropriate silencing or activation.

is also accompanied by a global increase in H3K9 methylation with differentiation. One additional key global change in histone modifications involves H3K27me3. This is a repressive histone modification associated with long-term gene silencing and mediated by the Polycomb group (PcG) of transcriptional repressor. H3K27me3 and DNA methylation undergo a curious inversely correlated wave of enrichment on a global level during embryonic development, resulting in a significant decrease in DNA methylation in both the zygote and the embryonic germ cells (Fig. 2) *(18)*. Several seminal studies of the epigenetic profiles of PcG genes in human ES and embryonic fibroblasts (EF) have been published. These studies identify PcG enrichment as a key regulator of genes essential for development, morphogenesis, and organogenesis and show that PcG proteins and/or the H3K27methylation mark are enriched at the promoters of between ~8% (ES cells) *(19)* and ~14% (EF cells) *(20)* of the annotated genome,

Although chromatin is generally considered to be either euchromatic or heterochromatic in somatic cells, "bivalent" chromatin is increasingly being recognized as a mechanism by which stem and progenitor cells may hold multilineage genes in a low level, steady state of transcription until activated or repressed permanently during development (Fig. 1). Bivalent chromatin is defined as consisting of the simultaneous presence at certain gene promoters of an active mark, H3K4me3, and, interestingly, the above discussed PcG mediated mark, H3K27me3. This pattern has recently been described in normal murine ES cells for a subset of developmental genes, which are maintained in a low expression state *(21–23)*. This bivalent state is a particularly important component of the above genome-wide characterization of chromatin and is resolved to a primarily active or repressive chromatin conformation with differentiation depending on which direction the transcription of the involved genes changes with differentiation cues. The degree of lineage commitment is thought to determine the balance of these chromatin modifications at gene promoters and the basal expression levels of involved genes *(21)*.

One might expect that similar to what has been observed for differentiating ES cells, the global chromatin state of a cell is also varied between adult differentiated cells and the adult tissue specific stem/precursor cells from which they derive. Most adult stem/precursor cells have already significantly committed to a specific lineage, and likely have programmed a considerable portion of their gene expression patterns through epigenetic packaging of the genome. We might still expect, however, that the extent to which adult tissue-derived stem/precursor cells retain the ability to differentiate into various differentiated lineages is reflective of their global chromatin structure and their ability to modify it. Bivalent chromatin structure has been identified in both mouse neural progenitor cells (NPC) and mouse embryonic fibroblasts (EF) *(23)* for a significant number of gene promoters. Although there is significant overlap between these adult, tissue-specific progenitor cells and ES cells, the subset of gene promoters with bivalent chromatin in NPC and EF cells are distinct from each other and from the mouse ES cells *(23)*. The advent of ChIP-on-ChIP and ChIP-sequencing technologies has opened huge new opportunities for the genome-wide study of histone modifications. These assays consist of immunoprecipitation with antibodies to various histone modifications or transcriptional activators and repressors, followed by microarray analysis or genomic sequencing *(20–26)*. ChIP-sequencing, in particular, because of its ability to handle relatively small numbers of cells and cover the genome with great density *(23, 25)*, will hopefully provide a platform to investigate the global chromatin signatures of various cell populations, including rare adult stem cells, adult precursor cells, and multiple types of differentiated cells, which constitute an adult tissue.

There are several instances in which DNA methylation is known to collaborate with chromatin configuration to stabilize key gene expression patterns, which emerge during normal development and adult tissue cell turnover. These include the long-term silencing of transposons and the permanent stabilization of silenced genes in the processes of imprinting and X-inactivation. Localized DNA methylation changes have also been observed at key cytokine target genes during embryonic and adult differentiation and maturation of lymphocytes *(27)*. Mammalian females use random x-chromosome inactivation to equalize the imbalance of X-chromosome gene expression created by females having two X chromosomes in contrast to the male XY. X inactivation is initiated in the epiblast or future embryo *(28)* in mammalian females. The inactivated X chromosome (Xi) acquires both H3K27me3 and H3K9me2, while the activating H3K4me3 histone modification is lost *(29, 30)*. These inactivating chromatin changes accompany the hallmark densely methylated regions of CpG dinucleotides, termed CpG islands, and discussed in great detail later below, which are observed along the entire Xi chromosome (31). This multifaceted collaboration of histone modifications, nucleosome remodeling, and DNA methylation provides an elegant control system to produce heritable patterns of gene expression to guarantee the complex functions of mammalian organisms.

Similar to random X chromosome inactivation, both H3K27me3 and H3K9me2 histone methylation and DNA methylation are involved in the normal silencing of approximately 100 known imprinted genes. Genomic imprinting allows for monoallelic expression from either the maternal or paternal allele, and most imprinted genes regulate placental and fetal growth (2). For detailed reviews of X-inactivation and genomic imprinting see references (2, 32).

The permanent silencing of important pluipotency-associated genes such as hTERT, Oct-4, and Nanog during stem and progenitor cell differentiation can also be attributed, at least in part, to the accumulation of DNA methylation at the promoters of these genes (2, 33–38). An increase in global de novo methylation and increases in both Dnmt1 and Dnmt3b proteins at the hTERT promoter midway through the differentiation process have been observed in teratocarcinoma cells (33). Additionally, silencing of Oct-4 in post-mitotic neurons has been shown to be associated with loss of the active H3K4me2 mark, an increase in the polycomb regulated H3K27me3 modification, and CpG dinucleotide DNA methylation (39), once again emphasizing how histone and DNA methylation work in concert to mediate transcriptional repression. Normal DNA methylation patterns differ for gene promoters lacking CpG islands vs. those which contain them. Thus, dense DNA methylation of promoter CpG islands is most often seen for a host of genes in cancers, and normally only on the inactive X chromosome of females and for the silenced alleles of selected imprinted genes. In contrast, the promoters of the embryogenesis regulating genes such as Oct-4 and Nanog have CpG poor promoters, and, for these pluripotency associated genes, there is normal differential methylation seen at a small number of CpG dinucleotides, which correlates to expression changes (33, 34). Extensive work will be required to understand how histone and DNA methylation, and the repressive complexes responsible for initiation and maintenance of the associated silencing, may similarly or divergently target alternating regions of dense or sparse CpG content.

PROGENITOR CELLS AS TUMOR INITIATING CELLS

Many groups have suggested that stem cells or early progenitor cells may be the precursors from which cancer cells are derived (40–42). All of these studies cite the fact that tumors harbor stem/ precursor cell population markers, have heterogeneous cell populations among which only cell subsets have tumor regeneration capacity, and are driven by the up-regulation of many pathways important to maintenance of normal stem/precursor cells including PcG proteins, and the Wnt, Shh, and Notch pathways (41). Drugs that target the rapidly proliferating bulk tumor population may leave the relatively quiescent cancer stem cells un-perturbed and allow for tumor regrowth (41). Similarly, both normal and malignant stem cells are known to be comparatively resistant to chemotherapy (43).

Despite the evidence for a potential stem cell of origin for cancer, this concept remains controversial, and there is no conclusive evidence to rule out the possibility that cancer is derived from more terminally differentiated cells that have acquired these characteristics of stem/progenitor cells by dedifferentiation (44). Detailed descriptions of the cancer stem cell theory and a discussion of the known characteristics of various cancer stem cells are included elsewhere in this book, but merits mention here as the similarities between epigenetic remodeling during both normal and malignant development implicate overlapping networks and pathways, and highlight the possibility that differentiating stem/progenitor cells are a leading candidate as tumor initiating cells, at least for some cancers. We hypothesize, from

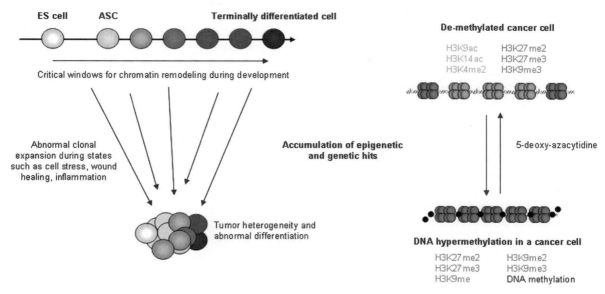

Fig. 3. Cancer stem cells, epigenetic gene silencing events, and tumorigenesis. For at least some pluripotency associated and alternate lineage genes, gene silencing is a normal event in stem/progenitor cells as adult cell renewal takes place. Silencing is mediated by repressive chromatin modifications, which are malleable such that the genes might be activated for transcription as required by cell maturation. This homeostasis allows stem/progenitor cells to move properly along the differentiation pathway for a given tissue or cell system (darkening blue color of cells along the *top left panel*). During chronic cell injury, stress, wound healing, or inflammation, the pressure for adaptive cell renewal draws from the stem/progenitor cell pool for ongoing repair. This pressure might allow for abnormal DNA methylation to be recruited to promoters of normally silenced genes by the chromatin which is in place (*lower right*, DNA hypermethylation, *black circles*). The result is a tight heritable silencing that cannot be easily reactivated as a cell clone expands, thereby channeling the cells toward the abnormal expansion, at the expense of differentiation. This entire scenario leads to benign precursor tumors that are at risk for progression. This progression would be fostered by subsequent genetic or epigenetic events. Chemically depleting DNA methylation using 5-aza-deoxy-cytidine can induce gene expression (upper right, demethylated cancer cell), but the gene does not return to the fully euchromatic state seen at a normally transcribed gene *(67)*. In this intermediate state, the histones contain the transcriptional activating marks (*green*) H3K4me2 and H3K9/14ac and HP1a is not present. However, several repressive modifications (*red*) including H3K27me3 and H3K9me3 remain and apparently need not change for significant transcription to occur *(see Color Plates)*.

recent of our data and the work of many others *(45)*, that failure of the stem cell epigenetic regulatory networks likely contributes to the diseased state in cancer - specifically, aberrant, promoter CpG island, DNA hypermethylation of developmental regulator genes and tumor suppressor genes. For the purposes of this chapter, we assume that both the cancer stem cell hypothesis and the dedifferentiation hypothesis may be true for different cancers and in different patients. The vast heterogeneity seen between different tumors may be reflective of the epigenetic state of differentiation of their cell of origin, and tumors may arise from cells at all points along a differentiation pathway (Fig. 3).

EPIGENETIC CHANGES DURING TUMOR INITIATION AND MALIGNANT PROGRESSION

Data are now emerging showing a striking link between the stem cell epigenetic regulatory pathways discussed in the preceding section and the aberrant silencing of tumor suppressor genes in cancer. There is now tantalizing evidence that the mechanisms responsible for normal epigenetic silencing in quiescent and differentiating stem/progenitor cells may have gone awry in a tumor cell of origin. The addition of abnormal DNA methylation to CpG islands within the promoters of groups of genes that should have been up-regulated with normal differentiation *(45–47)* may work in concert with repressive histone modifications to stabilize this gene silencing and facilitate tumor initiation and progression, thus converting transient gene silencing in normal development to permanent, heritable gene silencing in the malignant state.

The abnormal survival of stem/progenitor cells under chronic stress conditions, such as chronic wound healing and inflammation *(48, 49)* may be facilitated by increased epigenetic silencing of tumor suppressor genes (Fig. 3). These epigenetic changes are prevalent in all types of cancer, and their appearance may precede genetic changes in premalignant cells and foster the accumulation of additional genetic and epigenetic hits *(49)*. These epigenetically modified genes constitute important categories of tumor suppressor genes including cell cycle regulators, prodifferentiation factors, genes controlling key developmental pathways, and antiapoptotic genes *(15)*. Epigenetic gene silencing, and associated promoter CpG island DNA hypermethylation, is an alternative mechanism to mutations by which tumor suppressor genes may be inactivated within a cancer cell *(13–16, 50–52)*, and as above, many of these genes are known to play a role in normal development *(53–55)*.

In fact, compilation of a panel of genes that are particularly sensitive to methylation *(45)* as represented by their frequent targeting for this epigenetic change, indicates that many of these key proteins have known roles in tumorigenesis, and virtually all tied to normal differentiation and development. These genes encompass a wide range of tissue types including brain, breast, colon, esophageal, gastric, head and neck, hematopoetic, kidney/renal, liver, lung, ovarian, pancreatic, prostate, and uterine cancer and are expected to undergo remodeling of their chromatin in stem/progenitor cells during the normal differentiation of corresponding cell lineages. All of the genes were found to be hypermethylated in multiple tumor types, and hypermethylation of several of these genes (*CDH1*, *CDKN2A*, and *RASSF1*) has been observed in all of these tumor types. The high frequency of targeting of genes involved in normal development, including genes such as *CDKN2a (p16)*, which can regulate stem cell number and cell cycle functions *(56–61)*, *GATA* transcription factors, which regulate differentiation *(62)*, morphogenesis control genes such as *CDH1*, and antiapoptotic genes such as *DAP-kinase (15)* suggests that the underlying epigenetic mechanisms responsible for controlling expression of these genes in normal stem and progenitor cells may provide an explanation for the targeting of at least some genes for DNA hypermethylation and gene silencing during tumor initiation and progression.

Multiple groups *(45–47)* have recently compiled evidence that the bivalent transcriptionally repressive chromatin modifications inherent to important developmentally regulatory genes in normal embryonic stem cells (ES) are also associated with the more permanent, heritable silencing of these gene promoters in cancer cells. In the embryonic setting, these modifications may normally help prevent stem/precursor cells from conversion to committed cells until programmed to do so, and serve as temporary place holders as genes wait for external developmental cues. We have hypothesized *(45)* that this "transcription-ready" chromatin pattern is precisely what renders this group of genes vulnerable to errors, which result in recruitment of aberrant promoter DNA methylation during early progression of adult cancers and reducing the plasticity of these genes and their ability to alter their expression in responses to external stimuli.

Interestingly, both normal embryonic stem cells (ES) and embryonal carcinoma cells (EC; Tera-1 and Tera-2) generally lack the widespread gene promoter CpG island DNA methylation that is seen in adult cancer cells *(45)*. EC are malignant counterparts of normal embryonic germ cells, but in contrast to adult cancers, retain a marked ability to manifest spontaneous differentiation and multilineage commitment in vitro and in vivo *(63–66)*. Analysis of the histone modifications at the promoter regions of many of these important tumor suppressor genes in ES and EC cells reveals a mixture of active (H3K4me2) and repressive (H3K27me3) chromatin marks and demonstrates that the genes that get frequently hypermethylated in cancer are generally within the cluster of important developmental genes that are held in the bivalent, transcription ready state observed in ES and adult tissue-derived stem cells (Fig. 1b). Even though these genes in EC cells generally have the addition of the H3K9me3 silencing mark, when compared with the ES cells, the genes remain responsive to differentiation cues *(45)*. This plasticity of expression in EC cells is not seen for these same genes when they are DNA methylated and deeply, heritably repressed in adult cancers where these genes generally require that DNA methylation be removed to reactivate *(67)*.

The large numbers of epigenetically silenced genes that may be present in any given tumor, and the clustering of silenced genes within single cell pathways *(68)*, begs the question of whether gene silencing is a series of random events resulting in an enhanced survival of a premalignant clone, or whether silencing is the result of a directed, instructive program for silencing initiation reflective of the cell of origin for the tumors. Recent data have emerged implicating the Polycomb family of repressive proteins, key modulators of epigenetic control of normal development, in the establishment and maintenance of aberrant epigenetic patterns observed in cancer.

POLYCOMB REPRESSIVE COMPLEXES: AN EPIGENETIC BRIDGE BETWEEN NORMAL AND MALIGNANT DEVELOPMENT?

High steady-state levels of PcG complexes are especially present in stem and progenitor cells, as well as in tumor cells that have similar properties *(69–71)*. Recent research largely implicates the polycomb group (PcG) of transcriptional repressors as key players in DNA hypermethylation of tumor suppressor genes in cancer, primarily through the enrichment of the repressive H3K27me3 mark *(45–47)*. This histone modification is catalyzed by EZH2, a key component of the Polycomb group (PcG) complexes, which maintain long-term gene silencing from lower organisms to man and are essential for the normal state of stem/progenitor cells and their commitment to various tissue types *(69, 72–74)*. PcG regulation of gene silencing shows a dynamic and fascinating regulation during differentiation. Both the global and promoter specific levels of PcG complex related proteins, including SUZ12, EZH2, and SirT1, fall with in vitro differentiation for several genes that are frequently hypermethylated in cancer, such as GATA4 and CDKN2a (p16) *(45)*. Additionally, several PcG proteins, including Bmi1, Suz12, and Sfmbt, show a transient increase in expression at various points during the differentiation process, followed by a lowering of expression as cells enter a more differentiated state *(45)*. Such data support the extensive work of others in discerning a role for this family during normal differentiation *(69)*. While low level enrichment of the H3K27me3 mark appears to be nearly ubiquitous at the small subset of DNA hypermethylated cancer gene promoters we have studied to date *(67)*, direct global comparisons of PcG regulation between cancer cells and their proposed stem or progenitor cell of origin should help clarify and measure the full extent of the link between PcG regulation and DNA hypermethylation.

Recent studies have linked EZH2 to promoter recruitment of the enzymes that catalyze DNA methylation, the DNA methyltransferases (DNMT's), and have suggested a role for this protein during the induction and targeting of DNA methylation *(75)*. Interestingly, for many genes frequently hypermethylated in cancer, both normal embryonic stem (ES) cells and embryonal carcinomas (EC) demonstrate an enrichment of key PcG proteins including SUZ12, EZH2, and SirT1, plus the H3K27me3 mark to their promoters *(45)*. When compared with the above mentioned genome-wide studies of PcG enrichment at human gene promoters in ES and embryonic fibroblasts (EF), approximately 68% of the genes on our panel of genes frequently DNA hypermethylated in adult cancers were also associated with PcG in one or both of the PcG targeting studies of ES and/or EF cells *(45)*. These data were striking, particularly considering, as noted previously, that for each of the candidate genes we have studied in depth in adult cancer cells, DNA hypermethylation is accompanied by a low, but measurable enrichment of the H3K27 repressive mark *(67)*. Similar results were seen using 23 genes newly identified as hypermethylated in HCT-116 colon cancer cells *(76)* for which 56.5% were identified as PcG targets in either ES or EF cells, and is in agreement with data published simultaneously by two additional groups. Thus, Widschwendter et al. show that PcG targets are up to 12-fold more likely to have cancer-specific DNA hypermethylation than nontargets when comparing 177 genes identified as hypermethylated in primary human colorectal tumors *(46)*. Additionally, Schlesinger et al. demonstrate that of 24 genes identified as specifically DNA hypermethylated in the colon cancer line Caco-2, all also demonstrate concurrent enrichment of the H3K27me3 modification, which is generally lacking in unmethylated controls, and >60% of these genes are PcG regulated in the above studies of ES and EF cells *(47)*.

Although PcG regulation in stem/progenitor cells may leave developmental genes vulnerable to DNA hypermethylation in a cancer cell of origin, PcG is associated with a plethora of gene promoters in stem cells that are exquisitely responsive to differentiation cues and therefore assumed to be completely devoid of any DNA methylation. As a result, we fully expect that additional repressive marks are necessary for the transition of a gene promoter from a transient "transcription-ready" state to one of heritable, permanent gene silencing and recruitment of DNA hypermethylation in a premalignant cell. Although PcG complexes and the H3K27me marks have been associated with recruitment of DNA methylation *(67, 75)*, additional studies suggest that these PcG constituents are not required to maintain such methylation *(77)*. Recent studies showing the additional enrichment of two key repressive marks to the genes being discussed, H3K9me3, which is characteristic of silenced transcription in pericentromeric regions *(78)*, and to a lower and more variable extent, H3K9me2 in EC cells when compared with their normal ES cell counterparts *(45)* may provide us with some clues as to the initiation of dense promoter CpG island DNA methylation in cancer since both of these H3K9me marks are characteristic of DNA hypermethylated genes in adult cancers *(67, 79–84)*. Interestingly, in the EC cells, global levels of both of the H3K9me repressive marks are increased considerably when compared with ES cells *(45)*, suggesting a permissive background for the promoter changes in the neoplastic cells and/or a more differentiated cell of origin. In fact, in both Neurospora and Arabidopsis, mutations in histone methyltransferases, which catalyze H3K9 methylation, cause significant loss of genomic DNA methylation *(85–89)*. In adult cancers, the repressive chromatin present for DNA hypermethylated genes is initially more enriched for H3K9me2 *(67, 81)* than is seen in the EC cells, and this mark is the only repressive mark that we have studied which is uniformly reduced when DNA hypermethylated genes are chemically demethylated in adult cancer cells *(67)*. Perhaps most interesting, have been findings that these silenced cancer gene promoters, when reactivated by DNA demethylating agents, do not return to a fully euchromatic chromatin state *(67)*. Rather, while active marks are restored, most repressive histone modification marks remain, including H3K27me3, which is generally increased. The resulting chromatin absent of DNA methylation is remarkably similar to the bivalent state (McGarvey et al., Cancer Research 2008, manuscript in press) observed in ES, EF, and EC cells, bringing us full circle, and suggesting that a stem cell-like promoter "ground state" for these genes may be indicative of the contribution of stem cell and/or progenitor cells to the derivation of adult cancers.

In fact, the extensive normal epigenetic remodeling that is a hallmark of differentiating cells may be the very thing that leaves these cells especially at risk for cancer initiation if stalled in a state of continued expansion due chronic wound healing and inflammation *(48, 67)* (Fig. 3). Deregulation of this process in premalignant cells during this critical window for chromatin remodeling may result in the conversion of transient repression in stem/progenitor cells to one of heritable silencing via DNA hypermethylation and improper packaging of essential growth regulatory genes into regions of dense heterochromatin. The specific prodifferentiation, growth control properties of these genes may then enhance the likelihood, in these abnormal cell clones, of subsequent tumor initiation and progression in a stem/progenitor cell of origin.

REFERENCES

1. Horn PJ, Peterson CL. Molecular biology. Chromatin higher order folding-wrapping up transcription. Science 2002; 297:1824–7.
2. Kiefer JC. Epigenetics in development. Dev Dyn 2007; 236:1144–56.
3. Strahl BD, Allis CD. The language of covalent histone modifications. Nature 2000; 403:41–5.
4. Jenuwein T, Allis CD. Translating the histone code. Science 2001; 293:1074–80.
5. Kouzarides T. Chromatin modifications and their function. Cell 2007; 128:693–705.
6. Pruitt K, Zinn RL, Ohm JE, et al. Inhibition of SIRT1 reactivates silenced cancer genes without loss of promoter DNA hypermethylation. PLoS Genet 2006; 2:e40.
7. Tucker KL, Beard C, Dausmann J, et al. Germ-line passage is required for establishment of methylation and expression patterns of imprinted but not of nonimprinted genes. Genes Dev 1996; 10:1008–20.
8. Xie S, Wang Z, Okano M, et al. Cloning, expression and chromosome locations of the human DNMT3 gene family. Gene 1999; 236:87–95.
9. Bourc'his D, Xu GL, Lin CS, Bollman B, Bestor TH. Dnmt3L and the establishment of maternal genomic imprints. Science 2001; 294:2536–9.
10. Penterman J, Zilberman D, Huh JH, Ballinger T, Henikoff S, Fischer RL. DNA demethylation in the Arabidopsis genome. Proc Natl Acad Sci USA 2007; 104:6752–7.
11. Agius F, Kapoor A, Zhu JK. Role of the Arabidopsis DNA glycosylase/lyase ROS1 in active DNA demethylation. Proc Natl Acad Sci USA 2006; 103:11796–801.
12. Bruniquel D, Schwartz RH. Selective, stable demethylation of the interleukin-2 gene enhances transcription by an active process. Nat Immunol 2003; 4:235–40.
13. Jones PA, Laird PW. Cancer epigenetics comes of age. Nat Genet 1999; 21:163–167.
14. Feinberg AP, Tycko B. The history of cancer epigenetics. Nat Rev Cancer 2004; 4:143–53.
15. Herman JG, Baylin SB. Gene silencing in cancer in association with promoter hypermethylation. N Engl J Med 2003; 349:2042–54.
16. Jones PA, Baylin SB. The fundamental role of epigenetic events in cancer. Nat Rev Genet 2002; 3:415–28.
17. Meshorer E, Misteli T. Chromatin in pluripotent embryonic stem cells and differentiation. Nat Rev Mol Cell Biol 2006; 7:540–6.
18. Reik W. Stability and flexibility of epigenetic gene regulation in mammalian development. Nature 2007; 447:425–32.
19. Lee TI, Jenner RG, Boyer LA, et al. Control of developmental regulators by polycomb in human embryonic stem cells. Cell 2006; 125:301–13.
20. Bracken AP, Dietrich N, Pasini D, Hansen KH, Helin K. Genome-wide mapping of Polycomb target genes unravels their roles in cell fate transitions. Genes Dev 2006; 20:1123–1136.
21. Bernstein BE, Mikkelsen TS, Xie X, et al. A bivalent chromatin structure marks key developmental genes in embryonic stem cells. Cell 2006; 125:315–226.
22. Azuara V, Perry P, Sauer S, et al. Chromatin signatures of pluripotent cell lines. Nat Cell Biol 2006; 8:532–8.
23. Mikkelsen TS, Ku M, Jaffe DB, et al. Genome-wide maps of chromatin state in pluripotent and lineage-committed cells. Nature 2007; 448:553–60.
24. Ren B, Robert F, Wyrick JJ, et al. Genome-wide location and function of DNA binding proteins. Science 2000; 290:2306–9.
25. Barski A, Cuddapah S, Cui K, et al. High-resolution profiling of histone methylations in the human genome. Cell 2007; 129:823–37.
26. Lee TI, Jenner RG, Boyer LA, et al. Control of developmental regulators by Polycomb in human embryonic stem cells. Cell 2006; 125:301–313.
27. Sakashita K, Koike K, Kinoshita T, et al. Dynamic DNA methylation change in the CpG island region of p15 during human myeloid development. J Clin Invest 2001; 108:1195–204.

28. Allegrucci C, Thurston A, Lucas E, Young L. Epigenetics and the germline. Reproduction 2005; 129:137–49.

29. Plath K, Fang J, Mlynarczyk-Evans SK, et al. Role of histone H3 lysine 27 methylation in X inactivation. Science 2003; 300:131–5.

30. Valley CM, Pertz LM, Balakumaran BS, Willard HF. Chromosome-wide, allele-specific analysis of the histone code on the human X chromosome. Hum Mol Genet 2006; 15:2335–47.

31. Kratzer PG, Chapman VM, Lambert H, Evans RE, Liskay RM. Differences in the DNA of the inactive X chromosomes of fetal and extraembryonic tissues of mice. Cell 1983; 33:37–42.

32. Reik W, Lewis A. Co-evolution of X-chromosome inactivation and imprinting in mammals. Nat Rev Genet 2005; 6:403–10.

33. Lopatina NG, Poole JC, Saldanha SN, et al. Control mechanisms in the regulation of telomerase reverse transcriptase expression in differentiating human teratocarcinoma cells. Biochem Biophys Res Commun 2003; 306:650–9.

34. Hattori N, Nishino K, Ko YG, et al. Epigenetic control of mouse Oct-4 gene expression in embryonic stem cells and trophoblast stem cells. J Biol Chem 2004; 279:17063–9.

35. Deb-Rinker P, Ly D, Jezierski A, Sikorska M, Walker PR. Sequential DNA methylation of the Nanog and Oct-4 upstream regions in human NT2 cells during neuronal differentiation. J Biol Chem 2005; 280:6257–60.

36. Feldman N, Gerson A, Fang J, et al. G9a-mediated irreversible epigenetic inactivation of Oct-3/4 during early embryogenesis. Nat Cell Biol 2006; 8:188–94.

37. Hattori N, Imao Y, Nishino K, et al. Epigenetic regulation of Nanog gene in embryonic stem and trophoblast stem cells. Genes Cells 2007; 12:387–96.

38. Yeo S, Jeong S, Kim J, Han JS, Han YM, Kang YK. Characterization of DNA methylation change in stem cell marker genes during differentiation of human embryonic stem cells. Biochem Biophys Res Commun 2007; 359:536–42.

39. Aoto T, Saitoh N, Ichimura T, Niwa H, Nakao M. Nuclear and chromatin reorganization in the MHC-Oct3/4 locus at developmental phases of embryonic stem cell differentiation. Dev Biol 2006; 298:354–67.

40. Al-Hajj M, Wicha MS, Benito-Hernandez A, Morrison SJ, Clarke MF. Prospective identification of tumorigenic breast cancer cells. Proc Natl Acad Sci USA 2003; 100:3983–8.

41. Reya T, Morrison SJ, Clarke MF, Weissman IL. Stem cells, cancer, and cancer stem cells. Nature 2001; 414:105–11.

42. Clarke MF, Fuller M. Stem cells and cancer: two faces of eve. Cell 2006; 124:1111–5.

43. Harrison DE, Lerner CP. Most primitive hematopoietic stem cells are stimulated to cycle rapidly after treatment with 5-fluorouracil. Blood 1991; 78:1237–40.

44. Rapp UR, Ceteci F, Schreck R. Oncogene-induced plasticity and cancer stem cells. Cell Cycle 2007; 7.

45. Ohm JE, McGarvey KM, Yu X, et al. A stem cell-like chromatin pattern may predispose tumor suppressor genes to DNA hypermethylation and heritable silencing. Nat Genet 2007; 39:237–42.

46. Widschwendter M, Fiegl H, Egle D, et al. Epigenetic stem cell signature in cancer. Nat Genet 2007; 39:157–8.

47. Schlesinger Y, Straussman R, Keshet I, et al. Polycomb-mediated methylation on Lys27 of histone H3 pre-marks genes for de novo methylation in cancer. Nat Genet 2007; 39:232–6.

48. Beachy PA, Karhadkar SS, Berman DM. Tissue repair and stem cell renewal in carcinogenesis. Nature 2004; 432:324–31.

49. Baylin SB, Ohm JE. Epigenetic gene silencing in cancer - a mechanism for early oncogenic pathway addiction? Nat Rev Cancer 2006; 6:107–16.

50. Hahn WC, Counter CM, Lundberg AS, Beijersbergen RL, Brooks MW, Weinberg RA. Creation of human tumour cells with defined genetic elements. Nature 1999; 400:464–8.

51. Aaltonen LA, Peltomaki P, Leach FS, et al. Clues to the pathogenesis of familial colorectal cancer. Science 1993; 260:812–6.

52. Kinzler KW, Vogelstein B. Cancer-susceptibility genes. Gatekeepers and caretakers. Nature 1997; 386:761–3.

53. Gregorieff A, Clevers H. Wnt signaling in the intestinal epithelium: from endoderm to cancer. Genes Dev 2005; 19:877–90.

54. Furukawa Y. Cell cycle control genes and hematopoietic cell differentiation. Leuk Lymphoma 2002; 43:225–31.

55. Burch JB. Regulation of GATA gene expression during vertebrate development. Semin Cell Dev Biol 2005; 16:71–81.

56. Park IK, Qian D, Kiel M, et al. Bmi-1 is required for maintenance of adult self-renewing haematopoietic stem cells. Nature 2003; 423:302–5.

57. Sharpless NE, Alson S, Chan S, Silver DP, Castrillon DH, DePinho RA. p16(INK4a) and p53 deficiency cooperate in tumorigenesis. Cancer Res 2002; 62:2761–5.

58. Collado M, Blasco MA, Serrano M. Cellular senescence in cancer and aging. Cell 2007; 130:223–33.

59. Molofsky AV, Slutsky SG, Joseph NM, et al. Increasing p16INK4a expression decreases forebrain progenitors and neurogenesis during ageing. Nature 2006; 443:448–52.

60. Janzen V, Forkert R, Fleming HE, et al. Stem-cell ageing modified by the cyclin-dependent kinase inhibitor p16INK4a. Nature 2006; 443:421–6.

61. Krishnamurthy J, Ramsey MR, Ligon KL, et al. p16INK4a induces an age-dependent decline in islet regenerative potential. Nature 2006; 443:453–7.

62. Laverriere AC, MacNeill C, Mueller C, Poelmann RE, Burch JB, Evans T. GATA-4/5/6, a subfamily of three transcription factors transcribed in developing heart and gut. J Biol Chem 1994; 269:23177–84.

63. Andrews PW. Human teratocarcinomas. Biochim Biophys Acta 1988; 948:17–36.

64. Andrews PW. Retinoic acid induces neuronal differentiation of a cloned human embryonal carcinoma cell line in vitro. Dev Biol 1984; 103:285–93.

65. Mintz B, Illmensee K. Normal genetically mosaic mice produced from malignant teratocarcinoma cells. Proc Natl Acad Sci USA 1975; 72:3585–9.

66. Palmiter RD, Chen HY, Brinster RL. Differential regulation of metallothionein-thymidine kinase fusion genes in transgenic mice and their offspring. Cell 1982; 29:701–10.

67. McGarvey KM, Fahrner JA, Greene E, Martens J, Jenuwein T, Baylin SB. Silenced tumor suppressor genes reactivated by dna demethylation do not return to a fully euchromatic chromatin state. Cancer Res 2006; 66:3541–3549.

68. Jones PA, Baylin SB. The epigenomics of cancer. Cell 2007; 128:683–92.

69. Kuzmichev A, Margueron R, Vaquero A, et al. Composition and histone substrates of polycomb repressive group complexes change during cellular differentiation. Proc Natl Acad Sci USA 2005; 102:1859–1864.

70. Kleer CG, Cao Q, Varambally S, et al. EZH2 is a marker of aggressive breast cancer and promotes neoplastic transformation of breast epithelial cells. Proc Natl Acad Sci USA 2003; 100:11606–11.

71. Kirmizis A, Bartley SM, Farnham PJ. Identification of the polycomb group protein SU(Z)12 as a potential molecular target for human cancer therapy. Mol Cancer Ther 2003; 2:113–21.

72. LundAavL, M. Polycomb complexes and silencing mechanisms. Curr Opin Genet Dev 2004; 16:1–8.

73. Valk-Lingbeek ME, Bruggeman SW, van Lohuizen M. Stem cells and cancer; the polycomb connection. Cell 2004; 118:409–18.

74. Otte AP, Kwaks TH. Gene repression by Polycomb group protein complexes: a distinct complex for every occasion? Curr Opin Genet Dev 2003; 13:448–54.

75. Vire E, Brenner C, Deplus R, et al. The Polycomb group protein EZH2 directly controls DNA methylation. Nature 2006; 439:871–4.

76. Schuebel KE, Chen W, Cope L, et al. Comparing the DNA Hypermethylome with Gene Mutations in Human Colorectal Cancer. PLoS Genet 2007; 3:e157.

77. McGarvey KM, Greene E, Fahrner JA, Jenuwein T, Baylin SB. DNA methylation and complete transcriptional silencing of cancer genes persist after depletion of EZH2. Cancer Res 2007; 67:5097–102.

78. Schotta G, Lachner M, Sarma K, et al. A silencing pathway to induce H3-K9 and H4-K20 trimethylation at constitutive heterochromatin. Genes Dev 2004; 18:1251–62.

79. Lachner M, O'Sullivan RJ, Jenuwein T. An epigenetic road map for histone lysine methylation. J Cell Sci 2003; 116:2117–24.

80. Nguyen CT, Gonzales FA, Jones PA. Altered chromatin structure associated with methylation-induced gene silencing in cancer cells: correlation of accessibility, methylation, MeCP2 binding and acetylation. Nucleic Acids Res 2001; 29:4598–606.

81. Fahrner JA, Eguchi S, Herman JG, Baylin SB. Dependence of histone modifications and gene expression on DNA hypermethylation in cancer. Cancer Res 2002; 62:7213–8.

82. Kouzarides T. Histone methylation in transcriptional control. Curr Opin Genet Dev 2002; 12:198–209.

83. Briggs SD, Xiao T, Sun ZW, et al. Gene silencing: trans-histone regulatory pathway in chromatin. Nature 2002; 418:498.

84. Fischle W, Wang Y, Allis CD. Histone and chromatin cross-talk. Curr Opin Cell Biol 2003; 15:172–83.

85. Tamaru H, Selker EU. A histone H3 methyltransferase controls DNA methylation in Neurospora crassa. Nature 2001; 414:277–83.

86. Tamaru H, Zhang X, McMillen D, et al. Trimethylated lysine 9 of histone H3 is a mark for DNA methylation in Neurospora crassa. Nat Genet 2003; 34:75–9.

87. Johnson L, Cao X, Jacobsen S. Interplay between two epigenetic marks. DNA methylation and histone H3 lysine 9 methylation. Curr Biol 2002; 12:1360–7.

88. Malagnac F, Bartee L, Bender J. An Arabidopsis SET domain protein required for maintenance but not establishment of DNA methylation. Embo J 2002; 21:6842–52.

89. Jackson JP, Johnson L, Jasencakova Z, et al. Dimethylation of histone H3 lysine 9 is a critical mark for DNA methylation and gene silencing in Arabidopsis thaliana. Chromosoma 2004; 112:308–15.

8

Plasticity Underlying Multipotent Tumor Stem Cells

*Lynne-Marie Postovit, Naira V. Margaryan,
Elisabeth A. Seftor, Luigi Strizzi,
Richard E.B. Seftor, and Mary J.C. Hendrix*

ABSTRACT

Aggressive cancer cells manifest stem-cell-like qualities that allow them to self-renew and to derive a heterogeneous tumor. Ultimately, this multipotent phenotype facilitates metastasis and resistance to therapy. Cancer cells likely acquire and maintain multipotent phenotypes by aberrantly expressing embryonic factors, such as Nodal and Notch, which maintain pluripotency in normal embryonic stem cell types. Recent studies have shown that Nodal, an embryonic morphogen belonging to the transforming growth factor-beta (TGF-β) superfamily, is aberrantly expressed in melanoma and breast carcinoma cells. Moreover, Nodal facilitates breast cancer and melanoma tumorigenesis. During development, Nodal is regulated by the spatial and temporal expression of inhibitors such as Lefty. In aggressive cancer cells, this balance of regulatory mediators is disrupted, leading to unchecked Nodal expression. By exposing aggressive cancer cells to embryonic microenvironments, inclusive of Lefty, Nodal expression is decreased and tumorigenesis is suppressed. Embryonic stem cell-derived factors, such as Lefty, may provide therapeutic modalities that may be used to specifically differentiate and eradicate aggressive cancers.

Key Words: Nodal, Lefty, Microenvironment, Stem cells, Cancer

THE STEM-CELL-LIKE NATURE OF CANCER

Aggressive cancer cells are characterized by the ability to proliferate indefinitely and to generate a heterogeneous tumor inclusive of cells that can resist therapy and metastasize. Recent technological advances in microscopy and flow cytometry have allowed scientists to track and isolate such tumor-initiating stem cells, culminating in the establishment of the cancer stem cell theory. This theory was first validated for human leukemia when a subpopulation of leukemic cells was shown to be both required and sufficient to establish leukemia in mice *(1)*. Since this seminal discovery, cancer stem cells have been documented in malignancies as diverse as glioma, breast cancer, and melanoma *(2–4)*. In breast cancer, the stem cell population has been defined as CD44$^+$, CD24$^-$ *(3)*. These breast cancer initiating cells, which have been isolated from both patient tissue and breast cancer cell lines, are characterized by the ability to form proliferative nonadherent spherical clusters (mammospheres) in vitro and to initiate tumor formation in a mouse *(3, 5, 6)*. They are also radioresistant and highly

From: *Cancer Drug Discovery and Development: Stem Cells and Cancer,*
Edited by: R.G. Bagley and B.A. Teicher, DOI: 10.1007/978-1-60327-933-8_8,
© Humana Press, a part of Springer Science+Business Media, LLC 2009

invasive *(6, 7)*. Stem cells have also been shown to mediate melanomagenesis. For example, Frank and colleagues described a melanoma stem cell population delineated by the expression of the drug efflux transporter ABCB5. Moreover, they have shown that ABCB5 colocalizes with cells expressing the stem cell marker CD133, and that it can be targeted to specifically eradicate melanoma tumors in orthotopic mouse models *(8, 9)*. A melanoma stem cell population defined by the expression of CD20 with the propensity to differentiate into melanocyte, adipocyte, osteocyte, and chondrocyte lineages has also been described by Herlyn and coworkers *(4)*.

Although evidence suggests that the majority of cancers depend on the presence of a cancer stem cell population for tumorigenicity, the origins of such neoplastic progenitors have not been unequivocally demonstrated. Cancer stem cells may initiate from mutations and/or epigenetic modifications in normal stem cells that reside in organ-specific stem cell niches such as the basal layer of the epidermis, the crypts of the intestine, the bone marrow, or the mammary gland terminal end buds *(10–13)*. Alternatively, as has been proposed for gastric cancer, mesenchymal stem cells recruited to the sites of inflammation or injury may transform into cancer stem cells *(14)*. Finally, tumor cells may undergo genetic and/or epigenetic modifications that result in the manifestation of a plastic, multiipotent phenotype. For example, Fine and colleagues recently reported that glioblastoma tumor initiating cells can result from the epigenetic silencing of the bone morphogenic protein receptor 1B (BMPR1B) promoter, and that demethylation of this site prevents glioblastoma tumorigenesis *(15)*. In addition, committed myeloid progenitor cells have been shown to initiate mixed lineage leukemia by reactivating genes normally restricted to hematopoietic stem cells *(16)*.

Evidence suggests that multipotent cancer cells have a profound, perhaps essential role in tumor initiation. It is also likely that by facilitating cancer cell adaptability, they allow tumor cells to evade conventional therapies and to metastasize. In support of this concept, global gene analyses suggest that aggressive cancer cell lines express genes that are normally restricted to other cell lineages concomitant with a reduction in the expression of genes specific to their cell of origin *(17)*. For example, aggressive melanoma and breast cancer cells coexpress intermediate filaments characterizing epithelial (Keratin) and mesenchymal (Vimentin) lineages, and aberrantly express genes, including *Vascular Endothelial Cadherin (VE-Cadherin)*, normally associated with endothelial cells *(17–20)*. Collectively, this gene expression pattern confers upon aggressive cancer cells a functional plasticity that enables them to thrive and metastasize. For instance, in melanoma and breast carcinoma, the coexpression of Keratin and Vimentin is associated with enhanced invasion and metastasis *(18)*, and VE-Cadherin is essential for the formation of tumor-derived perfusion networks, a feature that provides the tumor with an auxiliary perfusion pathway (called vasculogenic mimicry) *(18, 20, 21)*. Of note, Frank and colleagues recently demonstrated that in melanoma, VE-Cadherin is preferentially expressed in the ABCB5+ tumor initiating fraction, thereby suggesting that these stem cells may contribute to the functional plasticity of aggressive melanomas *(9)*. Hence, by targeting the factors that sustain cancer stem cell populations, therapies could eradicate tumor initiating cells and/or mitigate the cellular plasticity that are directly involved in tumor progression.

It is likely that cancer cells sustain a pluripotent phenotype through the aberrant expression of stem cell associated factors. Indeed, numerous studies have demonstrated that cancer cells and stem cells implement similar molecular messengers to regulate self-renewal, proliferation, and cell fate. These factors, classically associated with developmental processes, include members of the Wingless (Wnt), Notch, transforming growth factor-beta (TGF-β), and Hedgehog signaling pathways *(17, 22–26)*. For example, the Notch receptors and Nodal, a member of the TGF-β superfamily, are aberrantly expressed in a number of cancers, and this expression has been shown to mediate tumorigenesis and metastatic progression. This review will describe the emerging roles of Notch and Nodal in melanoma and breast carcinoma progression, and will review recent data suggesting that the Nodal signaling pathway may be a target for the epigenetic reprogramming of aggressive cancer cells.

NODAL SIGNALING AND CELL FATE

Nodal, an embryonic morphogen belonging to the TGF-β superfamily, is a potent mediator of stem cell fate. During embryogenesis, Nodal acts as an organizing signal before gastrulation, to initiate axis formation (27–29). Studies in zebrafish and mice have demonstrated that Nodal is required for mesoderm and endoderm formation. In mice, *nodal*-null embryos fail to form a primitive streak and are deficient in endoderm and mesoderm. Moreover, these mice die shortly after gastrulation. Zebrafish similarly require Nodal-like proteins (cyclops and squint) for mesoderm and endoderm induction. Indeed, double mutants for *squint* (*sqt*) and *cyclops* (*cyc*) lack head and trunk mesoderm and fail to form a germ ring, which is similar to the primitive streak (28, 30–32). In addition, Nodal has been shown to induce secondary axis formation when ectopically engrafted into zebrafish blastulas (33). The Nodal signaling pathway is also involved in the establishment of the left/right (L/R) patterning. In mice, Nodal is expressed symmetrically before and during gastrulation but is restricted to the left side of the node and lateral plate mesoderm during early segmentation. Nodal proteins are similarly localized to the left side in the chick, frog, and zebrafish. This restriction is essential for L/R asymmetry as ectopic Nodal expression can cause defects in L/R asymmetry of the heart and gut in chick, *Xenopus*, and zebrafish (28). Moreover, in mouse hypomorphic mutants lacking *nodal* expression in the left lateral plate mesoderm, defects occur in left-right body patterning, resulting in organ anomalies including random heart looping (28).

In an apparent paradox, Nodal also maintains pluripotency in the epiblast and trophectoderm compartments (34, 35) of the murine embryo, and has been shown to sustain the totipotentiality of embryonic stem cells cultured in vitro. Indeed, Nodal is one of the first genes to be down-regulated as totipotent human ES cells (hESCs) differentiate during embryoid body formation; and inhibition of the Nodal signaling pathway, through pharmacological inhibition of its receptor, results in hESC differentiation (35–38). We recently demonstrated that Nodal similarly maintains the multipotent phenotype of metastatic melanoma cells (23). Specifically, we found that Nodal is present in tumorigenic melanoma cell lines. Moreover, inhibition of Nodal expression in a multipotent human metastatic melanoma cell line (C8161) resulted in the reexpression of the pigment enzyme Tyrosinase, concomitant with a reduction in the expression of Keratin 8/18 and VE-Cadherin (23). Functionally, these phenomena were associated with decreased invasion through an extracellular matrix and a loss of paravascular network formation (vasculogenic mimicry). Hence, in this melanoma cell line Nodal is required for the maintenance of a dedifferentiated phenotype.

To better characterize the role of Nodal in the maintenance of pluripotency and tumorigenicity, we have examined its expression in a panel of human normal, neoplastic and stem cell types (summarized in Table 1) (39). Our analyses have revealed that in a manner similar to hESCs, melanoma and breast

Table 1
Summary of nodal cripto and lefty expression in human normal, cancer, and stem cell lines

	Melanoma	Melanocytes	Breast cancer	hMEpCs	hESCs	Amniotic fluid MSCs	Cord blood MSCs	Adult MSCs
Nodal	+	−	+	−	+	+*	−	−
Cripto	+*	−	+	−	+	+	−	−
Lefty	−	−	−	−	+	+*	−	−

Summary of results from Western blot analyses and RT-PCR of melanoma cell lines (C8161, WM278) primary human melanocytes, breast carcinoma cells lines (MDA-MB-231, MCF7, T47D, MDA-MB-468, MDA-MB-330, ZR75-30), primary human mammary epithelial cells (hMEpC), human embryonic stem cells (hESCs; H9, H1, MEL-2), human amniotic fluid derived stem cells, human cord blood derived stem cells and adult bone marrow derived mesenchymal stem cells.+ indicates expression in the majority of cell lines examined; − indicates lack of expression and; +* indicates expression but at negligible levels relative to hESCs.

carcinoma cells express Nodal. This is in contrast to corresponding normal cell types such as melano-cytes, myoepithelial cells, and primary human mammary epithelial cells, in which Nodal was not detected (39). We have also determined that umbilical cord blood-derived mesenchymal stem cells, amniotic fluid-derived stem cells, and adult MSCs express negligible levels of this protein. Previous studies from other laboratories have reported that *Nodal* mRNA is present in placenta, testis, and ovar-ian tissues, and we have similarly found that Nodal is expressed in a cytotrophoblast cell line. In addi-tion, embryological studies in mice have shown that Nodal expression is absent after the 12–14 somite stage and SAGE analyses have determined that Nodal expression is restricted to embryonic tissues such as hESCs and to cancers. Hence, it appears as though Nodal expression is largely restricted to very early progenitor and reproductive cell types and that it reemerges during tumorigenesis.

Nodal propagates its signal by binding to heterodimeric complexes between type I (ALK 4/7) and type II (ActRIIB) activin-like kinase receptors. Assembly of this complex results in the phospho-rylation and activation of ALK 4/7 by ActRIIB, followed by the ALK 4/7 mediated phosphorylation of Smad-2 and possibly Smad-3 (outlined in Fig. 1). Phosphorylated Smad 2/3 subsequently associates with Smad-4 and then translocates to the nucleus where it regulates gene expression through an association with transcription factors such as FoxH1 and Mixer (29). Genetic studies in zebrafish and mice have defined an essential role for Cripto-1, an epidermal growth factor-Cripto-1/FRL1/cryptic (EGF-CFC) family member, in Nodal function. Indeed, embryological studies have determined that Cripto-1 directly associates with ALK 4 (with its CFC domain) and Nodal (with its EGF domain) and that these associations may be required for Nodal to propagate its signal (40, 41). This prerequisite is perhaps best exemplified in Cripto-1 null mice, which die at day 7.5 due to the inability to gastrulate (a Nodal-dependent phenomenon) (42, 43). Studies have determined that Nodal may also signal in a Cripto-1-independent fashion. For example, Reissmann and colleagues revealed that Nodal can bind to activate ALK 7 in the absence of Cripto-1, but that Cripto-1 markedly enhances this process (44). Another study determined that the Nodal precursor can bind to ALK 4 in the extraembryonic ectoderm of the developing mouse embryo in a Cripto-1-independent manner, and that this binding results in the expression of Nodal-responsive genes (45). Finally, using murine knock out models, Liguori and colleagues recently demonstrated that Nodal can signal extensively and control axis specification in the absence of Cripto-1, if its inhibitor Cerberus is also knocked out (46). Like Nodal, Cripto-1 is highly expressed in cancer but is rarely detected in normal adult tissues. Cripto-1 is associated with a poor prognosis for breast cancer patients and has recently been documented as a serological marker for both breast and colon cancer (47, 48). Furthermore, Cripto-1, also called teratocarcinoma derived growth factor (TDGF), is a stem cell marker that is associated with the pluripotency of hESCs (48–50). In addition, Cripto-1 expression promotes dedifferentiation, vascu-larization, and invasion in breast carcinoma cells (51, 52). Given its importance in canonical Nodal signaling as well as its expression in cancer, we have recently measured Cripto-1 levels in a panel of normal, cancer, and stem cells lines (summarized in Table 1) (39). Using Western blot analysis and immunofluorescence microscopy, we determined that hESCs uniformly express high levels of Cripto-1; however, only a low level of Cripto-1 was heterogeneously expressed in C8161 and MDA-MB-231 cells (39). Moreover, unlike Nodal, which was expressed in all of the tumorigenic cancer lines examined, Cripto-1 transcript was more heterogeneously detected. Of note, umbilical cord derived mesenchymal stem cells and adult MSCs did not express Cripto-1, and although amni-otic fluid-derived stem cells expressed very little Nodal, these cells expressed relatively high levels Cripto-1. Hence, it appears as though Cripto-1 is associated with stem cell phenotypes; however, its expression pattern does not necessarily mirror that of Nodal. Future studies will explore the role of Cripto-1 in the Nodal-induced maintenance of pluripotency.

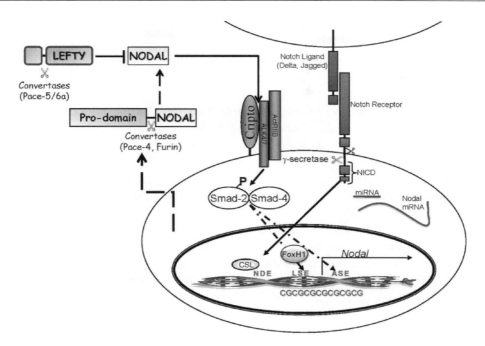

Fig. 1. The nodal signaling pathway. Nodal is secreted from the cell where it can act as an autocrine or paracrine factor. The Nodal precursor is cleaved and activated by the proprotein convertases (SPC), Pace-4 and Furin. This cleavage may occur inside the cell or in the extracellular space. Nodal binds to heterodimeric complexes between type I (ALK 4/7) and type II (ActRIIB) activin-like kinase receptors, resulting in the phosphorylation and activation of ALK 4/7 by ActRIIB, followed by the ALK 4/7 mediated phosphorylation of Smad-2 and possibly Smad-3. The epidermal growth factor-coreceptor (EGF-CFC), Cripto-1 (Cripto), is often a component of this receptor complex and can enhance Nodal signaling. Phosphorylated Smad-2/3 associates with Smad-4 and translocates to the nucleus where it regulates gene expression through the association with transcription factors such as FoxH1. Nodal up-regulates its own expression by stimulating transcriptional activation at the left side specific and asymmetric enhancers (LSE and ASE). Extracellular Nodal inhibitors, most notably Lefty-A and Lefty-B (Lefty), spatially and temporally restrict Nodal signaling levels through antagonism of Nodal and/or Cripto-1. The Lefty proteins are cleaved inside the cell (and likely in the extracellular space) by convertases, in particular Pace-5/6A. The Notch receptors become activated following binding to ligands, such as Delta and Jagged, expressed on adjacent cells. Once activated, the intracellular component of the Notch receptor (NICD) is released following a γ-secretase dependent cleavage. The NICD translocates to the nucleus where it interacts with CSL, a protein that binds to the DNA and inhibits transcription by associating with corepressor proteins. The NICD competes with these repressor proteins to form a NICD-CSL complex enabling the transcriptional activation of target genes, including Nodal, which has CSL binding domains in its node specific enhancer (NDE). Nodal levels may also be regulated by miRNA and possibly DNA methylation of a CpG island.

Nodal upregulates its own transcription via a positive feedback loop. To control the levels of this potent morphogen, hESCs also secrete Nodal inhibitors such as Lefty A, Lefty B, Cerberus, and Tomoregulin-1 (29, 53). Of these factors, the Lefty molecules, highly divergent members of the TGFβ superfamily, are expressed to the greatest extent. In fact, studies have demonstrated that in conjunction with Nodal and Oct 3/4, Lefty A and B are among the most enriched genes expressed in hESCs (53, 54). Like most members of the TGF-β superfamily, Lefty is cleaved by convertases. Proteolytic processing of the ~42 kDa Lefty precursor protein yields two forms of 34 kDa and 28 kDa (55). When compared with other convertases tested, Pace 5/6A has been found to be most efficient in cleavage of

Lefty A *(56)*; however, other convertases are also involved in Lefty processing *(53)*. The importance of this posttranslational modification was revealed in a recent study, in which Lefty processing was requisite for Nodal inhibition in a Xenopus model *(57)*. Lefty A and B specifically antagonize the Nodal signaling pathway by binding to and interacting with Nodal and/or with Cripto-1 in a manner that blocks ALK activation *(29, 58)*. This restriction of Nodal signaling can occur in the extracellular microenvironment, where Nodal and sometimes Cripto-1 are present, as well as at the cell surface. Of note, the Lefty proteins have not been found to bind ALK4 or ActRIIB; hence, these Lefty proteins are not competitive inhibitors of the ALK receptor complex. Furthermore, in embryological systems, the Lefty genes are often downstream targets of Nodal signaling, thereby providing a powerful negative-feedback loop for this pathway *(29, 58)*. We have recently analyzed Lefty expression in a panel of cell lines (summarized in Table 1). Our studies revealed that hESCs express Lefty protein, which is deposited into their microenvironment *(39)*. In contrast, Lefty is not expressed by metastatic breast carcinoma and melanoma cells or by corresponding normal somatic cell types. Of note, in contrast to hESCs, none of the other stem cell lines examined expressed an appreciable level of Lefty *(39)*. It should, however, be noted that these cells did not express Nodal. Indeed, the only cell types that expressed Nodal in the absence of Lefty were the cancer cells. We propose that this lack of feed-back inhibition allows Nodal signaling to go unchecked in tumor associated systems *(39, 59)*.

NODAL AS A MEDIATOR AND BIOMARKER OF TUMOR PROGRESSION

Our expression analyses indicate that Nodal is relatively restricted to tumorigenic and pluripotent stem cell lines. This raises an important question: Does Nodal regulate the tumor initiating/stem cell capacity of cancer cells? To this effect, studies in our laboratory have shown that Nodal is essential for tumorigenesis *(23, 39, 60)*. Using orthotopic mouse models, we have determined that knocking down Nodal expression in human melanoma (C8161) or breast carcinoma cells (MDA-MB-231) with Nodal targeting Morpholinos (MO[Nodal]) significantly mitigates the ability of these cells to form tumors (Table 2). For example, palpable subcutaneous tumors usually arise within 7 days following the injection of only 2.5×10^5 C8161 cells. However, when Nodal expression is knocked down in these cells, a 30% diminution of tumor incidence is observed and tumor growth is significantly inhibited *(23)*. To establish a mechanism for the reduction in tumorigenicity, we have since examined the effects of this treatment on in vivo tumor cell proliferation and apoptosis *(39)*. Using immunohistochemical staining for Ki67 as a measure of proliferation, and terminal deoxynucleotidyl transferase biotin-dUTP nick-end labeling (TUNEL) as a measure of apoptosis, we determined that inhibition of Nodal expression with MO[Nodal] decreases proliferation and increases apoptosis in orthotopic breast and melanoma tumors. These in vivo data support a role for Nodal in the maintenance of tumorigenicity

Table 2
Role of nodal expression in breast carcinoma and melanoma tumorigenesis

	MO[Control]	*MO[Nodal]*	*Control vector*	*Nodal*
MDA-MB-231 (4 weeks after injection)	907.94 ± 110.6	25.9 ± 12.9	N/A	N/A
C8161 (17 days after injection)	331 ± 71	67 ± 25.2	N/A	N/A
C81-61 (5 weeks after injection)	N/A	N/A	No tumors	72.1 ± 21.6

Summary of in vivo tumor formation in a mouse injected with MDA-MB-231 breast carcinoma and C8161 melanoma cells treated with either Control Morpholino or with Morpholino targeted against Nodal (MO[Control] or MO[Nodal]) or C81-61 cells transfected with either an empty vector or a Nodal expression construct. Values represent the mean tumor volume (mm³) ± standard error at the time of sacrifice. Tumor volumes were significantly different at the time points indicated ($p < 0.05$).

and implicate the potential involvement of apoptotic pathways. As a corollary to these studies, we have transfected non-tumorigenic, poorly invasive and well differentiated human melanoma cells (C81-61) with a vector encoding mature murine Nodal. In this cell line, overexpression of Nodal resulted in the acquisition of a tumorigenic phenotype (Table 2). Indeed, in contrast to control C81-61 cells, which are unable to form tumors, 100% of the animals injected with Nodal-expressing C81-61 cells formed palpable tumors within 5 weeks. It will be interesting to examine whether ectopic Nodal expression in poorly aggressive breast cancer cells will similarly promote tumor formation. In addition, future studies will involve the creation of transgenic animals that over-express the Nodal transgene driven by a mammary or melanocyte-specific promoter, so that the role of Nodal in tumor initiation may be deciphered.

Nodal expression is also positively correlated with melanoma and breast carcinoma progression clinically (Fig. 2). Immunohistochemical analysis has shown that Nodal protein is absent in normal skin and rare in poorly invasive RGP melanomas. This is in contrast to invasive VGP melanomas and melanoma metastases where Nodal expression is detectable in up to 60% of cases *(23)* (Fig. 2a). We have recently determined that Nodal correlates with clinical breast carcinoma progression *(39)*. Similar to normal skin, Nodal expression is absent in normal breast tissue. Moreover, Nodal is not detected in poorly invasive Ductal Carcinoma in situ (DCIS) but is observed later in more advanced

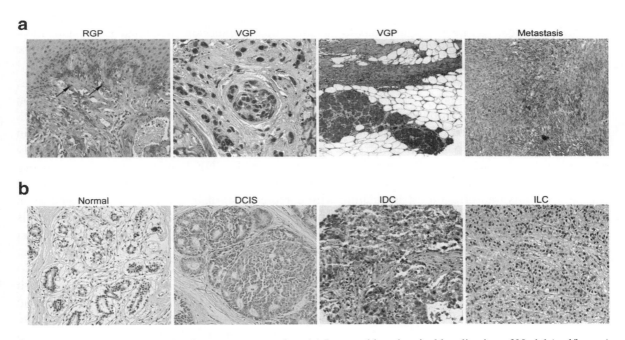

Fig. 2. Nodal as a new biomarker for tumor progression. (**a**) Immunohistochemical localization of Nodal (*red/brown*) in human melanoma. Sections (*left to right*) represent radial growth phase melanoma (RGP), vertical growth phase melanomas (VGP), and a melanoma metastasis in a lymph node biopsy. Note that RGP expresses relatively little Nodal; however, invasive cells begin to express Nodal as they leave the basal area and invade through the papillary dermis and dermal-epidermal junction toward the underlying reticular dermis (*arrows*). In contrast, strong expression of Nodal is seen in VGP melanoma cells that have invaded subcutaneous connective or adipose tissue. Nodal staining is also strong in melanoma cells that have metastasized to the lymph node. (**b**) Immunohistochemical localization of Nodal (*red/brown*) in human breast tissue. Sections (*left to right*) represent normal tissue from a reduction mammoplasty; localized ductal carcinoma in situ (DCIS); invasive ductal carcinoma (IDC) and invasive lobular carcinoma (ILC). Note that the normal tissue and DCIS do not express Nodal. In contrast, strong cytoplasmic staining for Nodal is detected in the invasive cancers (*see Color Plates*).

invasive carcinomas (IDC and ILC) and in metastatic lesions (Fig. 2b) *(39)*. Collectively, these results suggest that the acquisition of Nodal expression is associated with metastatic competence, which is obtained during the transition of a noninvasive cancer, such as DCIS or RGP melanoma, to an invasive lesion, such as IDC or VGP melanoma. Thus Nodal may be a biomarker of tumor progression – from a treatable local disease to a more aggressive invasive disease.

REGULATION OF NODAL EXPRESSION: CONVERGENCE WITH NOTCH

The Nodal signaling pathway is tightly regulated by a complex array of transcriptional regulators, posttranslational modifications, and extracellular factors (see Fig. 1 for summary). The human Nodal gene, containing 3 exons, is located on Chromosome 10q22.1. In mice, Nodal expression is enhanced by at least three separate transcriptional regulatory regions, the Node specific enhancer (NDE), approximately 10 kb upstream of the gene locus, the left side specific enhancer (LSE), approximately 4 kb upstream of the translational start site; and the asymmetric enhancer (ASE), located in the first intron *(61–63)*. Studies have determined that the LSE and the ASE are regulated by Nodal via a positive feedback loop that culminates in the activation of FoxH1. In contrast, the NDE has been shown to induce Nodal expression in response to Notch signaling *(64, 65)*. Gene alignments indicate that the human Nodal locus contains similar enhancer elements, so it is likely that human Nodal expression is regulated in a similar manner. Indeed, a positive feed-back loop, similar to that described for the LSE and ASE in mice, has been documented to sustain Nodal expression in human ESCs and, most recently, melanoma cell types *(23, 60, 66)*. Moreover, our preliminary studies indicate that like mouse Nodal, human Nodal is up-regulated by Notch signaling in cancer cells *(67)*.

There are four known mammalian Notch receptors (Notch1-4) and five ligands (Jagged1, Jagged2, Delta1, Delta3, and Delta4) *(68)*. The Notch receptors are activated by binding ligands expressed on adjacent cells. Upon activation, the Notch ectodomain is endocytosed by the ligand-bearing cell, exposing a site in the extracellular portion of the transmembrane domain for ADAM (A Disintegrin and Metalloproteinase) mediated cleavage *(69)*. the Notch intracellular domain (NICD) is subsequently released as a consequence of γ-secretase mediated cleavage. The NICD translocates to the nucleus where it interacts with CSL, a protein that binds to the DNA consensus sequence *CGTGGGAA* and normally inhibits transcription by associating with corepressor proteins. The NICD generated upon ligand-binding competes with these repressor proteins to form a NICD-CSL complex, which is recognized by Mastermind/Lag (MAML). This complex initiates transcriptional activation of target genes such as *Hes and Hey (64, 65, 68)* that have been shown to prevent the transcription of lineage specific genes including *Myo-D* and *Mash-1 (70)*. Of note, the NDE of the Nodal gene contains two CSL binding sites, and this region has been shown to respond to Notch signaling *(64, 65)*. Notch signaling has emerged as a major mediator of both melanoma and breast carcinoma progression *(71–74)*. Overexpression of Notch-4 inhibits the differentiation of breast epithelial cells and transgenic mice expressing constitutively active Notch-4 fail to develop mammary glands and eventually develop breast cancer *(75, 76)*. Notch has also been shown to sustain breast cancer tumor initiating cells *(71)*. Indeed, in a recent study, mammosphere formation by breast cancer cells was prevented by blocking Notch signaling with either a γ-secretase inhibitor (DAPT) or a Notch 4 neutralizing antibody *(75)*. Moreover, Notch 3 is enriched in CD44+ MCF-7 breast cancer initiating cells *(77)*. By preventing apoptosis, Notch has also been shown to maintain melanocyte stem cells, and constitutive Notch-1 expression is oncogenic in primary melanoma *(26, 72)*. We have recently determined that inhibiting Notch in metastatic melanoma cells with a γ-secretase inhibitor (DAPT) results in decreased Nodal expression. Moreover, using specific siRNAs, we have discovered that Notch-4 may preferentially regulate Nodal expression in these cells *(67)*.

Nodal expression is also governed by gene methylation and miRNA-directed degradation. For example, we have determined that there is a sizable CpG island (>1,300 bp) near the transcription start site (TSS) of the *Nodal* gene, and that this site may regulate Nodal expression *(59)*. Moreover, a novel miRNA (miR-430) has been shown to block the translation of a Nodal homolog, *squint*, in zebrafish *(78)*. MiR-430 target sites are also present in the mammalian *Nodal* gene; and so it is likely that Nodal expression is similarly affected by miRNA-mediated degradation in humans. Finally, posttranslational modifications by subtilisin-like proprotein convertases, including PACE-4 and Furin *(79)*, and by glycosylation also govern Nodal function. In a manner similar to most TGF-β family members, Nodal is synthesized as a proprotein that is activated following proteolytic processing by covertases *(29)*. Removal of the prodomain potentiates autocrine signaling but reduces Nodal stability and signaling range, thereby promoting autocrine signaling *(80)*. Conversely, glycosylation of mature Nodal increases the stability of this protein so that it can induce paracrine signaling events *(80)*.

The complexity of the Nodal signaling pathway likely underlies its propensity for aberrant expression in cancer. However, this complexity also affords a number of putative strategies for the inhibition of Nodal signaling and the circumvention of tumor progression. One such approach involves the epigenetic silencing of Nodal expression.

EPIGENETIC REPROGRAMMING OF MULTIPOTENT TUMOR CELLS

Although our studies provide correlative and functional evidence that Nodal is a regulator of tumor progression and plasticity, we do not understand how cancer cells acquire the ability to express this gene, which is normally restricted to embryonic lineages. Of note, the *Nodal* gene has been sequenced in hESCs and melanoma cells, and no differences or point mutations were detected *(39)*, suggesting that Nodal expression in cancer cells is acquired via epigenetic alterations. Epigenetic phenomena are theoretically reversible. Hence, the plastic, stem-cell-like phenotype of aggressive tumor cells should be receptive to reprogramming (i.e., redifferentiation) *(81)*. In support of this concept, embryonic microenvironments have been shown to inhibit the tumorigenicity of a variety of cancer cell lines *(81–83)*. For example, B16 murine melanoma cells were unable to form tumors and appeared to differentiate toward a neuronal phenotype following exposure to microenvironmental factors derived from the embryonic skin of a developing mouse *(81)*. In another set of experiments, Bissell and colleagues documented that Rous sarcoma virus, which causes a rapidly growing tumor when injected into hatched chicks, is nontumorigenic when injected into 4-day-old chick embryos, despite viral replication and v-src oncogene activation *(84)*.

More recently, we employed an in vitro 3D model to examine whether the microenvironment of human embryonic stem cells (hESCs) could similarly reprogram the multipotent phenotype of aggressive tumor cells *(39, 85)*. In this model, hESCs were allowed to "condition" a 3D matrix (CMTX), which would subsequently receive multipotent tumor cells. As such, the tumor cells are exposed to only the extracellular microenvironment of the hESCs, thereby removing the complexity of cell-cell interactions from the vast array of mechanisms that may be working to epigenetically modulate cell behavior. Utilizing this approach we determined that, similar to Nodal inhibition, exposure of melanoma cells to a hESC microenvironment results in the reexpression of Melan-A, a melanocyte specific marker, as well as a reduction in the expression of VE-Cadherin (Table 2) *(23, 60, 86)*. Moreover, aggressive melanoma (C8161) and breast carcinoma (MDA-MB-231) cells exposed to hESC microenvironments experienced a significant decrease in tumorigenicity concomitant with a marked reduction in Nodal expression *(39)*. For example, exposure to the hESC microenvironment significantly diminished anchorage-independent growth in the human tumor cells, a phenomenon that was partially rescued by the inclusion of rNodal (100 ng/mL) *(39)*. Moreover, exposure of these cells to hESC-derived CMTX resulted in an inhibition of tumor growth in an orthotopic mouse model (Fig. 3) *(39, 60)*. In a manner similar to Nodal inhibition, we found that exposure to hESC CMTX decreased proliferation and increased apoptosis in the orthotopic tumors *(39)*, implicating the potential involvement of apoptotic pathways in the tumor suppressive effects of the hESC microenvironment. Collectively, these findings illuminate the remarkable ability of hESC-derived factors to inhibit melanoma tumorigenicity and suggest that this tumor-suppressive phenomenon is at least partially mediated via an inhibition of Nodal expression and signaling. Of note, rNodal did not fully rescue the effects of the hESC microenvironment, suggesting that this milieu contains additional components that inhibit other protumorigenic factors.

The ability of hESCs to reprogram aggressive melanoma cells is reversible over time *(39, 59, 86)*. As such, this phenomenon is likely due to alterations in signaling. As summarized in Fig. 3, although aggressive cancer cells express Nodal and the coreceptor Cripto-1, they do not express Lefty-A/B: As a consequence, Nodal is allowed to signal in a deregulated manner in these tumor cells. This is in contrast to hESCs, which amply express all of the components of the Nodal signaling pathway, perhaps

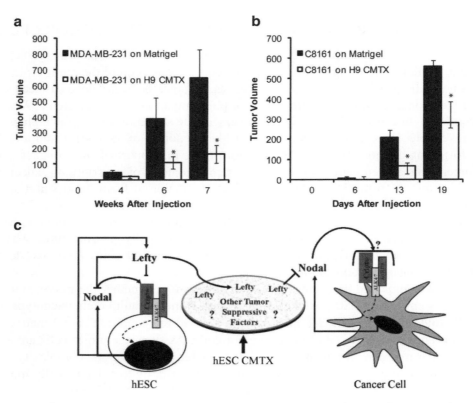

Fig. 3. Exposure of cancer cells to the hESC-derived Lefty decreases Nodal expression concomitant with reduced anchorage-independent growth and tumorigensis. In vivo tumor formation in a mouse injected with (**a**) MDA-MB-231 cells preexposed for 3 days to either a control matrix (Matrigel) or a matrix conditioned by hESCs (H9 CMTX) (*n* = 10) or (**b**) C8161 cells preexposed for 3 days to either a control matrix (Matrigel) or a matrix conditioned by hESCs (H9 CMTX) (*n* = 21). Values represent the mean tumor volume (mm^3) ± SE (**a**), or the median tumor volume (mm^3) ± interquartile range (**b**), and tumor volumes were significantly different at the time points indicated by an *asterisk* (*p* < 0.05). (**c**) Putative signaling model outlining how hESCs may reprogram metastatic cancer cells by inhibiting Nodal signaling. Nodal initiates a signaling cascade by binding to a receptor complex consisting of Cripto-1, type I (ALK 4/7).

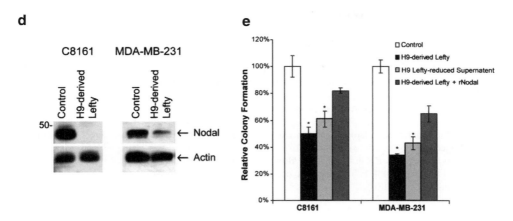

Fig. 3. (continued) and type II (ActRIIB) activin-like kinase receptors and is regulated via a positive feedback loop. hESCs secrete Nodal inhibitors, including Lefty, which antagonizes the Nodal signaling pathway by interacting with Nodal and/or Cripto. Like hESCs, cancer cells express Nodal while unlike hESCs they do not express Lefty. HESC-derived Lefty, found in hESC conditioned matrices (CMTX), may inhibit Nodal signaling in cancer cells and promote their reprogramming toward a less malignant phenotype. Other tumor suppressive factors may also be deposited by the hESCs. (**d**) Western blot analysis of Nodal protein in C8161 and MDA-MB-231 cells exposed for 3 days to either unconditioned control Matrigel or to Matrigel seeded with Lefty protein purified from hESCs (H9-derived Lefty). MDA-MB-231 cells were allowed to recover on fresh Matrigel for 2 days prior to analysis and Actin is used as a loading control. Exposure to Lefty reduced Nodal expression in the cancer cells. (**e**) Relative colony formation of C8161 and MDA-MB-231 cells cultured on soft agar for 14 days following 3 days of exposure to control Matrigel, Matrigel seeded with Lefty purified from hESCs (H9-derived Lefty), or Matrigel seeded with Lefty-reduced hESC supernatant. Assay was conducted in the presence or absence of rNodal (100 ng/mL). Bars represent mean normalized colony formation ± SD and values indicated by an *asterisk* are significantly different from the colony forming ability of control cells ($n = 6$, $p < 0.05$). Exposure to Lefty significantly reduced anchorage independent growth, and this effect was rescued by rNodal, suggesting that the effect of Lefty on clonogenicity is mediated via a reduction in Nodal expression.

enabling them to differentiate in response to microenvironmental cues. We, therefore, hypothesized that hESC-derived Lefty, found in hESC conditioned matrices (CMTX), may inhibit Nodal signaling in cancer cells and promote their reprogramming toward a less malignant phenotype. Utilizing Dynabeads covalently coupled to anti-Lefty antibody, we successfully isolated Lefty from hESC conditioned matrices. We then seeded this hESC-derived Lefty into an unconditioned matrix. Exposure of cancer cells to the "Lefty-spiked" microenvironment resulted in a diminution in Nodal expression associated with a significant reduction in anchorage-independent growth (Fig. 3) *(39)*. To further confirm these findings, we treated hESCs with MO[LEFTY] (to knock down Lefty-A/B) and demonstrated that Nodal expression was not inhibited in C8161 and MDA-MB-231 cells exposed to matrix derived from the "Lefty-deficient" hESCs. Collectively, these results revealed Lefty as a potent embryonic mediator that may be used to selectively reprogram multipotent tumor cells toward a nontumorigenic phenotype.

In summary, this review highlighted the challenging complexities underlying multipotent tumor stem cells, with a particular focus on the Nodal signaling pathway, its uncontrolled deregulation in aggressive melanoma and breast cancer cells, and molecular cross-talk with the Notch signaling pathway. The recent evidence summarized here regarding the aberrant expression by tumor cells of the embryonic morphogen Nodal illuminates a promising new avenue for therapeutic exploration and adds a new dimension to our understanding of cancer stem cells.

REFERENCES

1. Lapidot T, Sirard C, Vormoor J et al. A cell initiating human acute myeloid leukaemia after transplantation into SCID mice. Nature 1994; 367(6464):645–648.
2. Singh SK, Hawkins C, Clarke ID et al. Identification of human brain tumor initiating cells. Nature 2004; 432(7015):396–401.
3. Al-Hajj M, Wicha MS, ito-Hernandez A, Morrison SJ, Clarke MF. Prospective identification of tumorigenic breast cancer cells. Proc Natl Acad Sci USA 2003; 100(7):3983–3988.
4. Fang D, Nguyen TK, Leishear K et al. A tumorigenic subpopulation with stem cell properties in melanomas. Cancer Res 2005; 65(20):9328–9337.
5. Ponti D, Costa A, Zaffaroni N et al. Isolation and in vitro propagation of tumorigenic breast cancer cells with stem/progenitor cell properties. Cancer Res 2005; 65(13):5506–5511.
6. Sheridan C, Kishimoto H, Fuchs RK et al. CD44+/. Breast Cancer Res 2006; 8(5):R59.
7. Phillips TM, McBride WH, Pajonk F. The response of CD24(-/low)/CD44+ breast cancer-initiating cells to radiation. J Natl Cancer Inst 2006; 98(24):1777–1785.
8. Frank NY, Margaryan A, Huang Y et al. ABCB5-mediated doxorubicin transport and chemoresistance in human malignant melanoma. Cancer Res 2005; 65(10):4320–4333.
9. Schatton T, Murphy GF, Frank NY et al. Identification of cells initiating human melanomas. Nature 2008; 451(7176):345–349.
10. Toma JG, Akhavan M, Fernandes KJ et al. Isolation of multipotent adult stem cells from the dermis of mammalian skin. Nat Cell Biol 2001; 3(9):778–784.
11. Marshman E, Booth C, Potten CS. The intestinal epithelial stem cell. Bioessays 2002; 24(1):91–98.
12. Reya T, Morrison SJ, Clarke MF, Weissman IL. Stem cells, cancer, and cancer stem cells. Nature 2001; 414(6859):105–111.
13. Visvader JE, Lindeman GJ. Mammary stem cells and mammopoiesis. Cancer Res 2006; 66(20):9798–9801.
14. Houghton J, Stoicov C, Nomura S et al. Gastric cancer originating from bone marrow-derived cells. Science 2004; 306(5701):1568–1571.
15. Lee J, Son MJ, Woolard K et al. Epigenetic-mediated dysfunction of the bone morphogenetic protein pathway inhibits differentiation of glioblastoma-initiating cells. Cancer Cell 2008; 13(1):69–80.
16. Krivtsov AV, Twomey D, Feng Z et al. Transformation from committed progenitor to leukaemia stem cell initiated by MLL-AF9. Nature 2006; 442(7104):818–822.
17. Hendrix MJ, Seftor EA, Hess AR, Seftor RE. Vasculogenic mimicry and tumor-cell plasticity: lessons from melanoma. Nat Rev Cancer 2003; 3(6):411–421.
18. Hendrix MJ, Seftor EA, Chu YW et al. Coexpression of vimentin and keratins by human melanoma tumor cells: correlation with invasive and metastatic potential. J Natl Cancer Inst 1992; 84(3):165–174.
19. Hendrix MJ, Seftor EA, Hess AR, Seftor RE. Molecular plasticity of human melanoma cells. Oncogene 2003; 19;22(20):3070–3075.
20. Hendrix MJ, Seftor EA, Seftor RE, Trevor KT. Experimental co-expression of vimentin and keratin intermediate filaments in human breast cancer cells results in phenotypic interconversion and increased invasive behavior. Am J Pathol 1997; 150(2):483–495.
21. Hendrix MJ, Seftor EA, Meltzer PS et al. Expression and functional significance of VE-cadherin in aggressive human melanoma cells: role in vasculogenic mimicry. Proc Natl Acad Sci USA 2001; 98(14):8018–8023.
22. Hoek K, Rimm DL, Williams KR et al. Expression profiling reveals novel pathways in the transformation of melanocytes to melanomas. Cancer Res 2004; 64(15):5270–5282.
23. Topczewska JM, Postovit LM, Margaryan NV et al. Embryonic and tumorigenic pathways converge via Nodal signaling: role in melanoma aggressiveness. Nat Med 2006; 12(8):925–932.
24. Bittner M, Meltzer P, Chen Y et al. Molecular classification of cutaneous malignant melanoma by gene expression profiling. Nature 2000; 406(6795):536–540.
25. Weeraratna AT, Jiang Y, Hostetter G et al. Wnt5a signaling directly affects cell motility and invasion of metastatic melanoma. Cancer Cell 2002; 1(3):279–288.
26. Balint K, Xiao M, Pinnix CC et al. Activation of Notch1 signaling is required for beta-catenin-mediated human primary melanoma progression. J Clin Invest 2005; 115(11):3166–3176.
27. Smith WC, McKendry R, Ribisi S Jr, Harland RM. A nodal-related gene defines a physical and functional domain within the Spemann organizer. Cell 1995; 82(1):37–46.
28. Tian T, Meng AM. Nodal signals pattern vertebrate embryos. Cell Mol Life Sci 2006; 63(6):672–685.
29. Schier AF. Nodal signaling in vertebrate development. Annu Rev Cell Dev Biol 2003; 19:589–621.
30. Zhou X, Sasaki H, Lowe L, Hogan BL, Kuehn MR. Nodal is a novel TGF-beta-like gene expressed in the mouse node during gastrulation. Nature 1993; 361(6412):543–547.
31. Iannaccone PM, Zhou X, Khokha M, Boucher D, Kuehn MR. Insertional mutation of a gene involved in growth regulation of the early mouse embryo. Dev Dyn 1992; 194(3):198–208.
32. Conlon FL, Lyons KM, Takaesu N et al. A primary requirement for nodal in the formation and maintenance of the primitive streak in the mouse. Development 1994; 120(7):1919–1928.
33. Toyama R, O'Connell ML, Wright CV, Kuehn MR, Dawid IB. Nodal induces ectopic goosecoid and lim1 expression and axis duplication in zebrafish. Development 1995; 121(2):383–391.

34. Guzman-Ayala M, Ben-Haim N, Beck S, Constam DB. Nodal protein processing and fibroblast growth factor 4 synergize to maintain a trophoblast stem cell microenvironment. Proc Natl Acad Sci USA 2004; 101(44):15656–15660.
35. Mesnard D, Guzman-Ayala M, Constam DB. Nodal specifies embryonic visceral endoderm and sustains pluripotent cells in the epiblast before overt axial patterning. Development 2006; 133(13):2497–2505.
36. Vallier L, Reynolds D, Pedersen RA. Nodal inhibits differentiation of human embryonic stem cells along the neuroectodermal default pathway. Dev Biol 2004; 275(2):403–421.
37. Vallier L, Alexander M, Pedersen RA. Activin/Nodal and FGF pathways cooperate to maintain pluripotency of human embryonic stem cells. J Cell Sci 2005; 118:4495–4509.
38. James D, Levine AJ, Besser D, Hemmati-Brivanlou A. TGFbeta/activin/nodal signaling is necessary for the maintenance of pluripotency in human embryonic stem cells. Development 2005; 132(6):1273–1282.
39. Postovit LM, Margaryan NV, Seftor EA et al. Human embryonic stem cell microenvironment suppresses the tumorigenic phenotype of aggressive cancer cells. Proc Natl Acad Sci USA 2008; 105:4329–4334.
40. Yeo C, Whitman M. Nodal signals to Smads through Cripto-dependent and Cripto-independent mechanisms. Mol Cell 2001; 7(5):949–957.
41. Bianco C, Adkins HB, Wechselberger C et al. Cripto-1 activates nodal- and ALK4-dependent and independent signaling pathways in mammary epithelial Cells. Mol Cell Biol 2002; 22(8):2586–2597.
42. Liguori G, Tucci M, Montuori N et al. Characterization of the mouse Tdgf1 gene and Tdgf pseudogenes. Mamm Genome 1996; 7(5):344–348.
43. Ding J, Yang L, Yan YT et al. Cripto is required for correct orientation of the anterior-posterior axis in the mouse embryo. Nature 1998; 395(6703):702–707.
44. Reissmann E, Jornvall H, Blokzijl A et al. The orphan receptor ALK7 and the Activin receptor ALK4 mediate signaling by Nodal proteins during vertebrate development. Genes Dev 2001; 15(15):2010–2022.
45. Ben-Haim N, Lu C, Guzman-Ayala M et al. The nodal precursor acting via activin receptors induces mesoderm by maintaining a source of its convertases and BMP4. Dev Cell 2006; 11(3):313–323.
46. Liguori GL, Borges AC, D'Andrea D et al. Cripto-independent Nodal signaling promotes positioning of the A-P axis in the early mouse embryo. Dev Biol 2007; 315:280–289.
47. Gong YP, Yarrow PM, Carmalt HL et al. Overexpression of Cripto and its prognostic significance in breast cancer: A study with long-term survival. Eur J Surg Oncol 2006; 33(4):438–43.
48. Bianco C, Strizzi L, Mancino M et al. Identification of cripto-1 as a novel serologic marker for breast and colon cancer. Clin Cancer Res 2006; 12(17):5158–5164.
49. Adewumi O, Aflatoonian B, hrlund-Richter L et al. Characterization of human embryonic stem cell lines by the International Stem Cell Initiative. Nat Biotechnol 2007; 25(7):803–816.
50. Minchiotti G. Nodal-dependant Cripto signaling in ES cells: from stem cells to tumor biology. Oncogene 2005; 24(37):5668–5675.
51. Strizzi L, Bianco C, Normanno N et al. Epithelial mesenchymal transition is a characteristic of hyperplasias and tumors in mammary gland from MMTV-Cripto-1 transgenic mice. J Cell Physiol 2004; 201(2):266–276.
52. Normanno N, De LA, Bianco C et al. Cripto-1 overexpression leads to enhanced invasiveness and resistance to anoikis in human MCF-7 breast cancer cells. J Cell Physiol 2004; 198(1):31–39.
53. Tabibzadeh S, Hemmati-Brivanlou A. Lefty at the crossroads of "stemness" and differentiative events. Stem Cells 2006; 24(9):1998–2006.
54. Sato N, Sanjuan IM, Heke M, Uchida M, Naef F, Brivanlou AH. Molecular signature of human embryonic stem cells and its comparison with the mouse. Dev Biol 2003; 260(2):404–413.
55. Ulloa L, Creemers JW, Roy S, Liu S, Mason J, Tabibzadeh S. Lefty proteins exhibit unique processing and activate the MAPK pathway. J Biol Chem 2001; 276(24):21387–21396.
56. Tang M, Mikhailik A, Pauli I et al. Decidual differentiation of stromal cells promotes Proprotein Convertase 5/6 expression and lefty processing. Endocrinology 2005; 146(12):5313–5320.
57. Westmoreland JJ, Takahashi S, Wright CV. Xenopus Lefty requires proprotein cleavage but not N-linked glycosylation to inhibit nodal signaling. Dev Dyn 2007; 236(8):2050–2061.
58. Shen MM. Nodal signaling: developmental roles and regulation. Development 2007; 134(6):1023–34.
59. Postovit LM, Costa FF, Bischof JM et al. The commonality of plasticity underlying multipotent tumor cells and embryonic stem cells. J Cell Biochem 2007; 101(4):908–917.
60. Hendrix MJ, Seftor EA, Seftor RE, Kasemeier-Kulesa J, Kulesa PM, Postovit LM. Reprogramming metastatic tumor cells with embryonic microenvironments. Nat Rev Cancer 2007; 7(4):246–255.
61. Norris DP, Robertson EJ. Asymmetric and node-specific nodal expression patterns are controlled by two distinct cis-acting regulatory elements. Genes Dev 1999; 13(12):1575–1588.
62. Saijoh Y, Oki S, Tanaka C et al. Two nodal-responsive enhancers control left-right asymmetric expression of Nodal. Dev Dyn 2005; 232(4):1031–1036.
63. Vincent SD, Norris DP, Le Good JA, Constam DB, Robertson EJ. Asymmetric Nodal expression in the mouse is governed by the combinatorial activities of two distinct regulatory elements. Mech Dev 2004; 121(11):1403–1415.
64. Raya A, Kawakami Y, Rodriguez-Esteban C et al. Notch activity induces Nodal expression and mediates the establishment of left-right asymmetry in vertebrate embryos. Genes Dev 2003; 17(10):1213–1218.

65. Krebs LT, Iwai N, Nonaka S et al. Notch signaling regulates left-right asymmetry determination by inducing Nodal expression. Genes Dev 2003; 17(10):1207–1212.

66. Besser D. Expression of nodal, lefty-a, and lefty-B in undifferentiated human embryonic stem cells requires activation of Smad2/3. J Biol Chem 2004; 279(43):45076–45084.

67. Postovit LM, Seftor EA, Seftor RE, Hendrix MJ. Targeting Nodal in malignant melanoma cells. Expert Opin Ther Targets 2007; 11(4):497–505.

68. Bray SJ. Notch signalling: a simple pathway becomes complex. Nat Rev Mol Cell Biol 2006; 7(9):678–689.

69. Nichols JT, Miyamoto A, Olsen SL, D'Souza B, Yao C, Weinmaster G. DSL ligand endocytosis physically dissociates Notch1 heterodimers before activating proteolysis can occur. J Cell Biol 2007; 176(4):445–458.

70. Iso T, Kedes L, Hamamori Y. HES and HERP families: multiple effectors of the Notch signaling pathway. J Cell Physiol 2003; 194(3):237–255.

71. Farnie G, Clarke RB. Mammary stem cells and breast cancer-role of Notch signalling. Stem Cell Rev 2007; 3(2):169–175.

72. Pinnix CC, Herlyn M. The many faces of Notch signaling in skin-derived cells. Pigment Cell Res 2007; 20(6):458–465.

73. Nickoloff BJ, Osborne BA, Miele L. Notch signaling as a therapeutic target in cancer: a new approach to the development of cell fate modifying agents. Oncogene 2003; 22(42):6598–6608.

74. Callahan R, Egan SE. Notch signaling in mammary development and oncogenesis. J Mammary Gland Biol Neoplasia 2004; 9(2):145–163.

75. Farnie G, Clarke RB, Spence K et al. Novel cell culture technique for primary ductal carcinoma in situ: role of Notch and epidermal growth factor receptor signaling pathways. J Natl Cancer Inst 2007; 99(8):616–627.

76. Gallahan D, Jhappan C, Robinson G et al. Expression of a truncated Int3 gene in developing secretory mammary epithelium specifically retards lobular differentiation resulting in tumorigenesis. Cancer Res 1996; 56(8):1775–1785.

77. Shipitsin M, Campbell LL, Argani P et al. Molecular definition of breast tumor heterogeneity. Cancer Cell 2007; 11(3):259–273.

78. Choi WY, Giraldez AJ, Schier AF. Target protectors reveal dampening and balancing of Nodal agonist and antagonist by miR-430. Science 2007; 318(5848):271–274.

79. Beck S, Le Good JA, Guzman M et al. Extraembryonic proteases regulate Nodal signalling during gastrulation. Nat Cell Biol 2002; 4(12):981–985.

80. Le Good JA, Joubin K, Giraldez AJ et al. Nodal stability determines signaling range. Curr Biol 2005; 15(1):31–36.

81. Gerschenson M, Graves K, Carson SD, Wells RS, Pierce GB. Regulation of melanoma by the embryonic skin. Proc Natl Acad Sci USA 1986; 83(19):7307–7310.

82. Podesta AH, Mullins J, Pierce GB, Wells RS. The neurula stage mouse embryo in control of neuroblastoma. Proc Natl Acad Sci USA 1984; 81(23):7608–7611.

83. Pierce GB, Pantazis CG, Caldwell JE, Wells RS. Specificity of the control of tumor formation by the blastocyst. Cancer Res 1982; 42(3):1082–1087.

84. Dolberg DS, Bissell MJ. Inability of Rous sarcoma virus to cause sarcomas in the avian embryo. Nature 1984; 309(5968):552–556.

85. Postovit LM, Seftor EA, Seftor RE, Hendrix MJ. A 3-D model to study the epigenetic effects induced by the microenvironment of human embryonic stem cells. Stem Cells 2006; 24(3):501–505.

86. Abbott DE, Bailey CM, Postovit LM, Seftor EA, Margaryan NV, Hendrix MJ. The epigenetic influence of tumor and embryonic microenvironments: How different are they? Cancer Microenvironment. 2008; 1:13–21.

IV CANCER STEM CELLS IN SOLID TUMORS

9

Glioma Stem Cells in the Context of Oncogenesis

*Johan Bengzon, Elisabet Englund,
Leif G. Salford, and Xiaolong Fan*

ABSTRACT

Glioma is the most common primary tumor of adult central nervous system (CNS). Gliomas are hitherto classified according to morphological criteria, which is based on the assumption that relatively well-differentiated tumors are derived from mature glial cells, and poorly differentiated gliomas are derived from embryonic-like residual progenitor cells. Although the progression of grade I gliomas is seldomly observed, grade II gliomas often progress into grade III and IV gliomas, and grade IV glioma is also called glioblastoma (GBM) with dismal clinical outcomes. Recent studies have demonstrated that low as well as high-grade gliomas contain sphere initiating cells in neurosphere assays, a key property common to normal neural stem and progenitor cells. Glioma spheres can renew for multiple rounds and exhibit multilineage differentiation capacity. Sphere and xenograft-initiating glioma cells are operationally classified as glioma stem cells, and they represent a key target for glioma therapy. However, the relation between the putative glioma stem cells and the tumor initiating cells remains controversial. In this chapter, we review the evidence for the existence of glioma stem cells, and we discuss their relation to candidate glioma initiating cells using a glial cell ontogeny-based approach.

GLIOMAS CONTAIN HETEROGENEOUS TUMOR CELL POPULATIONS ACCORDING TO MORPHOLOGICAL CRITERIA

Gliomas represent the most common primary tumor in the adult human CNS. Classification of gliomas is, at present, based on morphological criteria. With the glial lineages as reference, gliomas are, according to the WHO classification, diagnosed into four major types: astrocytomas, oligodendrogliomas, mixed oligoastrocytomas, and ependymomas. Most gliomas are astrocytomas, and only about 10% of gliomas are of the oligodendro and oligoastrocytoma-type. Within the astrocytoma category, tumors are further subclassified into grade I to IV principally on the basis of extent of nuclear atypia, cell proliferation, microvascular density, and necrosis. Grade III gliomas are also termed anaplastic astrocytoma, and IV gliomas are termed glioblastoma multiforme (GBM). Oligodendrogliomas and mixed oligoastrocytomas are each divided into two grades (II and III) and ependymomas are classified into three grades (I–III). The part of the tumor showing the most malignant features determines the grade,

From: *Cancer Drug Discovery and Development: Stem Cells and Cancer,*
Edited by: R.G. Bagley and B.A. Teicher, DOI: 10.1007/978-1-60327-933-8_9,
© Humana Press, a part of Springer Science+Business Media, LLC 2009

which has implications for the therapy and prognosis. Grade I and II astrocytomas are relatively well differentiated, while grade III and IV tumors are anaplastic and highly invasive. It was traditionally assumed that low-grade gliomas arose from dedifferentiation of mature glial cells. However, since GBM cells are highly immature, it was presumed that they were derived from glial precursor cells with embryonic features *(1)*, so called glioblasts.

Compared with the well-established ontogeny-based classification of leukemias, the clinical significance of the current glioma classification is rather limited. Ideally, a classification of brain tumors would indicate the cell of origin, the lineage of origin, the stage of differentiation blockage, and even the driving genetic abnormalities. Such an "ideal" classification and diagnosis will provide guidance for improved and tailored treatment of brain malignancies. It can be envisaged that gliomas, in fact, are several distinct pathological entities. Grade I astrocytoma and grade II astrocytoma may arise from different cellular and genetic origins. Grade I astrocytomas seldomly progress into more malignant tumors, whereas most of the grade II astrocytomas do progress into high-grade gliomas (secondary GBMs). From the same glioma specimen, regions at grade II to IV progression stages can frequently be observed. The so-called de novo GBMs, which predominantly affects elder patients, are often diagnosed following a very short preceeding clinical history. Although the de novo and the secondary GBMs are morphologically similar, they may again have different cellular and molecular origins.

The clinical outcome for the vast majority of low-grade and high-grade gliomas has not been improved over the decades. The progression from low-grade to high-grade gliomas cannot be halted, and the 5-year survival rates of GBM are lower than 3% *(2)*. The identification of the tumor maintaining cell(s) is crucial for the development of more effective therapy. Although gliomas contain heterogeneous cell populations, genetic studies have firmly demonstrated their clonal origin. Thus, it is the initially transformed cell, which sustains the glioma development and generates the heterogeneous cell populations. However, it is challenging to identify the cell of origin in human glioma materials, because such cells are most likely rare, and their phenotype is likely drastically altered compared with their normal counterparts. Addressing this question in animal models will rely on introducing a candidate oncogene or a combination of oncogenes into a particular stem cell or progenitor cell type. Until now, most of the oncogenes identified in gliomas are common to other types of malignancies *(3)* and we are still awaiting the identification of specific glioma oncogenes, which can interfere with proliferation/survival and differentiation of neural stem cell or progenitor cells in the postnatal central nervous system.

In recent years, cancer stem cells have been identified as responsible for glioma initiation and maintenance, and they thus represent the key therapy target. Cancer stem cells were first identified in chronic myeloid leukemia (CML). In CML, the driving oncogene BCR-ABL, generated by 9:22 chromosomal translocation, is seeded in the long-term repopulating hematopoietic stem cells. However, CML is initially manifested in the overproduction of seemly mature granulocytes and the BCR-ABL positive CML stem cells represent only a minor fraction of the total population of neoplastic cells. With accumulation of more mutations, immature progenitor cells of either myeloid or lymphoid lineage are blocked with regard to further differentiation, which results in the end stage of disease. Thus, CML is initiated in stem cells, and its progression occurs in stem cells or its downstream progenitor cells *(4)*. The ability of leukemic stem cells to repopulate the entire tumor mass was demonstrated in acute myeloid leukemias. The malignancies are actually seeded in the true hematopoietic stem cells, and these transformed stem cells can regenerate leukemia, whereas their progenies cannot *(5)*. Motivated by the findings in leukemias, many research groups have identified stem cell-like subpopulations in solid tumors. Using the neurosphere assay, in combination with xenograft tumor initiation and gene expression analysis, putative cancer stem cells have been reported to exist in gliomas as well as in other types of brain tumors *(6–11)*.

EVIDENCE FOR THE EXISTENCE OF GLIOMA STEM CELLS

According to the traditional view, it is assumed that mutations occurring in mature glial cells results in oncogenic transformation. In such a model, the so-called stochastic model, although the glioma is composed of phenotypically heterogeneous cells, virtually all of them can function as tumor-initiating and maintaining cells. In contrast, the hierarchical model suggests that neoplastic transformation of one stem or glial precursor cell results in glioma initiation and development. The initiating cell is able to self-renew, and termed a cancer stem cell. The bulk of glioma cells, although heterogeneous in morphology, are unable to self-renew and to sustain glioma growth. Thus, only a subpopulation of cells within the tumor can produce neoplastic cells. The definition of a cancer stem cell bears resemblance to the definition of normal tissue stem cells. Strictly, cancer stem cells must fulfill the following criteria: (1) extensive self-renewal ability, (2) cancer-initiating ability upon orthotopic implantation, (3) aberrant differentiation properties and capacity to produce nontumorigenic progeny that recapitulates the cellular composition of the parental tumor, and (4) karyotypic and genetic alterations.

It is important to note that the term glioma stem cell does not take into account the cell of origin. Considering the limitation of the assays used to assess cancer stem cell features, these cells must be studied in the context of tumorigenesis. Without clarifying the lineage and differentiation stages of the heterogeneous glioma cell populations along the normal glial development hierachy, stem cell studies cannot resolve the issue whether reported stem cell features reflect true tumor-initiating capabilities or if they are merely assay dependent. We will first review the current literature on glioma stem cells based on the above-mentioned criteria. Subsequently, we will assess the relationship between brain cancer stem cells and normal neural stem and progenitor cells.

Glioma Stem Cell Self Renewal Capacity

Self-renewal capacity can be assayed by in vitro sphere-formation when a single cell suspension from glioma is grown in specialized serum free medium supplemented with epidermal growth factor and basic fibroblast growth factor *(12)*. However, as discussed by Singec et al. *(13)*, nearly all dividing cells form spheres when grown in serum free media on a nonadherent substrate. Furthermore, the commonly used neurosphere assay, which has been used as a surrogate assay to isolate and expand neural stem cells, neural progenitor cells, and cancer stem cells, have serious limitations. The majority of cells within a neurosphere are nonstem cells; in addition, neurospheres readily fuse into larger aggregates in vitro, which makes it difficult to measure the clonality of single cells *(13, 14)*. In spite of the potential flaws in the technical strategy, several research groups have investigated whether brain tumors, including gliomas, contain cells capable of forming self-renewing spheres. Following an initial report by Ignatova et al. *(8)*, the existence of sphere-forming cells in grade I as well as II–IV gliomas, in medulloblastomas and ependymomas has been reported by several groups *(6, 7, 9–11)*, thus suggesting the presence of self-renewing stem-cell-like cells in these tumors. The self-renewing cell population was subsequently demonstrated to exist in the fraction of primary brain tumor cells expressing CD133 *(9, 10)*. CD133 has been identified as a characteristic cell surface marker for several types of stem cells, including embryonic neural stem cells *(15, 16)*, hematopoietic stem cells *(17, 18)*, prostatic epithelial stem cells *(19)*, endothelial precursor cells *(20)*, and multipotent progenitor cells in adult human kidney *(21)*. CD133 expression can also be detected in primitive leukemia cells and tumor initiating colon cancer cells *(17, 22, 23)*. In the postnatal CNS, CD133 expression can only be detected in ependymal cells, but not in SVZ neurogenic astrocytes *(24)*. Within GBM, this cell fraction can constitute 0–90% of the tumor cells *(9, 10, 25)*. Following magnetic bead cell-sorting, single CD133-positive cells formed tumor spheres, whereas CD133-negative cells did not *(9, 10)*.

However, not every CD133-positive cell generated spheres in vitro in these studies. Different subtypes of GBM might have different cells of origin, and their cells may behave differently in neurosphere assays. For example, secondary GBM derived cells did not form spheres in a recent study, suggesting the absence of neural stem-cell-like tumor cells, whereas a majority of primary GBMs contained a significant CD133-positive subpopulation that displayed sphere growth and asymmetrical cell divisions *(26)*. Some cell lines derived from primary GBM in the same study were apparently generated by CD133-negative tumor cells that fulfilled stem cell criteria. Thus, CD133-positive cancer stem cells seem to maintain only a subset of primary GBMs *(26)*.

Most of the studies have focused on GBM, the self-renewal capacity of low-grade glioma cells, and the tumor cells following transition from low to high-grade gliomas is considerably less well studied. Low-grade gliomas contained fewer cells capable of generating self-renewable spheres compared with high-grade glioma cells *(9)*. The lower-grade astrocytomas typically had a lower CD133 fraction compared with high-grade gliomas, and the frequency of cells capable of sphere formation appeared to correlate with the clinical aggressiveness of the different tumor phenotypes *(9, 25)*. Importantly, CD133 expressing cells in low-grade gliomas might be predominantly of vessel origin, as demonstrated by the concomitant expression of vessel endothelial marker CD31 *(25)*.

Glioma Initiating Ability In Vivo

The cancer-initiating ability upon orthotopic implantation is tested in in-vivo grafting experiments. After enrichment of putative glioblastoma stem cells by sphere-culturing technique *(6)*, sphere-derived cells were capable of initiating and propagating glioma-like tumors in severe immune deficient mice (SCID) in serial transplantation trials, whereas nonsphere cultured populations did not form tumors. By using CD133 as a positive selection marker for primary tumor cells, Singh et al. first reported that CD133-positive GBM cells gave rise to serially transplantable xenograft tumors in the SCID mouse brain *(10)*. The tumor morphology and the assessed lineage marker expression resembled the original tumors and generated both CD133-positive and CD133-negative cells *(6, 10)*. CD133-negative tumors cells were not tumorigenic in SCID mice *(9, 10)*. However, more recent studies suggest that CD133 expression is not required for GBM initiation but that this protein may be involved in tumor progression *(25, 27)*. The ambiguous results using CD133 as a cancer stem cell marker might, at least in part, reflect the ability of transplanted human tumor cells to grow in a foreign environment (i.e., immunocompromised mice) rather than demonstrating cancer stem cell characteristics of these cells *(28)*. Alternatively, subgroups of GBMs exist, and each type of tumor may contain different tumor-initiating cells. Furthermore, although CD133 expression is used as a stem cell marker, the function of CD133 is not known and the relation between CD133 expression and "stemness" is uncertain. It can be envisaged that GBM cells not expressing CD133 are endowed with cancer stem cell activity *(25, 26)*.

Glioma Stem Cell Multilineage Differentiation Capacity

In several early studies, glioma-derived tumor cell spheres were shown to be multipotent and could differentiate into cells expressing neuronal and glial cell markers *(6, 7, 9–11)*. However, it is important to realize that GBMs are highly anaplastic and composed of heterogeneous cell populations at variable differentiation stages. In addition, glioma stem cell differentiation characteristics are influenced by the genetic instability and genome changes known to be present in these cells, as well as by the tumor microenvironment. Thus, glioma stem cell progeny phenotype likely displays highly aberrant protein expression patterns compared with normal neural lineages. Single markers from each lineage (β-III tubulin/TuJ1 or MAP-2 for neuronal lineage) cannot be used unambiguously in vitro or in vivo to evaluate multilineage potentiality *(6–11)*. Of note, the human A2B5-positive glial progenitor cells also express β-III tubulin, but such cells do not express other neuronal markers, and cannot generate neurons even under neuronal differentiating conditions *(29)*. Therefore, differentiation capacity of isolated putative glioma stem cells must be evaluated by the capacity to produce nontumorigenic progeny that recapitulate the cellular composition of the parental glioma, as is demonstrated by the generation of CD133-positive and negative cells following in vivo transplantation of CD133-positive GBM cells in SCID mice *(10)*. It is, however, not known if the CD133-positive tumor cell population constitutes a homogenous cell population and, consequently, the multilineage potentiality of individual cells within the CD133-positive fraction cannot be determined. It is likely that only a subset of cells within the CD133-positive population are true cancer stem cells with the potential to differentiate and produce all the tumor cell phenotypes within a human GBM. It is also important to assess whether the multilineage differentiation capacity can be directly demonstrated in gliomas in situ.

Karyotypic and Genetic Alterations

As demonstrated in murine glioma models *(30)*, transformed glioma cells can provide a niche environment recruiting normal stem cells or progenitor cells into the glioma mass. It is, therefore, necessary to demonstrate that the putative glioma stem cells are not normal CNS stem/progenitor cells recruited into the glioma. In accordance with this requisite, findings of abnormal karyotypes in GBM sphere cells has confirmed the neoplastic nature of the putative glioma stem cells *(6, 10, 11)*. However, one has to bear in mind that karyotype analysis does not allow the identification of detailed genetic alterations. Furthermore, constitutional aneuploidy has been observed in the normal human brain *(31)*.

In summary, the evidence supporting the glioma stem cell hypothesis have predominantly been generated in high-grade gliomas. Considering the progression of gliomas and the stepwise accumulation of multiple mutations required for tumorigenesis, the question will arise whether grade I and II gliomas also contain putative glioma stem cells. Despite that sphere-formation was demonstrated with low-grade glioma cells, the xenograft glioma initiating capacity as well as the genetic alterations of low-grade glioma cells are poorly characterized. We think that the major concern with previous studies on the identification of glioma stem cells is that tumor stem cell properties are predominantly demonstrated using analysis of serial sphere formation and multilineage differentiation in vitro. Because sphere assays to a substantial extent are influenced by the in vitro conditions, sphere assays can therefore not distinguish whether the initial input cells are multipotent stem cells, or lineage restricted progenitor cells. For most of the studies, it is a concern whether the stem-cell-like cells identified in sphere assays authentically represent the driving cell population in glioma.

GLIOMA STEM CELLS IN THE CONTEXT
OF GLIOMA ONCOGENESIS

By analyzing the polymorphic locus from the X chromosomal androgen receptor gene in histologically distinct regions of glioma specimens, the monoclonal origin of gliomas, irrespective of their astrocytoma, oligodendrocytoma, or oligoastrocytoma phenotype has been demonstrated *(32, 33)*. This conclusion is further supported by chromosomal and microsatellite analysis *(34, 35)*. Thus, gliomas are initiated from a single cell. The heterogeneous cell populations can theoretically be generated due to differentiation blockage at uncommitted differentiation stage(s) or at a lineage-commited differentiation stage. It is, therefore, possible to envisage that certain cell populations can be assessed as glioma stem cells in sphere forming assays, whereas others will not be detected. An absolute link between the hitherto identified glioma stem cells and the glioma initiating cells does therefore not exist. Below we discuss glioma oncogenesis in relation to cancer stem cells.

Gliomas are very likely generated due to subverted proliferation and differentiation in neural stem or progenitor-like cells in postnatal neural genesis. Multipotent neural stem cells exist in adult rodent and primate CNS *(36–38)*. The largest neurogenic niche in the adult rodent brain is the subventricular zone (SVZ). In the adult human brain, de novo neuronal genesis has been demonstrated in hippocampus and subventricular zone/rostral migratory stream *(39–42)*. In contrast to the restricted regions of neuronal progenitors, significant numbers of proliferating oligodendrocyte progenitors exist scattered in the cerebral hemispheres and such cells account for <0.5% of the total white matter cells *(43, 44)*. The oligodendrocyte lineage progenitor cells express A2B5, NG-2, and PDGFR-α as characteristic surface markers *(44–48)*. These NG2-positive cells continue to divide slowly throughout adult life, and they can, however, proliferate rapidly in response to CNS damage. Although these cells appear to only generate oligodendrocyte cells in transplantation assays *(49)*, they are endowed with a large extent of differentiation plasticity. When cultured under serum-containing media, they will generate type-2 astrocytes expressing A2B5 and GFAP and be further reprogrammed with multilineage differentiation capacity *(50)*. The astrocyte lineage restricted progenitor cells, which can be identified by A2B5 and CD44, but not PDGFR-α expression during the development *(51)*, have been less well studied in the adult human brain.

Accumulating evidence implies normal neural stem cells or neural progenitor cells as the glioma initiating cells *(52–57)*. It can be envisaged that oncogenic transformation of neural stem cells or noncommitted neural progenitor cells would generate and expand a great diversity of cell types, which are not, or rarely, observed in the normal CNS. Such a scenario would generate high grade gliomas without a preceeding clinical history. Putative glioma stem cells can be found within these diverse cell populations. If lineage committed progenitors, such as oligodendrocyte lineage-restricted progenitors or the astrocyte-lineage restricted progenitor cells are transformed, the resulting neoplastic growth would be more homogeneous with similarities to low-grade gliomas. In this scenario, the accumulation of genetic alternations will contribute to the progression of the glioma and emerging glioma stem cells are likely a result of the progressive transforming events. It can also be envisaged that the initial "seeding" mutation occurs in a neural stem cell or noncommitted progenitor cells, but such mutation is manifested in their progenies along the glial lineage.

In addition to the sphere formation capacity, the resemblance between putative glioma stem cells and primitive neural progenitor cells is also supported by shared gene expression patterns. Glioma cell gene expression is affected by transforming events, and its gene expression pattern will still maintain similarity to their normal counterparts. Although the role of CD133 expression in the maintenance of "stemness" is unknown and a causal link between CD133 expression and stem cell features has not been proven in cancer stem cells, CD133 expression was detected in cells from a substantial fraction of high-grade gliomas *(9, 25, 26, 44)*. In contrast to the heterogeneous CD133 expression between different gliomas and within the same glioma specimens, homogeneous expression of glial progenitor cells markers were found in these tumors at different grades. All gliomas express CD44 and A2B5 *(25)*. CD44 is a marker of astrocyte-restricted progenitor cells *(51)*, and A2B5 is expressed in glial restricted progenitor cells, oligodendrocyte progenitor cells, and astrocyte-restricted progenitor cells *(46–48)*. In addition to CD44 and A2B5, glioma cells can also express the oligodendrocyte-linage progenitor markers NG2, PDGFR-α, and O4 *(25, 58, 59)*. Our demonstration of concomitant expression of A2B5, O4 and other glial progenitor surface markers in freshly dissected living glioma cells without in vitro manipulation is in contrast to previous reports on astrocytomas using fixed specimens *(60, 61)*. Importantly, the transcription factor Olig2, which is critical for generation of

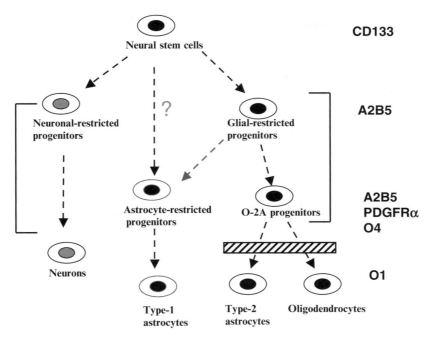

Fig. 1. Heterogeneous glioma cell populations in relation to glial genesis hierarchy. Glioma cells express a number of surface markers characterizing glial genesis hierarchy *(25)*, the pattern of glial progenitor marker expression implies that cells from the majority of gliomas are blocked at the differentiation stage between the O-2A progenitor cells and mature oligodendrocytes or type-2 astrocytes. In contrast to low-grade astrocytoma, high-grade gliomas show neuronal lineage differentiation potential, regardless of the level of CD133 expression.

oligodendrocyte progenitor cells from uncommitted progenitor cells, was found to be expressed in a large number of glioma cells *(62, 63)*. The concomitant expression of these markers appears not to be caused by genetic alterations. As depicted in Fig. 1, coexpression of glial progenitor cell markers indicates a common differentiation blockage stage. Interestingly, neuronal differentiation potential, as assessed by neuron specific enolase (NSE) immunolabelling, was not detected in low-grade gliomas (Fig. 2). In contrast, high-grade gliomas were frequently labeled by NSE and synaptophysin. Thus, although high-grade and low-grade gliomas share the expression pattern of glial progenitor cell surface markers, neuronal differentiation potential could only be detected in high-grade gliomas *(25)*. It remains to be established whether the in vivo multilineage differentiation capacity observed in high grade tumors can be gained following progression from low-grade to high-grade gliomas.

Most likely, low-grade gliomas are arrested at differentiation stages between the A2B5/O4 and O1 stage. However, immature cells with CD133 expression are few in low-grade gliomas. Although arrested at a differentiation level similar to the low-grade gliomas, high-grade gliomas can, in contrast to low-grade tumors, also express markers for putative stem cells and progenitor cells of neuronal and glial lineages (Fig. 1). In accordance with the shared glial progenitor surface marker expression, aberrant activation or inactivation of signaling pathways crucial for glial genesis can be detected in glioma cells. It has been demonstrated that normal adult human A2B5 cells are endowed with constitutively activated Notch signaling *(44)*. In normal neural stem cells or noncommitted primitive neural progenitor cells, activation of Notch signaling can drive the cell fate decision toward the glial lineage at the expense of neuronal lineage *(64)*. However, persistent Notch signaling activation blocks oligodendrocyte progenitor cell differentiation *(65)*. In concordance, the activation of Notch, Notch

Pilocytic
astrocytoma

GBM

GFAP

NSE

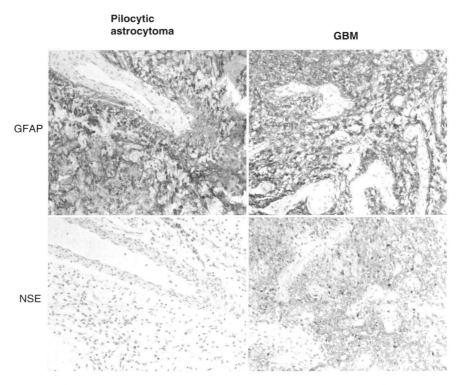

Fig. 2. Neuronal differentiation potential can be detected in high-grade, but not in low-grade gliomas. Archived glioma specimens were sectioned and stained for NSE, synaptophysin, and GFAP. GFAP can be detected in all cases of gliomas, whereas NSE and synaptophysin were only detected in high-grade glioma specimens *(25) (see Color Plates).*

ligand Delta-like-1, and Jagged-1 as well as their downstream signaling molecules are reported in gliomas *(66, 67)* and inhibition of Notch signaling resulted in diminished proliferation capacity of GBM cells *(68).*

CLINICAL IMPLICATIONS OF GLIOMA STEM CELLS

The classification of gliomas is currently based on histological criteria, which is less relevant than the cell-of-origin and the tumor cell differentiation status. Ideally, an ontogeny-based classification along the postnatal neural genesis shall be established, which will provide more precise diagnoses and potentially guide therapy. The identity and characterization of putative glioma stem cells regarding their potential in sustained proliferation, tumorigenic capacity and differentiation stages along the neural genesis hierarchy, will provide a new means for glioma classification.

The identification of glioma stem cells also suggests the importance of targeting these cells for glioma therapy. The sustained effect of any therapy will be dependent if such therapy can hit the stem cell population within the heterogeneous glioma cell population. The concept of glioma stem cells also implies that gliomas can be cured if the differentiation blockage of glioma stem cells or their progenies could be overcome. In fact, long-term survivors were observed in 3 out 10 GBM patients treated with the differentiation reagent retinoic acid *(69).* Along the same line, cell differentiation strategies have shown that bone morphogenetic proteins (BMPs) reduce the tumor-initiation capability of CD133-positive brain tumor cells *(70).* BMPs play a pivotal role in specification of neural stem cells during embryogenesis *(71)*, and Piccirillo et al. demonstrated the presence of BMP and their receptors on human GBM cells *(70)*. A significant reduction in stem-like, tumor-initiating precursors of human GBMs was seen after exposure to BMPs, amongst which BMP-4 elicited the strongest effect. In vivo delivery of BMP-4 resulted in abolished tumor growth after intracerebral grafting of human GBM cells. In another study, the effect of blockade of the Hedgehog pathway, a signaling pathway normally acting in nonneoplastic stem cells, was shown to deplete stem-like cancer cells in GBM *(72)*. GBM cells thus may retain a capability to respond to differentiation signals normally acting on neural precursor cells during embryogenesis. The issue of radiation resistance in GBM stem cells has been addressed by Bao et al. *(73)*. In this study, it was demonstrated that stem cells contribute to glioma radioresistance. The fraction of tumor cells expressing CD133 was enriched after radiation in gliomas in both cell culture experiments and in the brains of immunocompromised mice. Furthermore, it was demonstrated that CD133-expressing GBM cells preferentially activate the DNA damage checkpoint in response to radiation, and CD133 positive cells were shown to repair radiation-induced DNA damage more effectively than CD133-negative tumor cells. The authors proposed that targeting of the DNA damage checkpoint response in GBM cells may reduce the radioresistance.

Future studies that address the action of chemotherapy and radiotherapy on brain tumor stem cells are much warranted. In addition, efforts to elucidate the inherent immunological features of glioma stem cells needs to be performed. Furthermore, the relationship between glioma stem cells and the tumor microvasculature and the tumor stem cell niche needs to be further clarified to tailor future effective glioma treatments.

CONCLUDING REMARKS

Although a large body of knowledge on glioma has been generated over the decades, a cure for glioma still does not exist. Identifying the driving cell population among the heterogeneous glioma cell populations is of course important for clarifying the mechanisms of glioma oncogenesis as well as for therapy development. However, it remains controversial whether the putative glioma stem cells identified in sphere and/or xenograft tumor-initiating assay represent the authentic driving cell populations in human gliomas. Characterizing postnatal CNS stem cells and progenitor cells regarding their proliferation and differentiation capacity, and their potential of being transformed by relevant oncogenes in their proper brain microenvironment will be needed to resolve the current controversy.

REFERENCES

1. Kleihues P, Burger PC, Collins VP, Newcomb EW, Ohgaki H, Cavenee WK. Glioblastoma, in: Tumours of the Nervous System, Pathology and Genetics. World Health Organization Classification of Tumours. Lyon: IARC press; 2000.
2. Louis DN, Holland EC, Cairncross JG. Glioma classification: a molecular reappraisal. Am J Pathol 2001;159(3):779–86.
3. Maher EA, Furnari FB, Bachoo RM, et al. Malignant glioma: genetics and biology of a grave matter. Genes Dev 2001; 15(11):1311–33.
4. Faderl S, Talpaz M, Estrov Z, O'Brien S, Kurzrock R, Kantarjian HM. The biology of chronic myeloid leukemia. N Engl J Med 1999;341(3):164–72.
5. Bonnet D, Dick JE. Human acute myeloid leukemia is organized as a hierarchy that originates from a primitive hematopoietic cell. Nat Med 1997;3(7):730–7.
6. Galli R, Binda E, Orfanelli U, et al. Isolation and characterization of tumorigenic, stem-like neural precursors from human glioblastoma. Cancer Res 2004;64(19):7011–21.
7. Hemmati HD, Nakano I, Lazareff JA, et al. Cancerous stem cells can arise from pediatric brain tumors. Proc Natl Acad Sci USA 2003;100(25):15178–83.
8. Ignatova TN, Kukekov VG, Laywell ED, Suslov ON, Vrionis FD, Steindler DA. Human cortical glial tumors contain neural stem-like cells expressing astroglial and neuronal markers in vitro. Glia 2002;39(3):193–206.

9. Singh SK, Clarke ID, Terasaki M, et al. Identification of a cancer stem cell in human brain tumors. Cancer Res 2003; 63(18):5821–8.

10. Singh SK, Hawkins C, Clarke ID, et al. Identification of human brain tumour initiating cells. Nature 2004;432(7015):396–401.

11. Yuan X, Curtin J, Xiong Y, et al. Isolation of cancer stem cells from adult glioblastoma multiforme. Oncogene 2004; 23(58):9392–400.

12. Reynolds BA, Weiss S. Generation of neurons and astrocytes from isolated cells of the adult mammalian central nervous system. Science 1992;255(5052):1707–10.

13. Singec I, Knoth R, Meyer RP, et al. Defining the actual sensitivity and specificity of the neurosphere assay in stem cell biology. Nat Methods 2006;3(10):801–6.

14. Reynolds BA, Rietze RL. Neural stem cells and neurospheres–re-evaluating the relationship. Nat Methods 2005;2(5):333–6.

15. Uchida N, Buck DW, He D, et al. Direct isolation of human central nervous system stem cells. Proc Natl Acad Sci USA 2000;97(26):14720–5.

16. Weigmann A, Corbeil D, Hellwig A, Huttner WB. Prominin, a novel microvilli-specific polytopic membrane protein of the apical surface of epithelial cells, is targeted to plasmalemmal protrusions of non-epithelial cells. Proc Natl Acad Sci USA 1997;94(23):12425–30.

17. Miraglia S, Godfrey W, Yin AH, et al. A novel five-transmembrane hematopoietic stem cell antigen: isolation, characterization, and molecular cloning. Blood 1997;90(12):5013–21.

18. Yin AH, Miraglia S, Zanjani ED, et al. AC133, a novel marker for human hematopoietic stem and progenitor cells. Blood 1997;90(12):5002–12.

19. Collins AT, Habib FK, Maitland NJ, Neal DE. Identification and isolation of human prostate epithelial stem cells based on alpha(2)beta(1)-integrin expression. J Cell Sci 2001;114(Pt 21):3865–72.

20. Peichev M, Naiyer AJ, Pereira D, et al. Expression of VEGFR-2 and AC133 by circulating human CD34(+) cells identifies a population of functional endothelial precursors. Blood 2000;95(3):952–8.

21. Sagrinati C, Netti GS, Mazzinghi B, et al. Isolation and characterization of multipotent progenitor cells from the Bowman's capsule of adult human kidneys. J Am Soc Nephrol 2006;17(9):2443–56.

22. O'Brien CA, Pollett A, Gallinger S, Dick JE. A human colon cancer cell capable of initiating tumour growth in immunodeficient mice. Nature 2007;445(7123):106–10.

23. Ricci-Vitiani L, Lombardi DG, Pilozzi E, et al. Identification and expansion of human colon-cancer-initiating cells. Nature 2007;445(7123):111–5.

24. Pfenninger CV, Roschupkina T, Hertwig F, et al. CD133 is not present on neurogenic astrocytes in the adult subventricular zone, but on embryonic neural stem cells, ependymal cells, and glioblastoma cells. Cancer Res 2007;67(12):5727–36.

25. Rebetz J, Tian D, Persson A, et al.Glial progenitor-like phenotype in low-grade glioma and enhanced CD133-expression and neuronal lineage differentiation potential in high-grade glioma. PLoS ONE 2008;3(4):e1936.

26. Beier D, Hau P, Proescholdt M, et al. CD133(+) and CD133(−) glioblastoma-derived cancer stem cells show differential growth characteristics and molecular profiles. Cancer Res 2007;67(9):4010–5.

27. Wang J, Sakariassen PO, Tsinkalovsky O, et al. CD133 negative glioma cells form tumors in nude rats and give rise to CD133 positive cells. Int J Cancer 2008;122(4):761–8.

28. Kelly PN, Dakic A, Adams JM, Nutt SL, Strasser A. Tumor growth need not be driven by rare cancer stem cells. Science 2007;317(5836):337.

29. Dietrich J, Noble M, Mayer-Proschel M. Characterization of A2B5+ glial precursor cells from cryopreserved human fetal brain progenitor cells. Glia 2002;40(1):65–77.

30. Assanah M, Lochhead R, Ogden A, Bruce J, Goldman J, Canoll P. Glial progenitors in adult white matter are driven to form malignant gliomas by platelet-derived growth factor-expressing retroviruses. J Neurosci 2006;26(25):6781–90.

31. Rehen SK, Yung YC, McCreight MP, et al. Constitutional aneuploidy in the normal human brain. J Neurosci 2005; 25(9):2176–80.

32. Dong ZQ, Pang JC, Tong CY, Zhou LF, Ng HK. Clonality of oligoastrocytomas. Hum Pathol 2002;33(5):528–35.

33. Kattar MM, Kupsky WJ, Shimoyama RK, et al. Clonal analysis of gliomas. Hum Pathol 1997;28(10):1166–79.

34. James CD, Carlbom E, Dumanski JP, et al. Clonal genomic alterations in glioma malignancy stages. Cancer Res 1988; 48(19):5546–51.

35. Walker C, du Plessis DG, Joyce KA, et al. Phenotype versus genotype in gliomas displaying inter- or intratumoral histological heterogeneity. Clin Cancer Res 2003;9(13):4841–51.

36. Palmer TD, Takahashi J, Gage FH. The adult rat hippocampus contains primordial neural stem cells. Mol Cell Neurosci 1997;8(6):389–404.

37. Gould E, Tanapat P, McEwen BS, Flugge G, Fuchs E. Proliferation of granule cell precursors in the dentate gyrus of adult monkeys is diminished by stress. Proc Natl Acad Sci USA 1998;95(6):3168–71.

38. Gould E, Reeves AJ, Graziano MS, Gross CG. Neurogenesis in the neocortex of adult primates. Science 1999;286(5439):548–52.

39. Curtis MA, Kam M, Nannmark U, et al. Human neuroblasts migrate to the olfactory bulb via a lateral ventricular extension. Science 2007;315(5816):1243–9.

40. Eriksson PS, Perfilieva E, Bjork-Eriksson T, et al. Neurogenesis in the adult human hippocampus. Nat Med 1998; 4(11):1313–7.
41. Roy NS, Benraiss A, Wang S, et al. Promoter-targeted selection and isolation of neural progenitor cells from the adult human ventricular zone. J Neurosci Res 2000;59(3):321–31.
42. Roy NS, Wang S, Jiang L, et al. In vitro neurogenesis by progenitor cells isolated from the adult human hippocampus. Nat Med 2000;6(3):271–7.
43. Roy NS, Wang S, Harrison-Restelli C, et al. Identification, isolation, and promoter-defined separation of mitotic oligodendrocyte progenitor cells from the adult human subcortical white matter. J Neurosci 1999;19(22):9986–95.
44. Sim FJ, Lang JK, Waldau B, et al. Complementary patterns of gene expression by human oligodendrocyte progenitors and their environment predict determinants of progenitor maintenance and differentiation. Ann Neurol 2006;59(5):763–79.
45. Gregori N, Proschel C, Noble M, Mayer-Proschel M. The tripotential glial-restricted precursor (GRP) cell and glial development in the spinal cord: generation of bipotential oligodendrocyte-type-2 astrocyte progenitor cells and dorsal-ventral differences in GRP cell function. J Neurosci 2002;22(1):248–56.
46. Rao MS, Noble M, Mayer-Proschel M. A tripotential glial precursor cell is present in the developing spinal cord. Proc Natl Acad Sci USA 1998;95(7):3996–4001.
47. Scolding N, Franklin R, Stevens S, Heldin CH, Compston A, Newcombe J. Oligodendrocyte progenitors are present in the normal adult human CNS and in the lesions of multiple sclerosis. Brain 1998;121 (Pt 12):2221–8.
48. Scolding NJ, Rayner PJ, Compston DA. Identification of A2B5-positive putative oligodendrocyte progenitor cells and A2B5-positive astrocytes in adult human white matter. Neuroscience 1999;89(1):1–4.
49. Espinosa de los Monteros A, Zhang M, De Vellis J. O2A progenitor cells transplanted into the neonatal rat brain develop into oligodendrocytes but not astrocytes. Proc Natl Acad Sci USA 1993;90(1):50–4.
50. Kondo T, Raff M. Oligodendrocyte precursor cells reprogrammed to become multipotential CNS stem cells. Science 2000;289(5485):1754–7.
51. Liu Y, Han SS, Wu Y, et al. CD44 expression identifies astrocyte-restricted precursor cells. Dev Biol 2004;276(1):31–46.
52. Holland EC, Hively WP, DePinho RA, Varmus HE. A constitutively active epidermal growth factor receptor cooperates with disruption of G1 cell-cycle arrest pathways to induce glioma-like lesions in mice. Genes Dev 1998;12(23):3675–85.
53. Holland EC, Celestino J, Dai C, Schaefer L, Sawaya RE, Fuller GN. Combined activation of Ras and Akt in neural progenitors induces glioblastoma formation in mice. Nat Genet 2000;25(1):55–7.
54. Leonard JR, D'Sa C, Klocke BJ, Roth KA. Neural precursor cell apoptosis and glial tumorigenesis following transplacental ethyl-nitrosourea exposure. Oncogene 2001;20(57):8281–6.
55. Bachoo RM, Maher EA, Ligon KL, et al. Epidermal growth factor receptor and Ink4a/Arf: convergent mechanisms governing terminal differentiation and transformation along the neural stem cell to astrocyte axis. Cancer Cell 2002;1(3):269–77.
56. Wilhelmsson U, Eliasson C, Bjerkvig R, Pekny M. Loss of GFAP expression in high-grade astrocytomas does not contribute to tumor development or progression. Oncogene 2003;22(22):3407–11.
57. Zhu Y, Guignard F, Zhao D, et al. Early inactivation of p53 tumor suppressor gene cooperating with NF1 loss induces malignant astrocytoma. Cancer Cell 2005;8(2):119–30.
58. Armstrong RC, Dorn HH, Kufta CV, Friedman E, Dubois-Dalcq ME. Pre-oligodendrocytes from adult human CNS. J Neurosci 1992;12(4):1538–47.
59. Shoshan Y, Nishiyama A, Chang A, et al. Expression of oligodendrocyte progenitor cell antigens by gliomas: implications for the histogenesis of brain tumors. Proc Natl Acad Sci USA 1999;96(18):10361–6.
60. Bishop M, de la Monte SM. Dual lineage of astrocytomas. Am J Pathol 1989;135(3):517–27.
61. Xia CL, Du ZW, Liu ZY, Huang Q, Chan WY. A2B5 lineages of human astrocytic tumors and their recurrence. Int J Oncol 2003;23(2):353–61.
62. Bouvier C, Bartoli C, Aguirre-Cruz L, et al.Shared oligodendrocyte lineage gene expression in gliomas and oligodendrocyte progenitor cells. J Neurosurg 203;99(2):344–50.
63. Ligon KL, Alberta JA, Kho AT, et al. The oligodendroglial lineage marker OLIG2 is universally expressed in diffuse gliomas. J Neuropathol Exp Neurol 2004;63(5):499–509.
64. Morrison SJ, Perez SE, Qiao Z, et al. Transient Notch activation initiates an irreversible switch from neurogenesis to gliogenesis by neural crest stem cells. Cell 2000;101(5):499–510.
65. Wang S, Sdrulla AD, diSibio G, et al. Notch receptor activation inhibits oligodendrocyte differentiation. Neuron 1998;21(1):63–75.
66. Phillips HS, Kharbanda S, Chen R, et al. Molecular subclasses of high-grade glioma predict prognosis, delineate a pattern of disease progression, and resemble stages in neurogenesis. Cancer cell 2006;9(3):157–73.
67. Purow BW, Haque RM, Noel MW, et al. Expression of Notch-1 and its ligands, Delta-like-1 and Jagged-1, is critical for glioma cell survival and proliferation. Cancer Res 2005;65(6):2353–63.
68. Fan X, Matsui W, Khaki L, et al. Notch pathway inhibition depletes stem-like cells and blocks engraftment in embryonal brain tumors. Cancer Res 2006;66(15):7445–52.
69. See SJ, Levin VA, Yung WK, Hess KR, Groves MD. 13-cis-retinoic acid in the treatment of recurrent glioblastoma multiforme. Neuro Oncol 2004;6(3):253–8.

70. Piccirillo SG, Reynolds BA, Zanetti N, et al. Bone morphogenetic proteins inhibit the tumorigenic potential of human brain tumour-initiating cells. Nature 2006;444(7120):761–5.
71. Panchision DM, McKay RD. The control of neural stem cells by morphogenic signals. Curr Opin Genet Dev 2002;12(4):478–87.
72. Bar EE, Chaudhry A, Lin A, et al. Cyclopamine-mediated hedgehog pathway inhibition depletes stem-like cancer cells in glioblastoma. Stem Cells 2007;25(10):2524–33.
73. Bao S, Wu Q, McLendon RE, et al. Glioma stem cells promote radioresistance by preferential activation of the DNA damage response. Nature 2006;444(7120):756–60.

10

Mouse Mammary Tumor Virus: Stem Cells and Mammary Cancer

Gilbert H. Smith

ABSTRACT

The paradigm of mammary cancer induction by the mouse mammary tumor virus (MMTV) is used to illustrate the body of evidence that supports the hypothesis that mammary epithelial stem/progenitor cells represent targets for oncogenic transformation. It is argued that this is not a special case applicable only to MMTV-induced mammary cancer, because MMTV acts as an environmental mutagen producing random interruptions in the somatic DNA of infected cells by insertion of proviral DNA copies. In addition to disrupting the host genome, the proviral DNA also influences gene expression through its associated enhancer sequences over significant intergenomic distances. Genes commonly affected by MMTV insertion in multiple individual tumors include, the Wnt genes, the FGF gene family, and the Notch gene family. All of these gene families are known to play essential roles in stem cell maintenance and behavior in a variety of organs. The MMTV-induced mutations accumulate in cells that are long lived and possess the properties of stem cells, namely, self-renewal and the capacity to produce divergent epithelial progeny through asymmetric division. The evidence shows that epithelial cells with these properties are present in normal mammary glands, may be infected with MMTV, and become transformed to produce epithelial hyperplasia through MMTV-induced mutagenesis and progress to frank mammary malignancy. Retroviral marking via MMTV proviral insertion demonstrates that this process progresses from a single mammary epithelial cell that possesses all of the features ascribed to tissue-specific stem cells.

Key Words: Stem cell, MMTV, Mammary, Cancer, Transplantation, Mice

INTRODUCTION

In the sixth and seventh decades of the last millennium, interest was running very high regarding the role of viruses and the induction of cancer. Two types of oncogenic viruses were recognized, the "acute" tumor viruses, which caused cellular transformation and the onset of cancer rather quickly and the "nonacute" tumor viruses, which only produced cancer after very prolonged exposures. MMTV fell in this latter category *(1, 2)*. The discovery was subsequently made that "acute" tumor viruses actually carried a transforming gene in their genetic repertoire. These turned out to be acquired genetic sequences from the host and were subsequently dubbed "oncogenes" *(3)*. On the other hand "nonacute" tumor viruses were found to cause genetic changes by virtue of the insertion of their

From: *Cancer Drug Discovery and Development: Stem Cells and Cancer,*
Edited by: R.G. Bagley and B.A. Teicher, DOI: 10.1007/978-1-60327-933-8_10,
© Humana Press, a part of Springer Science+Business Media, LLC 2009

proviral DNA into the somatic DNA of the infected host. Since proviral DNA insertions occur randomly, the selection of a transforming event depended upon the response of the affected cell to these genetic events (insertions). With respect to MMTV insertions and mammary cancers, it was found that certain insertion sites commonly resulted in the clonal expansion of the affected cell and the subsequent development of a tumor. These commonly affected genes, i.e., "Int" genes were thus identified as genetic alterations that were instrumental in the process of malignant transformation of mammary epithelial cells. Further, it was recognized that the alteration of these Int genes were transforming because of their conscription in the clonal expansion of the cells bearing them to form a malignancy. Among the commonly affected "Int" genes are the Wingless (Wnt) genes, the fibroblast growth factor (FGF) genes, and the Notch genes. Recent evidence has implicated all of these genes as essential players in stem cell maintenance and function both during development and in adult organs *(4–8)*.

Before setting out on a discussion of the evidence for stem/progenitor cells as the likely targets for oncogenic transformation in the rodent mammary gland, a number of issues must be defined *(9–11)*. (a) All portions of a mammary gland are competent to regenerate a complete and functional gland upon transplantation to an epithelium-divested mammary fat pad. (b) This capacity is independent of age or reproductive history. (c) Dispersed mammary epithelial cells possess the same regenerative capacity. (d) Transplantation of limiting dilutions of dispersed mammary cells reveals the presence of duct-limited and lobule-limited multipotent stem/progenitor cells, signaling that a hierarchy of stem/progenitor cell exists in the rodent mammary gland. (e) All portions of a regenerated mammary outgrowth are likewise competent to recapitulate mammary gland growth upon serial passage, demonstrating that regenerative mammary niches are self-renewing. (f) Normal but not premalignant mammary tissue begins to show growth senescence beginning around the fourth transplant generation. The rate of the appearance of growth senescence is independent of the age or reproductive history of the original donor. (g) Growth senescence is not uniformly present in any outgrowth but appears at random among individual transplanted portions. (h) In pregnant hosts, senescence of duct morphogenesis and senescence of lobulogenesis were shown to develop independently from one another in serially transplanted outgrowths *(12)*. (i) Both lobule-predominant and duct-predominant outgrowth lines that fail to show growth senescence have been isolated. (j) Retroviral-tagging (MMTV) of normal, premalignant, and tumor outgrowths indicate that each is a clonal-dominant population most likely initiated from a single infected cell. (k) MMTV proviral insertions are random with respect to their location in the somatic cell DNA. Therefore, selection of a specific proviral insertion site and its fixation within a cellular population depends upon the proliferation of the cell bearing that particular insertion(s).

STEM/PROGENITOR CELL ACTIVITY IN MMTV-INDUCED TUMORS

The presence of MMTV proviral insertions and the clonal nature of tumor development allows for each tumor to be individually identified by its complement of MMTV DNA insertions via Southern blotting of its DNA. A study that emphatically makes this point was published by Sonnenberg et al. *(13)*, who demonstrate that three vastly different types of cell clones may be isolated from a single MMTV-induced mammary tumor that vary dramatically in their expression of epithelial, basal (myoepithelial), or stromal cellular markers but retain the original set of MMTV insertions representative of the original tumorigenic clone. These clones, variously described as polygonal, cuboidal, and elongated, share the same ancestral cell but express vastly different cellular and tumorigenic characteristics highlighting the plasticity in cell fate selection of the originally transformed cell. This, for some of us, was the first intimation that pluripotent cells may be the targets for MMTV-induced mammary tumorigenesis.

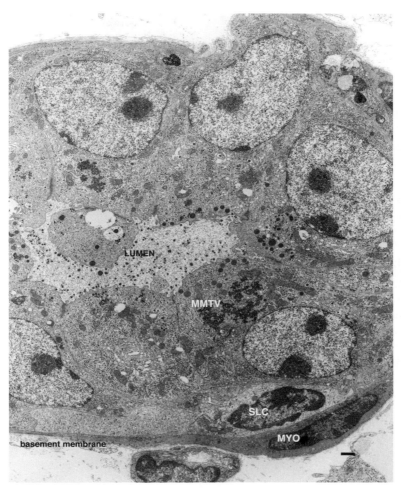

Fig. 1. This electron micrograph depicts an ultrathin section through one of the acini in an MMTV-induced alveolar hyperplasia. There is evidence of virus replication (MMTV), of secretory activity leading to secretory granule formation in the apical cytoplasm of the luminal cells and release into the lumen. An undifferentiated suprabasal cell (SLC) is present and proximal to it, a differentiated myoepithelial cell (*arrow*). Bar = 1 mm.

Subsequently, a morphologically distinct cell was recognized in the mammary tissue at all stages of mammary development in rodents and humans with characteristics reminiscent of an uncommitted (undifferentiated) epithelial cell *(14, 15)*. These cells were lightly staining and devoid of cellular organelles and other morphological signs of functional differentiation. They were found in two sizes, small light cells (SLC) and undifferentiated large light cells (ULLC). These cells also appeared in MMTV-induced mammary tumors and in premalignant mammary lesions and outgrowths (Fig. 1). Conversely, they were absent from growth senescent rodent mammary tissue *(16)*, an observation consistent with the interpretation that the presence of cells with the morphology of SLC and ULLC signifies the occurrence of mammary epithelial stem cell function. Human breast cells with corresponding attributes to SLC or ULLC, i.e., suprabasal location, epithelial antigen positive, smooth muscle actin negative, and sialomucin-low/negative, were isolated from human reduction mammoplasty tissue and found to display stem cell growth characteristics in cell culture *(17)*.

STEM/PROGENITOR CELL HIERARCHY

In mice, rats, and humans, evidence has accumulated that a hierarchy of mammary epithelial progenitor/stem cells exists *(18–20)*. At present, lobule-restricted, duct-restricted, and fully competent mammary stem cells are proposed to exist among the mammary epithelial population. In 1996, I demonstrated in the mouse that at least three distinct stem/progenitor epithelial cell activities were present in normal mammary glands by limiting dilution transplantation *(21)*. From cellular dilutions giving a nearly Poisson distribution of positive takes, three types of mammary outgrowths were recorded in full term pregnant hosts, outgrowths showing complete development, outgrowths capable of producing only mammary ducts, and outgrowths producing only secretory lobular structures without ductal branching (Fig. 2). All of these epithelial structures contain epithelial cells representing diverse epithelial cell phenotypes, including luminal, myoepithelial, and basal (SLC) cells. Premalignant and immortal mammary epithelial outgrowth populations, reflecting either ductal or lobular hyperplasia *(22, 23)* may be isolated from mouse mammary tissue, suggesting their origins began with the trans-formation of duct-limited or lobule-limited mammary epithelial stem/progenitors cells. These prema-lignant immortal populations also possess epithelial cells reflecting the full array of mammary epithelial cell types, basal, myoepithelial, and luminal (shown in Fig. 1). These populations, like the MMTV-induced mammary tumors, are clonal as determined by retroviral tagging *(24)*. Thus, the originally transformed cell surely possessed the capacity to produce epithelial cell progeny with diverse cellular fates, suggesting a stem/progenitor cell origin for MMTV-induced hyperplasia and tumors. To follow up on this hypothesis, we posed the question, "Are individual mammary outgrowths from implanted epithelial fragments clonally derived?" To address this question, we transplanted individual mammary gland fragments from multiparous MMTV-infected mice to gland-free mammary fat pads and 4 weeks after implantation impregnated the hosts to generate full and complete mammary growth.

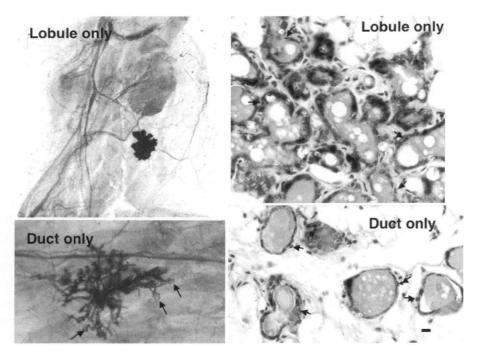

Fig. 2. Lobule only and duct only outgrowths in full term pregnant transplant hosts (*left panels*). Both lobule-only and duct-only outgrowths comprise both luminal and myoepithelial (*arrows*) cells. Bar = 10 mm.

We reasoned that if outgrowths clonally developed from MMTV-infected stem/progenitor epithelial cells, a specific and unique pattern of acquired proviral insertions would appear upon Southern Blot analysis of restriction enzyme-digested DNA from individual outgrowth populations. This would indicate that the majority, if not all, of the cells present in any given outgrowth were derived from a single MMTV-infected antecedent and further that this predecessor was capable of giving rise to progeny reflecting all the epithelial cell types present in a fully functional differentiated mammary gland *(25)*. This result was obtained in over 60% of outgrowths from random fragments dissected from multiparous females ($N = 6$) infected with MMTV whereas no outgrowths bearing a specific pattern of MMTV insertions was obtained when fragments were transplanted from MMTV-infected pubertal-aged females ($N = 6$). Outgrowths derived from MMTV-infected donors of intermediate age gave an intermediate range of retrovirus-tagged individual outgrowths. So expanding numbers of clonogenic mammary epithelial cells are infected with MMTV with increasing age and reproductive history. To confirm that individual outgrowths were comprised of single clones and not the result of the simultaneous expansion of two or more divergent clones, serial passages of random fragments from individual clonal-dominant outgrowths were carried out *(12)*. The results established the monoclonal nature of the tested outgrowth populations by demonstrating that all transplant generations of any given outgrowth containing MMTV insertions showed identical restriction patterns by Southern Blotting (Fig. 3). In addition to affirming the clonal nature of these populations, these experiments demonstrate the self-renewal capacity of the originally infected cell through multiple transplant generations while maintaining its multipotent properties. These results provide definitive proof that over time MMTV can infect mammary epithelial stem/progenitor cells and cause mutations in these cells through the random insertion of MMTV proviral DNA, thus, providing a basis for hypothesizing that mammary stem cells represent targets for oncogenesis in MMTV-infected mice.

The clonal expansion of mammary stem/progenitor cells containing MMTV insertional mutations may give rise to local premalignant hyperplasia (HAN) which upon transplantation produce hyperplastic growth comprised of both luminal epithelial and myoepithelial cell types, which fills the epithelium-divested mammary fat pad. The transplanted hyperplasia does not extend beyond the limits of the fat pad; ceases growth when confronted with fat occupied by normal mammary epithelial tissue and will not grow in ectopic transplantation sites otherwise permissive for mammary tumor cell proliferation. All of these properties are shared with outgrowths of normal mammary epithelium. In contrast to normal tissue, growth senescence is never attained upon serial transplantation of the hyperplastic populations and the frequency of focal mammary tumor formation is much greater, attesting to their premalignant nature. Like the hyperplasia, the tumors that arise often comprise both myoepithelial and luminal epithelial cell phenotypes (Fig. 4). The tumors and the hyperplasia within which they develop share the identical MMTV retroviral insertions indicating their lineal relationship, often the tumors have one or more additionally acquired proviral mutations. An example of this is shown in Fig. 5a, where DNA from two separate passages of an MMTV-induced hyperplastic outgrowth is compared with tumor DNA from lesions arising stochastically within these populations at different transplant generations. The original pattern of MMTV proviral insertion is maintained in all the tumors whether they possess new insertions or not. Individual metastatic lesions from the tumors also show a lineal relation to both the originating tumor and the hyperplastic population from which they sprung. Individual metastatic lesions from the same tumor are also clonally derived and may differ from one another by the number and the location of newly acquired proviral insertions (Fig. 5b). Taken together, these observations establish that individual cells among the mammary epithelium, capable of self-renewal and the production of epithelial progeny of divergent cellular phenotypes, biological attributes shared with stem cells, may be infected with MMTV to acquire transforming mutations and then expand clonally to give rise to premalignant and malignant epithelial colonies.

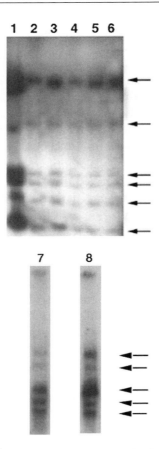

Fig. 3. Southern blot of DNA from five consecutive serial passages of a clonal-dominant normal mammary outgrowth (lanes 2–6), probed with the MMTV-LTR demonstrates that the original proviral insertion pattern is maintained in each passage. Lane 1 contains DNA from a tumor found in passage 4. In the Southern Blot (below) DNA from a lobule-limited outgrowth (lane 7) and a fully developed secretory outgrowth (lane 8) in the contralateral fat pad of the same female demonstrate the identical pattern for MMTV-host DNA restriction fragments demonstrating that each population arises from the same original MMTV-infected antecedent.

The role of epigenetic mechanisms in this progression has not been addressed except in those models where pregnancy has provided protection to malignant progression in chemical carcinogen and certain transgenic mammary tumorigenesis models *(23, 26)*.

SELECTIVE DNA SEGREGATION

Acquisition of new MMTV insertions and fixation in the genome (sic mutation) requires that the infected cell traverse the cell cycle. Nevertheless, new viral insertions have never been observed in these clonally expanding premalignant epithelial outgrowths (or in MMTV-tagged clonally expanding normal mammary outgrowths) despite the presence of replicating MMTV displaying a full vegetative life cycle including the synthesis of reverse transcriptase, pre-pronucleocapsids, unintegrated proviral DNA, and mature virions. The original retroviral insertion pattern is maintained throughout multiple transplant generations not withstanding the enormous expansion of the cellular population (Fig. 6; arrows). In addition, when one of these insertions occurs near a cellular gene, like Wnt-1, a new

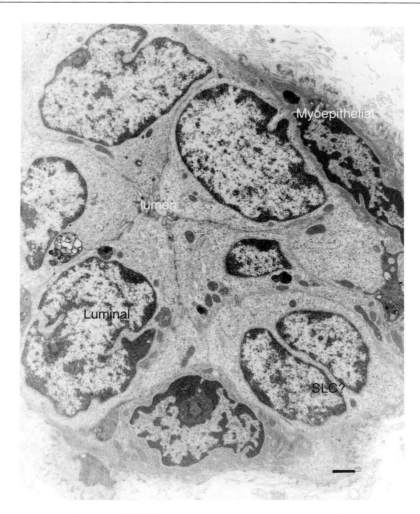

Fig. 4. An electron micrograph from an MMTV-induced primary mammary tumor shows that myoepithelial, luminal, and basal (SLC) epithelial phenotypes are present. Unlike the hyperplasia, the tumor cells show very little secretory activity, only a few mitochondria, sparse rough endoplasmic reticulum development and a collapsed lumen. Bar = 1 mm.

restriction fragment containing Wnt-1 sequence may be produced (Fig. 6; lower). This alteration is also maintained throughout malignant progression validating the clonal nature of this process. New MMTV insertions are only seen in the malignant clones arising stochastically within the premalignant outgrowth; although this also is not universally true (Figs. 5b and 6), suggesting that epigenetic mechanisms or mutations other than those caused by proviral insertion may promote malignant progression. In 1975, Cairns *(27)* proposed that somatic stem cells protect themselves from mutation by selectively retaining their template DNA strands during asymmetric divisions and pass the newly synthesized strands to their offspring. Such a mechanism in the MMTV-infected cells, which generate the hyperplasia at each transplant generation, might explain the absence of new MMTV insertions, as the insertion would occur in the new DNA strand and would subsequently be transmitted to the dispensable daughter cells. Cairns *(28)* also postulated that original somatic stem cells die and are replaced by an immediate daughter cell which may have acquired mutation during its inception (having selectively inherited the newly synthesized DNA strands) leading to a circumstance where a stem

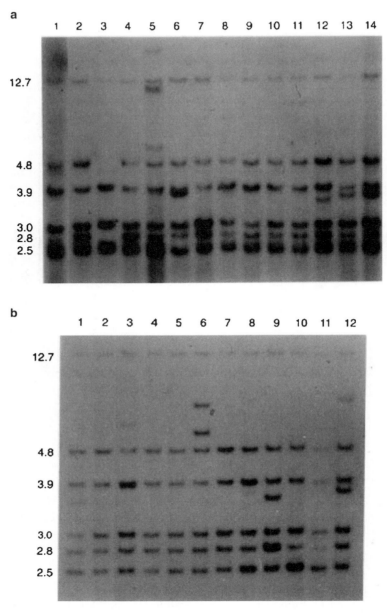

Fig. 5. (a) MMTV proviral restriction patterns are shown for DNA isolated from a premalignant hyperplastic mammary outgrowth (lanes 1 and 2) and from 12 independent mammary tumors (lanes 3–14) that arose focally within the hyperplastic population at various passages during its propagation in gland-free fat pads. The proviral content of the two different passages of the hyperplasia (lanes 1 and 2) are present in all of the tumors. New MMTV proviral insertions were detected in the tumors shown in lanes 5, 12, 13, and 14. A loss of one of the original insertions was noted in the tumor DNA shown in lane 3. The DNA was digested with EcoR1 and probed with the MMTV-LTR sequence. EcoR1 cuts within the provirus and the LTR is represented at both ends of the provirus. Therefore, each insertion produces two virus–host junction fragments detected by the LTR probe. In (**b**) the restriction enzymatic digestion and the probe were the same, however, DNA from a metastatic tumor (lane 1 in (**b**)) arising in the hyperplasia shown above in lanes1 and 2, gave 11 independent lung metastases in the same mouse (shown in lanes 2–12). The tumor and all the metastases bear the original proviral insertions from the hyperplasia. Additional MMTV insertions were detected in the metastatic nodule DNA shown in lanes 6, 8, 9, 10, and 12. This strongly suggests that each metastatic lesion is an individual clone.

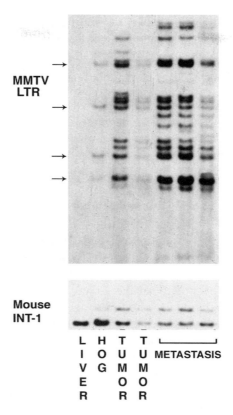

MMTV LTR

Mouse INT-1

L H T T
I O U U METASTASIS
V G M M
E O O
R R R

Fig. 6. A Southern Blot containing EcoR1 digested DNA from Czech mouse liver (Czech mice have no endogenous MMTV provirus), a Czech mammary hyperplastic outgrowth (HOG), two mammary tumors that developed in the contra-lateral mammary glands of the mouse bearing the hyperplastic implant and metastases from the lung of the same mouse were probed with MMTV-LTR and a probe specific for the Wnt-1 (INT-1) gene. No MMTV provirus is detected in the liver DNA, at least two insertions were evident in the HOG DNA and these were also represented in the two tumors. Additional MMTV insertions were present in the DNA from each tumor. By inspection of the proviral DNA content of the metastases, it can be determined that these most likely arose from the tumor in the 4th lane and not from the one in lane 3. In addition, the metastases contain additional MMTV insertions, which may tag mutations important to metastatic progression. One of the insertions in the cell producing the hyperplastic clone occurred near the Wnt-1 gene in one allele producing a larger restriction fragment detected by the Wnt-1 probe. This rearranged Wnt-1 sequence is also found in all the tumors and metastases arising within this hyperplasia validating the clonal nature of malignant progression.

cell with acquired mutations supplants its normal counterpart in the niche. This scenario might readily explain the appearance of the new proviral insertions observed in the DNA of the mammary tumors arising within the hyperplasia. Alternatively, local exponential, i.e., nonsymmetric, divisions of the stem/progenitor cells may result in fixation of new MMTV proviral insertions. Subsequent expansion of tumor populations from these newly mutated stem/progenitor cells will depend on the transforming nature of the newly acquired mutations.

Recent evidence has confirmed that long-label-retaining epithelial cells (LRCs) present among the mouse mammary epithelium selectively retained the labeled template DNA strands while traversing the cell cycle (29, 30). In addition, mammary transplants containing lacZ-positive lobule-limited progenitors contained long-label-retaining, lacZ-positive epithelial cells, which traversed the cell cycle and selectively retained their original DNA strands. Therefore, stem or progenitor cells and in some cases ERa and PR positive epithelial cells display the ability to selectively retain template DNA while undergoing asymmetric cell divisions. Mammary epithelial cells transformed by MMTV through insertion mutation exhibit the capacity for self-renewal, the ability to produce divergent epithelial cell progeny, and the capacity to selectively distribute newly synthesized DNA strands to their offspring while retaining their template copy, all properties of tissue stem cells. Therefore, it is likely that MMTV-induced mammary tumors arise from the mammary epithelial stem/progenitor cell subpopulation and are maintained by long-lived transformed cells capable of protecting their template DNA.

How does the conclusion that MMTV induces mammary cancer from mouse mammary epithelial stem/progenitor cells relate to the development of mammary cancer in general? This bridge is crossed when one considers the role that MMTV infection plays in the malignant transformation of mammary epithelial cells. MMTV is a nonacute oncogenic virus and indirectly brings about transformation through its role as a mutagen, i.e., causing mutations in the somatic cell DNA via insertion of its proviral DNA during its replicative cycle. Therefore, MMTV infection is comparable to other environmental mutagens, such as ionizing radiation, ultraviolet light, or chemical carcinogens, in the sense that they all randomly disrupt genomic structure. Thus, MMTV-induced carcinogenesis may be viewed as synonymous with sporadic mammary cancer induction, wherein accumulation of transforming mutations occurs over time, resulting eventually in the clonal expansion of the infected cell. MMTV is present from birth in an infected individual. A lifetime infection is established in the lymphatic system and infectious MMTV is associated with circulating lymphocytes *(31)*. MMTV is first detected in the mammary tissue around 2 weeks of age and spreads throughout the gland during duct development and lobulogenesis during successive pregnancies. When infected glands are dissociated and dispersed mammary cells are injected into the epithelium-divested mammary fat pads of syngeneic hosts, transformed epithelial cells are detectable as early as 1 month of age *(32)*. The frequency of these cells increases with age and their number and appearance is accelerated significantly by pregnancy *(33)*. Despite the presence of these "inapparent" transformed cells at an early age, the frank appearance of hyperplastic foci and/or tumors is delayed for several months indicating that clonal expansion of these cells requires a further alteration of their microenvironment. This is an indication that epigenetic mechanisms are manifest since the mutations resulting in the premalignant phenotype are already present before expansion. In addition, the transformed epithelial cells have already attained an "immortal" phenotype that is embodied in the absence of growth senescence upon serial transplantation.

ASYMMETRIC VERSUS SYMMETRIC CELL DIVISION IN CANCER

As mentioned earlier, symmetric divisions as opposed to asymmetric division (because of the selective retention of template DNA strands) will be required for the fixation of additional mutations in a stem/progenitor cell. It, therefore, seems reasonable to assume that the MMTV insertions are acquired during self-renewal and expansion of stem/progenitor cells during ductal morphogenesis and during the extensive increase (~25–30-fold) of the epithelium during pregnancy *(25)*. One might postulate that attenuation of the symmetric expansion of stem/progenitor cells, e.g., during pregnancy, should reduce the subsequent risk of hyperplasia and tumorigenesis in MMTV-infected mice. An opportunity to test this hypothesis developed in WAP-TGF-b1 mice. The whey-acidic-protein (WAP)-promoter targeted TGF-b1 expression to the secretory epithelium in pregnant females *(34)*. Expression of TGF-b1 caused the differentiating secretory cells to enter apoptosis but did not affect the epithelial cell proliferation, which was maintained at a significant level throughout pregnancy *(35)*. This resulted in lactation failure. In addition, transplantation of WAP-TGF-b1 mammary tissue indicated that growth senescence in the transplants was accelerated occurring in the first transplant generation from donors of only 6 weeks of age. Introduction of MMTV into these mice and their wild-type sisters at 6–8 weeks of age demonstrated that the WAP-TGF-b1 mice were protected from MMTV-induced mammary transformation compared to wild type, despite the presence of similar levels of MMTV infection *(36)*. However, if MMTV was introduced at birth, no protection for MMTV-induced mammary cancer was provided by the presence of WAP-TGF-b1 *(37)*. We concluded that the early senescence of mammary stem/progenitor cell self-renewal in the 6-week-old females was the basis for this tumor protection. This experimental result provides a "proof of principle," namely that reducing the replicative (self-renewing) longevity of stem/progenitor cells in the mammary glands markedly reduces the risk of mammary tumor development in MMTV-infected mice. This is consistent with the hypothesis that transformation by MMTV is suppressed in mammary glands containing stem/progenitor cells with a decreased ability to undergo expansion through symmetric divisions as determined by early growth senescence upon transplantation. A few years later, a new parity-induced mammary epithelial subpopulation (PI-MEC) was discovered in WAP-Cre/Rosa26-flStop-fl-LacZ mice following cre-lox recombinase removal of the Stop DNA fragment separating the Rosa26 promoter and the LacZ reporter gene *(38)*. This new ancillary epithelial population was found to be self-renewing, pluripotent, and responsible for the generation of new secretory epithelial lobules upon successive pregnancies *(39)*. Remarkably, when WAP-TGF-b1 was introduced into these mice, LacZ-positive PI-MEC appeared and was active in generating secretory lobules (asymmetric cell division kinetics) upon successive pregnancies despite the apoptosis of the differentiating secretory epithelium that resulted in lactation failure. However, when mammary fragments containing LacZ-positive PI-MEC from these females were transplanted, the PI-MEC was incapable of expansive self-renewal (symmetric cell division kinetics) and was absent from the resulting outgrowths *(39)*. Despite this, a new population of Lac-Z-positive cells appeared within these negative outgrowths in late pregnant hosts indicating that only those cells that had expressed WAP-TGF-b1 in the preceding pregnancy were incapable of mitotic expansion by symmetric division.

It seems likely that an early growth senescent phenotype in transplants may in part be related to the loss of this self-renewing population in WAP-TGF-b1 mammary tissue. The increased resistance to MMTV-induced mammary cancer in WAP-TGF-b1-positive females may also be the result of the disabling of the innate self-renewing capacity of PI-MEC by WAP-TGF-b1 expression. A result that implies that this long-lived, self-renewing, pluripotent, mammary cellular population may represent a primary target for MMTV tumorigenesis.

I have been discussing premalignant lesions and mammary tumors in MMTV-infected mice, which arose as the result of acquired MMTV proviral insertions that produced mutations that were transforming. When 7,12-dimethyl-[a]-benzanthracene (DMBA) was used to induce mammary cancer and premalignant lesions, the lesions arose primarily in ducts rather than alveoli. Despite this difference, when DMBA was employed in MMTV-infected mice, mammary tumors developed that were characterized by a specific set of acquired MMTV insertions indicating that these neoplasms also arose from individual cells within the mammary tissue of nulliparous females that had acquired MMTV provirus. This indicates that the same cellular subpopulation (sic stem/progenitor cells) was transformed by DMBA chemical carcinogenesis albeit through a different mutagenic mechanism. No differences were observed either in tumor incidence or in tumor latency between DMBA-treated C3H mice infected with MMTV and those uninfected, indicating that MMTV did not act synergistically with the carcinogen *(40–43)*.

STEM/PROGENITOR CELLS ARE TARGETS FOR MMTV TRANSFORMATION

The foregoing discussion was intended to enumerate and illuminate the reasons why we should consider stem/progenitor cells in the mammary glands of rodents and humans as the likely targets for neoplastic transformation irrespective of the environmental carcinogen. In summary, MMTV-induced mammary tumors arise from individual mammary epithelial cells within infected glands. Each tumor is characterized by its own unique set of acquired MMTV proviral insertions. In tissue culture, these tumors produce cell clones with widely disparate cellular features ranging from epitheloid to mesenchymal each of which bear the original proviral insertions *(13)*. Proviral insertions that commonly affect the same gene in multiple tumors have been identified and the affected genes are known as "Int" genes. Many of these Int gene mutations have been verified to possess transforming functions when expressed in the mammary glands of transgenic mice and many of these Int genes (Wnt, Notch, Fgf) have been linked to essential functions in tissue stem cell biology. Premalignant-transformed mammary cells are detectable in MMTV-infected glands long before the appearance of detectable focal lesions. Each of these appears capable of clonal expansion to produce hyperplasia characterized by the presence of multiple epithelial cell types including luminal, myoepithelial, and stem/progenitor (SLC, ULLC) cells. MMTV-infected epithelial cells in normal glands possess and extensive self-renewal capacity and the ability to give rise to daughters of diverse epithelial cell fates as determined by serial passage of MMTV-infected mammary tissue fragments. Complete functional mammary outgrowths from these implants are comprised of the progeny of a single MMTV-infected epithelial cell. Upon serial passage both premalignant and tumors develop within this clone and are characterized by the same unique set of MMTV proviral insertions as the original outgrowth. Taken together, these observations support the conclusion that pluripotent cells among the mammary epithelia become infected with MMTV, acquire mutations as a result and subsequently expand into clones, which variously exhibit hyperplasia and/or frank malignancy.

CONCLUSIONS

In summary, I have presented evidence supporting the conclusion that mammary stem/progenitor cells are the main targets for MMTV-induced transformation leading to mammary tumorigenesis. The main points of this argument are enumerated as follows: MMTV is an environmental mutagen targeting the mammary epithelium of susceptible mice; MMTV causes mutations in infected cells during its vegetative growth cycle by insertional mutation; these mutations are random and serve to specifically mark mammary epithelial cells that give rise to expanding clonal populations; these retrovirally marked populations may be normal, (i.e., subject to growth senescence), premalignant (i.e., not subject to growth senescence and possessing a higher risk for progression to frank malignancy) or fully tumorigenic and metastatic. The clones stably maintain their original proviral insertions during expansion through multiple passages suggesting that the cells that maintain these clones are capable of asymmetric divisions and selective retention of their original template DNA strands. The latter property has been established for LRCs in normal mouse mammary epithelium. The MMTV-tagged clones, whether normal, premalignant, or malignant, show the capacity for self-renewal upon transplantation and give rise to phenotypically heterogeneous cellular populations. All of these are properties that have been assigned to adult stem cells.

REFERENCES

1. Burmeister T. Oncogenic retroviruses in animals and humans. Rev Med Virol 2001;11(6):369–80.
2. Stehelin D, Varmus HE, Bishop JM. Detection of nucleotide sequences associated with transformation by avian sarcoma viruses. Bibl Haematol 1975(43):539–41.
3. Bishop JM. Retroviruses and cancer genes. Adv Cancer Res 1982;37:1–32.
4. Yamashita YM, Fuller MT, Jones DL. Signaling in stem cell niches: lessons from the Drosophila germline. J Cell Sci 2005;118(Pt 4):665–72.

5. Theodorou V, Boer M, Weigelt B, Jonkers J, van der Valk M, Hilkens J. Fgf10 is an oncogene activated by MMTV insertional mutagenesis in mouse mammary tumors and overexpressed in a subset of human breast carcinomas. Oncogene 2004;23(36):6047–55.

6. Eblaghie MC, Song SJ, Kim JY, Akita K, Tickle C, Jung HS. Interactions between FGF and Wnt signals and Tbx3 gene expression in mammary gland initiation in mouse embryos. J Anat 2004;205(1):1–13.

7. Farnie G, Clarke RB. Mammary stem cells and breast cancer – role of Notch signalling. Stem Cell Rev 2007;3(2):169–75.

8. Katoh M. Networking of WNT, FGF, Notch, BMP, and Hedgehog signaling pathways during carcinogenesis. Stem Cell Rev 2007;3(1):30–8.

9. Smith GH, Boulanger CA. Mammary epithelial stem cells: Transplantation and self-renewal analysis. Cell Proliferation 2003;Suppl. 1:I3–15.

10. Smith GH, Boulanger CA. Stem cells in mammary epithelium. In: Lanza R, Blau H., Melton D., Moore M., Thomas E.D., Verfaille C., Weissman I., West M., eds. Adult and Fetal Stem Cells: Handbook of Stem Cells. San Diego, CA: Elsevier Academic; 2004: 257–68.

11. Smith GH, Chepko G. Mammary epithelial stem cells. Microsc Res Tech 2001;52(2):190–203.

12. Smith GH, Boulanger CA. Mammary stem cell repertoire: New insights in aging epithelial populations. Mech Aging Dev 2002;123:1505–19.

13. Sonnenberg A, Daams H, Calafat J, Hilgers J. In vitro differentiation and progression of mouse mammary tumor cells. Cancer Res 1986;46(11):5913–22.

14. Smith GH, Medina D. A morphologically distinct candidate for an epithelial stem cell in mouse mammary gland. J Cell Sci 1988;90(Pt 1):173–83.

15. Chepko G, Smith GH. Three division-competent, structurally-distinct cell populations contribute to murine mammary epithelial renewal. Tissue Cell 1997;29(2):239–53.

16. Smith GH, Strickland P, Daniel CW. Putative stem cell loss corresponds with mammary growth senescence. Cell Tissue Res 2002;310:313–20.

17. Gudjonsson T, Villadsen R, Nielse HL, Ronnov-Jessen L, Bissell MJ, Petersen OW. Isolation, immortalization, and characterization of a human breast epithelial cell line with stem cell properties. Genes Dev 2002;16:693–706.

18. Kamiya K, Gould MN, Clifton KH. Quantitative studies of ductal versus alveolar differentiation from rat mammary clonogens. Proc Soc Exp Biol Med 1998;219(3):217–25.

19. Stingl J, Eaves CJ, Zandich I, Emerman JT. Characterization of bipotent mammary epithelial progenitor cells in normal adult human breast tissue. Breast Cancer Res Treat 2001;67:93–109.

20. Stingl J, Raouf A, Eirew P, Eaves CJ. Deciphering the mammary epithelial cell hierarchy. Cell Cycle 2006; 5(14):1519–22.

21. Smith GH. Experimental mammary epithelial morphogenesis in an in vivo model: evidence for distinct cellular progenitors of the ductal and lobular phenotype. Breast Cancer Res Treat 1996;39(1):21–31.

22. Medina D. The preoplastic phenotype in murine mammary tumorigenesis. J Mammary Gland Biol Neoplasia 2000;5(4):393–407.

23. Medina D. Mammary developmental fate and breast cancer risk. Endocr Relat Cancer 2005;12(3):483–95.

24. Callahan R, Smith GH. MMTV-induced mammary tumorigenesis: gene discovery, progression to malignancy and cellular pathways. Oncogene 2000;19(8):992–1001.

25. Kordon EC, Smith GH. An entire functional mammary gland may comprise the progeny from a single cell. Development 1998;125(10):1921–30.

26. Rajkumar L, Kittrell FS, Guzman RC, Brown PH, Nandi S, Medina D. Hormone-induced protection of mammary tumorigenesis in genetically engineered mouse models. Breast Cancer Res 2007;9(1):R12.

27. Cairns J. Mutation selection and the natural history of cancer. Nature 1975;255(5505):197–200.

28. Cairns J. Somatic stem cells and the kinetics of mutagenesis and carcinogenesis. Proc Natl Acad Sci USA 2002;99(16):10567–70.

29. Smith GH. Label-retaining mammary epithelial cells divide asymmetrically and retain their template DNA strands. Development 2005;132:681–7.

30. Booth BW, Smith GH. Estrogen receptor-alpha and progesterone receptor are expressed in label-retaining mammary epithelial cells that divide asymmetrically and retain their template DNA strands. Breast Cancer Res 2006;8(4):R49.

31. Ross SR, Schmidt JW, Katz E, et al. An immunoreceptor tyrosine activation motif in the mouse mammary tumor virus envelope protein plays a role in virus-induced mammary tumors. J Virol 2006;80(18):9000–8.

32. DeOme KB, Miyamoto MJ, Osborn RC, Guzman RC, Lum K. Detection of inapparent nodule-transformed cells in the mammary gland tissues of virgin female BALB/cfC3H mice. Cancer Res 1978;38(7):2103–11.

33. DeOme KB, Miyamoto MJ, Osborn RC, Guzman RC, Lum K. Effect of parity on recovery of inapparent nodule-transformed mammary gland cells in vivo. Cancer Res 1978;38(11 Pt 2):4050–3.

34. Jhappan C, Geiser AG, Kordon EC, et al. Targeting expression of a transforming growth factor beta 1 transgene to the pregnant mammary gland inhibits alveolar development and lactation. EMBO J 1993;12(5):1835–45.

35. Kordon EC, McKnight RA, Jhappan C, Hennighausen L, Merlino G, Smith GH. Ectopic TGF beta 1 expression in the secretory mammary epithelium induces early senescence of the epithelial stem cell population. Dev Biol 1995;168(1):47–61.

36. Boulanger CA, Smith GH. Reducing mammary cancer risk through premature stem cell senescence. Oncogene 2001;20(18):2264–72.

37. Buggiano V, Schere-Levy C, Abe K, et al. Impairment of mammary lobular development induced by expression of TGFbeta1 under the control of WAP promoter does not suppress tumorigenesis in MMTV-infected transgenic mice. Int J Cancer 2001;92(4):568–76.

38. Wagner KU, Boulanger CA, Henry MD, Sgagias M, Hennighausen L, Smith GH. An adjunct mammary epithelial cell population in parous females: its role in functional adaptation and tissue renewal. Development 2002;129(6):1377–86.

39. Boulanger CA, Wagner KU, Smith GH. Parity-induced mouse mammary epithelial cells are pluripotent, self-renewing and sensitive to TGF-b1 expression. Oncogene 2005;24:552–60.

40. Smith GH, Pauley RJ, Socher SH, Medina D. Chemical carcinogenesis in C3H/StWi mice, a worthwhile experimental model for breast cancer. Cancer Res 1978;38(12):4504–9.

41. Smith GH, Arthur LA, Medina D. Evidence of separate pathways for viral and chemical carcinogenesis in C3H/StWi mouse mammary glands. Int J Cancer 1980;26(3):373–9.

42. Drohan WN, Benade LE, Graham DE, Smith GH. Mouse mammary tumor virus proviral sequences congenital to C3H/Sm mice are differentially hypomethylated in chemically induced, virus-induced, and spontaneous mammary tumors. J Virol 1982;43(3):876–84.

43. Smith GH, Medina D. Re-evaluation of mammary stem cell biology based on in vivo transplantation. Breast Cancer Res 2008;10(1):203.

11

Tumor Dormancy, Metastasis, and Cancer Stem Cells

Alysha K. Croker, Jason L. Townson*,
Alison L. Allan, and Ann F. Chambers*

ABSTRACT

Metastatic cancer can recur months or even years after apparently successful treatment of the primary tumor. While the exact mechanisms leading to cancer recurrence remain poorly understood, failure to completely eliminate dormant micrometastases and solitary metastatic cells is believed to be a major contributor. Thus, while not of initial clinical concern, metastatic dormancy is still of significant clinical importance. The discovery of cancer stem cells (CSCs) in several solid tumor types may provide insight into better understanding the process of metastatic dormancy. In this chapter, we review the metastasis process and metastatic dormancy and discuss the parallels that exist between dormant metastatic cells and CSCs. Finally, we consider the therapeutic implications of CSCs and tumor dormancy on the treatment of metastatic disease.

Key Words: Breast cancer, Recurrence, Metastasis, Dormancy, Cancer stem cells, Microenvironment

INTRODUCTION

While significant progress has been made in the areas of early detection and treatment, breast cancer remains the most commonly diagnosed cancer among women and is a leading cause of morbidity and mortality *(1)*. This is largely due to breast cancer's propensity to metastasize to several vital organs including lung, bone, liver, and brain *(2)*. It is well documented that the presence of metastatic cancer discovered at or near the time the primary tumor is diagnosed is an indicator of poor prognosis *(3)*. Intriguingly, however, breast cancer has been observed to recur, even in patients originally diagnosed with early stage breast cancer, years to decades following apparently successfully primary tumor treatment *(4, 5)*. Such recurrence has been attributed to the delayed growth of previously dormant solitary cells or micrometastases *(6–8)*. Assuming successful removal of the primary tumor, this delayed recurrence is the result of growth of malignant cells that had previously spread from the primary tumor and remained dormant within the secondary site. While recent research has begun elucidating the

---

* These two authors contributed equally to the book chapter.

From: *Cancer Drug Discovery and Development: Stem Cells and Cancer,*
Edited by: R.G. Bagley and B.A. Teicher, DOI: 10.1007/978-1-60327-933-8_11,
© Humana Press, a part of Springer Science+Business Media, LLC 2009

mechanisms responsible for metastatic dormancy, much is still left to be understood. The identification of cancer stem cells (CSCs) in several types of solid tumors raises many interesting questions and possibilities. Here we describe the striking similarities between dormant metastatic cells and CSCs, and consider possible therapeutic implications of the CSC hypothesis on metastatic disease.

METASTASIS AND DORMANCY

Despite the fact that metastasis (the process by which cancer cells spread) is often lethal, it is an extremely inefficient process. The majority of cells shed from a primary tumor behave in a nonmetastatic fashion, failing to form a tumor in the secondary site *(9, 10)*. For a cancer cell to successfully form a metastatic tumor, it must leave the primary tumor, intravasate into a blood or lymphatic vessel, survive transit within the vasculature, arrest in a secondary site, extravasate into the secondary tissue, and commence and continue growth in this new microenvironment *(2)*. As failure at any step during this process will result in failure of the cell to form a metastatic tumor, it is not surprising that metastasis is such an inefficient process. In fact, despite more than 80% of cells successfully extravasating in an experimental model of hematogenous metastasis, only a small proportion (~0.02% in this model) of cells successfully form large vascularized metastases *(10, 11)*. A number of similar metastatic models have also revealed the presence of an often substantial proportion of cancer cells that extravasate into a secondary organ and remain as solitary dormant cells for prolonged periods *(10, 12)*. Initial metastatic inefficiency is thus not solely due to the loss of cells via apoptosis, but due to both apoptosis and failure of cells to initially form metastases due to dormancy.

Following extravasation into a secondary site, metastatic cells undergo one of the three possible fates (Fig. 1): they begin proliferating, undergo cell death (apoptosis), or remain dormant. However, commencing proliferation does not necessarily destine a cell to become a large vascularized metastasis, as most micrometastases either die off or become dormant. Dormancy, therefore, may occur at both the single cell and micrometastasis stages of metastasis formation. These two types of metastatic dormancy are, however, dissimilar in several important ways, including differences in the mechanisms controlling their dormancy, their proliferation status, and likely their response to treatment. Solitary dormant metastatic cells are believed to be quiescent cells and are currently defined by their lack of proliferation and apoptosis as well as by retention of inert fluorescent or other markers that are diluted and unobservable after a few cycles of cell division *(12)*. In contrast, micrometastasis dormancy is characterized by a balanced rate of proliferation and apoptosis, not by their absence *(13)*. Although cells that immediately commence proliferating and continue growing as metastases may be of primary concern clinically, dormant single cells and micrometastases also have clinical implications, as they can be a source of cells responsible for recurrence.

While it has long been known that primary tumors preferentially metastasize to certain organs, the exact reasons why they grow preferentially in these organs are not understood. Differences in blood flow patterns, as well as homing, "seed and soil," and heterogeneous tumor population theories have all been proposed to explain this phenomenon *(14–16)*. While it is likely that each of these play some role in differential growth in separate organs, the situation becomes more confusing when differential growth within the same secondary organ is considered. The discovery of CSCs in many solid tumors suggests another theory to explain the differential behavior of metastatic cells. It is with the previously described principles of metastasis and dormancy in mind that we consider the nature of CSCs and their striking parallels with metastatic cells and dormant metastatic cells in particular.

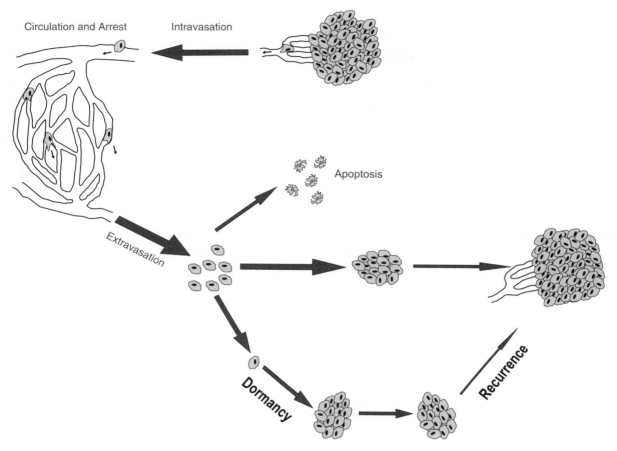

Fig. 1. The metastatic process begins with cells leaving a primary tumor, intravasating and disseminating through the vasculature. Following arrival in a secondary site, the majority of metastatic cells extravasate and carry on to one of the three possible fates: they can undergo cell death (apoptosis); remain dormant; or begin proliferating. Cells must begin and continue proliferating as well as acquire a vasculature in order to become a large, clinically relevant metastatic tumor. Dormant single cells and micrometastases are possible sources of recurrent cancer.

THE CSC HYPOTHESIS

Two theories have been proposed that attempt to explain how tumors develop *(17, 18)*. The stochastic model suggests that every cell within a tumor is a potential tumor-initiator, but that entry into the cell cycle is governed by a low probability of stochastic events. According to this model, all cells have the same ability to initiate tumorigenic growth since each cell has an equal ability to be tumorigenic. This is in contrast to the hierarchy theory, which proposes that only a small subset of cells in a tumor are capable of initiating tumorigenic growth, but that these cells all do so at a high frequency. According to this theory, it should be possible to identify the cells responsible for tumor formation because not all the cells have the same phenotypic characteristics. This latter idea is what is now known as the "cancer stem cell (CSC) hypothesis".

In 1855, Rudolph Virchow suggested that cancer cells behaved in a similar manner to embryonic-like cells *(19)*. However, it was not until 1994 that the first solid evidence supporting the CSC hypothesis emerged *(20)*. Bonnet and Dick *(21)* discovered that AML (acute myeloid leukemia) originated from a hierarchy of tumor-initiating stem-like cells, where only the most primitive cells (CD34$^+$CD38$^-$ cells) were able to initiate and sustain the leukemia. After isolating these CSCs and the non-CSCs (CD34$^-$CD38$^-$ cells) and injecting them into NOD/SCID mice, they found that only the CSCs were able to initiate and sustain the leukemia *(21, 22)*. These findings sparked tremendous interest in discovering stem-like cells in solid tumors, and there is now evidence supporting the existence of CSC populations in brain, breast, prostate, colon, and pancreatic tumors, as well as in melanoma *(23–30)*.

In breast cancer, stem-like cells were identified based on CD44$^+$CD24$^{-/low}$lin$^-$ cell surface marker phenotype. When these cells were isolated from primary tumors or pleural effusions from breast cancer patients and injected into the mammary fat pad of immunocompromised mice, as few as 100 CD44$^+$CD24$^{-/low}$lin$^-$ cells were sufficient to cause a tumor in these mice, whereas injections of tens of thousands of cells that did not express that phenotype failed to cause tumor formation *(24)*. Similar results have been observed in brain, pancreatic, and colon cancer, where the CD133-expressing cells are able to form tumors; however, the CD133$^-$ cells were consistently unable to form tumors *(23, 27–29)*. In prostate cancer, CD44$^+$ stem-like cells have been identified, and have been shown to express higher mRNA levels of several "stemness" genes (i.e., SMO and Oct 3/4) compared to the CD44$^-$ cells, as well as being able to undergo asymmetric division in clonal analysis *(25)*. CD44$^+$CD24$^+$ESA$^+$ cells in pancreatic tumors display a 100-fold increase in tumorigenic potential compared to the rest of the cells of the tumor. Additionally, tumors that formed from these CD44$^+$CD24$^+$ESA$^+$ cells were indistinguishable from the human tumors in which they originated, demonstrating their ability to self-renew and give rise to heterogeneous cell populations *(28)*.

The CSC has been clearly defined by Clarke et al. as "a cell within a tumor that possesses the capacity to self-renew and to cause the heterogeneous lineages of cancer cells that comprise the tumor" *(31)*. Contrary to this clear definition, the most elusive and highly debated question surrounding the CSC hypothesis is related to the cellular origin of the CSC (i.e., from a differentiated mature cell, progenitor cell, or primitive stem cell). Given the limited lifespan of mature cells, it is difficult to comprehend how a differentiated mature cell could somehow accumulate enough mutations to de-differentiate and become more stem-cell like. Alternatively, normal, primitive stem cells stay relatively dormant and protected throughout their lifespan *(32–34)*, so accumulating enough mutations to become cancerous would seem rather difficult. Progenitor cells, however, are actively dividing and participating in cellular events within a tissue. Since these cells (albeit protected from damaging stimuli due to inherent self-protection mechanisms) have an inherently increased resistance for apoptosis and senescence over normal cells *(35, 36)*, then accumulating mutations would make them very dangerous. Furthermore, since these cells survive in the tissue for prolonged periods of time (i.e., much longer than normal, more differentiated cells), they have an increased exposure to potentially damaging stimuli, and an increased chance of accumulating enough mutations to become cancerous. In further support of this idea, microarray analyses have demonstrated that the gene signatures of CSCs are more similar to the stem cells of that particular tissue than to the non-CSCs of the cancer *(37–39)*.

Populations of stem-like cells have been identified in primary tumors and have been shown to be able to initiate and sustain tumorigenic growth *(20–30)*. Although two recently published studies have demonstrated a potential link between CSCs and successful metastatic behavior in breast *(40)* and pancreatic *(29)* cancer, the functional contribution of CSCs to metastasis remains very poorly understood. However, there are several parallels among normal stem cells, CSCs, and metastatic cells that provide strong rationale for considering that successful metastatic cells may in fact be CSCs *(41, 42)*.

STEM CELLS, CANCER STEM CELLS, AND METASTATIC CELLS

As discussed earlier, metastasis is a highly inefficient process with only a small subset of disseminated cells actually able to form clinically relevant macrometastases *(10)*. The rate-limiting steps in the metastatic cascade include the ability of disseminated cells to initiate and sustain growth in the secondary site *(2, 10, 43, 44)*. This inefficiency has been attributed to the inability of disseminated cells to find the proper microenvironment to support metastatic growth *(45–48)*. However, with the emergence of the CSC hypothesis, there may be an alternative explanation; one that suggests that only CSCs are capable of metastatic growth *(41, 42)*. This makes intuitive sense, since evidence suggests that CSCs are the only cells capable of initiating and sustaining tumorigenic growth in primary tumors. In primary breast tumors, the CSC population is quite small, ranging from ~1 to 2% of the cells comprising the tumor *(24)*. Many cells may escape the primary tumor, but only a small proportion of them will be CSCs since they are believed to represent such a small percentage of the primary tumor. When these rare cells disseminate, however, they could have a high capacity for initiating metastatic growth. To date, there is only minimal evidence linking CSCs to metastasis. However, there are several striking similarities among normal stem cells, CSCs, and metastatic cells, including the requirement for a niche or microenvironment to grow; enhanced resistance to apoptosis and protection from cellular insult; and cellular dormancy.

The Niche/Microenvironment

It is well documented that normal stem cells require a particular protective microenvironment, or "niche," in which to reside *(32–34)*. This environment effectively protects stem cells from molecules that could cause differentiation or damage, allows the stem cells to remain dormant until they are needed for tissue repair, and can also regulate the growth activation and symmetric vs. asymmetric cell division *(32–34)*. Putative mammary stem and progenitor cells, for example, are sequestered from both the basement membrane and the lumen in structurally defined spaces *(33)*.

Metastatic cells also appear to require a particular "niche" or microenvironment which actively contributes to the growth and invasion of metastatic tumors *(14, 49–51)*. This was elegantly demonstrated by Kaplan et al. *(49)* who were able to show that bone marrow derived VEGFR1[+] hematopoietic cells can home to tumor-specific premetastatic sites and form cellular clusters before the arrival of metastatic tumor cells in mice. These cells alter the local microenvironment such that it can promote tumor cell attraction, survival, and growth. When treated with an anti-VEGFR1 antibody, the premetastatic cell clusters were eliminated, and metastasis was prevented *(49)*.

Although still under debate, there is some evidence that CSCs also require a particular stem-cell niche. For example, it has been shown that leukemic stem cells (LSCs) occupy the perioendosteal region (the normal HSC niche) *(52)*. Additionally, when immunocompromised mice affected with AML were treated with a monoclonal antibody targeting CD44, LSCs were completely eradicated. This effect was due to disruption of CD44-mediated communication between the LSCs and their niche, leading ultimately to LSC differentiation and/or death *(53)*. Furthermore, TGF-β has been shown to inhibit the proliferation of quiescent hematopoietic stem cells (HSCs) *(54)*, so perhaps in malignancy, niche cells may control TGF-β secretion to dysregulate CSC division, thus influencing the delicate balance between CSC proliferation, differentiation, and senescence. In solid cancers, it could be hypothesized that CSCs in metastatic sites are similarly regulated by inappropriate signaling from the metastatic niche that drives the dormancy vs. proliferation decision-making process *(55, 56)*. Currently, the similarities between stem cell niches in different tissues remain poorly understood, in particular with regards to whether tissue-specific stem cells can be regulated by stem cell niches in other organs. This knowledge will have important implications for understanding metastatic growth in secondary sites, including the possibility that some CSCs (i.e., breast) may favor survival and/or growth in the bone marrow because it provides a particularly rich stem cell niche *(57)*.

Resistance to Apoptosis and Protection from Cellular Insult

Resistance to apoptosis is another key property shared by normal stem cells, CSCs, and metastatic cancer cells. Stem cells can resist apoptosis by a number of mechanisms, including via TGF-β signalling or activation of the Hedgehog (HH) pathway *(58)*. Additionally, stem cells express higher levels of antiapoptotic proteins than differentiated cells, including members of the Bcl-2 family *(59)*. Stem cells must also resist early senescence in order to maintain the stem cell pool, a process facilitated by Bmi-1 expression. Interestingly, Bmi-1, Bcl-2, TGF-β, and HH pathway components have all been shown to be upregulated in cancer cells *(58–62)*. Furthermore, despite their limitless self-renewal capacity, normal stem cells are relatively quiescent and divide infrequently unless activated *(61, 63–65)*. Similarly, CSCs and metastatic cells may cycle through long periods of quiescence/dormancy and short bursts of proliferation, and since most chemotherapeutic anticancer agents are designed to target rapidly dividing cells, this may be one mechanism by which CSCs and metastatic cells escape cytoxicity from these drugs *(66)*.

From an evolutionary point of view, normal stem cells have a number of unique properties that help protect them from cellular insult and ensure their long lifespan. For instance, normal stem cells express high levels of ABC transporters that facilitate rapid efflux of toxins and drugs, but these genes get turned off in committed mature cells *(64)*. These transporters include *ABCB1*, which encodes P-glycoprotein, and *ABCG2*, which encodes a protein called breast cancer resistance protein (BCRP). These two transporter proteins can help a cell efflux a large number of different chemotherapeutic agents, including doxorubicin and paclitaxel. Along with *ABCC1*, *ABCB1* and *ABCG2* represent the three principal multi-drug resistance (MDR) genes overexpressed in tumor cells *(63, 67–69)*. This drug resistance could be an inherent feature of CSCs, and could help explain the high level of drug resistance in metastatic disease *(57, 64)*.

Finally, stem cells are also thought to be more resistant to DNA damaging agents than differentiated cells because of their ability to undergo asynchronous DNA synthesis and their enhanced capacity for DNA repair. During asynchronous DNA synthesis, the parental "immortal" DNA strand always segregates with the new stem cell rather than with the differentiating progeny, thus helping to protect the stem cell population from DNA damage *(61, 70–73)*. Similarly, CSCs are believed to be resistant to radiation therapy by preferentially upregulating their DNA proofreading mechanisms in order to avoid cellular death due to DNA damage *(74, 75)*. Studies have shown that treating a tumor with radiation can deplete the non-CSC population and increase the CSC population by threefold to fivefold, thus rendering the tumor even more aggressive and resistant to treatment *(75)*.

Cell Dormancy

As discussed earlier, an interesting characteristic of metastatic cells is their ability to remain dormant for months, or even years after arriving in a secondary site. In fact, it is not uncommon for a breast cancer patient to be in seemingly complete remission from their primary tumor, only to present years later with metastatic disease. Interestingly, the behavior of these dormant metastatic cells is in many ways similar to stem cell quiescence. If it is indeed true that successful metastatic cells are CSCs, then perhaps metastatic cell dormancy can be better understood by taking into consideration some of the mechanisms that regulate the balance between quiescence and activation/ growth in stem cells.

Many adult tissues maintain a stem cell pool which is needed to sustain tissue homeostasis and ensure rapid response to injury. One way in which this pool is maintained is through tight control of the number of cell divisions undertaken by stem cells within the pool. Thus, stem cells go through long periods of quiescence, and only proliferate when needed for production of differentiated progeny and/or replenishment of the stem cell pool *(76)*. Several molecular mechanisms have been identified that contributed to this process. For example, stem cell quiescence has been associated with the Kruppel, FoxO, and Rb families of transcriptional regulators that induce reversible arrest in various lineages *(77)*. Microarray data has also shown that during stem cell quiescence, there is active suppression of differentiation-related housekeeping genes, and a higher expression of Notch and its downstream molecules, which are important in maintaining the stem cell pool in some tissues *(77, 78)*. During quiescence, expression of Lrig1 ensures that stem cells are less responsive to growth factor stimulation than their differentiated progeny. It has been proposed that Lrig1 expression maintains skin stem cells in a quiescent, nonproliferative state in part by negatively regulating Myc transcription. It has also been suggested that Myc-induced differentiation acts as a fail-safe device to prevent uncontrolled proliferation of stem cells when Lrig1 is downregulated *(79)*. Interestingly, a soluble form of LRIG1 has been shown to inhibit proliferation of some cancers *(80)*. A similar situation has been observed in a Myc inducible transgenic mouse model of cancer, where Myc inactivation resulted in tumor dormancy, cell differentiation, and expression of cytokeratin 19 in a subset of cells. This effect however was reversible, and upon Myc reactivation tumors continued growing *(81)*. Although relatively little is known about what controls solitary metastatic cell dormancy, several key molecules and pathways, including p21, p27, p38, uPAR, ERK, and Myc, have been implicated in maintaining this dormancy *(7, 82)*. As these molecules are known as cell cycle regulators or upstream signaling pathways, it is logical that the niche or microenvironment, much in the same way it regulates stem cells, is regulating these dormant metastatic cells.

Interestingly, recent evidence has indicated that the stem cell pool itself can be comprised of a heterogeneous cell population. For example, in the murine hematopoietic system, two subtypes of HSCs have been identified, a large proportion that are capable of activation for homeostasis purposes, and a smaller proportion of protected, dormant HSCs which are needed for critical response to injury and absolute maintenance of the stem cell pool. These "dormant" HSCs have the highest repopulating and self-renewing capacity of all HSCs, and are only activated in response to injury. Once repair is complete, 100% of the previously dormant HSCs return to their niche microenvironment and their dormant state *(83)*. HSCs have also been shown to be heterogeneous in terms of their differentiation capacity and migratory ability *(84–86)*. This observed stem cell heterogeneity implies that this is perhaps also the case in the CSC hierarchy. It is possible that there are primitive CSCs that remain relatively dormant, and that these cells, once activated, will have the highest self-renewing and tumor repopulating activity of all the CSCs. If this is the case, then targeting the dormant metastatic cells would be very important. This observation of stem cell heterogeneity could explain why, in the majority of metastasis models, cells are simultaneously observed at the single cell, micrometastasis and macrometastasis stages *(10, 12)*.

Chronic wound healing has been suggested as a mechanism of cancer initiation, where the dormant stem cells repeatedly become activated for tissue repair, but eventually lose the ability to differentiate and become CSCs [reviewed in *(87)*]. In support of this, small populations of "primed" cells within tumors have an increased ability to grow due to epigenetic silencing of the p16 promoter. This silencing leads to an increase in proliferation, invasion, and angiogenesis and a decrease in apoptosis and immune surveillance. Furthermore, loss of p16 holds cells in a primitive state, increasing stem cell self-renewal and preventing differentiation *(88)*. It is possible that activation of dormant metastatic cells occurs in much the same way (illustrated in Fig. 2). When the most primitive of CSCs disseminate

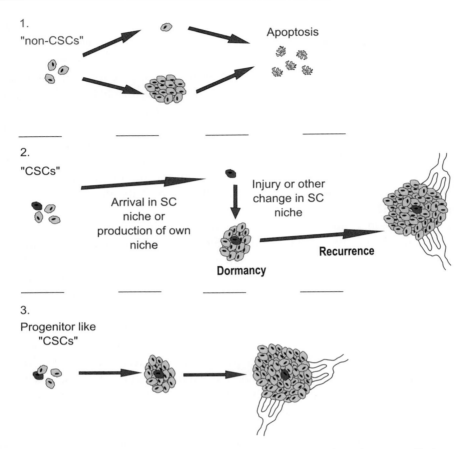

Fig. 2. The cancer stem cell (CSC) hypothesis applied to the fate of disseminated cancer cells in a secondary site. Upon arriving in the secondary site, cells may undergo apoptosis, remain dormant or begin proliferating. The fate of each cell is likely due to both the cell population (CSC or non-CSC) and the microenvironment or niche. Non-CSCs that disseminate to a secondary tissue may remain dormant, eventually undergo apoptosis and fail to form tumors (1). In contrast, primitive CSCs may migrate to a stem cell (SC) niche in a secondary tissue, or alternatively, make their own niche and become dormant at the solitary cell or micrometastasis stage (2). These cells could then remain dormant until the niche becomes activated by aging, injury, or mechanical trauma; and once activated, the CSCs begin dividing in a dysregulated manner, forming a secondary tumor. Finally, less primitive, more progenitor-like CSCs may begin proliferating immediately when in a secondary tissue, receiving signals to proliferate (3). In this case, a metastatic tumor could develop relatively quickly.

from the primary tumor, they may stay in their proper niche (i.e., breast CSCs would stay in the mammary stem cell niche), or alternatively, migrate to a niche that meets the cells' requirements (i.e., the bone marrow). The CSCs then remain "quiescent" or "dormant" for long periods of time, perhaps enabling them to escape from prolonged cancer therapy. It may be that they stay dormant, in fact, until such a time as the normal stem cells in that niche are stimulated due changes in the microenvironment and/or injury related to aging, toxins, or mechanical damage. The stem cells (along with the CSCs) are then activated and migrate toward the site of the injury, and the CSC, due to its previous mutations, begins dividing in a dysregulated manner, ultimately forming a metastatic tumor. Alternatively, CSCs may escape from a primary tumor and form their own niche via differentiated progeny in the secondary tissue of their choosing. In this way, the non-CSC niche (much like a normal stem cell niche) would protect the CSCs from damaging and differentiating molecules, and relay signals to keep the CSCs in a dormant state until such a time that some stimuli awaken the CSCs and a metastatic tumor is initiated. Of course, sometimes dormancy does not occur and metastatic cells form secondary tumors while a patient is still being treated for the primary tumor. In this case, it is possible that these metastatic events are caused by a less primitive, more progenitor-like CSC population that does not travel to any stem cell niche at all, and instead travels right to an active tissue, receiving signals to proliferate. In this case, a metastatic tumor could develop relatively quickly.

THERAPEUTIC IMPLICATIONS

The idea that CSCs are involved in metastasis has many important implications for the way in which we currently treat cancer. There is evidence to suggest that CSCs are resistant to both radiation and chemotherapy *(64, 65, 74, 75)*. In response to radiation, the CSC population has been shown to upregulate DNA damage checkpoint proteins to ensure less DNA damage, and in this way, the CSC population is actually enriched following radiation therapy *(74, 75)*. In the case of chemotherapy, it is possible that by expressing more ABC pumps to pump out chemotherapeutic agents, the CSC population is preferentially spared *(64, 65)*. Additionally, the CSCs may in fact be dormant; cycling more slowly than their differentiated progeny; and/or hidden away in their protective niche, thus giving the chemotherapeutic agents less of a chance to target the cells responsible for cancer progression and recurrence *(89)*. Therefore, current cancer therapies may shrink the bulk of the tumor (i.e., kill off the more differentiated cells), leaving the tumor-initiating CSCs behind to eventually rebuild the tumor, or worse, disseminate to a new location and initiate metastatic growth.

The therapeutic dilemma is that while a therapy may be effective against primary tumors, and even initially against metastases after they form, the ultimate goal would be successfully target dormant/quiescent cancer cells and avoid metastases before they even get a chance develop. However, dormant cancer cells clearly present a substantial therapeutic problem, since it is nearly impossible to target a dormant cell. Taking into account the parallels between stem cells, CSCs, and dormant metastatic cell discussed here, perhaps new therapeutic approaches will evolve. For example, if dormant CSCs could be first forced into an activated state (potentially by the same mechanistic pathways that activate normal dormant stem cells) it may be possible to successfully employ a more conventional therapy (i.e., chemotherapy) aimed at killing and/or differentiating the elusive dormant CSCs. However, this approach would need to be undertaken with caution, in order to ensure that only CSCs, and not normal stem cells, become activated and targeted. Understanding the signals that trigger activation of both CSCs and dormant metastatic cells will be important for working toward this approach.

CONCLUDING REMARKS

Elucidation of the mechanisms regulating metastasis and clinical tumor dormancy remain two of the most important and provocative challenges in cancer biology. Metastasis is a lethal yet entirely inefficient process. This inefficiency largely lies in the ability of only a small proportion of metastatic cells to initiate and sustain metastatic growth in a secondary site. Additionally, once disseminated, many tumor cells become dormant and may activate to form metastases months or even years after removal of the primary tumor. Metastatic inefficiency and tumor dormancy have been attributed to inability to grow in certain microenvironments; however, with the emergence of the CSC hypothesis, it is possible to add a new dimension to this concept. The possible conceptual application of the CSC hypothesis to metastasis and dormancy is diagrammed in Fig. 2. Since CSCs have a high ability to initiate and sustain tumorigenic growth, then it is probable that the CSCs within the primary tumor also represent the successful metastatic cells. Normal stem cells, CSCs, and metastatic cells demonstrate strikingly similar characteristics, including the requirement for a particular niche or microenvironment in which to survive and grow; enhanced resistance to apoptosis; and cell dormancy as a mechanism of survival and self-protection. In particular, the CSC hypothesis and the idea that the most primitive CSCs may undergo periods of quiescence has major therapeutic implications for treatment of both primary and metastatic disease. Understanding the functional and mechanistic role that CSCs may play in determining tumor dormancy and metastatic potential will therefore have significant implications for the way we currently study, diagnosis, and treat cancer.

ACKNOWLEDGMENTS

We thank members of our laboratory and our collaborators for helpful discussions during preparation of this book chapter. The authors' work on dormancy and cancer stem cells is supported in part by grants from the London Regional Cancer Program (A.L.A., A.F.C.) and by grants from the Canadian Institutes of Health Research (grant #42511 to A.F.C.) and the US Department of Defense Breast Cancer Research Program (#W81XWH-06-2-0033 to A.F.C.). A.K.C. is the recipient of a Canadian Institute of Health Research Strategic Training Program Scholarship, a Translational Breast Cancer Scholarship through the London Regional Cancer Program, and a Fellowship from the Canadian Breast Cancer Foundation-Ontario Chapter. J.L.T is supported by a Doctoral Research Award from the Canadian Institute of Health Research. A.L.A. is supported by the Imperial Oil Foundation and A.F.C. is the recipient of a Canada Research Chair in Oncology.

REFERENCES

1. Jemal A, Siegel R, Ward E, et al. Cancer statistics. CA Cancer J Clin 2007;57:43–66.
2. Chambers AF, Groom AC, MacDonald IC. Dissemination and growth of cancer cells in metastatic sites. Nat Rev Cancer 2002;2:563–72.
3. Greenberg PA, Hortobagyi GN, Smith TL, Ziegler LD, Frye DK, Buzdar AU. Long-term follow-up of patients with complete remission following combination chemotherapy for metastatic breast cancer. J Clin Oncol 1996;14:2197–205.
4. Fisher B, Jeong J-H, Dignam J, Anderson S, et al. Findings from recent National Surgical Adjuvant Breast and Bowel Project adjuvant studies in stage 1 breast cancer. J Natl Cancer Inst Monogr 2001;30:62–6.
5. Wallgren A, Bonetti M, Gelber RD, et al. Risk factors for locoregional recurrence among breast cancer patients: Results from international breast cancer study group trials I through VII. J Clin Oncol 2003;21:1205–13.
6. Townson JL, Chambers AF. Dormancy of solitary metastatic cells. Cell Cycle 2006; 5:1744–50.
7. Brackstone M, Townson JL and Chambers AF. Tumour dormancy in breast cancer: an update. Breast Cancer Res 2007;9:208–14.
8. Aguirre-Ghiso JL. Models, mechanisms and clinical evidence for cancer dormancy. Nat Rev Cancer 2007;7:834–46.
9. Weiss L. Metastatic inefficiency: intravascular and intraperitoneal implantation of cancer cells. Cancer Treat Res 1996;82:1–11
10. Luzzi KJ, MacDonald IC, Schmidt EE, et al. Multistep nature of metastatic inefficiency: dormancy of solitary cells after successful extravasation and limited survival of early micrometastases. Am J Pathol 1998;153:865–73.
11. Koop S, MacDonald IC, Luzzi K, et al. Fate of melanoma cells entering the microcirculation: over 80% survive and extravasate. Cancer Res 1995;55:2520–23.
12. Naumov GN, MacDonald IC, Weinmeister PM, et al. Persistence of solitary mammary carcinoma cells in a secondary site: a possible contributor to dormancy. Cancer Res 2002;62:2162–68.
13. Holmgren L, O'Reilly MS, Folkman J. Dormancy of micrometastases: balanced proliferation and apoptosis in the presence of angiogenesis suppression. Nat Med 1995;1:149–53.
14. Psaila B, Kaplan RN, Port ER, Lyden D. Priming the "soil" for breast cancer metastasis: the pre-metastatic niche. Breast Dis 2006–2007;26:65–74.
15. Ramaswamy S, Ross KN, Lander ES, Golub TR. A molecular signature of metastasis in primary solid tumors. Nat Genet 2003;33:49–54.

16. Poste G, Fidler IJ. The pathogenesis of cancer metastasis. Nature 1980;283:139–46.
17. Reya T, Morrison SJ, Clarke MF, Weissman IL. Stem cells, cancer, and cancer stem cells. Nature 2001;414:105–11.
18. Dick JE. Breast cancer stem cells revealed. Proc Natl Acad Sci USA 2003;100:3547–9.
19. Virchow R. Editorial. Virchows Arch Pathol Anat Physiol Klin Med 1855;3:23.
20. Lapidot T, Sirard C, Vormoor J, et al. A cell initiating human acute myeloid leukemia after transplantation into SCID mice. Nature 1994;367:645–48.
21. Bonnet D, Dick JE. Human acute myeloid leukemia is organized as a hierarchy that originates from a primitive hematopoietic cell. Nat Med 1997;3:730–7.
22. Hope KJ, Jin L, Dick JE. Acute myeloid leukemia originates from a hierarchy of leukemic stem cell classes that differ in self-renewal capacity. Nat Immunol 2004;5:738–43.
23. Singh SK, Hawkins C, Clarke ID, et al. Identification of human brain tumour initiating cells. Nature 2004;432:396–401.
24. Al-Hajj M, Wicha MS, Benito-Hernandez A, et al. Prospective identification of tumorigenic breast cancer cells. Proc Natl Acad Sci USA 2003;100:3983–88.
25. Patrawala L, Calhoun T, Schneider-Broussard R, et al. Highly purified CD44+ prostate cancer cells from xenografts human tumors are enriched in tumorigenic and metastatic progenitor cells. Oncogene 2006;25:1696–1708.
26. Collins AT, Berry PA, Hyde C, et al. Prospective identification of tumorigenic prostate cancer stem cells. Cancer Res 2005;65:10946–51.
27. O'Brien CA, Pollett A, Gallinger S, Dick JE. A human colon caner cell capable of initiating tumour growth in immuno-deficient mice. Nature 2007;445:106–10.
28. Li C, Heidt DG, Dalerba P, et al. Identification of pancreatic cancer stem cells. Cancer Res 2007;67:1030–37.
29. Hermann PC, Huber SL, Herrler T, Aicher A, et al. Distinct populations of cancer stem cells determine tumor growth and metastatic activity in human pancreatic cancer. Cell Stem Cell 2007;1:313–23.
30. Schatton T, Murphy GF, Frank NY, et al. Identification of cells initiating human melanomas. Nature 2008;451:345–49.
31. Clarke MF, Dick JE, Dirks PB, et al. Cancer stem cells – Perspectives on current status and future directions: AACR workshop on cancer stem cells. Cancer Res 2006;66:9339–44.
32. Scadden DT. The stem cell niche in health and leukemic disease. Clin Hematol 2007;20:19–27.
33. Chepko G, Dickson RB. Ultrastructure of the putative stem cell niche in rat mammary epithelium. Tissue Cell 2003;35:83–93.
34. Hendrix MJC, Seftor, EA, Seftor REB, et al. Reprogramming metastatic tumor cells with embryonic microenvironments. Nature 2007;7:246–55.
35. Johansson I, Destefanis S, Aberg DN, et al. Proliferative and protective effects of growth hormone secretagogues on adult rat hippocampal progenitor cells. Endocrinology 2008;149:2191–9; Epub ahead of print, PMID: 18218693.
36. Inoue A, Seidel MG, Wu W, et al. Slug, a highly conserved zinc finger transcriptional repressor, protects hematopoietic progenitor cells from radiation-induced apoptosis in vivo. Cancer Cell 2002;2:279–88.
37. Gal H, Amariglio N, Trakhtenbrot L, et al. Gene expression profiles of AML derived stem cells; similarity to hematopoietic stem cells. Leukemia 2006;20:2147–54.
38. Sperger JM, Chen X, Draper JS, et al. Gene expression patterns in human embryonic stem cells and human pluripotent germ cell tumors. Proc Natl Acad Sci USA 2003;100:13350–55.
39. Jones RJ, Matsui WH, Smith BD. Cancer stem cells: are we missing the target? J Natl Cancer Inst 2004;96:583–85.
40. Yu F, Yao H, Zhu P, et al. let-7 regulates self renewal and tumorigenicity of breast cancer cells. Cell 2007;131:1109–23.
41. Croker AK, Allan AL. Cancer stem cells: implications for the progression and treatment of metastatic disease. J Cell Mol Med 2008;12:374–90; Epub ahead of print, PMID: 18182063.
42. Li F, Tiede B, Massagué J, Kang Y. Beyond tumorigenesis: cancer stem cells in metastasis. Cell Res 2002,17:3–14.
43. Pantel K, Brakenhoff RH. Dissecting the metastatic cascade. Nat Rev Cancer 2004;4:448–56.
44. Weiss L. Metastatic inefficiency. Adv Cancer Res 1990;54:159–211.
45. Ewing J. A treatise on tumors. In: Neoplastic Diseases. London: W.B. Saunders, 1928, pp. 77–89.
46. Paget S. The distribution of secondary growths in cancer of the breast (re-publication of the original 1889 Lancet article). Cancer Met Rev 1989;8:98–101.
47. Fidler IJ. Seed and soil revisited: contribution of the organ microenvironment to cancer metastasis. Surg Oncol Clin N Am 2001;10:257–69, vii–viii.
48. Weiss L. Comments on hematogenous metastatic patterns in humans as revealed by autopsy. Clin Exp Metastasis 1992;10:191–9.
49. Kaplan RN, Riba RD, Zacharoulis S, et al. VEGFR1-positive haematopoietic bone marrow progenitors initiate the pre-metastatic niche. Nature 2005;438:820–26.
50. Kaplan RN, Raffi S, Lyden D. Preparing the "soil": the premetastatic niche. Cancer Res 2006;66:11089–93.

51. Wang W, Eddy R, Condeelis J. The cofilin pathway in breast cancer invasion and metastasis. Nature 2007;7:429–40.

52. Ishikawa F, Yoshida S, Saito Y, et al. Chemotherapy-resistant human AML stem cells home to and engraft within the bone-marrow endosteal region. Nat Biotechnol 2007;25:1315–21.

53. Jin L, Hope KJ, Zhai Q, et al. Targeting of CD44 eradicates human acute myeloid leukemic stem cells. Nat Med 2006;12:1167–74.

54. Isufi I, Seetharam M, Zhou L, et al. Transforming growth factor-b signaling in normal and malignant hematopoiesis. J Interferon Cytokine Res 2007;27:543–52.

55. Wicha MS, Liu S, Dontu G. Cancer stem cells: an old idea – a paradigm shift. Cancer Res 2006;66:1883–90; discussion 95–6.

56. Li L, Neaves WB. Normal stem cells and cancer stem cells: the niche matters. Cancer Res. 2006;66:4553–7.

57. Allan AL, Vantyghem SA, Tuck AB, Chambers AF. Tumor dormancy and cancer stem cells: implications for the biology and treatment of breast cancer metastasis. Breast Dis 2007;26:87–98.

58. Thayer SP, Pasca di Magliano M, Heiser PW, et al. Hedgehog is an early and late mediator of pancreatic cancer tumori-genesis. Nature 2003;425:851–6.

59. Wang S, Yang D, Lippman ME. Targeting Bcl-2 and Bcl-XL with nonpeptidic small-molecule antagonists. Semin Oncol 2003;30:133–42.

60. Liu S, Dontu G, Mantle ID, et al. Hedgehog signaling and Bmi-1 regulate self-renewal of normal and malignant human mammary stem cells. Cancer Res 2006;66:6063–71.

61. Park Y, Gerson SL. DNA repair defects in stem cell function and aging. Annu Rev Med 2005;56:495–508.

62. Berman DM, Karhadkar SS, Maltra A, et al. Widespread requirement for hedgehog ligand stimulation in growth of digestive tract tumours. Nature 2003;425:846–51.

63. Pardal R, Clarke MF, Morrison SJ. Applying the principles of stem-cell biology to cancer. Nat Rev Cancer 2003;3:895–902.

64. Dean M, Fojo T, Bates S. Tumour stem cells and drug resistance. Nat Rev Cancer 2005;5:275–84.

65. Dean M. Cancer stem cells: Redefining the paradigm of cancer treatment strategies. Mol Interv 2006;6:140–8.

66. Naumov GN, Townson JL, MacDonald IC, et al., Ineffectiveness of doxorubicin treatment on solitary dormant mammary carcinoma cells or late-developing metastases. Breast Cancer Res Treat 2003;82(3):199–206.

67. Scharenberg CW, Harkey MA, Torok-Storb B. The ABCG2 transporter is an efficient Hoechst 33342 efflux pump and is preferentially expressed by immature human hematopoietic progenitors. Blood 2002;99:507–12.

68. Kim M, Turnquist H, Jackson J, Sgagias M, et al. The multidrug resistance transporter ABCG2 (breast cancer resistance protein 1) effluxes Hoechst 33342 and is overexpressed in hematopoietic stem cells. Clin Cancer Res 2002;8:22–8.

69. Doyle LA, Yang W, Abruzzo LV, et al. A multidrug resistance transporter from human MCF-7 breast cancer cells. Proc Natl Acad Sci USA 1998;95:15665–70.

70. Cairns J. The cancer problem. Sci Am 1975;233:64–72.

71. Cairns J. Somatic stem cells and the kinetics of mutagenesis and carcinogenesis. Proc Natl Acad Sci USA 2002;99:10567–70.

72. Potten CS, Owen G, Booth D. Intestinal stem cells protect their genome by selective segregation of template DNA strands. J Cell Sci 2002;115:2381–8.

73. Cai J, Weiss ML, Rao MS. In search of "stemness". Exp Hematol 2004;32:585–98.

74. Phillips TM, McBride WH, Pajonk F. The response of CD24$^{-/low}$/CD44$^+$ breast cancer-initiating cells to radiation. J Natl Cancer Inst 2006;98:1777–85.

75. Bao S, Wu Q, McLendon RE, et al. Glioma stem cells promote radioresistance by preferential activation of the DNA damage response. Nature 2006;444:756–60.

76. Komarova NL, Wodarz D. Stochastic modeling of cellular colonies with quiescence: an application to drug resistance in cancer. Theor Popul Biol 2007;72:523–38.

77. Nishikawa S-I, Osawa M. Generating quiescent stem cells. Pigment Cell Res 2007;20:263–70.

78. Kawamata S, Du C, Lavau C. Overexpression of the Notch target genes Hes in vivo induces lymphoid and myeloid alterations. Oncogene 2002;21:3855–63.

79. Jensen KB, Watt FM. Single-cell expression profiling of human epidermal stem and transit-amplifying cells: Lrig1 is a regulator of stem cell quiescence. Proc Natl Acad Sci USA 2006;103:11958–63.

80. Goldoni S, Iozzo RA, Kay P, et al. A soluble ectodomain of LRIG1 inhibits cancer cell growth by attenuating basal and ligand-dependent EGFR activity. Oncogene 2007;26:368–81.

81. Shachaf CM, Kopelman AM, Arvanitis C, et al. MYC inactivation uncovers pluripotent differentiation and tumour dor-mancy in hepatocellular cancer. Nature 2004;431:1112–7.

82. Aguirre-Ghiso JA. The problem of cancer dormancy: understanding the basic mechanisms and identifying therapeutic opportunities. Cell Cycle 2006;5:1740–3.

83. Wilson A, Oser GM, Jaworski M, et al. Dormant and self-renewing hematopoietic stem cells and their niches. Ann N Y Acad Sci 2007;1106:64–75.
84. Sieburg HB, Cho RH, Dykstra B, et al. The hematopoietic stem compartment consists of a limited number of discrete stem cell subsets. Blood 2006;107:2311–16.
85. McKenzie JL, Gan OI, Doedens M, et al. Individual stem cells with highly variable proliferation and self-renewal properties comprise the human hematopoietic stem cell compartment. Nat Immunol 2006;7:1225–33.
86. Holyoake TL, Nicolini FE, Eaves CJ. Functional differences between transplantable human hematopoietic stem cells from fetal liver, cord blood, and adult marrow. Exp Hematol 1999;27:1418–27.
87. Widera D, Kaus A, Kaltschmidt C, Kaltschmidt B. Neural stem cells, inflammation and NF-kappaB: basic principle of maintenance and repair or origin of brain tumours? J Cell Mol Med 2008;12:459–70; Epub ahead of print, PMID: 18182066.
88. Reynolds PA, Sigaroudinia M, Zardo G, et al. Tumor suppressor p16INK4A regulates polycomb-mediated DNA hypermethylation in human mammary epithelial cells. J Biol Chem 2006;281:24790–802.
89. Graham SM, Jorgensen HG, Allan E, et al. Primitive, quiescent, Philadelphia-positive stem cells from patients with chronic myeloid leukemia are insensitive to ST1571 in vitro. Blood 2002;99:319–25.

12

Cancer Stem Cells: Gastrointestinal Cancers

Hideshi Ishii, Naotsugu Haraguchi, Keisuke Ieta,
Koshi Mimori, and Masaki Mori

ABSTRACT

The multistep model of tumor progression emphasizes the accumulation of genetic alterations as the central mechanism driving tumorigenesis. It is indicated that the normal stem/progenitor cells are an almost passive recipient of the mutations, and its cancer-associated heterogeneity are governed largely by somatic mutations and cancer stem cell-specific signaling, which are detectable by marker analysis during the course of tumor progression. Here we update our knowledge of esophagus, stomach, colon and liver, which would help our better understanding gastrointestinal cancer stem cells.

INTRODUCTION

Cancer stem cells (CSCs) are a subpopulation of cancer cells that possess characteristics normally associated with tissue stem cells. Normal stem cells are characterized as having: *(1)* the capability of self-renewal, *(2)* the potential to divide and differentiate to generate all functional elements of a particular tissue, and *(3)* strict control over stem cell numbers *(1, 2)*. CSCs are defined as cells within the tumor with tumor-initiating potential *(2, 3)*, so they are believed to have no control over cell numbers *(2)*. CSCs are present in very small numbers in whole tumors and are responsible for the growth *(2)*. CSCs are tumorigenic, in contrast to the bulk of cancer cells, which are thought to be nontumorigenic. A hypothesis suggests CSCs persist in tumors as a distinct population and might cause relapse and metastasis by giving rise to new tumors. Thus, development of therapeutic therapies targeted at CSCs holds hope for improvement of survival and quality of life of cancer patients, especially for sufferers of metastasis. The clinicopathological process is driven by the mechanism of cell death, growth, and differentiation, which are altered in CSCs. Here we note our recent knowledge regarding CSCs of gastrointestinal organs.

CANCER GENOMICS AND BIOLOGY IN GASTROINTESTINAL CANCERS

Generally it is accepted that cancer is a disease with genetic and epigenetic alterations, which could lead to the disorder of developmental program in somatic cells *(4, 5)*. In tumors, so-called heterogeneity is noted, and the CSC model could explains why the biological heterogeneity of tumors could occur *(3, 6)*.

From: *Cancer Drug Discovery and Development: Stem Cells and Cancer,*
Edited by: R.G. Bagley and B.A. Teicher, DOI: 10.1007/978-1-60327-933-8_12,
© Humana Press, a part of Springer Science+Business Media, LLC 2009

Complicated and Overlapping Cancer Genomics

Over the last decade, evidence has mounted for cancer genetics that they are fundamentally genomic diseases, which associate genetic and epigenetic alterations, requiring the accumulation of genomic alterations that inactivate tumor suppressors and activate protooncogenes *(5, 7)*. The accumulation occurs in a stepwise manner, which progress from very early stage with a few or several alterations to advanced stages with numerous alterations leading to aggressive characteristics. Classical tumor suppressors such as RB1 and TP53 and oncogenes such as RAS and MYC have been extensively studied *(8, 9)*. Epigenetic changes are associated with the spatial arrangement and three-dimensional structure of DNA by the interdigitation of DNA-binding proteins such as histones and their modifiers, the Polycomb-Trithorax proteins, the DNA methyltransferase, and histone deacethylase enzymes *(4)*.

But recent studies also implicate that numerous alterations, such as alterations of nonprotein-coding RNAs expression and DNA damage checkpoint responses, are associated to structural aberrations of tumor suppressor and oncogene loci *(10)*. Those are involved in complicated and overlapping pathways that regulate the biologically important processes including cell-cycle progression, gene expression, DNA damage response, and apoptosis *(11)*.

Cancer Heterogeneity and Stem Cell Hypothesis

Genomic alterations could result in variations of cancer cell genome, but also in the biological response of the surrounding tissue components including stroma and vessels of the host. Eventually, the extreme biological heterogeneity leads to a lack of consistency in treatment planning, since similar cases under a clinico-pathological point of view may differ widely in prognosis in gastrointestinal cancers *(12)*.

The CSC model could explain why the biological heterogeneity of tumors could occur *(3, 6)*. There is a small subset of cancer cells, the CSCs, which constitute a reservoir of self-sustaining cells with the exclusive ability to self-renew and maintain the tumor *(6)*. The CSCs have the capacity to both divide and expand the CSC pool and to differentiate into the heterogeneous non or less tumorigenic cancer cell types that in most cases appear to constitute the bulk of the cancer cells within the tumor. If CSCs are relatively refractory to therapies to eradicate the rapidly dividing cells within the tumor that constitute the majority of the nonstem cell component of tumors, then they are unlikely to be curative and relapses would be expected. If correct, the CSC hypothesis would require that we rethink the way we diagnose and treat tumors. It is suggested that our objective would have to turn from eliminating the bulk of rapidly dividing but terminally differentiated components of the tumor to targeting CSCs, and we should refocus on the minority CSC population that possesses the dormancy and fuels tumor growth *(6)*.

Molecular Markers

Little is known about the molecular markers characterizing the stem and transit amplifying populations of the gastrointestinal tract *(13)*, although Musashi-1 *(14)*, hairy and enhancer of split homolog-1 (Hes-1) *(15)*, CD133 (prominin-1, PROM1) *(16, 17)*, EpCAM *(18)*, Claudin-7 *(18)*, CD44 variant isoforms *(18)*, Lgr5 *(19)*, Hedgehog (Hh) *(20)*, bone morphogenic protein (Bmp) *(21, 22)*, Notch *(23)*, and Wnt *(13)* have been proposed.

Stem Cell Signaling

As the mammalian gastrointestinal tract develops from the embryonic gut, it is made up of an endodermally-derived epithelium surrounded by cells of mesoderm origin *(13)*. Cell signaling between these two tissue layers plays a critical role in coordinating patterning and organogenesis of the gut and its derivatives *(13)*. Many lines of evidence have revealed that the critical signal transduction pathways, including Bmp/Tgf-beta, Hh, fibroblast growth factor (Fgf), Wnt and Notch, constitute the stem cell signaling network, which plays a key role in a variety of processes, such as embryogenesis, maintenance of adult tissue homeostasis, tissue repair during chronic persistent inflammation, and carcinogenesis. In gastrointestinal stem cell signaling, the following issues are reported: *(1)* Wnt signaling is the most dominant force in controlling cell proliferation, differentiation, and apoptosis along the crypt-villus axis *(13)*; *(2)* Hh signaling is frequently activated in esophageal cancer, gastric cancer, and pancreatic cancer due to transcriptional up-regulation of Hh ligands and epigenetic silencing of inhibitory molecules, Hhip1, and Hh signaling is rarely activated in colorectal cancer due to negative regulation by the Wnt signaling pathway *(24)*; *(3)* Gastric mucosal repair and parietal cell proliferation during chronic *Helicobacter pylori* infection is associated with Shh signaling *(25)*.

Hh

The Hh family of signaling proteins, Hedgehog ligands, Sonic (Shh), Indian (Ihh), and Desert (Dhh), are secreted proteins, which signal through autocrine and paracrine mechanisms to control cell proliferation, differentiation, and morphology *(20)*. The Hh proteins exert their function by binding to a 12-pass transmembrane protein called Patched (Ptch) *(26)*, which relieves the inhibitory affect of Ptch on a serpentine protein called Smoothened (Smo), leading to hyper-phosphorylation of Smo *(27, 28)*. The signal pathway induces the activation and repression of target genes through the Gli family of transcription factors, Gli-1, Gli-2, Gli-3, which regulate the transcription of target genes.

Bmp

Bmps, members of the Tgf-ß family of signaling proteins, are secreted ligands that signal via autocrine and paracrine mechanisms to regulate cell proliferation and differentiation *(21, 22)*. Bmp ligands bind to cell surface-associated proteins called bone morphogenic receptors type I and type II *(21, 22)*.

Notch

Notch signaling is critical for cell-cell communication and regulates a broad spectrum of cell fate decisions during embryonic development and in the adult organism via stem cell proliferation, differentiation and cell death *(23)*. Notch is instrumental in regulating processes such as neurogenesis, somitogenesis, and angiogenesis *(29)*. Notch proteins are members of the conserved transmembrane receptor family including four members, Notch 1–4 *(23)*. The Notch genes encode transmembrane receptors, which contain a large extracellular domain, composed of a variable number of epidermal growth factor (Egf)-like repeats and an intracellular signaling domain, which consists of six ankyrin/cdc10 motifs and nuclear localization signals *(30)*. Notch receptors interact through their extracellular domain with other membrane-associated ligands, the Delta and Serrate/Jagged families, which are composed of five proteins, Jagged 1 and 2, and Delta-like 1, 3, and 4 *(30)*. Notch signaling is activated by ligand-receptor interaction and triggers proteolytic cleavages by the g-secretase complex, which releases the Notch intracellular domain (NICD) into the nucleus. NICD binds to the CBF1 DNA-binding protein of the transcriptional activator complex, the activation of which can lead to the expression of target genes, such as Hes family genes, involved in cell growth and differentiation. Notch signals are transduced to the canonical pathway (CSL-NICD-Mastermind signaling cascade) or the non-canonical pathway (NF-kappaB-NICD and CSL-NICD-Deltex signaling cascades) based on the expression profile of Notch ligands, Notch receptors, and Notch signaling modifiers *(31)*.

Epithelial-to-Mesenchymal Transition (EMT)

Recent studies indicate that embryonic pathways have been shown to affect the survival of tumor initiating or stem cells and to orchestrate a complex microenvironment, i.e., niche that promotes tumor survival and progression *(32)*. Increased motility and invasiveness of certain cancer cells is associated with the process, the EMT, which occurs during embryonic development *(33)*. EMT is an important change in cell phenotype, which allows the escape of epithelial cells from the structural constraints imposed by tissue architecture *(34)*. Although the observations of morphology of various tumors had indicated epithelial and mesenchymal components of tumors as metaplasia *(35, 36)*, the EMT phenomenon was recognized by Elizabeth Hay in the early to mid 1980s to be a central process in early embryonic morphogenesis *(33)* and the phrase of epithelial to mesenchymal transition appear in 1980s with reference to the study of a cellular change elicited by extracellular matrix *(37)*, and this phenomenon was further characterized by Hay *(33)*. The EMT can be affected by Shh *(38)*, Bmp2 *(39)*, and Notch signaling *(40)*.

COLORECTAL CANCER

Although there is increasing evidence that a rare CSC population of undifferentiated cells is responsible for tumor formation and maintenance, it remains to be explored for colorectal cancer. Recently, the high-density CD133+ population was isolated from tumorigenic cells in colon cancer, which accounts for about 2.5% of the tumor cells *(41)*. The study indicates: *(1)* Subcutaneous injection of colon cancer CD133+ but not CD133– cells readily reproduced the original tumor in immunodeficient mice; *(2)* Serially transplantation for several generations of CD133+ colon cancer cells resulted in exponential growing tumors for more than one year; *(3)* They reproduce the same morphological and antigenic pattern of the original tumor *(41)*, suggesting the candidacy of CD133 as a marker of CSCs. Recently, by using clinical samples, Mori's team was able to show that CD133+ cells were detected in 5 of 12 colon cancer cell lines *(42)*. A higher tumorigenic potential was shown in isolated CD133+ cells from the HT29 colon cancer cell line *(42)*. Furthermore, CD133+ cells are more proliferative, and have high colony-forming and invasive abilities compared with CD133– cells *(42)* (Fig. 1). These data show that colorectal cancer is created and propagated by a small number of undifferentiated tumorigenic CD133+ cells, which possess high proliferation potential *(41, 42)*.

Nevertheless, the biological characteristics of CD133+ CSCs remain to be elucidated. Previous studies of CD133+ cells suggest the association of the mechanism of DNA damage repairs *(43)*, hypoxia *(44)* and chemokine SDF-1-CXCR4 axis *(45)*. As to repairs *(43)*, the study of CD133+ glioma stem cells indicated that the radioresistance of CD133+ CSCs can be reversed with a specific inhibitor of the Chk1 and Chk2 checkpoint kinases, indicating CD133+ cells confers glioma radioresistance and could be the source of tumor recurrence after radiation. It is known that the Chk1 and Chk2 proteins play roles in the execution of checkpoint response to delay or arrest of cell cycle, which elicits repair of DNA damage response *(11)*. It is suggested that the activity might be involved in aberrant repairs of damaged cells to survive and might contribute to the accumulation of further genomic alterations during carcinogenesis scenario. Taken together with the observation of an increased proliferation in CD133+ colon cancer cells *(42)*, the uncoupling of repair and cell cycle control might be the critical feature of CD133+ CSCs. Studies suggest that the elucidation of DNA damage response in isolated CSCs and targeting DNA damage checkpoint response in CSCs may open an avenue to overcome the current chemo or radiation therapy, and it would provide a new model for cancer medicine.

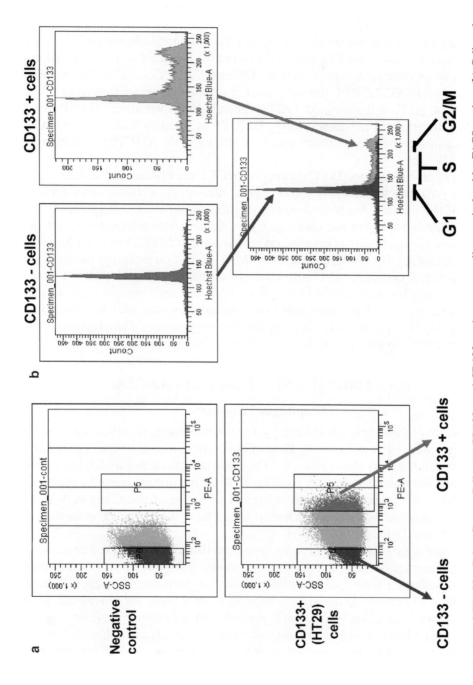

Fig. 1. Characterization of CD133+ Colon Cancer Cells. (**a**) CD133+ and CD133− colon cancer cells were isolated by FACS sorting. (**b**) Cell cycle analysis of CD133+ and CD133− colon cancer cells. CD133+ fraction exhibits cell cycling proliferation, compared with CD133− fraction. Note, in the *upper part*, the scale of the cell count on *Y*-axis indicates ~2-times accumulation of the G1 phase in CD133− cells, compared with CD133+ cells (*see Color Plates*).

HEPATOCELLULAR CARCINOMA

Liver stem cells, or oval cells, have been put forth as a possible target for hepatocarcinogens *(46)*. Genetically modified and in vitro transformed oval cells have been shown to be tumorigenic in animals *(46)*. Chemical carcinogenesis can induce various degrees of oval cell proliferation in liver models. Preliminary evidence has been shown that hepatocellular carcinoma (HCC) may maintain a bipotential phenotype consistent with an oval cell origin *(46)*. Markers that have aided in the identification of oval cells in mammalian liver include: OV-6; OC.2, OC.3, OC.4, OC.5, OC.10; BDS7; Thy-1; *c*-kit; CD34; ABCG2/BCRP1 (breast cancer resistance protein); Connexin 43; cytokeratin (CK) 7, CK19, CK14; AFP (α-fetoprotein); GGT (γ-glutamyltranspeptidase); GST-P (placental form of glutathione-S-transferase); Flt-3 ligand/Flt-3; DMBT1 (deleted in malignant brain tumour *(1)*; NCAM-1/CD56 (neural cell adhesion molecule *(1)*; Chromogranin A; PTHrP (parathyroid hormone related peptide) *(47)*.

Upon induction of protooncogene MYC expression, HCCs quickly develop and the mice die within a matter of weeks *(48)*. Inactivation of the MYC gene subsequent to tumor development promotes rapid regression of the tumors. Analysis demonstrates that tumor cells undergo apoptosis, whereas some differentiate into hepatocytes and cholangiocytes. Some tumor cells enter a state of dormancy and quickly reacquire the neoplastic phenotype on reactivation of MYC. The study suggests two possible mechanisms regarding MYC-induced HCC: *(1)* MYC activation promotes tumor formation from a population of liver stem cells; *(2)* MYC activation affects the dedifferentiation of terminally differentiated hepatocytes to a bipotential neoplastic phenotype. Although both of these explanations are possible, the former is arguably less complicated than the latter moving back and forth through levels of differentiation *(46)*. The recent study supports the first explanation; a small stem cell population, i.e., CSC, which gives rise to the bulk of the tumor *(46)*.

ESOPHAGEAL AND STOMACH CANCER

Esophageal Cancer

The luminal surface of the esophagus is lined by a non-keratinising, stratified squamous epithelium that has a highly complex organization *(49)*. The lamina propria invaginates the epithelium at regular intervals, producing tall papillary structures *(49)*. The basal layer is further divisible anatomically into two components: one flat (the interpapillary basal layer, IBL) and one covering the papillae (the papillary basal layer, PBL). Cellular proliferation is limited to the basal zone, and cells are thought to migrate from this area toward the esophageal lumen *(49)*. The molecular markers include b1 integrin, CK13, CK14, CK15, and Egfr *(49, 50)*.

In the study of esophageal CSCs, the following issues are included: *(1)* Egf receptor and signaling in proliferation and transformation in squamous cell carcinoma (SCC); *(2)* possibly transdifferentiation into an intestinal metaplastic phenotype that defines Barrett's esophagus; *(3)* epithelial-stromal interactions. Notch signaling to promote keratinocyte differentiation is likely anti-oncogenic in SCC of the esophagus, although Notch signaling is activated in normal stem or progenitor domain of gastrointestinal epithelium, such as basal layer in esophagus and lower part of the crypt in colon, and Notch signaling to inhibit cell differentiation possesses oncogenic property in gastric and colorectal cancers *(31)*.

Stomach Cancer

Shh regulates growth and differentiation within gastric mucosa through autocrine loop and epithelial-mesenchymal interaction *(51)*. Shh is implicated in stem and progenitor cell restitution of damaged gastric mucosa during chronic infection with *Helicobacter pylori*. Up-regulation of Shh and Ihh and down-regulation of inhibitory Hhip lead to aberrant activation of Hh signaling through Ptch1 to Gli1 in gastric cancer.

Canonical Notch signaling is activated in the stem or progenitor domain of gastric epithelium *(31)*. Notch signaling to inhibit cell differentiation is oncogenic in gastric cancer. It is proposed that single nucleotide polymorphism (SNP), epigenetic change, and genetic alteration of genes encoding Notch signaling-associated molecules will be utilized as biomarkers for gastrointestinal cancer *(31)*; g-secretase inhibitors, functioning as Notch signaling inhibitors, will be applied as anti-cancer drugs for gastric cancer cancer *(31)*.

PERSPECTIVE

Gastrointestinal epithelium possesses a high rate of cell turnover, which is similar to the skin, where cancers are common *(52)*. Although stem cells are believe to be the only cells that live long enough to acquire genetic abnormalities for carcinogenesis, more differentiated cancer cells or damaged progenitors might acquire properties of "stemness," because of unstableness of the genome. Recent researches have indicated several CSC markers, which are hallmarks of high tumorigenicity and less apoptosis. Although the role of somatic mutations has been extensively documented in determining tumor phenotype and many of the observed differences have been explained among different tumors *(53)*, undoubtedly the detection and biological regulation of CSCs during the course of carcinogenesis would be critical issues for the development of the efficient prevention, diagnosis, and novel therapeutic approach to gastrointestinal cancers.

REFERENCES

1. Bixby S, Kruger GM, Mosher JT, Joseph NM, Morrison SJ. Cell-intrinsic differences between stem cells from different regions of the peripheral nervous system regulate the generation of neural diversity. Neuron 2002:35:643–56.
2. Sagar J, Chaib B, Sales K, Winslet M, Seifalian A. Role of stem cells in cancer therapy and cancer stem cells: a review. Cancer Cell Intern 2007:7:9.
3. Reya T, Morrison SJ, Clarke MF, Weissman IL. Stem cells, cancer, and cancer stem cells. Nature 2001:414:105–11.
4. Waterland RA. Epigenetic mechanisms and gastrointestinal development. J Pediatr 2006:149(5 Suppl): S137–42.
5. Nowell PC. Chromosomes and cancer: the evolution of an idea. Adv Cancer Res 1993:62:1–17.
6. Clarke M, DJ, Dirks PB, Eaves CJ, Jamieson CH, Jones DL, Visvader J, Weissman IL, Wahl GM. Cancer stem cells-perspectives on current status and future directions: AACR Workshop on cancer stem cells. Cancer Res 2006:66:9339–44.
7. Vogelstein B, Kinzler KW. The multistep nature of cancer. Trends Genet 1993:9:138–41.
8. Hickman ES, Moroni MC, Helin K. The role of p53 and pRB in apoptosis and cancer. Curr Opin Genet Dev 2002:12:60–6.
9. Malumbres M, Barbacid M. RAS oncogenes: the first 30 years. Nat Rev Cancer 2003:3:459–65.
10. Calin GA, Croce CM. MicroRNAs and chromosomal abnormalities in cancer cells. Oncogene 2006:25:6202–10.
11. Sancar A, Lindsey-Boltz LA, Unsal-Kacmaz K, Linn S. Molecular mechanisms of mammalian DNA repair and the DNA damage checkpoints. Annu Rev Biochem 2004:73:39–85.
12. Almadori G, Bussu F, Paludetti G. Should there be more molecular staging of head and neck cancer to improve the choice of treatments and thereby improve survival? Curr Opin Otolaryngol Head Neck Surg 2008:16:117–26.
13. Yen TH, Wright NA. The gastrointestinal tract stem cell niche. Stem Cell Rev 2006:2:203–12.
14. Nakamura M, Okano H, Blendy J, Montell C. Musashi, a neural RNA-binding protein required for Drosophila adult external sensory organ development. Neuron 1994:13:67–81.
15. Ishibashi M, Ang SL, Shiota K, Nakanishi S, Kageyama R, Guillemot F. Targeted disruption of mammalian hairy and Enhancer of split homolog-1 (HES-1) leads to up-regulation of neural helix-loop-helix factors, premature neurogenesis, and severe neural tube defects. Genes Dev 1995:9:3136–48.
16. Lin EH, Hassan M, Li Y, Zhao H, Nooka A, Sorenson E, Xie K, Champlin R, Wu X, Li D. Elevated circulating endothelial progenitor marker CD133 messenger RNA levels predict colon cancer recurrence. Cancer 2007:110:534–42.

17. Mehra N, Penning M, Maas J, Beerepoot LV, van Daal N, van Gils CH, Giles RH, Voest EE. Progenitor marker CD133 mRNA is elevated in peripheral blood of cancer patients with bone metastases. Clin Cancer Res 2006:12:4859–66.

18. Kuhn S, Koch M, Nübel T, Ladwein M, Antolovic D, Klingbeil P, Hildebrand D, Moldenhauer G, Langbein L, Franke WW, Weitz J, Zöller M. A complex of EpCAM, claudin-7, CD44 variant isoforms, and tetraspanins promotes colorectal cancer progression. Mol Cancer Res 2007:5:553–67.

19. Barker N, van Es JH, Kuipers J, Kujala P, van den Born M, Cozijnsen M, Haegebarth A, Korving J, Begthel H, Peters PJ, Clevers H. Identification of stem cells in small intestine and colon by marker gene Lgr5. Nature 2007:449:1003–7.

20. Ingham PW, McMahon AP. Hedgehog signaling in animal development: Paradigms and principles. Genes Dev 2001:15:3059–87.

21. Koenig BB, Cook JS, Wolsing DH, Ting J, Tiesman JP, Correa PE, Olson CA, Pecquet Al, Ventura F, Grant RA. Characterization and cloning of a receptor for BMP-2 and BMP-4 from NIH 3T3 cells. Mol Cell Biol 1994:14:5961–74.

22. ten Dijke P, Yamashita H, Sampath TK, Reddi AH, Estevez M, Riddle DL, Ichijo H, Heldin CH, Miyazono K. Identification of type I receptors for osteogenic protein-1 and bone morphogenetic protein-4. J Biol Chem 1994:269:16985–8.

23. Bray S. Notch signalling: a simple pathway becomes complex. Nat Rev Mol Cell Biol 2006:7:678–89.

24. Katoh Y, Katoh M. Hedgehog signaling pathway and gastrointestinal stem cell signaling network. Int J Mol Med 2006:18:1019–23.

25. Nishizawa T, Suzuki H, Masaoka T, Minegishi Y, Iwasahi E, Hibi T. Helicobacter pylori eradication restored sonic hedgehog expression in the stomach. Hepatogastroenterology 2007:54:697–700.

26. Pepinsky RB, Rayhorn P, Day ES, Dergay A, Williams KP, Galdes A, Taylor FR, Boriack-Sjodin PA, Garber EA. Mapping sonic hedgehog-receptor interactions by steric interference. J Biol Chem 2000:275:10995–1001.

27. Murone M, Rosenthal A, de Sauvage FJ. Sonic hedgehog signaling by the patched-smoothened receptor complex. Curr Biol 1999:9:76–84.

28. Corbit KC, Aanstad P, Singla V, Norman AR, Stainier DY, Reiter JF. Vertebrate Smoothened functions at the primary cilium. Nature 2005:437:1018–21.

29. Bolos V, Grego-Bessa J, de la Pompa JL. Notchsignaling in development and cancer. Endocr Rev 2007:28:339–63.

30. Artavanis-Tsakonas S, Rand MD, Lake RJ. Notch signaling: Cell fate control and signal integration in development. Science:1999:284:770–6.

31. Katoh M, Katoh M. Notch signaling in gastrointestinal tract. Int J Oncol 2007:30:247–51.

32. Bailey JM, Singh PK, Hollingsworth MA. Cancer metastasis facilitated by developmental pathways: Sonic hedgehog, Notch, and bone morphogenic proteins. J Cell Biochem 2007:102:829–39.

33. Hay ED. An overview of epithelio-mesenchymal transformation. Acta Anat (Basel) 1995:154:8–20.

34. Hugo HA, ML, Blick T, Lawrence MG, Clements JA, Williams ED, Thompson EW. Epithelial-mesenchymal and mesenchymal-epithelial transitions in carcinoma progression. J Cell Physiol 2007:213:374–83.

35. Kahn LB, Uys CJ, Dale J, Rutherfoord S. Carcinoma of the breast with metaplasia to chondrosarcoma: A light and electron microscopic study. Histopathology 1978:2:93–106.

36. Ishikawa S, Kaneko H, Sumida T, Sekiya M. Ultrastructure of mesodermalmixed tumor of the uterus. Acta Pathol Jpn 1979:29:801–9.

37. Krug EL, Mjaatvedt CH, Markwald RR. Extracellular matrix from embryonic myocardium elicits an early morphogenetic event in cardiac endothelial differentiation. Dev Biol 1987:120:348–55.

38. Feldmann G, Dhara S, Fendrich V, Bedja D, Beaty R, Mullendore M, Karikari C, Alvarez H, Iacobuzio-Donahue C, Jimeno A, Gabrielson KL, Matsui W, Maitra A. Blockade of hedgehog signaling inhibits pancreatic cancer invasion and metastases: A new paradigm for combination therapy in solid cancers. Cancer Res 2007:67:2187–96.

39. Ma L, Lu MF, Schwartz RJ, Martin JF. Bmp2 is essential for cardiac cushion epithelial-mesenchymal transition and myocardial patterning. Development 2005:132:5601–11.

40. Timmerman LA, Grego-Bessa J, Raya A, Bertran E, Perez-Pomares JM, Diez J, Aranda S, Palomo S, McCormick F, Izpisua-Belmonte JC, de la Pompa JL. Notch promotes epithelial-mesenchymal transition during cardiac development and oncogenic transformation. Genes Dev 2004:18:99–115.

41. Ricci-Vitiani L, Lombardi DG, Pilozzi E, Biffoni M, Todaro M, Peschle C, De Maria R. Identification and expansion of human colon-cancer-initiating cells. Nature 2007:445:111–5.

42. Ieta K, Tanaka F, Haraguchi N, Kita Y, Sakashita H, Mimori K, Matsumoto T, Inoue H, Kuwano H, Mori M. Biological and genetic characteristics of tumor-initiating cells in colon cancer. Ann Surg Oncol 2008:15:638–48.

43. Bao S, Wu Q, McLendon RE, Hao Y, Shi Q, Hjelmeland AB, Dewhirst MW, Bigner DD, Rich JN. Glioma stem cells promote radioresistance by preferential activation of the DNA damage response. Nature 2006:444:756–60.

44. Blazek ER, Foutch JL, Maki G. Daoy medulloblastoma cells that express CD133 are radioresistant relative to CD133-cells, and the CD133+ sector is enlarged by hypoxia. Int J Radiat Oncol Biol Phys 2007:67:1–5.

45. Czarnowska E, Gajerska-Dzieciatkowska M, Ku mierski K, Lichomski J, Machaj EK, Pojda Z, Brudek M, Beresewicz A. Expression of SDF-1-CXCR4 axis and an anti-remodelling effectiveness of foetal-liver stem cell transplantation in the infarcted rat heart. J Physiol Pharmacol. 2007:58:729–44.

46. Shupe T, Petersen BE. Evidence regarding a stem cell origin of hepatocellular carcinoma. Stem Cell Rev 2005:1:261–4.

47. Alison MR. Liver stem cells: implications for hepatocarcinogenesis. Stem Cell Rev 2005:1:253–60.

48. Shachaf CM, Kopelman AM, Arvanitis C, Karlsson A, Beer S, Mandl S, Bachmann MH, Borowsky AD, Ruebner B, Cardiff RD, Yang Q, Bishop JM, Contag CH, Felsher DW. MYC inactivation uncovers pluripotent differentiation and tumour dormancy in hepatocellular cancer. Nature 2004:431:1112–7.

49. Seery JP. Stem cells of the oesophageal epithelium. J Cell Sci 2002:115:1783–9.

50. Rustgi AK. Models of esophageal carcinogenesis. Semin Oncol 2006: 33(6 Suppl 11):S57–8.

51. Katoh Y, Katoh M. Hedgehog signaling pathway and gastric cancer. Cancer Biol Ther 2005:4:1050–4.

52. Wershil BK, Furuta GT. Gastrointestinal mucosal immunity. J Allergy Clin Immunol 2008:121(2 Suppl):S380–3;quiz S415.

53. Ince TA, Richardson AL, Bell GW, Saitoh M, Godar S, Karnoub AE, Iglehart JD, Weinberg RA. Transformation of different human breast epithelial cell types leads to distinct tumor phenotypes. Cancer Cell 2007:12:160–70.

13

Cancer Stem Cells: Hepatocellular Carcinoma

Thomas Shupe and Bryon E. Petersen

ABSTRACT

It has been hypothesized that cancer stem cells result from the initiation of normal tissue stem cells by mutagens. These cells give rise to a population of growth and differentiation dysregulated transient amplifying cells that represent the bulk of the tumor. Fifty years of research has provided a relatively large knowledge base on adult liver stem cells termed "oval cells" in rodents and hepatic progenitor cells in humans. Despite this fact, information regarding liver cancer stem cells remains scarce. Abundant circumstantial evidence suggests that bipotential liver progenitor cells may act as targets for carcinogens, giving rise to liver cancer. Evidence is also beginning to indicate that these mutated progenitor cells, or their derivatives, may act as cancer stem cells. These cells maintain themselves through self-renewal and give rise to the transient amplifying cells that comprise a majority of the liver tumor volume. Putative liver cancer stem cells likely escape chemotherapeutic treatment, both by limiting time in the cell cycle, and by up-regulating membrane transporters. It is also likely that the ability to establish metastasis is limited to the liver cancer stem cell population. Because regrowth of tumors following unsuccessful cytoreductive therapy is mediated by tumor stem cells, careful consideration must be paid to this cell population when developing future liver cancer therapies. Several potential markers for the identification of liver cancer stem cells are currently under investigation. CD133 and CD90 show particular promise as discriminators of human liver cancer stem cells. These markers are being used to help unravel the mystery of tumor reoccurrence following treatment of the original tumor by surgery and cytoreductive drug/radio therapy, and may someday lead to a true cure for this ominous form of cancer. The following chapter presents evidence for both the stem cell origin of liver tumors, and the presence of altered stem cells within the tumors themselves.

Key Words: Stem cells, Oval cells, Hepatic progenitor cells, Hepatocellular carcinoma, Liver cancer stem cells, CD90, CD133, Side population cells

INTRODUCTION

Cancer stem cells represent the self-renewing, transplantable elements within a tumor. These cells give rise to the transient amplifying population that represents the bulk of the tumor and are able to establish metastasis at distant sites. As an asymmetrically dividing population, at least one of the daughter cells retains the undifferentiated phenotype and maintains indefinite proliferation potential. These

From: *Cancer Drug Discovery and Development: Stem Cells and Cancer,*
Edited by: R.G. Bagley and B.A. Teicher, DOI: 10.1007/978-1-60327-933-8_13,
© Humana Press, a part of Springer Science+Business Media, LLC 2009

properties render the cancer stem cell virtually immortal. As with normal stem cells, cancer stem cells enter the cell cycle only occasionally, allowing this population to escape most chemotherapeutics, which target rapidly the dividing cell populations. These surviving cells are then responsible for regrowth of the tumor following unsuccessful cytoreductive therapy.

The general idea of tumor stem cells has evolved over decades, if not centuries. As pointed out by Stewart Sell, the current iteration of this theory began to take shape in the early 1950s when researchers discovered that tumors contain a subpopulations of cells able to transfer the tumor following transplant to laboratory animals (1–3). It was also noted that the number of stem cells within a tumor is roughly equivalent to the number of cancer cells that survive following chemical or radio therapy (4). By the 1990s biomedical research techniques had developed sufficiently to allow the identification of cancer stem cells in human leukemia (5). The transplantable elements within the leukemic cell population displayed a specific surface marker profile, and were able to give rise to differentiated progeny that were phenotypically identical to the original cancer. Subsequent studies have described cancer stem cells within a myriad of tumor types including: breast, brain, colon, head and neck, and pancreas (6–11). It is ironic that little is known about liver cancer stem cells, given the wealth of literature available on normal liver stem cells. However, the following data indicate that liver tumors do indeed contain a stem cell component.

A STEM CELL ORIGIN OF LIVER TUMORS

Liver Development, Hepatoblasts, and Oval Cells

The concepts of tumor stem cells and the stem cell origin of tumors are intimately intertwined. If tumors arise from undifferentiated tissue stem cells, then the cancer stem cells are likely the direct descendants of this initiated population. During the latter half of the nineteenth century, Julius Conheim hypothesized that tumors may arise from embryonic cells that remain dormant throughout the life of an organism…tissue stem cells (12). Conheim recognized that embryonic and neoplastic tissue shared similar morphologic and functional characteristics, and postulated that a relationship may exist between the two. During the subsequent decades, variations of the stem cell origin hypothesis were entertained by various research pathologists. However, no histological evidence for "embryonal rests" was forthcoming, and enthusiasm for this theory waned. Technological advances allowing for the immunophenotypic characterization of cell lineages and the tracking of transplanted cells eventually enabled the discovery of stem cells within virtually every adult tissue (13–23). The identification of these "embryonic remnants" reopened the possibility of a stem cell origin of tumors.

The embryonic liver is derived from a population of ventral fore-gut cells, which intimately contact the precardiac mesoderm (24). These cells bud off from the developing gastrointestinal tract as hepatoblasts, bipotential cells with the capability to give rise to both the hepatic parenchyma and the biliary tree (25–28). Bipotential progenitor cells present within the adult liver are referred to as "oval cells" in rodents and liver progenitor cells in human. These cells likely represent vestigial hepatoblasts or their derivatives that remain dormant in the liver following development of the organ (29). These cells, like their embryonic ancestors, are able to differentiate into either hepatocytes or cholangiocytes (30–32). Unlike differentiated cells from most organs, mature hepatocytes maintain a robust proliferative potential throughout the lifespan of the cell. Following chemical or physical injury to the liver, hepatocyte division is usually able to affect restoration of liver mass (33–35). Under experimental conditions where hepatocyte division is chemically inhibited or in situations of chronic injury, oval cells are recruited to compensate for insufficient hepatocyte proliferation (30, 36–39). These cells begin to proliferate at several niches within or adjacent to the canal of Hering in the portal zone, migrate across the liver lobule, and commit to either the hepatocyte or cholangiocyte lineage (32, 40–42). More recent research demonstrates that oval cells may derive from the bone marrow, though the extent to which these cells play a role under physiologic conditions remains unclear *(22, 23, 43)*. Preliminary studies conducted in our own laboratory indicate that bone marrow derived cells, under extreme circumstances, may give rise to liver tumors (unpublished data).

Chemical Carcinogenesis

Most liver carcinogens are taken up in a procarcinogenic form, requiring metabolic activation to the ultimate carcinogen. As a general rule, CYPs associated with the endoplasmic reticulum are responsible for activation to the electrophilic metabolite. These enzymes are robustly expressed by mature hepatocytes, but not oval cells. However, activated carcinogens may passively diffuse into neighboring cells. Data from our own laboratory indicate that the procarcinogen aflatoxin B_1, when administered in a single bolus dose, forms DNA adducts within oval cells (Unpublished Data). Additionally, as oval cells begin to differentiate into hepatocytes, they begin to express CYPs *(44)*. Therefore, transitional hepatocytes may act as targets for hepatocarcinogens, perhaps before completely committing to the hepatocyte lineage.

Following the development of the cyclic 2-acetylaminofluorene and Solt-Farber models for rapid induction of pre-neoplastic nodules, thinking temporarily shifted to a hepatocyte origin of hepatocellular carcinoma *(45–47)*. Each of these models appeared to demonstrate the progression of altered hepatocyte foci to nodules to persistent nodules to cancer. Later work offered an alternative explanation for the origin of tumors in these models. By using an ultra sensitive radioimmunoassay for the oncofetal protein, alphafetoprotein (AFP), it was demonstrated that serum AFP levels correlated not with the number of altered hepatocytes, but with the number of oval cells situated peripheral to, or within the nodules *(32)*. Immunohistochemical analysis of the nodules confirmed that the oval cell population was the source of serum AFP. The resulting tumors were also AFP positive, suggesting that they likely were derived from the oval cell population associated with the nodules

It has been speculated that while the altered hepatocytes within the nodules do not directly give rise to tumors, they may play a supportive role in the development of liver cancer from the oval cell population *(48)*. In the cyclic 2-acetylaminofluorene model, developing nodules will regress and no tumors will develop if treatment is discontinued after the second cycle *(45)*. Having already been exposed to the carcinogenic compound twice, it is reasonable to assume that initiated oval cells are present at this time. A possible explanation may involve modification of the local microenvironment by the altered hepatocytes that make up the nodule. In this scenario, the expanding nodules, which have somehow avoided mitotic inhibition by 2-acetylaminofluorene, would bathe the local area in autocrine growth signals and induce modifications to the extracellular matrix. These changes may provide a growth promoting microenvironment in which the oval cells may freely proliferate. It is only later, after individual oval cells gain additional mutations that allow for autonomous proliferation, that the developing tumor is able to thrive independent of the nodule.

In Vitro Initiation of Oval Cells

Although concrete evidence for a progenitor cell origin of hepatocellular carcinoma has yet to be presented, an abundance of circumstantial evidence suggests that this is probably the case. The absolute potential of oval cells to give rise to liver cancer has been established by two studies. In the first study, the putative rat oval cell line WB344 was treated with the chemical carcinogen *N*-methyl-*N*'-nitro-*N*-nitrosoguanidine *(49, 50)*. Several immortal cell lines were developed from this protocol, many of which were able to form aggressively growing tumors following subcutaneous transplant into recipient animals. Interestingly, these lines proved to be much less aggressive when transplanted directly into the liver, suggesting that the local microenvironment of the liver was able to bring these cells under some degree of growth control.

Quail and coworkers isolated oval cells from mice that were deficient for the well characterized tumor suppressor gene *p53 (51)*. These mice had been fed a chemically modified diet that was deficient in choline and supplemented with ethionine. This regimen has been proven to be a potent inducer of oval cell proliferation in rats, and the mice described in this study did appear to develop an oval cell response. The livers of treated animals were disassociated, and the oval cell population was purified by cell density. Immunohistochemical characterization of these cells indicated that the intended population was collected. The cells were propagated in culture and survived long term. Subclones of the cultured cells were subcutaneously transplanted into athymic, Swiss nude mice. Over the next 100 days, a significant number of transplanted mice developed tumors at the site of inoculation. These tumors displayed immunophenotypic and morphologic characteristics, which were consistent with hepatocellular carcinoma. This may not seem surprising, given that oval cells possess the potential to differentiate into hepatocytes, and the oval cells used in this study were lacking one of the most critical tumor suppressor genes identified to date. It does, however, provide solid evidence that a pathway from oval cell to liver cancer is possible.

Human Hepatocellular Carcinoma

Histological evidence of progenitor cell proliferation may be seen in a variety of liver pathologies including hemochromatosis, alcoholic liver disease, and viral hepatitis *(52–56)*. Each of these diseases carries with it a heightened risk for the development of hepatocellular carcinoma. It is possible that progenitor cell activity accompanying these diseases provides an increased number of cellular targets on which carcinogens may act. The most relevant example of increased risk of hepatocellular carcinoma on the background of chronic disease is, perhaps, chronic viral hepatitis infection. This condition is responsible for a majority of the world's incidence of liver cancer, particularly in regions with high exposure to aflatoxin $B_1(57)$.

Additional evidence for a stem cell origin of human liver cancer is the uncommon occurrence of liver tumors with mixed hepatocyte/cholangiocyte phenotype *(58, 59)*. Although rarely reported in the literature, these tumors would seem to suggest that the original initiating events occurred in a single, bipotential cell. At some point early in the development of the tumor, individual cells may alternatively commit to either the hepatocyte or cholangiocyte lineage. This explanation seems much more likely than the alternative; i.e., hepatocellular and cholangiocarcinoma developing simultaneously, adjacent to one another and presenting as a single tumor. If all liver tumors arose from oval cells, one would expect more of this type of tumor. It is, however, possible that differentiation signals within the liver favor commitance to the hepatocyte lineage.

The origin of liver tumors remains equivocal. However, it does appear that some, if not all, liver tumors develop from the stem cell population. Taking into account the recently discovered similarities between normal stem cells and cancer stem cells within the same tissue, a stem cell origin for tumors seems increasingly probable. If liver cancers do, indeed, arise from the stem cell population, dysregulation of the normal process of asymmetric division may amplify the number of altered stem cells, and a tumor is born *(60, 61)*.

LIVER CANCER STEM CELLS

MYC Transgenic Mice and Liver Cancer Stem Cells

The advent of transgenic mice along with the development of conditional expression constructs has allowed the expression of oncogenes in specific tissues during defined periods of time. A recent study utilized a line of transgenic mice, which conditionally over-express the oncogene MYC within the liver *(62)*. Upon activation of MYC expression, aggressive hepatocellular carcinomas developed over a 12-week period. Inactivation of the MYC gene subsequent to tumor development promoted a rapid and complete regression of all tumors. Analysis of cell fate within the regressing tumors demonstrated that while a majority of the tumor cells underwent apoptosis, many differentiated into hepatocytes, integrating normally into liver cords. Additionally, many of the tumor cells adopted a morphology and immunophenotype consistent with the cholangiocyte lineage. Of particular relevance to the topic at hand, the authors describe a small population of tumor cells that enter a state of dormancy. Following the reactivation of MYC, these cells immediately begin to generate new tumors. These results may indicate that MYC activation induces dysregulation of the growth and differentiation programs of uncommitted cells derived from liver resident stem cells. Inactivation of the MYC oncogene restores these regulations, allowing cells to either initiate programmed cell death or terminally differentiate. The cells that become dormant may be considered a cancer stem cell, able to regrow the tumor upon subsequent MYC activation. It is unclear from this study whether MYC expression has an effect on the partially differentiated cell population, the cancer stem cell or both. The latter seems most likely, as MYC is known to play a strong role in both tissue growth and differentiation. A plausible scenario is that MYC induces dysregulation of the normal stem cell regeneration program while simultaneously interfering with the differentiation process of the resulting transient amplifying population. This would explain why MYC is such a potent oncogene. By causing continual proliferation of the stem cell while imparting a neoplastic phenotype onto the differentiating daughter cells, both requirements for tumor growth are met.

Side Population Cells

In 2006, Chiba et al. published the results of a study conducted on liver cancer cell lines derived from human liver tumors *(63)*. This study was based on the known up-regulation of ATP binding cassette membrane transporters by hematopoietic stem cells. The authors hypothesized that a similar up-regulation may occur in liver cancer stem cells, and that this property may allow for the isolation of a side population from liver cancer cell lines, which efficiently efflux Hoechst 33342 dye. Such a side population was found to be present in two of the four cell lines tested, occurring at a frequency of less than 1/100 cells. Side population cells demonstrated both increased proliferation and resistance to apoptosis when compared with the remaining cells in the line. Immunophenotypically, the side population cells proved to be greatly enriched for the expression of both AFP and cytokeratin 19. Both of these markers are frequently used to identify oval cells in regenerating rodent livers. Transplant experiments showed that the side population cells were able to establish tumors in immunocompromised recipient mice at a cell dosage more than three logs below that of nonside population cells. The report concludes with differential gene expression microarray analysis of the side population and nonside population cells. A significant difference in expression profiles was noted between these two groups of cells. Many of the genes that were reported as being highly expressed in the side population were genes that are known to be associated with the stem cell phenotype. Although this study does appear to be the first demonstration of liver tumor stem cells, two facts detract from the strength of the results. First, and most obvious, is the fact that the study was conducted strictly on cell lines. Primary culture of human liver tumor cells is extremely difficult, even in the most experienced hands *(64)*. It is doubtful that primary cultures would survive long enough to conduct studies similar to the one described above. The second, and potentially most significant, problem that needs to be considered is the well documented cytotoxicity of the Hoechst 33342 dye *(65)*. This fact is of particular concern in studies involving cell sorting as the excitation laser used during the sort appears to potentiate the cytotoxic effect of Hoechst 33342 *(65)*. It is unclear what effect the concentrations of Hoechst 33342 used in this study may have had on the viability of cells unable to efflux the dye. The nonside population cells do appear to proliferate in culture. However, toxic effects of the dye must be considered when evaluating these results.

CD133 as a Potential Liver Cancer Stem Cell Marker

CD133 was first identified as a human hematopoietic stem cell marker, and has since been shown to identify stem cells and tumors from several tissues (66–69). Analysis of liver cancer cell lines indicated that one line (Huh-7) contained a subpopulation of cells that expressed CD133 (70). The CD133 positive cells demonstrated a marginal, though significant increase in proliferation rate. These cells are also more likely to express markers associated with a less differentiated phenotype. Not surprisingly, the CD133 positive population proved to be more tumorigenic upon transplant to immunocompromised mice. Subsequent studies identified a CD133 positive population in several additional liver cancer cell lines and human liver tumor sections. These cells showed greater invasiveness in soft agar colony formation assays (71, 72). Most recently, CD133 positive cells from human cancer cell lines were shown to possess a much higher resistance to the chemotherapeutic agents doxorubicin and fluorouracil. This effect was proven both in vitro and in vivo following transplant to immunocompromised mice. Mechanisms underlying the noted chemoresistance were shown to involve the Akt/PKB and Bcl-2 apoptosis survival pathway. Chemical inhibition of the Akt pathway showed a concomitant reduction in Bcl-2 protein. Cells treated with the inhibitor both in vitro and in vivo became sensitive to the chemotherapeutic agents, often to a surprising degree.

These studies also suffer from the shortcomings associated with the use of cell lines. However, unlike the side population studies, CD133 positive cells were clearly demonstrated in primary human liver tumors. Additionally, functional demonstration of mechanism both in culture and following transplant to recipient mice elevate the potential value of these studies above previous liver cancer stem cell research.

CD90 as a Potential Liver Cancer Stem Cell Marker

Most recently, CD90 has emerged as a very promising marker for human liver cancer stem cells. In what may prove to be a seminal study, cells positive for CD90 and negative for the leukocyte antigen CD45 were identified in primary human liver tumors (including both hepatocellular carcinomas and cholangiocarcinomas), but not in normal liver tissue (73, 74). As was the case in the previously described studies, the CD90 positive fraction of several liver cancer cell lines easily established tumors in immunocompromised mice at cell doses on the order of 10^3. CD90 positive cells isolated from these tumors proved to be serially transplantable into secondary and tertiary recipients. The CD90 negative population failed to establish tumors, even at cell doses two logs higher.

Closer analysis of primary human liver tumors revealed that the CD90 positive cells coexpressed several markers associated with the stem cell phenotype, including CD133. As with the human cell lines, CD90 positive cells from the primary tumors were able to establish tumors in immunocompromised mice, and were serially transplantable. CD44, an adhesion molecule that contributes to tumor invasiveness, was also shown to be highly expressed by the CD90 positive cells. Blockage of this molecule by neutralizing antibody significantly induced apoptosis of the CD90 positive cells in vitro. The most intriguing aspect of these studies was the discovery that the blood of liver cancer patients contained a population of CD45 negative, CD90 positive cells. These cells were isolated, and were shown to give rise to tumors following transplant to mice. Furthermore, the tumor forming potential of these cells could be blocked with anti-CD44 antibody. This strongly suggests that CD90 positive cells may be responsible for establishment of metastasis, and the metastatic potential of these cells may be partially dependant on functional CD44. Taken together, these data indicate that CD90 may potentially be used clinically as a prognostic marker, and CD44 as a therapeutic target.

A Possible Liver Cancer Stem Cell...Stem Cell?

TGF- b family proteins play a critical role in the developmental regulation of embryonic stem cells *(75)*. Analysis of regenerating human liver following single lobe transplant demonstrated a very small number of cells $(1/10^5)$ that express the embryonic stem cell marker Oct4 *(76)*. The presence of this marker suggests an extremely undifferentiated phenotype. Human hepatocellular carcinomas were screened for the presence of cells with a similar immunophenotype, and rare clusters of Oct4 positive cells were found *(76)*. Interestingly, TGF-b receptor II and ELF, two critical components of the TGF-b signaling pathway, were not expressed by the Oct4 positive cells. TGF-b signaling is required for appropriate regulation of the early developmental program of embryonic stem cells. Through elegant transgenic mouse studies, the authors show that dysregulation of the TGF- b pathway is also a critical

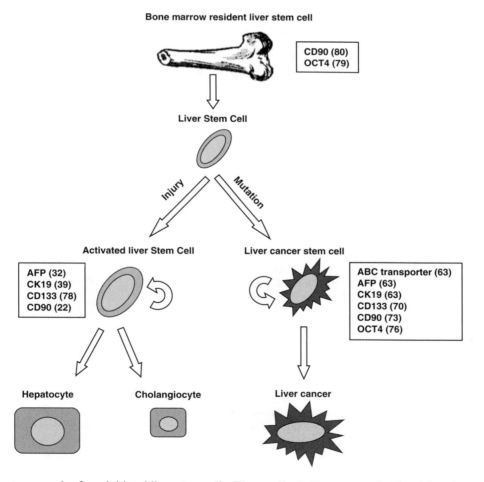

Fig. 1. Liver tumors arise from initiated liver stem cells. These cells divide asymmetrically, giving rise to a transient amplifying population which represents the bulk of the tumor. Markers for bone marrow liver stem cells, liver resident cells, and liver cancer stem cells are presented within the *black boxes*.

component of liver carcinogenesis. These data indicate that liver tumor stem cells may derive from a very immature cell within the liver that has lost the ability to maintain growth control through disruption of TGF- b responsiveness.

CONCLUSION

Hepatocellular carcinoma remains one of the most frequent human tumors worldwide, and the prognosis is usually abysmal. The incidence of hepatocellular carcinoma in the United States is approaching 3 cases per 100,000 per year and is expected to continue to climb with the rising incidence of hepatitis C infection *(77)*. The cellular origin of hepatocellular carcinoma has been under debate for over a half century, but the collective body of evidence indicates that liver progenitor cells are very likely suspects. Liver cancer stem cells most likely arise from normal liver stem cells, which, due to genetic mutation, have initiated dysregulated development or regeneration programs. Amplification of an altered stem cell population is probably responsible for giving rise to the huge volume of cells with impaired differentiation capacity that make up the bulk of the tumor. Recently identified markers for liver tumor cells with stem-like properties afford us the possibility to isolate and study liver cancer at its root. Such studies may lead to the development of therapies with the potential to bring liver cancer stem cells back under control, or eradicate them entirely.

REFERENCES

1. Hewitt HB. (1952) Transplantation of mouse sarcomas with small numbers of single cells. Nature; 170:622–623.
2. Reinhard MC, Goltz HL, Warner SG, Mirand EC. (1952) Growth rate and percentage takes following inoculation of known numbers of viable mouse tumor cells. Exp Med Surg; 10:254.
3. Sell S. (2009) In: Rajasekhar VK and Vemuri M (eds.) History of cancer stem cells. Regulatory networks in stem cells, Humana Press, Totowa NJ.
4. Salmon S. (1952) In vitro effects of drugs on human tumor stem cell assays, in Cloning of Human Tumor Stem Cells. S. Salmon, Ed. AR Liss, New York; 197–312.
5. Bonnet D, Dick JE. (1997) Human acute myeloid leukemia is organized as a hierarchy that originates from a primitive hematopoietic cell. Nature Med; 3:730–737.
6. Al-Hajj M, Wicha MS, Benito-Hernandez A, Morrison SJ, Clarke MF. (2003) Prospective identification of tumorigenic breast cancer cells. Proc Natl Acad Sci USA; 100:3983–3988.
7. Singh SK, Hawkins C, Clarke ID, Squire JA, Bayani J, Hide T, Henkelman RM, Cusimano MD, Dirks PB. (2004) Identification of human brain tumour initiating cells. Nature; 432:396–401.
8. Ricci-Vitiani L, Lombardi DG, Pilozzi E, Biffoni M, Todaro M, Peschle C, De Maria R. (2007) Identification and expansion of human colon-cancer-initiating cells. Nature; 445:111–115.
9. O'Brien CA, Pollett A, Gallinger S, Dick JE. (2007) A human colon cancer cell capable of initiating tumour growth in immunodeficient mice. Nature; 445:106–110.
10. Prince ME, Sivanandan R, Kaczorowski A, Wolf GT, Kaplan MJ, Dalerba P, Weissman IL, Clarke MF, Ailles LE. (2007) Identification of a subpopulation of cells with cancer stem cell properties in head and neck squamous cell carcinoma. Proc Natl Acad Sci USA; 104:973–978.
11. Li C, Heidt DG, Dalerba P, Burant CF, Zhang L, Adsay V, Wicha M, Clarke MF, Simeone DM. (2007) Identification of pancreatic cancer stem cells. Cancer Res; 67:1030–1037.
12. Conheim J. (1875) Congenitales, quergestreiftes Muskelsarkon der Nireren. Virchows Arch 65:64.
13. Lagasse, E, Connors, H, Al-Dhalimy, M. (2000) Purified hematopoietic stem cells can differentiate into hepatocytes in vivo. Nat Med; 6:1229–1234.
14. Alison, MR, Poulsom, R, Jeffery, R. (2000) Hepatocytes from non-hepatic adult stem cells. Nature (London); 406:257.
15. Theise, N, Nimmakalayu, M, Gardner, R. (2000) Liver from bone marrow in humans. Hepatology; 32:11–16.
16. Lagaaij, E, Cramer-Knijnenburg, G, van Kemenade, F, van Es, L, Bruijn, J, van Krieken, J. (2001) Endothelial cell chimerism after renal transplantation and vascular rejection. Lancet; 357:33–37.
17. Poulsom, R, Forbes, SJ, Hodivala-Dilke, K, Ryan E, Wyles S, Navaratnarasah S, Jeffery R, Hunt T, Alison M, Cook T, Pusey C, Wright NA. (2001) Bone marrow contributes to renal parenchymal turnover and regeneration. J Pathol; 195:229–235.

18. Orlic, D, Kajstura, J, Chimenti, S (2001) Bone marrow cells regenerate infarcted myocardium. Nature (London); 410:701–704.
19. Woodbury, D, Schwartz, E, Prockop, D and Black, I. (2000) Adult rat and human bone marrow stromal cells differentiate into neurons. J Neurosci Res; 61:364–370.
20. Krause, D. Theise, N. Collector, M. (2001) Multi-organ, multi-lineage engraftment by a single bone marrow-derived stem cell. Cell; 105:369–377.
21. Mezey, E, Chandross, K, Harta, G, Maki, R, McKercher, S. (2000) Turning blood into brain: cells bearing neuronal antigens generated in vivo from bone marrow. Science; 290:1779–1782.
22. Petersen BE, Bowen WC, Patrene KD, Mars WM, Sullivan AK, Murase N, Boggs SS, Greenberger JS, Goff JP. (1999) Bone marrow as a potential source of hepatic oval cells. Science; 284:1168–1170.
23. Theise ND, Badve S, Saxena R, Henegariu O, Sell S, Crawford JM, Krause DS. (2000) Derivation of hepatocytes from bone marrow cells in mice after radiation-induced myeloablation. Hepatology; 31:235–240.
24. Duncan SA. (2003) Mechanisms controlling early development of the liver. Mech Dev; 120:19–33.
25. Shiojiri N, Lemire JM, Fausto N. (1991) Cell lineages and oval cell progenitors in rat liver development. Cancer Res; 51:2611–2620.
26. Shiojiri N. (1984) The origin of intrahepatic bile duct cells in the mouse. J Embryol Exp Morphol; 79:25–39.
27. Germain L, Blouin MJ, Marceau N. (1988) Biliary epithelial and hepatocytic cell lineage relationships in embryonic rat liver as determined by the differential expression of cytokeratins, alpha-fetoprotein, albumin, and cell surface-exposed components. Cancer Res; 48:4909–4918.
28. Rogler LE. (1997) Selective bipotential differentiation of mouse embryonic hepatoblasts in vitro. Am J Pathol; 150:591–602.
29. Shiojiri N, Lemire JM, Fausto N. (1991) Cell lineages and oval cell progenitors in rat liver development. Cancer Res; 51:2611–220.
30. Evarts RP, Nagy P, Nakatsukasa H, Marsden E, Thorgeirsson SS. (1989) In vivo differentiation of rat liver oval cells into hepatocytes. Cancer Res; 49:1541–1547.
31. Sell S, Leffert HL. (1982) An evaluation of cellular lineages in the pathogenesis of experimental hepatocellular carcinoma. Hepatology; 2:77–86.
32. Sell S, Osborn K, Leffert HL. (1981) Autoradiography of "oval cells" appearing rapidly in the livers of rats fed N-2-fluorenylacetamide in a choline devoid diet. Carcinogenesis; 2:7–14.
33. Higgins GM, Andersen RM. (1931) Experimental pathology of the liver, restoration of the liver of the white rat following partial surgical removal. AMA Arch Pathol; 12:186–202.
34. Grisham JW. (1962) A morphologic study of deoxyribonucleic acid synthesis and cell proliferation in regenerating rat liver; autoradiography with thymidine-H3. Cancer Res; 22:842–849.
35. Overturf K, al-Dhalimy M, Ou CN, Finegold M, Grompe M. (1997) Serial transplantation reveals the stem-cell-like regenerative potential of adult mouse hepatocytes. Am J Pathol; 151:1273–1280.
36. Solt DB, Medline A, Farber E. (1977) Rapid emergence of carcinogen-induced hyperplastic lesions in a new model for the sequential analysis of liver carcinogenesis. Am J Pathol; 88:595–618.
37. Novikoff PM, Yam A, Oikawa I. (1996) Blast-like cell compartment in carcinogen-induced proliferating bile ductules. Am J Pathol; 148:1473–1492.
38. Bisgaard HC, Nagy P, Santoni-Rugiu E, Thorgeirsson SS. (1996) Proliferation, apoptosis, and induction of hepatic transcription factors are characteristics of the early response of biliary epithelial (oval) cells to chemical carcinogens. Hepatology; 23:62–70.
39. Petersen BE, Goff JP, Greenberger JS, Michalopoulos GK. (1998) Hepatic oval cells express the hematopoietic stem cell marker Thy-1 in the rat. Hepatology; 27:433–45.
40. Sell S, Salman J. (1984) Light- and electron-microscopic autoradiographic analysis of proliferating cells during the early stages of chemical hepatocarcinogenesis in the rat induced by feeding N-2-fluorenylacetamide in a choline-deficient diet. Am J Pathol; 114:287–300.
41. Onoe T, Dempo K, Kaneko A, Watabe H. (1973) Significance of Alpha-fetoprotein appearance in the early stage of azo-dye carcinogenesis. Gann; 14:233–243.
42. Kuwahara R, Kofman AV, Landis CS, Swenson ES, Barendswaard E, Theise ND. (2008) The hepatic stem cell niche: Identification by label-retaining cell assay. Hepatology; 47:1994–2002.
43. Oh SH, Witek RP, Bae SH, Zheng D, Jung Y, Piscaglia AC, Petersen BE. (2007) Bone marrow-derived hepatic oval cells differentiate into hepatocytes in 2 acetylaminofluorene/partial hepatectomy-induced liver regeneration. Gastroenterology; 132:1077–1087.
44. Kaplanski C, Pauley CJ, Griffiths TG, Kawabata TT, Ledwith BJ. (2000) Differentiation of rat oval cells after activation of peroxisome proliferator-activated receptor alpha43. Cancer Res; 60:580–587.

45. Teebor GW, Becker FF. (1971) Regression and persistence of hyperplastic hepatic nodules induced by *N*-2-fluorenyl-lacetamide and their relationship to hepatocarcinogenesis; 31:1–3.

46. Solt D, Farber E. (1977) Persistence of carcinogen-induced initiated hepatocytes in liver carcinogenesis. Proc Am Assoc Cancer Res; 18:52.

47. Solt DB, Medline A, Farber E. (1977) Rapid emergence of carcinogen-induced hyperplastic lesions in a new model for the sequential analysis of liver carcinogenesis. Am J Pathol; 88:595–609.

48. Sell S. (2002) Cellular origin of hepatocellular carcinomas. Semin Cell Dev Biol; 13:419–424.

49. Coleman WB, Wennerberg AE, Smith GJ, Grisham JW. (1993) Regulation of the differentiation of diploid and some aneuploid rat liver epithelial (stemlike) cells by the hepatic microenvironment. Am J Pathol; 142:1373–1382.

50. Tsao MS, Grisham JW, Nelson KG, Smith JD. (1985) Phenotypic and karyotypic changes induced in cultured rat hepatic epithelial cells that express the "oval" cell phenotype by exposure to *N*-methyl-*N'*-nitro-*N*-nitrosoguanidine. Am J Pathol; 118:306–315.

51. Dumble ML, Croager EJ, Yeoh GC, Quail EA. (2002) Generation and characterization of p53 null transformed hepatic progenitor cells: oval cells give rise to hepatocellular carcinoma. Carcinogenesis; 23:435–445.

52. Su Q, Zerban H, Otto G, Bannasch P. (1998) Cytokeratin expression is reduced in glycogenotic clear hepatocytes but increased in ground-glass cells in chronic human and woodchuck hepadnaviral infection. Hepatology; 28:347–359.

53. Fotiadu A, Tzioufa V, Vrettou E, Koufogiannis D, Papadimitriou CS, Hytiroglou P. (2004) Progenitor cell activation in chronic viralhepatitis. Liver Int; 24:268–274.

54. Lowes KN, Brennan BA, Yeoh GC, Olynyk JK. (1999) Oval cell numbers in human chronic liver diseases are directly related to disease severity. Am J Pathol; 54:537–541.

55. Roskams TA, Libbrecht L, Desmet VJ. (2003) Progenitor cells in diseased human liver. Semin Liver Dis; 23:385–396.

56. Thorgeirsson SS. (1995) Target cell populations in virus-associated hepatocarcinogenesis. Princess Takamatsu Symp; 25:163–170.

57. Omata M, Yoshida H. (2004) Prevention and treatment of hepatocellular carcinoma. Liver Transpl 10(S2):S111–S114.

58. Kim H, Park C, Han KH, Choi J, Kim YB, Kim JK, Park YN. (2004) Primary liver carcinoma of intermediate (hepatocyte-cholangiocyte) phenotype. J Hepatol; 40:298–304.

59. Theise ND, Yao JL, Harada K, Hytiroglou P, Portmann B, Thung SN, Tsui W, Ohta H, Nakanuma Y. (2003) Hepatic 'stem cell' malignancies in adults: four cases. Histopathology; 43:263–271.

60. Caussinus E, Hirth F. (2007) Asymmetric stem cell division in development and cancer. Prog Mol Subcell Biol; 45:205–225.

61. Wicha MS. (2008) Cancer stem cell heterogeneity in hereditary breast cancer. Breast Cancer Res; 10:105.

62. Shachaf CM, Kopelman AM, Arvanitis C, Karlsson A, Beer S, Mandl S, Bachmann MH, Borowsky AD, Ruebner B, Cardiff RD, Yang Q, Bishop JM, Contag CH, Felsher DW. (2004) MYC inactivation uncovers pluripotent differentiation and tumour dormancy in hepatocellular cancer. Nature; 431:1112–1117.

63. Chiba T, Kita K, Zheng YW, Yokosuka O, Saisho H, Iwama A, Nakauchi H, Taniguchi H. (2006) Side population purified from hepatocellular carcinoma cells harbors cancer stem cell-like properties. Hepatology; 44:240–251.

64. Zhu H, Dong H, Eksioglu E, Hemming A, Cao M, Crawford JM, Nelson DR, Liu C. (2007) Hepatitis C virus triggers apoptosis of a newly developed hepatoma cell line through antiviral defense system. Gastroenterology; 133:1649–1659.

65. Erba E, Ubezio P, Broggini M, Ponti M, D'Incalci M. (1988) DNA damage, cytotoxic effect and cell-cycle perturbation of Hoechst 33342 on L1210 cells in vitro. Cytometry; 9:1–6.

66. Tong QS, Zheng LD, Tang ST, Ruan QL, Liu Y, Li SW, Jiang GS, Cai JB. (2008) Expression and clinical significance of stem cell marker CD133 in human neuroblastoma. World J Pediatr; 4:58–62.

67. Miki J, Furusato B, Li H, Gu Y, Takahashi H, Egawa S, Sesterhenn IA, McLeod DG, Srivastava S, Rhim JS. (2007) Identification of putative stem cell markers, CD133 and CXCR4, in hTERT-immortalized primary nonmalignant and malignant tumor-derived human prostate epithelial cell lines and in prostate cancer specimens. Cancer Res; 67:3153–3161.

68. Yamada Y, Yokoyama S, Wang XD, Fukuda N, Takakura N. (2007) Cardiac stem cells in brown adipose tissue express CD133 and induce bone marrow nonhematopoietic cells to differentiate into cardiomyocytes. Stem Cells; 25:1326–1333.

69. Mizrak D, Brittan M, Alison MR. (2008) CD133: molecule of the moment. J Pathol; 214:3–9.

70. Suetsugu A, Nagaki M, Aoki H, Motohashi T, Kunisada T, Moriwaki H. (2006) Characterization of CD133+ hepatocellular carcinoma cells as cancer stem/progenitor cells. Biochem Biophys Res Commun; 351:820–824.

71. Yin S, Li J, Hu C, Chen X, Yao M, Yan M, Jiang G, Ge C, Xie H, Wan D, Yang S, Zheng S, Gu J. (2007) CD133 positive hepatocellular carcinoma cells possess high capacity for tumorigenicity. Int J Cancer; 120:1444–1450.

72. Ma S, Chan KW, Hu L, Lee TK, Wo JY, Ng IO, Zheng BJ, Guan XY. (2007) Identification and characterization of tumorigenic liver cancer stem/progenitor cells. Gastroenterology; 132:2542–2556.

73. Yang ZF, Ngai P, Ho DW, Yu WC, Ng MN, Lau CK, Li ML, Tam KH, Lam CT, Poon RT, Fan ST. (2008) Identification of local and circulating cancer stem cells in human liver cancer. Hepatology; 47:919–928.

74. Yang ZF, Ho DW, Ng MN, Lau CK, Yu WC, Ngai P, Chu PW, Lam CT, Poon RT, Fan ST. (2008) Significance of CD90+ cancer stem cells in human liver cancer. Cancer Cell; 13:153–166.

75. Mishra L, Derynck R, Mishra B. (2005) Transforming growth factor-beta signaling in stem cells and cancer. Science; 310:68–71.

76. Tang Y, Kitisin K, Jogunoori W, Li C, Deng CX, Mueller SC, Ressom HW, Rashid A, He AR, Mendelson JS, Jessup JM, Shetty K, Zasloff M, Mishra B, Reddy EP, Johnson L, Mishra L. (2008) Progenitor/stem cells give rise to liver cancer due to aberrant TGF-beta and IL-6 signaling. Proc Natl Acad Sci USA; 105:2445–2450.

77. Marrero JA. (2005) Hepatocellular carcinoma. Curr Opin Gastroenterol; 21:308–312.

78. Yovchev MI, Grozdanov PN, Joseph B, Gupta S, Dabeva MD. (2007) Novel hepatic progenitor cell surface markers in the adult rat liver. Hepatology; 245:139–149.

79. Kucia M, Reca R, Campbell FR, Zuba-Surma E, Majka M, Ratajczak J, Ratajczak MZ. (2006) A population of very small embryonic-like (VSEL) CXCR4(+)SSEA-1(+)Oct-4+ stem cells identified in adult bone marrow. Leukemia; 20:857–869.

80. Okumoto K, Saito T, Hattori E, Ito JI, Adachi T, Takeda T, Sugahara K, Watanabe H, Saito K, Togashi H, Kawata S. (2003) Differentiation of bone marrow cells into cells that express liver-specific genes in vitro: implication of the Notch signals in differentiation. Biochem Biophys Res Commun; 304:691–695.

Color Plates

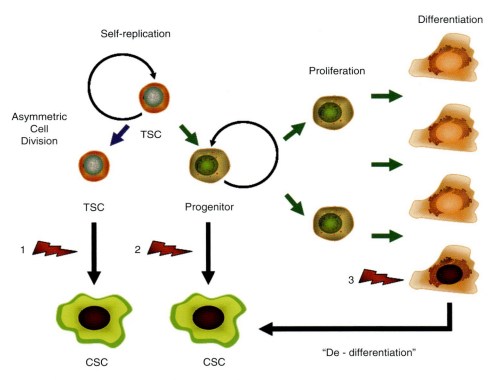

Chapter 1, Fig. 2. Possible origins of CSCs. Three different but not mutually exclusive models are schematically presented. "Lightning" symbols indicate transforming mutations. CSCs may originate exclusively from the transformation of primitive tissue stem cells (TSC, model 1), or from the transformation of either TSC or progenitor cells (model 2). Alternatively, CSCs may originate from the transformation and dedifferentiation of more mature cells, which reacquire stem cell properties as a consequence of transforming mutations (model 3).

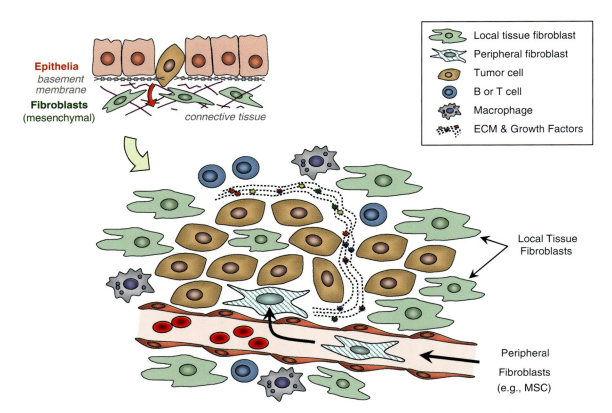

Chapter 3, Fig. 1. Similar to an organ, solid tumor masses are composed of a complex mixture of cellular and acellular components, which together comprise the tumor microenvironment. Following loss of basement membrane integrity, tumor cells invade into the underlying connective tissue and interact directly with local mesenchymal fibroblasts. Subsequent tumor and fibroblast cell expansion promotes recruitment of immune cells, peripheral mesenchymal fibroblasts, and *de novo* production and remodeling of extracellular matrix (ECM).

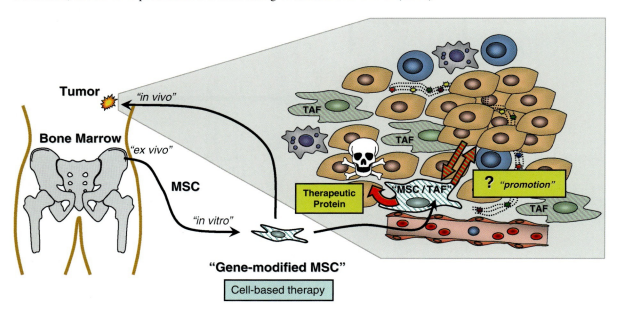

Chapter 3, Fig. 2. A "Trojan Horse" anticancer therapy. Bone marrow MSC are isolated from bone marrow and expanded in tissue culture. MSC, *in vitro*, are gene-modified to produce a given antitumor protein and are then reintroduced back into the cancer patient. Given the strong affinity for tumors, MSC selectively engraft and expand within the tumor microenvironment and produce locally concentrated levels of select antitumor proteins.

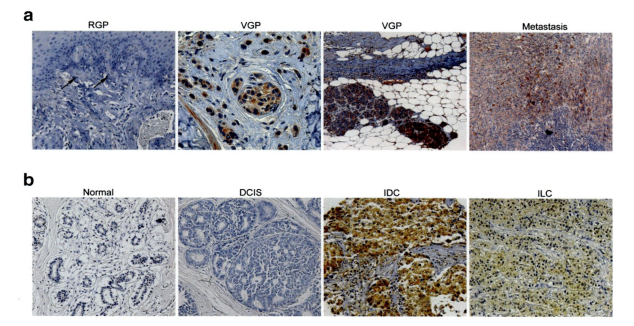

Chapter 8, Fig. 2. Nodal as a new biomarker for tumor progression. (**a**) Immunohistochemical localization of Nodal (*red/brown*) in human melanoma. Sections (*left to right*) represent radial growth phase melanoma (RGP), vertical growth phase melanomas (VGP), and a melanoma metastasis in a lymph node biopsy. Note that RGP expresses relatively little Nodal; however, invasive cells begin to express Nodal as they leave the basal area and invade through the papillary dermis and dermal-epidermal junction toward the underlying reticular dermis (*arrows*). In contrast, strong expression of Nodal is seen in VGP melanoma cells that have invaded subcutaneous connective or adipose tissue. Nodal staining is also strong in melanoma cells that have metastasized to the lymph node. (**b**) Immunohistochemical localization of Nodal (*red/brown*) in human breast tissue. Sections (*left to right*) represent normal tissue from a reduction mammoplasty; localized ductal carcinoma in situ (DCIS); invasive ductal carcinoma (IDC) and invasive lobular carcinoma (ILC). Note that the normal tissue and DCIS do not express Nodal. In contrast, strong cytoplasmic staining for Nodal is detected in the invasive cancers.

Chapter 7, Fig. 3. Cancer stem cells, epigenetic gene silencing events, and tumorigenesis. For at least some pluripotency associated and alternate lineage genes, gene silencing is a normal event in stem/progenitor cells as adult cell renewal takes place. Silencing is mediated by repressive chromatin modifications, which are malleable such that the genes might be activated for transcription as required by cell maturation. This homeostasis allows stem/progenitor cells to move properly along the differentiation pathway for a given tissue or cell system (darkening blue color of cells along the *top left panel*). During chronic cell injury, stress, wound healing, or inflammation, the pressure for adaptive cell renewal draws from the stem/progenitor cell pool for ongoing repair. This pressure might allow for abnormal DNA methylation to be recruited to promoters of normally silenced genes by the chromatin which is in place (*lower right*, DNA hypermethylation, *black circles*). The result is a tight heritable silencing that cannot be easily reactivated as a cell clone expands, thereby channeling the cells toward the abnormal expansion, at the expense of differentiation. This entire scenario leads to benign precursor tumors that are at risk for progression. This progression would be fostered by subsequent genetic or epigenetic events. Chemically depleting DNA methylation using 5-aza-deoxy-cytidine can induce gene expression (upper right, demethylated cancer cell), but the gene does not return to the fully euchromatic state seen at a normally transcribed gene *(67)*. In this intermediate state, the histones contain the transcriptional activating marks (*green*) H3K4me2 and H3K9/14ac and HP1a is not present. However, several repressive modifications (*red*) including H3K27me3 and H3K9me3 remain and apparently need not change for significant transcription to occur.

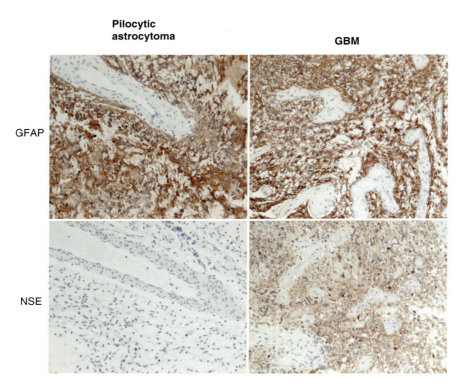

Chapter 9, Fig. 2. Neuronal differentiation potential can be detected in high-grade, but not in low-grade gliomas. Archived glioma specimens were sectioned and stained for NSE, synaptophysin, and GFAP. GFAP can be detected in all cases of gliomas, whereas NSE and synaptophysin were only detected in high-grade glioma specimens *(25)*.

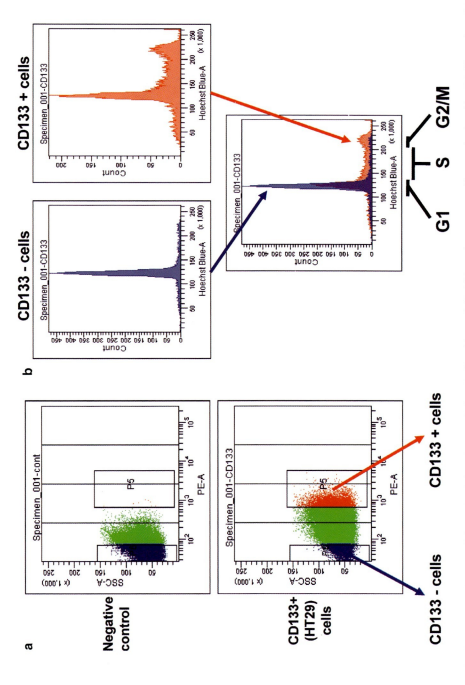

Chapter 12, Fig. 1. Characterization of CD133+ Colon Cancer Cells. (**a**) CD133+ and CD133– colon cancer cells were isolated by FACS sorting. (**b**) Cell cycle analysis of CD133+ and CD133– colon cancer cells. CD133+ fraction exhibits cell cycling proliferation, compared with CD133– fraction. Note, in the *upper part*, the scale of the cell count on *Y*-axis indicates ~2-times accumulation of the G1 phase in CD133– cells, compared with CD133+ cells.

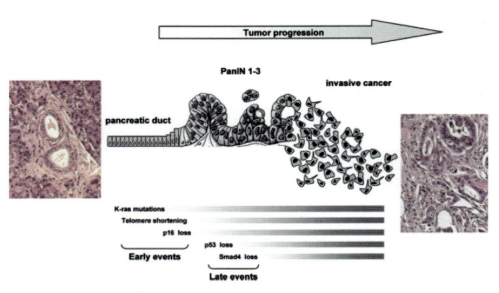

Chapter 15, Fig. 1. Progression of PanIN lesions to invasive pancreatic disease *(8)*.

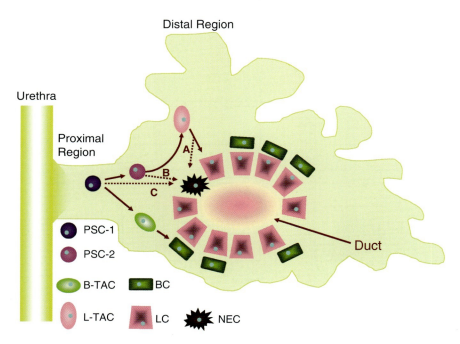

Chapter 16, Fig. 2. The branching differentiation model of stem cell differentiation in the prostate. In this model the prostate stem cell (PSC-1) give rise to at least two different lineages; the luminal cell lineage, in which luminal transit amplifying cells (L-TAC) give rise to the more differentiated luminal cells; and the basal lineage, in which basal transit amplifying cells (B-TAC) give rise to more to differentiated basal cells (BC). Luminal cells surround the ducts into which they secrete various proteins. Neuroendocrine cells may differentiate from L-TAC (A), a stem/progenitor cell with a more restricted differentiation potential and common with that for luminal epithelium (PSC-2) (B), directly from PSC-1 (C) or from an independent precursor altogether.

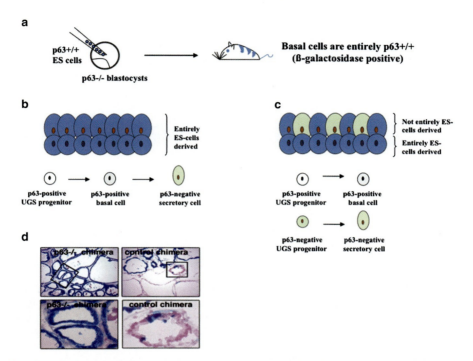

Chapter 18, Fig. 1. p63-deficient blastocyst complementation. (**a**) Chimeric mice were created by injecting p63−/− blastocysts with p63+/+ ES cells constitutively expressing the β-galactosidase gene. As expected, the prostate of the rescued chimeras contained entirely ES-cell-derived basal cells. Insights on prostate cell lineages could be achieved by evaluating the relative contribution of the p63+/+ and p63−/− cells to the secretory cell compartment. (**b, c**). Models of epithelial development based on possible outcomes of blastocyst complementation experiments. In one scenario (**b**), both secretory cells and basal cells originate from the p63+/+ (β-galactosidase-positive) ES cells, indicating that the secretory cell compartment is derived from the p63-positive basal cell layer. In the alternative scenario (**c**), the secretory compartment is composed of both p63+/+ and p63−/− cells, implying that the basal and secretory cell compartments are not hierarchically related. (**d**) The results of our experiments show that only p63+/+ (β-galactosidase-positive) cells are present in the prostate epithelium (*left panels*) of rescued chimeras. In contrast, both β-galactosidase-positive and β-galactosidase-negative cells are detected in the prostate of control chimeras generated by injecting p63+/+ β-galactosidase-positive ES cells into p63+/+ blastocysts (*right panels*). Figure modified from Signoretti et al. *(36)*.

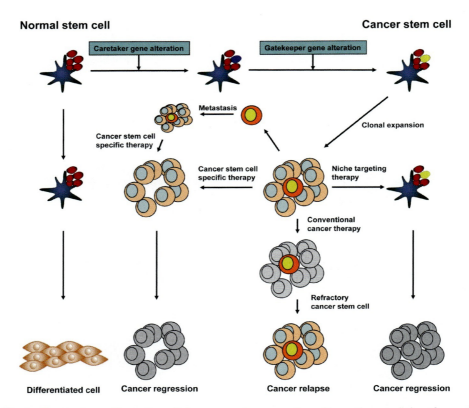

Normal stem cell

Cancer stem cell

Caretaker gene alteration

Gatekeeper gene alteration

Metastasis

Clonal expansion

Cancer stem cell specific therapy

Cancer stem cell specific therapy

Niche targeting therapy

Conventional cancer therapy

Refractory cancer stem cell

Differentiated cell   Cancer regression   Cancer relapse   Cancer regression

Chapter 20, Fig. 1. Cancer stem cells are the cellular source of cancer cells and have characteristics of somatic stem cells. Normal stem cells renew themselves under the support of specialized microenvironment (niche) and differentiate into differentiated tissue cells (*left panel*). When genetic alterations involving caretaker and gatekeeper genes accumulate in the stem cell, a cancer stem cell may form (*upper right*). Subsequently, the cancer stem cells form a cancer through clonal expansion. The overall cellular population of a cancer consists of 1–4% cancer stem cells and 97–99% differentiated cancer cells. Only cancer stem cells are tumorigenic and form metastases. Conventional cancer therapy kills differentiated cancer cells but refractory cancer stem cells remain due to chemotherapy and radiation resistance. Cancer relapse occurs because of clonal expansion of surviving cancer stem cells. However, when cancer stem cell specific therapy is applied, the cancer stem cells are depleted and the differentiated cancer cells will die soon thereafter. Another option for therapy is to target the cancer stem cell microenvironment, niche. When the niche is interrupted the cancer stem cell cannot undergo self-renewal or clonal expansion.

Chapter 23, Fig. 2. Cellular events associated with the initiation and progression of epithelial cancer mediated through tumorigenic and migrating cancer stem/progenitor cells. The asymmetric division of cancer stem cells localized in the basal compartment into transit-amplifying cancer progenitor cells that, in turn, may regenerate the further differentiated cancer cells is illustrated. The oncogenic transformation of tumorigenic stem/progenitor cells into migrating cancer progenitor cells, which may be induced by the sustained activation of distinct growth factor signaling during the epithelial-mesenchymal transition (EMT) program is also shown. The invasion of tumorigenic and migrating cancer stem/progenitor cells in the bloodstream, which may lead to their dissemination at distant sites and metastases, is also indicated. This model of carcinogenesis supports the therapeutic interest of targeting tumorigenic and migrating cancer stem/progenitor cells to counteract the cancer progression and metastases at distant sites. *ECM* extracellular matrix, *MMPs* matrix metalloproteinases, and *uPA* urokinase type-plasminogene activator.

EPITHELIAL CANCER DERIVED FROM A HIERARCHICAL ORGANIZATION OF CANCER STEM/PROGENITOR CELLS

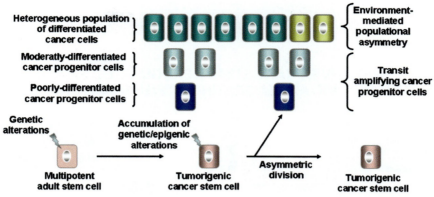

Chapter 23, Fig. 1. New concept on epithelial cancer formation derived from the malignant transformation of adult stem cells into tumorigenic cancer stem/progenitor cells. This scheme shows the malignant transformation of adult stem cells into tumorigenic cancer stem cells (CSCs), which may be induced through the genetic and/or epigenetic alterations. More specifically, an asymmetric division of a CSC that gives rise to one CSC daughter and one poorly-differentiated cancer progenitor cell termed early transit-amplifying (TA)/intermediate cancer progenitor cell is indicated. Moreover, the possibility that early poorly-differentiated TA cells, which possess a high proliferative potential, may in turn, generate the moderately-differentiated cancer progenitor cells and subsequently the bulk mass of well-differentiated cancer cells is also illustrated. This hierarchical model of carcinogenesis also implicates that the changes in the local environmental of early and late TA cancer progenitor cells during the amplification process and their migration at distant sites from niche may influence the phenotype of their further and terminally differentiated progenies, and thereby contribute to the populational asymmetry and cellular diversity characterizing cancer subtype.

CANCER PROGRESSION MEDIATED THROUGH TUMORIGENIC AND MIGRATING STEM/PROGENITOR CELLS

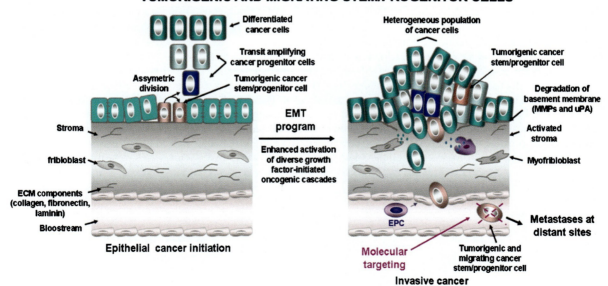

NOVEL CANCER THERAPY BY TARGETING DEREGULATED SIGNALING ELEMENTS IN TUMORIGENIC AND MIGRATING STEM/PROGENITOR CELLS

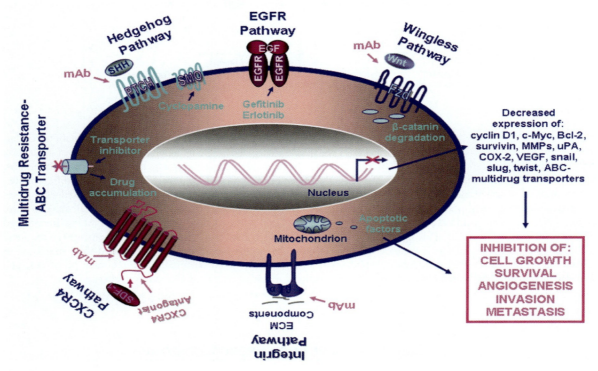

Chapter 23, Fig. 3. Novel therapeutic strategies against aggressive and invasive cancers by targeting distinct deregulated signaling cascades in tumorigenic and migrating cancer progenitor cells. The inhibitory effects on the tumorigenic signaling cascades induced by using pharmacological agents such as the selective inhibitors of smoothened (SMO) hedgehog signaling element (cyclopamine) and epidermal growth factor receptor (EGFR) tyrosine kinase activity (gefitinib or erlotinib) are indicated. Moreover, the anti-carcinogenic effects induced by a CXC chemokine receptor 4 (CXCR4) antagonist or monoclonal antibody (mAb) directed against stromal cell-derived factor-1 (SDF-1), CXCR4, Wingless ligand (Wnt) or integrin are also indicated. Particularly, the anti-proliferative, anti-invasive and apoptotic effects induced by these pharmacological agents in cancer stem/progenitor cells through the down-regulation of the expression levels of numerous gene products are also indicated. In addition, the potent inhibitory effect mediated by a specific inhibitor of ATP-binding cassette (ABC)-multidrug transporter on drug efflux is also indicated. *COX-2* cyclooxygenase 2, *ECM* extracellular matrix, *EGF* epidermal growth factor, *Fzd* Frizzled receptor, *MMPs* matrix metalloproteinases, *PTCH* hedgehog-patched receptor, *uPA* urokinase type-plasminogene activator, and *VEGF* vascular endothelial growth factor.

14 Cancer Stem Cells: Lung Cancer

Jaclyn Y. Hung

Key Words: Lung cancer, Side population, Stem-like

Lung cancer is today the most common cause of cancer death worldwide with a mortality rate exceeding that of colon, cervical, breast, and prostate cancers combined. The estimated global burden for 2002 is 1.35 million new cases diagnosed (incidence) and 1.18 million deaths (mortality) *(1)*. The causal link between smoking and lung cancer is well established. The World Health Organization (WHO) has estimated that tobacco will cause about 10 million deaths per annum by the year 2030; about a quarter of these deaths will be from lung cancer *(2)*. Many people commonly perceive that cessation of smoking will prevent the onset lung cancer; however, unlike heart disease, stroke, and chronic obstructive pulmonary disease, the risk of lung cancer remains significantly elevated among long-term heavy smokers despite cessation of smoking *(3, 4)*. Fifty percent of new lung cancer cases are former smokers, many of whom have stopped smoking for five or more years. In the United States, there are currently about 50 million smokers and 50 million former smokers; about half of the former smokers are above 45 years of age and hence at risk for lung cancer. With this large reservoir of current and former smokers and the increasing incidence of lung cancer among women, lung cancer will remain a major health issue for several decades even if the current strategies to eliminate tobacco smoking are completely successful. There would still be lung cancer cases for 50 years due to damage already caused.

Lung cancer is classified clinically into two major groups, small cell lung carcinoma (SCLC), accounting for 13% of lung cancer, and nonsmall cell lung carcinoma (NSCLC), which accounts for almost all of the remaining cases of primary lung cancers. NSCLC has three major subtypes: squamous cell carcinoma, adenocarcinoma, and large cell carcinoma. Despite the advances in diagnosis and the treatment of cancer, lung cancers remain nearly uniformly fatal; 85% of the people in United States who are diagnosed with lung cancer die of the disease within five years *(5)*. The average survival in Europe is 10% and in the developing countries is 8.9% *(1)*. This poor cure rate, in part is because at the time of diagnosis, majority of the patients are already beyond cure by surgery or radiotherapy, and a large percentage of those diagnosed with resectable early-stage disease eventually experience recurrence of metastatic disease. Moreover, there is a 1–3% chance per year of developing a second primary lung cancer after curative treatment of the first cancer.

Although chemotherapy offers hope to control systemic disease in patients with inoperable lung cancer, treatment outcomes are still disappointing. Median survival of patients with advanced inoperable disease has improved only modestly over the last 20 years *(6, 7)*: 4–6 months with best supportive

From: *Cancer Drug Discovery and Development: Stem Cells and Cancer,*
Edited by: R.G. Bagley and B.A. Teicher, DOI: 10.1007/978-1-60327-933-8_14,
© Humana Press, a part of Springer Science+Business Media, LLC 2009

care *(8)*, 8–11 months with Cisplatin-based doublet chemotherapy *(9)*. Although these aggressive, treatment-intense protocols do prolong median survival, the overall impact has been mainly on palliation rather than reduction in mortality, with total cure remaining elusive. Moreover, the treatment regimes have a nonspecific toxicity profile that exceeds its therapeutic profile. These sobering data have led to a greater emphasis on public health and research strategies to prevent lung cancer, either by removing tobacco carcinogens through cessation of smoking or through developing rational approaches aimed at the multistep carcinogenic process. Several targeted biological agents have been approved for use in the clinic for NSCLC, including targeting of the epidermal growth factor (EGFR) with gefitinib and targeting of vascular endothelial growth factor (VEGF) with bevacizumab in combination with paclitaxel-carboplatin for the initial systemic treatment of patient with locally advance, inoperable, recurrent, or metastatic disease. Emerging data suggest that most cancers, if not all, rely on the "cancer stem cells" for the continued growth of their mass. As well, relapse and metastasis are likely orchestrated by the posttherapy residual cancer stem cells that escape treatment. Therefore, selective targeting of cancer stem cells is believed to offer radical advances in cancer treatment and diagnosis, by attacking the disease at its root.

The purification and characterization of cancer stem cells has been reported in many cancers *(10– 20)*. These cancer stem cells have been enriched on the basis of the expression of their unique cell surface marker(s). However, in human lung cancer, the purification of cancer stem cells has been hampered by the lack of definitive cell-surface marker(s). An alterative approach to surface antigens is to identify putative stem cells based primary on their stem cell functionality, notably the ability to efflux the Hoechst 33342 dye *(21, 22)*.

Cells subject to Hoechst 33342 dye staining and fluorescence-activated cell sorting (FACS) analysis can give a profile such that those cells that actively efflux the dye appear as a distinct population of cells on the side of the dual-color emission spectra (blue vs. red) FACS profile on a density plot; hence the name "side population" (SP) has been given to these cells. The dye efflux is due to the activity of various members of the adenosine triphosphate (ATP)-binding cassette (ABC) transporters family. By using the energy of ATP hydrolysis, these transporters (~49 in human) actively efflux toxin from cells, thus protecting them from cytotoxic agents. Of note various members such as ABCB (MDR1), ABCC1 (MRP1), and ABCG2 (BCRP1) have been shown to mediate multidrug resistance. Interestingly, hematopoietic stem cells express high levels of ABCG2, but the gene is turned off in most committed progenitor and mature blood cells. The Hoechst staining profile is a continuum, with no clear-cut separation line between the SP and the non-SP. As a result the SP is defined, according to convention, by depletion using Hoechst transporter-inhibitors such as reserpine or verapamil.

The SP phenotype is initially used to isolate murine stem hematopoietic cells *(23)*. In the bone marrow, these SP cells are enriched approximately 1,000-fold in hematopoietic stem cell activity in repopulation experiments, which can protect murine recipients from lethal irradiation at low cell doses, thus establishing their functional capacity as hematopoietic stem cells. In addition, SP cells also contribute to both myeloid and lymphoid lineages in the transplant recipients. The SP population is present in bone marrow at a low level (0.02–0.08%) and express the cell surface markers characteristic Sca-1^{+}/lin$^{-/low}$ of hematopoietic stem cells. Subsequent studies have demonstrated that the hematopoietic SP is conserved across species. ABCG2 has been identified as a molecular determinant for bone marrow stem cells and proposed as a universal marker for stem cells, although not all reports agree *(24)*. However, the SP phenotype might be a way to identify stem cell populations from various sources independently of cell-type specific markers, thus making it an important tool in stem cell characterization and research.

Since its initial application in murine bone marrow hematopoietic stem cells, the Hoechst 33342 dye-efflux SP phenotype has been extended to sort out putative somatic stems cells and progenitors in a diverse range of normal tissues across species including the pancreas *(25)*, prostate *(26)*, lung *(27, 28)*, mammary glands *(29, 30)*, arteries *(31)*, as well as embryonic stem cells. In many of these studies, it is reported that the SP cells are enriched for stem cell markers and in some studies the SP cells can behave as clonogenic stem cells. These SP are rare and heterogeneous, varying with tissue type, stage of development, and method of preparation. Parallel studies have demonstrated the SP phenotype in human cancers of different origins, including acute myeloid leukemia *(32, 33)* neuroblastoma *(34)*, glioma *(35)*, retinoblastoma *(36)*, prostate *(37)*, head and neck *(38)*, liver *(39)*, ovarian *(40)*, thyroid *(41)*, and gastrointestinal *(42)* cancers.

We have recently identified an enriched population of cells with stem-like phenotype based primary on their ability to efflux the Hoechst 33342 dye from various human lung cancer cell lines and lung tissues from surgical resection *(43)*. The SP fraction is composed of 0.023–1.08% of cells from human lung cancer tissues, and 1.5–6.1% of cells from cell lines. The majority of these cells have lower expression of MCM7, an essential component of the replication helicase complex required for DNA replication. Its expression is required during the cell cycle, but in quiescent cells (G0) it is found to be absent suggesting that these cells are mainly outside the active cell cycle. These SP cells from human lung cancer cell lines are also more drug resistant against a number of chemotherapeutic drugs, a number of which, notably cisplatin, gemcitabine, and vinorelbine, are commonly used as first-line therapy for lung cancer. The increase in drug resistance in part is due to the elevated expression of several ABC transporters associated with multidrug resistance *(43–45)* and their lower proliferation rate. Therefore, in nontargeted therapies such as chemotherapy, the coadministration of chemotherapeutics and inhibitors to ABC transporters to sensitize cancer stem cells could be employed as a good defensive measure to multidrug resistance.

The SP cells have a higher capacity for regenerating tumors in vivo. When injected into NOD-SCID mice, SP cells are found to be more tumorigenic than non-SP, thus indicating a significant enrichment of cancer-initiating cells in this small population. Even though the non-SP forms the majority of cells, the tumors initiated from SP cells are larger, very vascular, and required much fewer cells for initiation of the tumor. Hence, the functional importance of the SP are twofold: they are more significantly enhanced in tumorigenicity and are also more resistant to existing chemotherapeutic agents, possibly due to heightened expression of a range of drug resistance transporters. This suggests the SP will have survival advantage under chemotherapy and can regenerate a tumor leading to refractory/relapsed disease, and is likely an important target for more effective therapy.

Similar findings have been obtained for CD133+ stem-like cells within spheres that are serially propagated from primary lung cancer tissue *(46)*. By applying the same conditions that are use for the isolation of human neural stem cells *(47)*, a putative cancer stem-like cell is identified from human lung cancer tissues. These "tumor spheres" are significantly enriched in neuronal stem cell marker CD 133, able to grow indefinitely in serum-free medium supplemented with hrEGF and hrbFGF, have drug resistant phenotype after multiple passage in vitro, demonstrated enhanced tumorigenicity, and are also resistant to DNA-damaging agent – chemotherapeutic drug.

Current lung cancer chemotherapy regimens include a platinum compound in combination with taxane analogues, gemcitabine, or vinorelbine. Most of the patients that respond will relapse following initial remission after therapy, with a median survival of 8–11 months *(9)*. The failure of these therapies suggests that relapse and/or disease progression is likely the result of clonal expansion of drug resistant malignant stem cells in the original heterogeneous tumor cell population. Whether or not such resistant clones are present de novo or are induced by chemotherapy is not known. A premise proposed more than 20 years ago posits that a small percentage of cells in a tumor harbor intrinsic characteristics that make them resistant to treatment *(48)*. If the drug resistance clones are indeed orchestrated by the posttherapy residual cancer stem cells that escape treatment, then strategies to identify the "drug resistance clones" may provide the experimental tool to investigate the molecular properties of the clinically relevant malignant cell population.

Interestingly, the lung cancer SP cells are more invasive than non-SP, suggesting that "stemness" may relate to invasiveness. Possibly, there exists a virulent population of stem-like cells within a lung tumor that is involved in the initiation of invasion. It is known that one of the crucial events to malignancy that occurs before metastasis is the gain of migratory phenotype at the expense of epithelial-cell properties. This is referred as the epithelial to mesenchymal transition (EMT). Likely the cancer stem cells undergo EMT and hence attain migratory and other properties that promote metastasis. This notion is proposed as a two-phase process in which "stationary" lung cancer stem cells acquire mesenchymal characteristics and become migrating cancer stem cells. A recent study show that ABCG2 expression and SP fraction in MCF7 human breast cancer cells is depleted during a transforming growth factor beta (TGFb)-directed EMT and is restored upon the removal of TGFb and reversal from mesenchymal back to an epithelial phenotype (MET) *(49)*. A study by Kaplan et al. investigating the relationship of niche formation and metastasis shows that communication between cancer stem cells and target tissue microenvironment at distant sites occurs before the cancer cells even arrived at its target *(50)*. Cancer stem cells drive both initiation of tumorigenesis and metastasis can explain the formation of tumor at distinct sites *(51–53)*. The tumor is fuelled and sustained by the initial pool of cancer stem cells, and eventually secrete factors that form the premetastatic niche at distinct sites. The metastatic cancer stem cells are guided toward the niche at these distinct sites through chemoattractants and other homing factors. When the cancer stem cells arrive, they are able to proliferate into a metastatic lesion, or enter a quiescent phase until reactivated to promote expansion into a secondary tumor. The concept of migrating cancer stem cells has many important implications. The combination of migratory and "stemness" properties integrates both tumor metastasis and initiation concepts into one cell, and potentially provides an explanation to tumorigenic progress. Since the putative cancer stem cell has enhanced tumorigenic capacity, their added increase in mobility enables them to initiate secondary tumors at distant sites from the primary tumor, adds to the importance of developing therapeutics that target these cells.

The SP cells preferentially express stem cell-associated genes such as BMI-1 and NOTCH1 (unpublished data). In lung cancer activated Notch, Wnt, Hedgehog, and Bmi-1 may be important. Thus, canonical signaling pathways that regulate self-renewal and stem cell properties are candidate "druggability" targets for successful molecular therapy of cancer. These targets may synergize with preclinical agents such as gamma-secretase and cyclopamine to increase efficacy. However, targeting the cancer stem cells without harming the somatic stem cells may not be trivial.

These putative stem-like SP cells also expressed elevated level of telomerase (hTERT). This is consistent with the work of Keshet et al. *(54)* that showed elevated levels of hTERT in the stem-like MDR1+ cell fraction of primary cultures of human melanoma. Emerging data suggest that normal stem cells may have longer telomeres compared with cancer stem cell *(55)*, thus there may be a window of opportunity to potentially target both lung cancer stem cells and more mature cancer cells using telomerase-based therapies, either alone or in combination with tumor debulking agents hopefully sparing the normal stem cell *(56, 57)*.

Lung cancer is the end-stage of a multistep process, in most cases, driven by accumulative genetic and epigenetic damage caused by chronic carcinogen exposure to a large surface area with a range of normal respiratory epithelial cell populations. Two distinct hypotheses have been proposed to explain the simultaneous and/or sequential development of multiple foci of preinvasive lesions as well as occurrence of multiple primary and secondary tumors in the respiratory epithelium. The monoclonal neoplasia hypothesis holds that progeny from a single transformed cell can spread to produce multiple preinvasive lesions and tumors. The second hypothesis posit that exposure of the respiratory epithelium to tobacco smoke carcinogens predisposes the entire epithelium to develop multiple, independent preinvasive lesions that can be develop into cancers. This concept is referred to "field cancerization," which implies that the entire epithelium is mutagenized *(58)*.

Likely, the accumulation of key mutations is in the expanding clones of cells originating from multipotent resident lung stem cells. Because of its extensive and lifelong turnover, stem cell can serve as a tissue reservoir for the slow acquisition of oncogenic mutations and aberrant epigenetic changes that perturb intrinsic mechanisms regulation normal cell proliferation and differentiation leading ultimately to the acquisition of a full-blown malignant phenotype. These slowly renewing somatic stem cells are located within specific microenvironments (niches) in tissue and chronic irritation and mucosal injury caused by exposure to cigarette smoke might facilitate trapping of stem cells in a state of perpetual activation in an attempt to repair tissue damage, and subsequent genetic changes in the cells or the inability to return to a quiescent may result in the stem cell progressing to a cancer stem cell *(59, 60)*. Significant numbers of multipotent cells/progenitor cells exist in the lung of rodent and human. Experimental models have identified several types of resident stem cells in the normal lung with proliferative and regenerative potential *(61–67)*. In the mouse model, SP cells composed of ~0.03–0.07% are sca1$^+$/lin$^-$, heterogeneous at CD45 locus and express the vascular CD31 had been reported *(28)*. Another report suggests a CD45$^-$/sca1$^+$ SP from mouse lung had a molecular phenotype similar to neuroepithelial body-associated variant Clara cells. The variant Clara cell is label-retaining cell of multipotent differentiation capacity and is pollutant resistant *(68)*. Bromodeoxyurdine labeling and ^{3}H-thymidine incorporation techniques have demonstrated that these lung stem cells are located in the niche and continue to replicate throughout the adult life. Several stem cell niches that are key in maintaining the epithelial lining of lung tissues have been identified in the proximal and distal airways of mice *(69)*. Recent studies from a transgenic mouse model that conditionally express *K-ras* implicate a population of cells at the region of the bronchioalveolar duct junction that exhibits self-renewal and differentiation, properties characteristics of stem cells *(70)*. Introduction of *K-ras* causes these putative stem cells to expand, suggesting that these cells are precursors of adenocarcinoma of the lung.

The lung can be divided into conducting and respiratory parts. The bronchi and bronchioles constitute the conducting parts, while the alveoli form the respiratory surfaces. Although controversial, the putative stem cell population of the human lung likely includes the basal cells of the bronchi, which is believed to give rise to the neuroendocrine cells and the differentiated ciliated mucous cells, Clara cells of the bronchioles, and the surfactant secreting type II pneumocytes of the alveoli. The major histological types of lung cancer arise in the different anatomical compartments of the lung. Small cell lung cancer is considered to arise from the neuroendocrine cells of the central airway compartment (bronchi) and squamous cell carcinoma from the basal cells. Adenocarcinomas appear to be predominantly from the peripheral airways *(71)*. The cell types that are exposed to and in which metabolic activation of tobacco-derived carcinogens take place in the respiratory tract are likely the target cells for DNA damage, tumor initiation, and subsequent development of lung cancer. It is noteworthy that both Clara cells and type II alveolar pneumocytes are the primary sites of xenobiotic metabolism involving the P450 cytochrome enzyme activity in the respiratory epithelium. Implicitly, most known carcinogens in tobacco smoke require metabolic activation for binding to DNA to cause mutations. Tobacco smoke derived nitrosamines, such as 4(methylnitrosamino)-1-(3-pyridyl)-1-butanone (NNK), are metabolized to potentially carcinogenic derivatives by phase I enzymes of the cytochrome P450s including CYP2A6, CYP2D6, and CYP2E1. PAH, including benzo(a)Pyrene also are metabolized by cytochrome p450s enzymes, particularly CYP1A1 and 1B1. Activation of the ubiquitous procarcinogen, benzo(a)Pyrene to the carcinogenic BP-7,8-Diol-9,10-epoxide derivatives requires expression of both CYP1A1 enzyme and microsomal epoxide hydrolase (mEH). When cells express CYP1A1 activity but no mEH activity, benzo(a)Pyrene is metabolized primarily to non-carcinogenic 7,8 benzophenolic products. It has been shown that benzo(a)pyrenediolepoxide preferentially forms DNA adduct at guanine positions in codon 157, 248, and 273 of p53 *(72)*.

Alternatively, the lung cancer stem cells could be the result of transformation events that involve progenitors (transit-amplifying cells) or the more mature differentiated cancer cells that acquired stem cell-like functions through a process of dedifferentiation as described for other cancers *(73–76)*. It is difficult to definitively determine the numerous factors that can cause the emergence of cancer stem cells, yet the fact remains that these cells are malignant cells displaying stem-like cell properties. Hence, irrespective of the origin of cancer stem cells, this rare population displays stem cell properties, notably, the ability to self-renew and to differentiate into a functional hierarchy of tumorigenic and non-tumorigenic cells.

However, lung cancer stem cells have not yet been identified directly, although they can be enriched for and propagated in vitro. Nevertheless, for now, the distinct SP phenotype and the lung cancer "tumor sphere" culture provide attractive testing models for studying lung cancer-initiating cell biology and a framework for testing potential lung cancer stem cell markers. As well, these models are important tools for developing selective therapies targeting lung cancer stem cells and predictor of response to treatment.

In conclusion, the ability to isolate enriched cancer stem populations is a big first step forward, which could open the door to future targeted biological studies, which, hopefully, will yield new diagnostic markers, and targets. Eliminating the lung cancer stem cells may be the new measure for all future treatments. Validation and adoption of the cancer stem cell concept should offer a real possibility of long-term cure rather than current palliative therapy for this challenging disease. Lung cancer therapy needs to add a new aspect to its already huge scope – mechanisms to kill cancer stem cells.

ACKNOWLEDGMENTS

I recognize the support from the Canadian Institute of Health Research, British Columbia Lung Association, and the British Columbia Cancer Agency. These sources have no role in the preparation of this chapter. I thank Alvin V. Ng and Maria Ho for their hard work in characterizing the lung SP cells. I apologize to colleagues whose work I could not cite due to space limitation.

REFERENCES

1. Parkin DM, Bray F, Ferlay J, Pisani P. Global cancer statistics, 2002. CA Cancer J Clin 2005;55:74–108.
2. Proctor RN. Tobacco and the global lung cancer epidemic. Nat Rev Cancer 2001;1:82–6.
3. Halpern MT, Warner KE. Motivations for smoking cessation: a comparison of successful quitters and failures. J Subst Abuse 1993;5:247–56.
4. Tong L, Spitz MR, Fueger JJ, Amos CA. Lung carcinoma in former smokers. Cancer 1996;78:1004–10.
5. Jemal A, Siegel R, Ward E, et al. Cancer statistics, 2008. CA Cancer J Clin 2008;58:71–96.
6. Breathnach OS, Freidlin B, Conley B, et al. Twenty-two years of phase III trials for patients with advanced non-small-cell lung cancer: sobering results. J Clin Oncol 2001;19:1734–42.
7. Jemal A, Siegel R, Ward E, et al. Cancer statistics, 2006. CA Cancer J Clin 2006;56:106–30.
8. Scagliotti GV, De Marinis F, Rinaldi M, et al. Phase III randomized trial comparing three platinum-based doublets in advanced non-small-cell lung cancer. J Clin Oncol 2002;20:4285–91.
9. Schiller JH, Harrington D, Belani CP, et al. Comparison of four chemotherapy regimens for advanced non-small-cell lung cancer. N Engl J Med 2002;346:92–8.
10. Bonnet D, Dick JE. Human acute myeloid leukemia is organized as a hierarchy that originates from a primitive hematopoietic cell. Nat Med 1997;3:730–7.
11. Al-Hajj M, Wicha MS, Benito-Hernandez A, Morrison SJ, Clarke MF. Prospective identification of tumorigenic breast cancer cells. Proc Natl Acad Sci USA 2003;100:3983–8.
12. Singh SK, Hawkins C, Clarke ID, et al. Identification of human brain tumour initiating cells. Nature 2004;432:396–401.
13. Collins AT, Berry PA, Hyde C, Stower MJ, Maitland NJ. Prospective identification of tumorigenic prostate cancer stem cells. Cancer Res 2005;65:10946–51.

14. Dalerba P, Dylla SJ, Park IK, et al. Phenotypic characterization of human colorectal cancer stem cells. Proc Natl Acad Sci USA 2007;104:10158–63.

15. Gibbs CP, Kukekov VG, Reith JD, et al. Stem-like cells in bone sarcomas: implications for tumorigenesis. Neoplasia 2005;7:967–76.

16. Li C, Heidt DG, Dalerba P, et al. Identification of pancreatic cancer stem cells. Cancer Res 2007;67:1030–7.

17. Ma S, Chan KW, Hu L, et al. Identification and characterization of tumorigenic liver cancer stem/progenitor cells. Gastroenterology 2007;132:2542–56.

18. Prince ME, Sivanandan R, Kaczorowski A, et al. Identification of a subpopulation of cells with cancer stem cell properties in head and neck squamous cell carcinoma. Proc Natl Acad Sci U S A 2007;104:973–8.

19. Ricci-Vitiani L, Lombardi DG, Pilozzi E, et al. Identification and expansion of human colon-cancer-initiating cells. Nature 2007;445:111–5.

20. Fang D, Nguyen TK, Leishear K, et al. A tumorigenic subpopulation with stem cell properties in melanomas. Cancer Res 2005;65:9328–37.

21. Hadnagy A, Gaboury L, Beaulieu R, Balicki D. SP analysis may be used to identify cancer stem cell populations. Exp Cell Res 2006;312:3701–10.

22. Challen GA, Little MH. A side order of stem cells: the SP phenotype. Stem Cells 2006;24:3–12.

23. Goodell MA, Brose K, Paradis G, Conner AS, Mulligan RC. Isolation and functional properties of murine hematopoietic stem cells that are replicating in vivo. J Exp Med 1996;183:1797–806.

24. Zhou S, Schuetz JD, Bunting KD, et al. The ABC transporter Bcrp1/ABCG2 is expressed in a wide variety of stem cells and is a molecular determinant of the side-population phenotype. Nat Med 2001;7:1028–34.

25. Zhang L, Hu J, Hong TP, Liu YN, Wu YH, Li LS. Monoclonal side population progenitors isolated from human fetal pancreas. Biochem Biophys Res Commun 2005;333:603–8.

26. Bhatt RI, Brown MD, Hart CA, et al. Novel method for the isolation and characterisation of the putative prostatic stem cell. Cytometry A 2003;54:89–99.

27. Reynolds SD, Shen H, Reynolds PR, et al. Molecular and functional properties of lung SP cells. Am J Physiol Lung Cell Mol Physiol 2007;292:L972–83.

28. Summer R, Kotton DN, Sun X, Ma B, Fitzsimmons K, Fine A. Side population cells and Bcrp1 expression in lung. Am J Physiol Lung Cell Mol Physiol 2003;285:L97–104.

29. Alvi AJ, Clayton H, Joshi C, et al. Functional and molecular characterisation of mammary side population cells. Breast Cancer Res 2003;5:R1–8.

30. Clarke RB, Spence K, Anderson E, Howell A, Okano H, Potten CS. A putative human breast stem cell population is enriched for steroid receptor-positive cells. Dev Biol 2005;277:443–56.

31. Sainz J, Al Haj Zen A, Caligiuri G, et al. Isolation of "side population" progenitor cells from healthy arteries of adult mice. Arterioscler Thromb Vasc Biol 2006;26:281–6.

32. Feuring-Buske M, Hogge DE. Hoechst 33342 efflux identifies a subpopulation of cytogenetically normal CD34(+) CD38(-) progenitor cells from patients with acute myeloid leukemia. Blood 2001;97:3882–9.

33. Wulf GG, Wang RY, Kuehnle I, et al. A leukemic stem cell with intrinsic drug efflux capacity in acute myeloid leukemia. Blood 2001;98:1166–73.

34. Hirschmann-Jax C, Foster AE, Wulf GG, et al. A distinct "side population" of cells with high drug efflux capacity in human tumor cells. Proc Natl Acad Sci USA 2004;101:14228–33.

35. Kondo T, Setoguchi T, Taga T. Persistence of a small subpopulation of cancer stem-like cells in the C6 glioma cell line. Proc Natl Acad Sci USA 2004;101:781–6.

36. Seigel GM, Campbell LM, Narayan M, Gonzalez-Fernandez F. Cancer stem cell characteristics in retinoblastoma. Mol Vis 2005;11:729–37.

37. Patrawala L, Calhoun T, Schneider-Broussard R, Zhou J, Claypool K, Tang DG. Side population is enriched in tumorigenic, stem-like cancer cells, whereas ABCG2+ and ABCG2- cancer cells are similarly tumorigenic. Cancer Res 2005;65:6207–19.

38. Chen JS, Pardo FS, Wang-Rodriguez J, et al. EGFR regulates the side population in head and neck squamous cell carcinoma. Laryngoscope 2006;116:401–6.

39. Chiba T, Kita K, Zheng YW, et al. Side population purified from hepatocellular carcinoma cells harbors cancer stem cell-like properties. Hepatology 2006;44:240–51.

40. Szotek PP, Pieretti-Vanmarcke R, Masiakos PT, et al. Ovarian cancer side population defines cells with stem cell-like characteristics and Mullerian Inhibiting Substance responsiveness. Proc Natl Acad Sci USA 2006;103:11154–9.

41. Mitsutake N, Iwao A, Nagai K, et al. Characterization of side population in thyroid cancer cell lines: cancer stem-like cells are enriched partly but not exclusively. Endocrinology 2007;148:1797–803.

42. Haraguchi N, Utsunomiya T, Inoue H, et al. Characterization of a side population of cancer cells from human gastrointestinal system. Stem Cells 2006;24:506–13.

43. Ho MM, Ng AV, Lam S, Hung JY. Side population in human lung cancer cell lines and tumors is enriched with stem-like cancer cells. Cancer Res 2007;67:4827–33.
44. Dean M, Fojo T, Bates S. Tumour stem cells and drug resistance. Nat Rev Cancer 2005;5:275–84.
45. Donnenberg VS, Donnenberg AD. Multiple drug resistance in cancer revisited: the cancer stem cell hypothesis. J Clin Pharmacol 2005;45:872–7.
46. Eramo A, Lotti F, Sette G, et al. Identification and expansion of the tumorigenic lung cancer stem cell population. Cell Death Differ 2008;15:504–14.
47. Reynolds BA, Weiss S. Generation of neurons and astrocytes from isolated cells of the adult mammalian central nervous system. Science 1992;255:1707–10.
48. Goldie JH, Coldman AJ. A mathematic model for relating the drug sensitivity of tumors to their spontaneous mutation rate. Cancer Treat Rep 1979;63:1727–33.
49. Yin L, Castagnino P, Assoian RK. ABCG2 expression and side population abundance regulated by a transforming growth factor beta-directed epithelial-mesenchymal transition. Cancer Res 2008;68:800–7.
50. Kaplan RN, Riba RD, Zacharoulis S, et al. VEGFR1-positive haematopoietic bone marrow progenitors initiate the pre-metastatic niche. Nature 2005;438:820–7.
51. Brabletz T, Jung A, Spaderna S, Hlubek F, Kirchner T. Opinion: migrating cancer stem cells - an integrated concept of malignant tumour progression. Nat Rev Cancer 2005;5:744–9.
52. Li F, Tiede B, Massague J, Kang Y. Beyond tumorigenesis: cancer stem cells in metastasis. Cell Res 2007;17:3–14.
53. Tu SM, Lin SH, Logothetis CJ. Stem-cell origin of metastasis and heterogeneity in solid tumours. Lancet Oncol 2002;3:508–13.
54. Keshet GI, Goldstein I, Itzhaki O, et al. MDR1 expression identifies human melanoma stem cells. Biochem Biophys Res Commun 2008;368:930–6.
55. Shay JW, Keith WN. Targeting telomerase for cancer therapeutics. Br J Cancer 2008;98:677–83.
56. Harley CB. Telomerase and cancer therapeutics. Nat Rev Cancer 2008;8:167–79.
57. Sun S, Schiller JH, Spinola M, Minna JD. New molecularly targeted therapies for lung cancer. J Clin Invest 2007;117:2740–50.
58. Slaughter DP, Southwick HW, Smejkal W. Field cancerization in oral stratified squamous epithelium; clinical implications of multicentric origin. Cancer 1953;6:963–8.
59. Beachy PA, Karhadkar SS, Berman DM. Tissue repair and stem cell renewal in carcinogenesis. Nature 2004;432:324–31.
60. Beachy PA, Karhadkar SS, Berman DM. Mending and malignancy. Nature 2004;431:402.
61. Emura M. Stem cells of the respiratory tract. Paediatr Respir Rev 2002;3:36–40.
62. Giangreco A, Groot KR, Janes SM. Lung cancer and lung stem cells: strange bedfellows? Am J Respir Crit Care Med 2007;175:547–53.
63. Giangreco A, Reynolds SD, Stripp BR. Terminal bronchioles harbor a unique airway stem cell population that localizes to the bronchoalveolar duct junction. Am J Pathol 2002;161:173–82.
64. Gomperts BN, Strieter RM. Stem cells and chronic lung disease. Annu Rev Med 2007;58:285–98.
65. Griffiths MJ, Bonnet D, Janes SM. Stem cells of the alveolar epithelium. Lancet 2005;366:249–60.
66. Kotton DN, Fine A. Lung stem cells. Cell Tissue Res 2008;331:145–56.
67. Lane S, Rippon HJ, Bishop AE. Stem cells in lung repair and regeneration. Regen Med 2007;2:407–15.
68. Giangreco A, Shen H, Reynolds SD, Stripp BR. Molecular phenotype of airway side population cells. Am J Physiol Lung Cell Mol Physiol 2004;286:L624–30.
69. Engelhardt JF. Stem cell niches in the mouse airway. Am J Respir Cell Mol Biol 2001;24:649–52.
70. Kim CF, Jackson EL, Woolfenden AE, et al. Identification of bronchioalveolar stem cells in normal lung and lung cancer. Cell 2005;121:823–35.
71. Sun S, Schiller JH, Gazdar AF. Lung cancer in never smokers-a different disease. Nat Rev Cancer 2007;7:778–90.
72. Denissenko MF, Pao A, Tang M, Pfeifer GP. Preferential formation of benzo[a]pyrene adducts at lung cancer mutational hotspots in P53. Science 1996;274:430–2.
73. Cozzio A, Passegue E, Ayton PM, Karsunky H, Cleary ML, Weissman IL. Similar MLL-associated leukemias arising from self-renewing stem cells and short-lived myeloid progenitors. Genes Dev 2003;17:3029–35.
74. Jamieson CH, Ailles LE, Dylla SJ, et al. Granulocyte-macrophage progenitors as candidate leukemic stem cells in blast-crisis CML. N Engl J Med 2004;351:657–67.
75. Krivtsov AV, Twomey D, Feng Z, et al. Transformation from committed progenitor to leukaemia stem cell initiated by MLL-AF9. Nature 2006;442:818–22.
76. Passegue E, Jamieson CH, Ailles LE, Weissman IL. Normal and leukemic hematopoiesis: are leukemias a stem cell disorder or a reacquisition of stem cell characteristics? Proc Natl Acad Sci USA 2003;100 Suppl 1:11842–9.

15

Cancer Stem Cells: Pancreatic Cancer

Joseph Dosch, Cheong Jun Lee,
and Diane M. Simeone

ABSTRACT

Pancreatic cancer is a devastating disease that usually presents at a late stage that is not amenable to curative treatments. It is notoriously resistant to chemotherapy and radiation, and it is clear that new treatment strategies are needed to positively impact the dismal outcomes associated with this disease. While the initial dogma of tumor biology viewed all tumor cells as equal, recent findings in the field have lead to the discovery of heterogeneous populations of tumor cells, first in blood-borne derived cancers and now within multiple solid tumor organ systems that display a differential ability to repopulate the original tumor. Conceptualized from this finding was the stem-cell hypothesis for cancer, which suggests that only a specific subset of cancer cells within each tumor is responsible for tumor initiation and propagation, termed tumor initiating cells or cancer stem cells (CSCs). By using specific cell surface marker analysis, we have identified distinct populations of tumor cells from primary pancreatic adenocarcinomas that express the surface markers CD44, CD24, and ESA, which are responsible for the initiation of new tumor growth and exhibit characteristics that support the CSC hypothesis. The identification of these cells has opened up an exciting new paradigm on how we might view and devise new patient treatments for this devastating disease. Current investigations of these pancreatic CSCs have identified such signaling pathways as the Hedgehog and BMI-1 signaling pathways which are aberrantly regulated in this select population of cells. Further study of these CSCs and the important signaling pathways that control their function will provide us with powerful information on targeting new therapies to improve patient outcomes.

Key Words: Pancreatic cancer, Cancer stem cells, Cell sorting, Xenografts

PANCREATIC CANCER OVERVIEW

Pancreatic cancer is a highly lethal disease, usually diagnosed at late stages for which there are little or no effective therapies. Approximately 37,000 patients will be diagnosed with pancreatic adenocarcinoma in the year 2008, making it the fourth leading cause of cancer death in the United States *(1)*. Additionally, a National Cancer Database Report on pancreatic cancer found that of the 17,490 patients surveyed, at least 50% of patients presented with locally advanced, unresectable lesions and 35% had metastatic disease at the time of diagnosis *(2)*. Unfortunately, even in the small number of patients who undergo surgical intervention a vast majority of them eventually succumb to recurrent

From: *Cancer Drug Discovery and Development: Stem Cells and Cancer,*
Edited by: R.G. Bagley and B.A. Teicher, DOI: 10.1007/978-1-60327-933-8_15,
© Humana Press, a part of Springer Science+Business Media, LLC 2009

and metastatic disease. These sobering statistics underscore the need for new ways to combat this disease and improve the long term prognosis for these patients.

While pancreatic cancer can arise from cystic neoplasms and in tumors derived from the endocrine compartment of the gland, greater than 95% of patients present with pancreatic ductal adenocarcinoma (PDA). The cell of origin for this disease is a much debated topic, as mouse models of pancreatic cancer have pointed to both cells in the exocrine region, ductal epithelium, and centroacinar cells as sources of progenitors for tumor initiation *(3–5)*. An evolving hypothesis in the tumor biology field is the possibility that solid tumors in many organ systems develop from accumulated mutations in the normal resident stem cell of that tissue. Since normal stem cell populations are thought to be long-lived and quiescent, these cells would be more likely to develop and accumulate mutations over time that would eventually transform them into tumor initiating cells. This theory has emerged from research in tumors arising in the mammary gland, brain, skin, and intestinal tract where there are supporting data for defined normal stem/progenitor cell populations. While there has been little evidence for a normal stem cell population in the adult pancreas, there are cells termed centroacinar cells situated at the base of the acinar glands and the epithelial cells lining the pancreatic ducts that have purported stem cell-like characteristics *(6, 7)*. Whether or not these cells are the targets for mutations that lead to pancreatic cancer is still to be defined by ongoing research, but clearly future studies into the nature and function of these cells may give us new insight into how PDA is initiated.

SIGNALING PATHWAYS CONTROLLING
PANCREATIC CANCER DEVELOPMENT

Regardless of the cell of origin, animal models of pancreatic cancer using transgenic mice to mimic the mutations and aberrant pathways commonly found in human pancreatic tumors including activated KRAS, p53 deficiency, and Hedgehog pathway stimulation have provided important data on how these tumors develop. The first step in the progression of pancreatic cancer is the formation of small epithelial lesions, termed pancreatic intraepithelial neoplasms (PanINs). PanINs begin as flat atypical lesions and take on a tall columnar shape with accumulating supranuclear mucin (Fig. 1) *(8)*. Progression of these lesions leads to nuclear abnormalities with a characteristic papillary dysplasia of

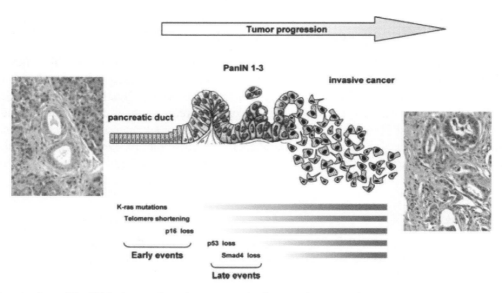

Fig. 1. Progression of PanIN lesions to invasive pancreatic disease *(8) (see Color Plates)*.

the ducts, however, at this stage the lesions are not locally invasive *(9)*. The steps between a benign PanIN lesion and invasive disease can be marked by several events including activation of the Hedgehog signaling pathway, loss of the tumor suppressor p53, and aberrant TGFβ signaling among others. Accumulation of these factors in transgenic mouse models leads to the ability of these lesions to spread and infiltrate the surrounding tissue leading to invasive PDA.

Kras

The most common mutation found in PDA, with an incidence in approximately 90% of patients, is an activating mutation of KRAS. The RAS signaling pathway includes a number of GTPases that control signaling for a variety of important cell functions including proliferation, cell migration and adhesion, and apoptosis. Transgenic mice using the PDX-1 promoter, a transcription factor expressed in all pancreatic subtypes in the embryonic stages, but restricted to the endocrine cells in the adult animal, can be used to specifically target the expression of a mutated KRAS allele in the developing pancreas. This mutation, a modification of the first exon from glycine to aspartic acid that mimics a mutation commonly observed in patients, renders the KRAS protein in a constitutively active form that results in the activation of RAS downstream pathways *(10)*. Animals expressing the mutated KRAS transgene form PanIN lesions in the small, intralobular ducts, mirroring what is often seen in patients with similar diagnosis. As the mice age, these lesions progress to more advanced disease, with higher grade PanIN lesions, accompanied by a robust desmoplastic reaction which is characteristic of histological features of the human disease. However, only 2 out of 29 mice surveyed with this KRAS^{G12D} mutation using the PDX-1 or p48 promoters to target pancreas-specific expression, progressed to invasive pancreatic adenocarcinoma. While this demonstrates that activated KRAS alone is sufficient to drive PDA formation, complete penetrance of invasive PDA likely requires the cooperation of other pathways to mediate the transition of the disease from PanINs to invasive cancer.

Hedgehog Signaling Pathway

Another signaling network, which is now emerging as one of the most important pathways involved in the progression of pancreatic cancer is the Hedgehog signaling pathway. This regulatory pathway is critical for the development and specification of embryonic tissues, along with the roles for self-renewal and differentiation of adult stem cells across many different animal systems. Activation of this pathway is stimulated by three known ligands: Sonic Hedgehog (SHH), Indian Hedgehog (IHH), and Desert Hedgehog (DHH). In the absence of Hedgehog signaling, the ligand receptor Patched (PTCH) represses the signaling receptor Smoothened (SMO) and prevents it from releasing transcriptional activators. Ligand binding to PTCH releases its repression of SMO and signals the disruption of a repression complex that allows the GLI family of transcriptional activators to translocate to the nucleus and activate downstream target genes. Depending on the cellular context, there is evidence that these downstream targets include cell proliferation and differentiation factors like Wnt, TGFβ, and FGF pathway components, as well as cell cycle regulators like p21 and cyclinD1 *(11)*.

In the normal adult pancreas, there is little if any active Hedgehog pathway signaling; however, tissue samples from patients with PanINs and advanced PDA often express high amounts of Hedgehog pathway ligands, specifically SHH and display activation of pathway signaling by GLI1 expression *(12)*. This phenotype has been recapitulated in transgenic animal models by ectopically expressing SHH in the pancreatic epithelium using a PDX-1 promoter. These animals displayed lesions that closely resembled human PanINs and showed elevated expression of HER2/neu and altered KRAS seen typically in pancreatic cancers *(12)*. Alternatively, aberrant activation of the Hedgehog pathway by using a constitutively active GLI2 (CLEG2) and PDX-1 promoter resulted in animals developing pancreatic tumors described as undifferentiated carcinomas, but not progressing through initiation of PanIN lesions. However, crossing these mice, PDX1-Cre;CLEG2, with animals that have a conditional KRAS mutation, KRAS^{G12D}, resulted in animals that rapidly developed advanced PanIN lesions and invasive pancreatic cancer (13). Interestingly, there was elevated expression of Hedgehog ligands, SHH and IHH in the PanIN lesions of the triple transgenic animals but not in the PDX-Cre;CLEG2 animals alone. This suggests a model for pancreatic cancer development in which cells in the pancreas acquire mutations to KRAS and begin to develop PanIN lesions, but require further "hits" which may include loss of p53 function along with activation of the Hedgehog pathway in order to develop a more advanced disease.

ISOLATION OF PANCREATIC CANCER STEM CELLS

While much has been learned by the study of mouse models of cancer, there is little substitute for working with primary human tumors and having the tools necessary to expand and analyze these patient samples. The groundwork for these types of studies was started in hematopoietic malignancies, using similar techniques that were developed to isolate the normal adult stem cells of the hematopoietic system. The first study exhibiting a CSC population was first reported by the identification of specific subpopulations of acute myeloid leukemia (AML) cells that demonstrated differential host engraftment in NOD-SCID animals (14). While this work was exciting, it was not clear whether or not this hypothesis would hold up for solid tumors, which have a much more complex pathology. However, work by Al-Hajj et al. validated this hypothesis with the identification of CD44$^+$/CD24$^{-/low}$/ESA$^+$ cells in tumors from human breast cancer patients that were able to recapitulate the original patient tumor and were able to be serially transplanted in multiple animals without loss of tumorigenicity (15).

To identify whether or not a similar CSC population resided in primary human pancreatic adeno-carcinoma, we utilized the same techniques pioneered by our colleagues in the breast cancer field. We obtained primary human PDA samples and established xenografts from multiple patient samples by inserting small pieces of patient tumor in a subcutaneous pocket in the abdomen of NOD-SCID animals. After expansion of these tumor samples, we then harvested the tumor and used mechanical and enzymatic dissociation with collagenase to process the tumor into a single cell suspension. As a starting point for identifying prospective cell surface markers, we stained these cells with fluorescently conjugated antibodies to CD44, CD24, and epithelial surface antigen (ESA) all of which have been studied in the analysis of CSC populations in both solid tumor and hematopoietic malignancies. We then analyzed these cell populations by fluorescence-activated cell sorting (FACS), which is a method that allows us to separate a heterogeneous mixture of cells into up to four separate populations at a time, one cell at a time, based upon the specific light scattering and fluorescent characteristics of each cell.

FACS analysis of primary or low passage (1–2) xenograft primary human PDA tumors using the CD44, CD24, and ESA markers alone or in combination allowed us to develop a staining profile that identified multiple subpopulations of tumor cells. To test which populations were responsible for tumor initiation in pancreatic cancer, each population alone or in combination with other markers were sorted and implanted subcutaneously into mice to assess their tumorigenic potential (Table 1). Initial observations using ESA$^+$ cells and either CD44$^+$ or CD24$^+$ in combination with ESA revealed a populations of cells that had a tumor initiation rate of 1 in 4 animals even with as few as 100 viable human cells injected (16). To identify a more enriched CSC population we utilized all three markers in combination and identified a population of CD44$^+$CD24$^+$ESA$^+$ cells comprising only 0.2–0.8% of all human pancreatic cancer cells in the ten pancreatic tumors examined. As few as 100 CD44$^+$CD24$^+$ESA$^+$ cells injected in NOD-SCID mice were able to generate tumors in 50% of the

Table 1
Tumor formation ability of sorted pancreatic cancer cells

Number of cells injected	10^4	10^3	500	100
Unsorted	4/6	0/6	0/3	0/3
CD44+	8/16	7/16	5/16	4/16
CD44−	2/16	1/16	1/16	0/16
P	0.022*	0.014*	0.07	0.03*
ESA+	12/18	13/18	8/18	0/18
ESA−	3/18	1/18	1/18	0/18
P	0.002*	0.0001*	0.007*	N/A
CD24+	11/16	10/16	7/16	1/16
CD24−	2/16	1/16	0/16	0/16
P	0.001*	0.001*	0.003*	0.31
CD44+ESA+	9/16	10/16	7/16	4/16
CD44−ESA−	3/16	2/16	0/16	0/16
P	0.03*	0.004*	0.003*	0.033*
CD24+ESA+	6/8	5/8	5/8	2/8
CD24−ESA−	2/8	1/8	0/8	0/8
P	0.05*	0.04*	0.007*	0.13
CD44+CD24+	6/8	5/8	4/8*	2/8
CD44−CD24−	1/8	1/8	0/8	0/8
P	0.01*	0.04*	0.02*	0.13
CD44+CD24+ESA+	10/12	10/12	7/12	6/12
CD44−CD24−ESA−	1/12	0/12	0/12	0/12
P	0.0002*	0.0001*	0.001*	0.004*

*$P < 0.05$

animals (6 of 12), while conversely CD44−CD24−ESA− cells did not form tumors until at least 10,000 cells were injected. In this case, only one of 12 animals formed a tumor from these marker negative cells, reflecting at least a 100-fold greater tumor-initiating potential in the CD44+CD24+ESA+ population. Additionally, FACS analysis of CD44+CD24+ESA+-derived tumors displayed a staining profile with CSCs and nontumorigenic cells represented in populations equivalent to the staining levels in the primary tumor. These populations remained stable in subsequent passages into NOD-SCID animals with up to four passages tested. These data as a whole provide strong evidence of a self-renewing, multipotent population of pancreatic tumor initiating cells in human pancreatic adenocarcinoma.

ALTERNATIVE CSC MARKERS?

While this CD44+CD24+ESA+ cell surface marker profile has been successful for our group in identifying highly tumorigenic PDA cancer cells, it is still not clear if this cell population is the best marker profile for isolating a pure population of pancreatic cancer stem cells (CSCs). There have been reports by others utilizing other cell surface markers along with internal protein activity to isolate highly tumorigenic pancreatic cancer cells from primary patient tumors and pancreatic cancer cell lines. Does this mean that there are different populations of CSCs in pancreatic tumors or is there just overlap between multiple different markers? Here we speculate on two markers, which have recently been linked to CSC and pancreatic cancer and consider what role they might have improving our ability to isolate pancreatic CSCs.

CD133

In brain and colon cancer, studies have demonstrated that cancer cells expressing the surface marker CD133+ exhibited properties of CSCs (17–19). CD133 is a glycoprotein also known as Prominin 1 (PROM1), which, in the pancreas, is normally expressed on the apical surface of pancreatic ductal epithelial cells and has been reported to distinguish cells with stem cell-like properties in embryonic mouse pancreas (20). Recently, Hermann et al. found that CD133+ cells in primary human pancreatic cancers and pancreatic cancer cell lines also discriminate for cells with enhanced tumorigenic capacity (21). They found that CD133+ cells comprised 1–3% of PDA tumor cells and as few as 500 cells implanted into NOD-SCID animals gave rise to tumors that recapitulated the primary tumor of origin. Additionally, histological staining of primary tumor sections with antibodies against CD133 localized these cells to the leading edge of the tumor. The authors also reported an overlap of 14% between CD44+CD24+ESA+ and CD133+ pancreatic cancer cells. Further in vivo tumorigenicity experiments will need to be performed to determine if CD44+CD24+ESA+ and CD133+ pancreatic cancer cells represent distinct CSC populations, or if a combination of all four markers improves enrichment for the most highly tumorigenic CSCs.

Aldehyde Dehydrogenase

An additional marker being utilized is the analysis of cells for high aldehyde dehydrogenase (ALDH) activity as a marker for stem cell populations. ALDH isoforms are intracellular enzymes responsible for oxidizing aldehydes to carboxylic acids with specific activity in the conversion of vitamin A to retinoic acid. Gene expression studies of hematopoietic stem cells pointed to high expression and enzymatic activity of these enzymes compared to differentiated progenitors. Commercially available kits (Aldefluor) have been optimized to use a fluorescent ALDH substrate, BODIPY aminoacetaldehyde (BAAA) which includes contains an aminoacetaldehyde moiety that when processed by ALDH enzymes, becomes charged and remains trapped within the cell. Using this method to characterize ALDH activity, several normal stem cell populations in the hematopoietic and neuronal systems (22, 23) and CSC populations in the breast and pancreas (24, 25) have been examined. ALDH+ cells in our limited experience include tumor initiating cells; however, this population encompasses a larger percentage of cancer cells (5–15%) than published CSC populations, and therefore may represent a "less enriched" population (unpublished observations). Further characterization of the utility of ALDH as a pancreatic CSC marker or in concert with previously identified cell surface markers is currently being assessed in our laboratory along with several others.

IN VITRO CULTURE OF PANCREATIC CANCER STEM CELLS

In addition to serial propagation assays in NOD-SCID animals, in vitro cell culture assays have also been developed to identify and expand CSC populations. Initially pioneered by studies in the neuronal stem cell field, it was found that stem cells from these organ systems were able to be cultured in special low-attachment plates in defined serum-free media. These cells, when cultured in these defined conditions, developed floating clonal sphere-like colonies while the differentiated cell populations did not. These studies have now been extended to the study of CSC populations from brain, mammary, and colon cancer (18, 26, 27).

Using this assay with defined media including B27 and N2 supplements along with bFGF, we have confirmed that visually inspected and plated single CD44+CD24+ESA+ cells form clonal colonies similar to mammospheres and gliomaspheres, which we term pancreatic cancer tumorspheres, while CD44−CD24−ESA− fail to form these colonies (Fig. 2). These CD44+CD24+ESA+ tumorspheres can be

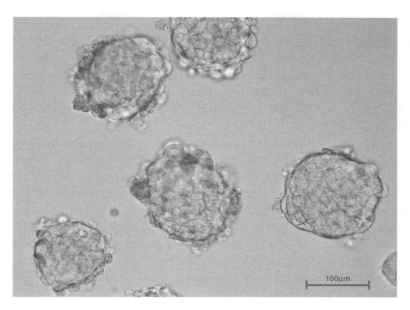

Fig. 2. In vitro culture of pancreatic cancer tumorspheres derived from CD44+CD24+ESA+ pancreatic cancer cells.

maintained in culture with >30 self-renewing passages (and still counting). Additionally, reanalysis of the tumorspheres by FACS analysis following 7–10 days in culture revealed that the spheres contain both CSC and marker negative cell populations. This demonstrates that the CSCs are able to self-renew in culture along with giving rise to differentiated progeny. One could envision using such an assay to screen for other potential cell surface markers to identify pancreatic CSCs, or even to perform high throughput drug or small interfering RNA screening, as the tumorsphere assays can be done quickly and more cheaply than the in vivo tumor xenograft studies, the latter of which are considered the gold standard for studies of CSC function.

PATHWAYS INVOLVED IN CONTROLLING PANCREATIC CSC FUNCTION

Distinct populations of highly tumorigenic cancer cell populations have now been isolated from breast, brain, colon, skin, and pancreas with surely other solid tumor types to follow. While we now know much about what these cells are capable of, we know very little about what cellular pathways are at work in these cells that make them different from their differentiated counterparts. As it has been shown in many other cancer systems that embryonic gene pathways as well as pathways that affect normal stem cell function are aberrantly regulated, so is the case for pancreatic cancer and pancreatic CSCs. We have identified two proteins, SHH and BMI-1, which are upregulated in pancreatic CSCs which may give us some clues as to how these cells acquire and maintain their unique functions.

Hedgehog Signaling Pathway

While normally suppressed in the adult pancreas, the Hedgehog signaling pathway is frequently found to be upregulated in pancreatic cancer. The Hedgehog pathway has also been found to play an important role in the proliferation and self-renewal of normal stem cell populations in the hematopoietic system, mammary glands, skin, and brain *(27–30)*. To learn if this pathway is differentially regulated in pancreatic CSC populations, we isolated RNA from directly FACS sorted CD44+CD24+ESA+ along with companion marker negative cells, prepared cDNA, and performed quantitative PCR for SHH transcript. We found that the expression of SHH transcript was upregulated over 40-fold compared to nontumorigenic cells and normal pancreatic epithelial cells *(16)*. Current research is focused on determining what role SHH upregulation in pancreatic CSCs plays in the function of these cells, however, we can speculate from work done in other CSC systems.

Our colleagues in the breast cancer field have observed that adding soluble SHH to cultures of normal mammary stem cells, grown as clonal floating mammosphere colonies, is a potent mitogen, and upregulates self-renewal pathways including expression of the polycomb gene BMI-1[27]. These treated mammospheres show increased secondary sphere formation, an assay that measures self-renewal, along with an increase in the amount of multipotent cells following differentiation. This enhancement could also be reversed by the addition of the Hedgehog pathway inhibitor, cyclopamine. Additionally, breast CSC populations were found to have 30-fold higher level of expression of GLI1 along with significant upregulation of PTCH1 and GLI2 compared to nontumorigenic cells. While there is still much to learn about the nature of Hedgehog signaling in the CSC population, clearly this pathway is a vital part of the maintenance and function of these cells.

BMI-1

BMI-1 is a polycomb gene family member that has been found to be a potent regulator of self-renewal in both normal and CSC systems. It was initially characterized as an oncogene that induced neoplastic proliferation when overexpressed in the hematopoietic system. Conversely, BMI-1 null mice display a severe defect in hematopoiesis, growth retardation, and short life spans compared to control animals *(31)*. While further studies are needed to understand how BMI-1 exerts this action on stem cell populations, it has been shown that expression of BMI-1 is important in suppressing p16^{Ink4a}, a cyclin-dependent kinase inhibitor *(32)*. Further evidence showing that the defect in self-renewal of neural stem cell populations in BMI-1 null mice is partially restored by p16^{Ink4a} provides some insight into how BMI-1 functions in these cells.

However, there was previously no evidence as to the role BMI-1 plays in pancreatic cancer. To learn if BMI-1 was differentially expressed in pancreatic CSC populations, we performed qRT-PCR on tumorigenic and nontumorigenic pancreatic tumor cells. We identified a fivefold increase in BMI-1 expression in CD44+CD24+ESA+ cells compared to the nontumorigenic population. BMI-1 was also seen to be activated early in pancreatic cancer progression, as a significant proportion of pancreatic cancer precursor PanIN lesions were found to express BMI-1 (unpublished observations). On going studies utilizing the in vitro tumorsphere model will allow us to further test the role of BMI-1 in the maintenance and function of the pancreatic CSC population.

PANCREATIC CANCER STEM CELLS AND METASTASIS

A hot topic in the CSC field is the hypothesis that CSCs are the specific cells that act as seeds in the formation of metastases in solid tumor systems. This theory in part comes from the fact that these cells are defined by their ability to initiate tumors in xenograft models compared to other populations of tumor cells. But is there something different about these cells that would enable them with the ability to migrate and form new sites of tumor growth? Recent work in the study of epithelial to mesenchymal (EMT) transition, a key step in the formation of metastasis, has provided clues as to how CSCs may be involved.

EMT is a cellular process that is characterized by the downregulation of cell adhesion proteins, loss of cell-cell junction connections like E-cadherin, and an increase in overall cell mobility. While normally involved during the development of tissues and organs in embryogenesis as well as wound healing, this cellular process has found to be increasingly important in the development of cancer. Many cancer subtypes have been found to overexpress a number of important EMT-related transcription factors including Twist, Snail, and Slug *(33–35)*. These transcription factors play an important role in suppressing E-cadherin and mediating the transition to highly proliferative and motile cells.

Little is known, however, on the relationship between EMT and stem cell populations, but recent work by Mani et al. *(36)* examined changes that occurred in normal epithelial cells forced to undergo EMT and showed how these cells acquired stem cell-like characteristics. In these experiments, normal immortalized human mammary epithelial cells were induced to EMT by the ectopic expression of either Twist or Snail. Subsequent FACS analysis of these induced cells for the cell surface markers CD44 and CD24 showed that the vast majority of cells displayed a CD44^{high}/CD24^{low} expression pattern that mimicked what is seen in breast CSCs. In addition, these EMT-induced cells had a 30-fold higher rate of mammosphere formation compared to normal epithelial cells. These factors were also used to demonstrate that overexpressing Twist or Snail in transformed mammary epithelial cells resulted in greater tumor initiation in xenograft models. These data as a whole provide strong new evidence that CSCs may indeed be specialized tumor cells that have undergone EMT.

There is also evidence from pancreatic cancer xenograft models that pancreatic CSCs are responsible for metastasis. A recent study by Hermann and colleagues explored the relationship between a pancreatic CSC population isolated from an aggressive pancreatic cancer cell line that was characterized by CD133 expression, and CXCR4, a chemokine receptor for the ligand stromal derived factor-1 *(21)*. Using this metastatic pancreatic cancer cell line, L3.6pl, as a model system, the authors' isolated separate populations of CD133$^+$/CXCR4$^+$ and CD133$^+$/CXCR4$^-$ cells and implanted these cells orthotopically in the pancreas of immune compromised animals. While both populations of cells were able to form appreciable tumors, only the animals in which CD133$^+$/CXCR4$^+$ cells were implanted were found to have tumor cells in the circulating blood. Additionally these tumors were found to give rise to local metastases to the liver, surrounding lymph nodes and spleen while the CD133$^+$/CXCR4$^-$ negative tumors remained restricted to the site of injection. Further evidence supporting the role of this population in metastasis was shown by pharmacological blockade of CXCR4 which significantly reduced the ability of these cells to become metastatic in this tumor model. In a similar study, Feldmann et al. *(25)* utilized a known metastatic pancreatic cancer cell line, E3LZ10.7, and examined its invasion capability following treatment with the specific Hedgehog pathway inhibitor, cyclopamine. Following 30 days of cyclopamine treatment, the authors observed no remarkable change in tumor volume compared to control; however, only 14% of animals were found with metastatic lesions compared to 100% of the animals in the control group. This reduction in metastatic potential corresponded with a threefold decrease in ALDH$^+$ cells, a prospective pancreatic CSC marker. While there is still much work to be done in the characterization of pancreatic CSCs, finding ways to target these cells may have dramatic implications for developing more effective treatments along with safeguarding a relapse of this devastating disease.

PANCREATIC CANCER STEM CELLS AND RESISTANCE TO THERAPY

One of the most troubling aspects of initiating therapy for pancreatic cancer is its unwavering ability to resist standard chemotherapy and ionizing radiation. Even in the event of successful surgical resection and chemotherapy, the rate of relapse is extremely high. A possible explanation for this finding is the hypothesis that CSCs residing in tumors are resistant to these therapies and recurrence of the disease is inevitable unless these cells are specifically destroyed. Evidence of this resistance is now emerging from studies of CSCs in blood, brain, and from our own observations in pancreas.

The idea that CSC populations would be resistant to therapy is not hard to imagine, given that their normal stem cell counterparts are equipped with tools to help them resist environmental insults with programmed quiescence, expression of ATP-associated transporters to shuttle out toxins, along with mechanisms to withstand multiple apoptotic stimuli. In xenograft models of AML, the leukemic stem cell population (CD34$^+$CD38$^-$) displays marked resistance to arabinoside (Ara-C) treatment, a common chemotherapy agent for the treatment of AML, compared to non-CSC populations (37). These animal models of AML show that while chemotherapy treatments provide an initial relief of disease burden, the AML will eventually relapse due to the rebounding of the chemoresistant leukemia stem cell population.

There is also evidence of the resistance of brain CSC populations to standard therapies in xenograft models of human gliomas. This class of brain tumors is highly vascularized, invasive, resistant to standard therapies, and has a relatively poor long-term patient prognosis. These tumors contain a highly tumorigenic stem cell population characterized by the expression of CD133 and a lack of expression of neural differentiation markers (38). While it was known that these tumors and CSC populations were resistant to traditional therapies, there were few clues as to what mechanisms these cells use to evade these treatment regimens. Recent evidence points to the upregulation of DNA damage checkpoint response activation and an increase in DNA repair capacity in the brain CSC population in response to therapy (39). In these studies, the authors demonstrated that the CSC population expressing CD133$^+$ in both primary tumors and xenografts increased twofold to fourfold after ionizing radiation. These CD133$^+$ cells survive due to more efficient and robust activating phosphorylation of ataxia-telangiectasia-mutated (ATM), Rad17, Chk1 and Chk2 checkpoint proteins which are critical to the DNA damage response. Additionally, alkaline comet assays which measure DNA repair showed that CD133$^+$ cells decrease comet tails 4–9 times that of companion CD133$^-$ cells. In order to counteract this resistance to therapy, use of inhibitors against the DNA damage checkpoint protein Chk1 in synergy with ionizing radiation proved effective in combating the radioresistance of these CD133$^+$ brain CSCs.

Some recently published data suggests that pancreatic CSCs may also be resistant to chemotherapy and radiation. In a study mentioned previously, the authors found that CD133$^+$ populations in L3.6pl pancreatic cancer cell line derived tumors were enriched after exposure to gemcitabine (21). In our own observations, we have found that treatment with ionizing radiation and the chemotherapeutic agent gemcitabine results in enrichment of the CD44$^+$CD24$^+$ESA$^+$ population in human primary pancreatic cancer xenografts (unpublished observations), indicating that novel therapies that target CSCs or sensitize them to traditional therapies may significantly improve patient outcomes. Ongoing work, utilizing microarray gene profiling systems to analyze pancreatic CSC populations isolated from tumors before and after chemotherapy and/or radiation treatments will give us clues as the mechanisms by which these cells protect themselves from these therapies.

CANCER STEM CELL-BASED THERAPEUTICS

An important aspect of testing potential CSC therapeutics will be the utilization of an optimal preclinical model system. We consider the primary pancreatic cancer orthotopic xenograft model system as optimal for testing potential therapeutics, as this model system best reflects the tumor heterogeneity that is observed in actual patients and represents the real challenges of therapy delivery to the tumor site. The validity of this model system may be further strengthened by cotransfer of appropriate human pancreatic stromal cells, as many cancer model systems have demonstrated the importance of the cellular signaling cross-talk in the local microenvironment to the biology of the tumor (40).

While there is much yet to be learned about the function of pancreatic CSCs, clinical trials with agents designed to target CSCs will soon be upon us. In fact, the first clinical trial to target CSCs in human cancer, specifically breast cancer, using a gamma secretase inhibitor to block Notch signaling is underway. Many pharmaceutical companies are investing heavily in developing new therapeutics to target CSCs, and more efficient inhibitors of several developmental signaling pathways are currently being developed or in early phases of testing (41). An important issue that will need to be sorted out before embarking on clinical trials to target pancreatic CSCs will be determining the best way to measure efficacy of these new therapies.

Traditionally, the effectiveness of cancer agents is measured by tumor shrinkage. Tumor response is usually defined as tumor shrinkage by at least 50%. If CSCs are resistant to therapy and comprise a very small percentage of cells within the tumor, the effect of therapeutics may reflect the effect on the differentiated, nontumorigenic cancer cells, rather than CSCs. For clinical trials testing pancreatic CSC therapeutics, new measures of efficacy will need to be devised. What will be the best cell surface markers to use to measure CSC burden? Can we utilize immunohistochemistry of biopsy samples to measure CSC content, or will cell sorting be needed, and if so, how difficult will it be to perform these assays on small tissue samples? Alternatively, perhaps measurement of circulating CSCs in patients can be used as a readout of treatment effect. Several recent reports using microfluidics-based technology and spectral imaging suggest that this may be possible, avoiding the potential need to biopsy the pancreas to assess treatment response (42–44). It may be that combination therapies that target both the pancreatic CSC population and the differentiated, nontumorigenic bulk population of pancreatic cancer cells will be most efficacious in treating patient symptoms associated with tumor mass and resulting in long-term cure. Upcoming clinical trials will help us determine if this indeed is the case.

CONCLUSION

The identification of CSCs in solid tumor cancers has provided a bright new outlook on how we will view and treat these devastating diseases. While the discovery of these cells has provided some answers into what cells we need to target for curative treatments, we still have a long way to go in identifying the signaling pathways and understanding the mechanisms by which these cells function to sustain and manipulate the tumor environment. In the case of human pancreatic adenocarcinoma, we have identified a select population of cells that are enriched for tumor initiating ability and exhibit self-renewal and multipotent differentiation. These cells express high levels of genes related to embryonic development and stem cell function, as well as display the ability to resist traditional chemotherapy and ionizing radiation. Furthermore, evidence suggests that metastatic potential may be conferred to these cells through EMT mechanisms with assistance from signaling pathway cross-talk in the tumor microenvironment. Future experiments will be aimed to develop a genetic and molecular profile of these cells that will direct us in ways to answer questions about how these cells function and how to target this cell population with effective treatments. It is an exciting frontier for pancreatic cancer research that will hopefully lead to a breakthrough in developing desperately needed new therapies for this disease.

REFERENCES

1. Jemal A, Siegel R, Ward E, Murray T, Xu J, Thun MJ. Cancer statistics, 2007. CA Cancer J Clin 2007;57:43–66.
2. Niederhuber JE, Brennan MF, Menck HR. The National Cancer Data Base report on pancreatic cancer. Cancer 1995;76:1671–7.
3. Carriere C, Seeley ES, Goetze T, Longnecker DS, Korc M. The Nestin progenitor lineage is the compartment of origin for pancreatic intraepithelial neoplasia. Proc Natl Acad Sci USA 2007;104:4437–42.

4. Grippo PJ, Nowlin PS, Demeure MJ, Longnecker DS, Sandgren EP. Preinvasive pancreatic neoplasia of ductal phenotype induced by acinar cell targeting of mutant Kras in transgenic mice. Cancer Res 2003;63:2016–9.

5. Stanger BZ, Stiles B, Lauwers GY, et al. Pten constrains centroacinar cell expansion and malignant transformation in the pancreas. Cancer Cell 2005;8:185–95.

6. Jensen JN, Cameron E, Garay MV, Starkey TW, Gianani R, Jensen J. Recapitulation of elements of embryonic development in adult mouse pancreatic regeneration. Gastroenterology 2005;128:728–41.

7. Bonner-Weir S, Taneja M, Weir GC, et al. In vitro cultivation of human islets from expanded ductal tissue. Proc Natl Acad Sci USA 2000;97:7999–8004.

8. Kleeff J, Beckhove P, Esposito I, et al. Pancreatic cancer microenvironment. Int J Cancer 2007;121:699–705.

9. Klein WM, Hruban RH, Klein-Szanto AJ, Wilentz RE. Direct correlation between proliferative activity and dysplasia in pancreatic intraepithelial neoplasia (PanIN): additional evidence for a recently proposed model of progression. Mod Pathol 2002;15:441–7.

10. Hingorani SR, Petricoin EF, Maitra A, et al. Preinvasive and invasive ductal pancreatic cancer and its early detection in the mouse. Cancer Cell 2003;4:437–50.

11. Pasca di Magliano M, Hebrok M. Hedgehog signalling in cancer formation and maintenance. Nat Rev Cancer 2003;3:903–11.

12. Thayer SP, di Magliano MP, Heiser PW, et al. Hedgehog is an early and late mediator of pancreatic cancer tumorigenesis. Nature 2003;425:851–6.

13. Pasca di Magliano M, Sekine S, Ermilov A, Ferris J, Dlugosz AA, Hebrok M. Hedgehog/Ras interactions regulate early stages of pancreatic cancer. Genes Dev 2006;20:3161–73.

14. Bonnet D, Dick JE. Human acute myeloid leukemia is organized as a hierarchy that originates from a primitive hematopoietic cell. Nat Med 1997;3:730–7.

15. Al-Hajj M, Wicha MS, Benito-Hernandez A, Morrison SJ, Clarke MF. Prospective identification of tumorigenic breast cancer cells. Proc Natl Acad Sci USA 2003;100:3983–8.

16. Li C, Heidt DG, Dalerba P, et al. Identification of pancreatic cancer stem cells. Cancer Res 2007;67:1030–7.

17. O'Brien CA, Pollett A, Gallinger S, Dick JE. A human colon cancer cell capable of initiating tumour growth in immunodeficient mice. Nature 2007;445:106–10.

18. Ricci-Vitiani L, Lombardi DG, Pilozzi E, et al. Identification and expansion of human colon-cancer-initiating cells. Nature 2007;445:111–5.

19. Singh SK, Hawkins C, Clarke ID, et al. Identification of human brain tumour initiating cells. Nature 2004;432:396–401.

20. Sugiyama T, Rodriguez RT, McLean GW, Kim SK. Conserved markers of fetal pancreatic epithelium permit prospective isolation of islet progenitor cells by FACS. Proc Natl Acad Sci USA 2007;104:175–80.

21. Hermann PC, Huber SL, Herrler T, et al. Distinct populations of cancer stem cells determine tumor growth and metastatic activity in human pancreatic cancer. Cell Stem Cell 2007;1:313–23.

22. Fallon P, Gentry T, Balber AE, et al. Mobilized peripheral blood SSCloALDHbr cells have the phenotypic and functional properties of primitive haematopoietic cells and their number correlates with engraftment following autologous transplantation. Br J Haematol 2003;122:99–108.

23. Corti S, Locatelli F, Papadimitriou D, et al. Identification of a primitive brain-derived neural stem cell population based on aldehyde dehydrogenase activity. Stem Cells 2006;24:975–85.

24. Ginestier C, Hur MH, Charafe-Jauffret E, et al. ALDH1 is a marker of normal and malignant human mammary stem cells and a predictor of poor clinical outcome. Cell Stem Cell 2007;1:555–67.

25. Feldmann G, Dhara S, Fendrich V, et al. Blockade of hedgehog signaling inhibits pancreatic cancer invasion and metastases: a new paradigm for combination therapy in solid cancers. Cancer Res 2007;67:2187–96.

26. Yuan X, Curtin J, Xiong Y, et al. Isolation of cancer stem cells from adult glioblastoma multiforme. Oncogene 2004;23:9392–400.

27. Liu S, Dontu G, Mantle ID, et al. Hedgehog signaling and BMI-1 regulate self-renewal of normal and malignant human mammary stem cells. Cancer Res 2006;66:6063–71.

28. Bhardwaj G, Murdoch B, Wu D, et al. Sonic hedgehog induces the proliferation of primitive human hematopoietic cells via BMP regulation. Nat Immunol 2001;2:172–80.

29. Ahn S, Joyner AL. In vivo analysis of quiescent adult neural stem cells responding to Sonic hedgehog. Nature 2005;437:894–7.

30. Paladini RD, Saleh J, Qian C, Xu GX, Rubin LL. Modulation of hair growth with small molecule agonists of the hedgehog signaling pathway. J Invest Dermatol 2005;125:638–46.

31. van der Lugt NM, Domen J, Linders K, et al. Posterior transformation, neurological abnormalities, and severe hematopoietic defects in mice with a targeted deletion of the bmi-1 proto-oncogene. Genes Dev 1994;8:757–69.

32. Molofsky AV, Pardal R, Iwashita T, Park IK, Clarke MF, Morrison SJ. BMI-1 dependence distinguishes neural stem cell self-renewal from progenitor proliferation. Nature 2003;425:962–7.

33. Yang J, Mani SA, Donaher JL, et al. Twist, a master regulator of morphogenesis, plays an essential role in tumor metastasis. Cell 2004;117:927–39.

34. Barbera MJ, Puig I, Dominguez D, et al. Regulation of Snail transcription during epithelial to mesenchymal transition of tumor cells. Oncogene 2004;23:7345–54.

35. Hajra KM, Chen DY, Fearon ER. The SLUG zinc-finger protein represses E-cadherin in breast cancer. Cancer Res 2002;62:1613–8.
36. Mani SA, Guo W, Liao MJ, et al. The epithelial-mesenchymal transition generates cells with properties of stem cells. Cell 2008;133:704–15.
37. Ishikawa F, Yoshida S, Saito Y, et al. Chemotherapy-resistant human AML stem cells home to and engraft within the bone-marrow endosteal region. Nat Biotechnol 2007;25:1315–21.
38. Singh SK, Clarke ID, Terasaki M, et al. Identification of a cancer stem cell in human brain tumors. Cancer Res 2003;63:5821–8.
39. Bao S, Wu Q, McLendon RE, et al. Glioma stem cells promote radioresistance by preferential activation of the DNA damage response. Nature 2006;444:756–60.
40. Tuxhorn JA, Ayala GE, Rowley DR. Reactive stroma in prostate cancer progression. J Urol 2001;166:2472–83.
41. Garber K. Notch emerges as new cancer drug target. J Natl Cancer Inst 2007;99:1284–5.
42. Balic M, Lin H, Young L, et al. Most early disseminated cancer cells detected in bone marrow of breast cancer patients have a putative breast cancer stem cell phenotype. Clin Cancer Res 2006;12:5615–21.
43. Zheng S, Lin H, Liu J Q, et al. Membrane microfilter device for selective capture, electrolysis and genomic analysis of human circulating tumor cells. J Chromatogr A 2007;1162:154–61.
44. Nagrath S, Sequist LV, Maheswaran S, et al. Isolation of rare circulating tumour cells in cancer patients by microchip technology. Nature 2007;450:1235–9.

16

Prostate Stem Cells and Cancer in Animals

*Alexander Yu. Nikitin, Melia G. Nafus,
Zongxiang Zhou, Chun-Peng Liao,
and Pradip Roy-Burman*

ABSTRACT

The mouse prostate has been the primary focus of research in regards to both normal stem cells and cancer stem cell-like cell populations in the animal prostate. The proximal region is the probable location of stem cells because it contains a high number of label-retaining cells, which express stem-cell specific markers, that are resistant to androgen ablation and have a greater capacity to regenerate prostate tissue in growth assays as compared to cells located in the distal regions. Stem cell growth assays include both in vivo and cell culture techniques. However, in vivo growth assays are better suited toward assessing full stem cell potential. Stem cells reside in a specialized microenvironment, in which their quiescence and proliferation is regulated by factors such as TGF-β, EGF, and IGF. Currently, two models of differentiation exist, the traditional linear model and the more recent branching differentiation model. Transgenic mice with activation or deficiency of genes such as androgen receptor, fibroblast growth factor 8, c-*Myc*, *Akt, Pten, Nkx3.1, Rb, p53, Apc*, or some of their combinations demonstrate gene-dependent development of the various stages of prostate cancer. Preliminary findings suggest that different genetic events have unequal transforming effects on stem cells and their progeny, and mouse models do have the potential to increase our understanding of the relevance of fundamental processes governing the control of stem cells to cancer. Additionally, they allow for the investigation of a stem cell-like cancer cell population, which may be responsible for maintaining growth after androgen ablation therapy.

Key Words: Growth assays for prostate stem cells, Prostate stem cell niche, Mouse prostate stem cell markers, Stem cell differentiation models, Mouse models for prostate cancer stem cells, Androgen depletion-independent prostate cancer, Origins of prostate cancer stem/progenitor cells

INTRODUCTION

The prostate gland is developmentally formed from the embryonic urogenital sinus (UGS), with the largest part of its development being postnatal. Proliferation of primordial prostatic epithelial cells occurs in a manner that generates multiple separate, subanatomically defined compartments in the mature gland. The murine prostate, in specific, can be divided into four pairs of lobes: ventral, dorsal,

From: *Cancer Drug Discovery and Development: Stem Cells and Cancer,*
Edited by: R.G. Bagley and B.A. Teicher, DOI: 10.1007/978-1-60327-933-8_16,
© Humana Press, a part of Springer Science+Business Media, LLC 2009

lateral, and anterior. Each lobe is composed of a series of branching ducts, and each duct can be divided into proximal, intermediate, and distal regions in relation to the urethra *(1–3)*. In the rodent, the prostate develops along the proximal–distal axis, with the proximal region appearing the most primitive *(4)*.

In organisms studied so far, there are three epithelial cell types from which the prostate is composed (a) luminal cells, (b) neuroendocrine cells, and (c) basal cells. Luminal cells are functionally active, differentiated secretory cells, constituting the major cell type in the normal rodent and dog prostate *(5)*. Neuroendocrine cells are rare, morphologically heterogeneous cells present in both the basal and luminal cell layers. They secrete neuroendocrine specific peptides and proteins, and are marked by the expression of synaptophysin and chromogranin A. Their function is not well understood, but they appear to be involved in regulating epithelial cell growth and differentiation in an androgen-independent manner. Basal cells present in murine and canine prostates appear as undifferentiated cells *(6)*. They are typically described as nonsecretory epithelial cells, and have been hypothesized to contain the progenitor cells of the prostate *(7)*.

Evidence that stem cells are present in the prostate originates from studies done mostly on rats, which have demonstrated that the rat prostate has an extensive ability to regenerate. When the rodent or dog prostate is deprived of androgen, it undergoes extensive apoptotic death of androgen-dependent cells, concomitant with rapid atrophy *(7–12)*. However, in spite of massive cell loss, the androgen-deprived prostate retains the ability to regenerate completely following exposure to androgens. Importantly, the involution-regeneration cycle can occur repeatedly *(13)*. A reasonable, and well-accepted, explanation for this phenomenon is that the regressed prostate has a reserve of stem cells resistant to death from androgen deprivation but which could become activated to proliferate and differentiate when stimulated by androgen.

By extending this scenario to prostate cancer, it may also be reasonable to ask if stem cell-like cells resident in the tissue are the source for growth, regrowth, or recurrence of prostate cancer. For example, the clinical course of prostate cancer is generally grouped into two broad phases. The first phase, conventionally described as androgen-dependent cancer is responsive to castration, antiandrogen therapy, therapy with drugs that block synthesis of relevant androgens, or combinations of these modalities *(14)*. The second phase, which is not responsive to such treatments, has been termed variously as androgen-independent, androgen-refractory, hormone-refractory, androgen-resistant, or androgen-insensitive prostate cancer; although, more recent terminology references it as "androgen depletion-independent" cancer, and is considered more accurate since the androgen environment is not nullified and androgen receptor-mediated signaling continues to operate *(15)*. A critical question is what cellular reserve in the cancer may be activated to give rise to recurrent cancer. Like the stem cells of the normal prostate, could there be stem cell-like cells in the cancer that are resistant to therapy? While the origin of such "prostate cancer stem cell" remains unclear, these cells may bear or carry the potential for a complete set of mutations responsible for the carcinogenic properties *(16)*, and may differ from their differentiated progeny by epigenetic or other types of controls *(17)*. According to this postulation, primary tumors may mainly consist of neoplastic cells that underwent genetic and epigenetic changes incompatible with the cancer stem or progenitor cell properties and do not contribute to the persistent growth of the tumor. Such cells will be responsible for the initial response to chemotherapy or androgen deprivation therapy. However, since this therapy is not designed to target cancer stem cells that possess the capacity to be quiescent while still retaining the potential for self-renewal, the disease is likely to relapse later as recurrent cancer *(18–21)*.

GROWTH ASSAYS FOR STEM CELLS FROM THE NORMAL PROSTATE

There are two basic cell growth assays used to test for the presence of stem cell populations in the mouse prostate, their ability to grow in cell culture and in immunodeficient mice (Table 1). Though there have been a number of growth techniques developed, the efficiency of standard cell culture technology is limited in regards to defining the properties of the prostate epithelial stem cell populations. When combined with irradiated mouse 3T3 fibroblasts and grown in agar plates approximately 1–2% of the plated cells form colonies reflecting some stem cell properties *(22, 23)*. Prostate epithelial cells cultured in serum supplemented with EGF and FGF, and without dihydrotestosterone (DHT), form free floating spheres of cells. These conditions also seem to have some success in maintaining stem cell properties *(24)*. However, prostate epithelial cells have been grown relatively more successful in three-dimensional culture conditions using Matrigel *(23, 25)*. When mixed with fetal stromal cells and suspended in Matrigel and PrEGM media, sphere-like structures grow, generating the so-called prostaspheres. Spheres are apparently clonal in origin, express both luminal and basal cell-specific cytokeratins (CK), and are able to withstand serial passaging for up to six generations *(23)*. However, though cell culture colonies appear to be derived from prostate progenitor cells, they are often limited to a low passage generation. One possible reason might be that culture conditions promote differentiation.

In vivo growth was initially shown to be possible when adult rodent prostate tissue fragments were combined with UGS mesenchyme, and implanted under the renal capsule of mice. In these experiments, tissue fragments were able to regenerate prostate morphology *(26)*. Xin and colleagues further modified the tissue recombination method of growth by the use of dissociated cells, rather than tissue fragments *(27)*. Prospective stem cells (combined with UGS mesenchymal cells) are typically suspended in either Matrigel or collagen and then inserted under the renal capsule *(23, 25, 27–30)*. Additionally, subcutaneous injections of suspended stem cell/UGS mesenchyme have successfully regenerated prostatic tissue structure *(25)*. The tissue graft is usually left in place for several weeks before the animal is sacrificed. If transplanted tissues/cells are able to reconstitute prostate morphology by forming branching ductal structures that contain both luminal and basal cells, then the implanted materials is considered to contain cells with stem cell properties *(3, 27, 31)*. Several groups

Table 1
A summary of the animal models used for studies with relevance to prostate stem cells

Animal	Cell lineages	Indication of stem cell reserve[a]	Growth assays	Putative markers identified
Canine	Basal Luminal Neuroendocrine	Yes	No	No
Mouse	Basal Luminal Neuroendocrine	Yes	**Cell Culture** Agar assays Free floating spheres Prostaspheres in Matrigel **In vivo** Renal capsule transplantation Subcutaneous injection	Sca-1, Prominin, α6 integrin, BCL-2, BCRP, Notch1
Rat	Basal Luminal Neuroendocrine	Yes	No	No

[a]Assessed by androgen ablation-reintroduction cycles

have shown the viability of this method; in that (a) regenerated tubules are rarely chimeric, indicating regenerated tissue is clonal; (b) regenerated prostate tubules contain both basal and luminal cell phenotypes, indicating cells are capable of multilineage differentiation potential, and (c) tissue growths can be passaged for multiple generations (25, 29, 31). Therefore, in vivo growth assays appear to be better suited for assessing and estimating stem cell potential in cells from the prostate.

A PLACE CALLED HOME: STEM CELL LOCALIZATION AND NICHE

Localization

The location of prostate epithelial stem cells is still somewhat controversial, though recent research has begun to enhance clarity. Initially, prostate stem cells were proposed to be located in the distal tips of murine prostates, due to the high proliferative activity of the cells located in this region (33–35). However, subsequent studies have implicated distal cells to be more likely transit amplifying cells; whereas, stem cells may actually reside in the proximal region. Proximal cells not only have a higher capacity than distal cells to regenerate prostatic tissue in growth assays, but are also programmed to replicate prostate structure (25, 30, 36). Tsujimura and colleagues found that cells located in the proximal region of the mouse prostate had markedly increased abilities to retain BrdU as compared to cells from other regions of the prostate. Though generally quiescent, these cells were able to proliferate in reponse to the reintroduction of androgen into a castrated male (36). In this regard, BrdU labeling has been used successfully to identify stem cells in the skin and hematopoietic systems (37, 38). Proximal region cells were able to form large glandular structures in collagen gel. Consistently, Azuma and colleagues found that even single cells from the proximal region were able to give rise to ductal branching structures that were significantly larger and much more developed than the colonies produced by the distal cells. Proximal cells were also found to have a higher capacity to regenerate functional prostate tissues than distal cells when they were subcutaneously grafted in Matrigel suspensions; the efficiency was 44% and 21%, respectively (25).

Previous studies have shown that telomerase activity is associated with germinative compartments in several self-renewing tissues (39–41). In the normal rat prostate, telomerase activity was reported to be low or not detectable. However, after castration and involution the remaining population of cells had high levels of telomerase activity and were capable of regenerating the prostate after androgen reintroduction (42). Therefore, it is likely that cells demonstrating telomerase activity in the prostate may comprise prostatic stem cells. Interestingly, there exists a gradient of telomerase activity in which the proximal region has the greatest activity (43), supporting the hypothesis that prostatic stem cells are located in the proximal region of the rodent prostate.

Finally, androgenic response is not uniform throughout the prostate. Distal ducts are more dependent on androgen for morphological maintenance, and atrophy caused by castration is most intense in the distal region; whereas, the proximal region remains relatively unaffected (2, 10, 34, 44). In fact, after castration approximately 35% of the distal tips and branching points are lost, but more proximally located ducts experience minimal loss (33). Moreover, cells isolated from the proximal region and implanted in castrated animals maintained full regenerative capacity even after 8 weeks of androgen deprivation. In contrast, cells from the intermediate and distal regions had impaired abilities to regenerate prostatic tissue after androgen deprivation (30). Additionally, after castration, the number of cells in proximal segments staining positive for capthepsin D, a marker associated with cell death was reduced, as compared to staining prior to castration (2). This suggests the existence of a proximal population of cells whose survival is not necessarily dependent on androgen. Functionally, this is important because of the role the prostatic stem cell is presumed to play in the regeneration of the prostate upon reintroduction of androgen, and which therefore, cannot be dependent on androgen for survival.

Niche

It is becoming increasingly clear that stem cells are localized in a defined microenvironment, otherwise known as their "niche." The existence of a niche probably provides stem cells with specific factors necessary for the maintenance of the stem cell properties via a combination of intracellular and inter-cellular signaling. There are a complex array of cytokines, chemokines, and adhesive molecules known to be capable of altering the balance between proliferation, differentiation, and quiescence in stem cell populations *(45, 46)*. One can probably assume that this is equally true for prostatic stem cells as it is for other stem cell populations.

The evidence that transforming growth factor-β (TGF-β) functions as a regulatory molecule in the prostatic stem cell niche, most particularly as a promoter of stem cell quiescence and differentiation, is strong. TGF-β has been demonstrated to be involved in the regulation of stem cell quiescence in numerous tissues *(47–51)*. In the mouse prostate, proximal cells activate significantly more latent TGF-β (32%) than do distal cells (4%), and also produce more TGF-β than distal cells *(32)*; therefore, it is likely that stem cell quiescence is maintained by TGF-β in the prostate stem cell niche. Consistently, expression of a dominant-negative form of the TGF-β receptor in the prostate is associated with increased proliferation of prostatic epithelial cells located in the proximal region *(52)*. TGF-β also appears to regulate, in part, the decision of daughter cells to self-renew or differentiate. For example, TGF-β promoted the luminal phenotype and suppressed the basal cell phenotype when mitogens, such as, insulin-like growth factor-1 (IGF-1) and epithelial growth factor (EGF) were depleted in the rat NRP-152 cell line *(53)*. Additionally, a TGF-β expression gradient exists in the prostatic stroma, such that TGF-β expression is highest in the stroma surrounding the proximal region and lowest in the distal region (the site of the highest cell proliferation), The above studies in combination with the fact that the proximal region of the mouse prostate is surrounded by a thick band of smooth muscle cells that produces high levels of TGF-β *(54, 55)*, suggests that prostatic stem cells exist in a specialized microenvironment in which TGF-β is an important regulatory molecule.

TGF-β's apparent importance in relation to the microenvironment's ability to promote prostate stem cell quiescence and differentiation, raises an interesting question as to whether other factors are needed to overcome TGF-β-mediated inhibition of proliferation and promote self-renewal. Most of the qualifying candidates identified so far are mitogenic factors, such as EGF, fibroblast growth factor-2 (FGF), and stem cell factor. Addition of these mitogens has been shown to alleviate the inhibitory effect of TGF-β on proximal cell proliferation *(32)*. In particular, EGF has been shown not only to counteract TGF-β-mediated inhibition of proliferation, but also to inhibit TGF-β-mediated cell death *(56)*. Additionally, repletion of IGF-1 and EGF decreased the extent of luminal differentiation of NRP-152 cells *(53)*. Notably, proximal basal cells have also been found to be more resistant to differentiation inducing effects of TGF-β than distal basal cells *(32)*.

Interestingly, DHT exposure causes the production and release of stromal growth factors. Binding of androgen to stromal androgen receptors mediates the release of growth factors that include TGF, IGF, and FGF *(57)*. This indicates that the addition of androgen into the prostate has the potential to induce the niche to produce factors that not only promote stem cell division, but also inhibit their differentiation, two features that would be important for rapid tissue regeneration to occur.

There is a strong indication that the microenvironment in which prostate stem cells reside is also regulated by androgens. For example, following castration, TGF-β signaling increases distally and decreases proximally. Furthermore, castration results in dramatically increased activation of TGF-β receptors in the distal region, with a contrasting decrease in activation in the proximal region *(32)*. Interestingly, exposure to DHT is also associated with decreased expression of CK5 and p63, two basal cell markers, and increased expression of CK8, a luminal cell marker *(58)*, indicating that DHT may promote the differentiation of luminal instead of basal cells. The latter experiments were done using prostaspheres grown in cell culture and, therefore do not address whether this is a regional event. However, regional variation between the proximal and distal regions in response to androgen exposure has been demonstrated to occur *(10)*. Thus, a possibility exists that DHT exposure induces differentiation of progenitor cells in the distal regions while at the same time promoting self-renewal of stem cells in the proximal regions.

SEARCHING FOR THE INVISIBLE: ENRICHING FOR PROSTATIC PROGENITOR CELLS VIA STEM CELL MARKERS

Developing techniques for isolation of stem cells is an important first step for better identification and understanding of stem cell characteristics and function. Traditional isolation techniques have employed the use of cell surface markers, differential gene expression, and cell sorting technology. Currently there is a small group of differentially expressed genes and surface markers that has gained popularity as plausible prostate epithelial stem cell markers in mice (Table 1).

Stem cell antigen-1 (Sca-1) is a marker that has been demonstrated to enrich for stem cells in hematopoietic, skin, cardiac and testicular tissues *(59–62)*, though the function of Sca-1 is not well understood. When Sca-1$^+$ and Sca-1$^-$ mouse prostate cells were grafted into the renal capsule, the grafts of Sca-1$^+$ cells were larger and weighed more than Sca-1$^-$ grafts. Additionally, Sca-1$^+$ grafts were able to undergo differentiation into both luminal and basal cells *(29)*. Furthermore, Burger and colleagues found that cells with high Sca-1 expression (Sca-1^{+high}) had considerably more growth potential and proliferative capabilities than cells expressing low or no Sca-1 antigen *(28)*. Sca-1$^+$ cells were also concentrated in the proximal region, in a pattern similar to BrdU label-retaining cells *(27, 29)*. Interestingly, Sca-1$^+$ cell assortments contained both more quiescent cells and more cycling cells than Sca-1 negative cells. Additionally, androgen ablation enriches for Sca-1$^+$ cells *(29)*. In summary, Sca-1$^+$ cell fractions contain a higher proportion of cells demonstrating progenitor cell characteristics, which include replication quiescence, androgen independence, and multilineage differentiation potentials, indicating that Sca-1 is a prostate stem cell marker. However, the Sca-1 antigen is present on a much larger population of cells (10–15%) than what can be true stem cells *(31)*; therefore, Sca-1 is most likely expressed by more differentiated progenitor cells as well.

Another candidate that has demonstrated strong potential is α6 integrin (CD49f). Integrins are a large family of membrane receptors that are important for the interaction of cells with the extracellular matrix. These interactions are important in that they regulate organization during tissue and organ development, differentiation, and proliferation *(63)*. Stem cells in keranocytes have been shown to express α6 integrin, and anti-α6 integrin antibodies have been used successfully to enrich for spermatogonial stem cells in the mouse testis and mammary gland *(64–66)*. Cells enriched for α6 integrin expression alone formed approximately fourfold more prostatic tissue than did cells not expressing the antigen *(30)*, indicating α6 integrin-expressing cells have greater regenerative potential than those cells lacking the antigen. Similar to Sca-1, α6 integrin expressing cell subpopulations were also found to increase after castration. In analogy, a structurally related integrin, namely α$_2$ subunit, is expressed in higher levels in putative human prostate stem cells than in other cells of the basal layer *(67)*.

A third strong contender is BCL-2, a mitochondrial oncoprotein that functions as an antiapoptotic protein. BCL-2 expression is usually confined to long-lived or proliferating cell zones, typical sites of putative stem cells *(68)*. It is known to be expressed in the stem cells of the hematopoietic system and colon *(69, 70)*. In mouse prostates, cells with the highest BCL-2 levels are predominately located in the proximal region *(32, 71)*. Interestingly, downregulation of BCL-2 in secretory luminal cells is correlated with differentiation, reduced proliferation capacity, and reduced lifespan *(72)*. Over expression of BCL-2 has been shown to increase stem cell number and prevent apoptosis in hematopoietic stem cells *(70, 73)*. Therefore, it is possible that BCL-2 has a similar role in the prostate stem cells, serving to regulate proliferation as well as to protect cells from apoptosis in states of androgen depletion.

Recently, the murine homolog of CD133 (prominin) has been shown to be a potential stem cell marker in the prostate. Prominin is a pentaspan membrane protein typically found on membrane protrusions on the surface of neuroepithelial cells *(74)*. Prominin function is not well understood. However, prominin is considered a stem cell marker for hematopoietic and neural cells, and prominin staining in the prostate is pronounced in the proximal segment of the dorsal lobe *(75, 76)*. Additionally, prominin positive cells have been shown to give rise to numerous, large-branched ducts, whereas prominin negative cells form fewer such structures. Furthermore, localization of prominin positive cells was similar to that of label-retaining cells. Additionally, TERT staining correlates to prominin staining, in that approximately 96% of cells that stain negative for prominin also stain negative for TERT *(76)*. As discussed previously, telomerase activity is thought to be indicative of stem cells. Since TERT expression levels correlate with telomerase activity; prominin's association with TERT activity strengthens its candidacy as a prostate stem cell marker.

Cells expressing a combination of two or more of the above markers have been found to be enriched in the proximal region of the mouse prostate. Certainly cells that coexpress Sca-1, BCL-2, and α6 integrin are expressed in much higher proportions in the proximal than in the distal regions of the prostate. In fact, Sca-1$^+$high/α6 integrin$^+$/BCL-2$^+$ based sorting appear to select for cells that are 98-fold more concentrated in proximal regions as compared to other prostatic regions *(28)*. In agreement to this, Lawson and colleagues also found that Sca-1$^+$/α6 integrin$^+$ populations are higher in the proximal than in the distal region. Interestingly, castration results in an increase in the proportion of cells coexpressing Sca-1, BCL-2, and α6 integrin *(30)*.

Though there is very little known about which gene functions are important for prostate stem cell maintenance, at least three genes have been implicated to have stem cell maintenance roles. NOTCH1 expression is localized to the basal cell compartment in which stem cells are thought to reside. Ablation of NOTCH1 signaling in transgenic mice severely impairs prostate stem cell function, resulting in reduced proliferation, impaired differentiation, and regeneration of branching morphogenesis following reintroduction of androgen in castrated mice. Additionally, NOTCH1 was shown to be upregulated immediately after castration, though the regional distribution of that upregulation is not specified *(77)*. Therefore, one possible function of NOTCH1 is protection of stem cells from apoptosis during periods of androgen depletion. PTEN has also been implicated to be important to stem cell function. *Pten* deletion is associated with an increase in the density of the progenitor cell population as well as increased numbers of differentiated progeny *(78)*. The breast cancer gene BCRP/ABCG2 also appears to localize on stem cells of the mouse prostate. Cells positive for BCRP and negative for androgen receptor (AR) are label-retaining cells. BCRP was mechanistically linked to maintenance of the prostate stem cell by preventing AR-mediated differentiation inducing effects of DHT *(79)*. BCRP is a demonstrated hepatic progenitor cells marker in rats *(80)*. Therefore, expression of NOTCH1, PTEN and BCRP genes may represent putative stem cell markers in the prostate.

MODELS OF DIFFERENTIATION

The traditional model of prostate epithelial cell differentiation relies on the hypothesis that a subpopulation of the basal cell population represents the stem cell population of the prostate. In this linear differentiation model, basal cells give rise to transit amplifying cells, which have an intermediate phenotype expressing both luminal, basal, and intermediate cell markers, migrate distally, and

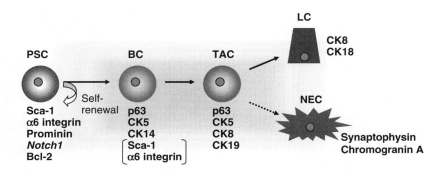

Fig. 1. Traditional (linear) model of stem cell differentiation in the prostate. In this model the prostate stem cells (PSC) gives rise to basal cells (BC), which in turn give rise to the transit amplifying cell (TAC) population. TAC differentiate into luminal cells (LC) and, perhaps, into neuroendocrine cells (NEC). Each stage of differentiation appears to be characterized by a unique combination of markers identifying individual cell types. BC markers in parenthesis (Sca-1 and α 6 integrin) are only known to be associated with basal cell marker CK5 when cells are located in the proximal region.

undergo further differentiation into luminal cells (Fig. 1) *(13, 36, 81)*. There is a reasonable amount of evidence that is consistent with this hypothesis. For instance, the prostatic stem cell population is hypothesized to be androgen independent. In both the canine and the rodent prostate, basal cells are independent of androgen for survival *(7, 12, 82)*. Furthermore, increase in *Bcl-2* mRNA concentrations in the rat prostate after castration is limited to the basal cell layer *(83)*. Additionally, immunohistochemical techniques have demonstrated that the majority of cells in the pre-prostatic UGS epithelium and developing prostatic epithelium coexpress luminal (CK8, CK18) and basal (CK14, CK5, p63) cell markers, as well as the intermediate marker CK19. This phenotype was observed to be retained by a small fraction of adult basal cells *(84)*. Interestingly, immunohistochemical staining has also shown that Sca-1$^+$/α6 integrin$^+$ cells in the proximal region coexpressed the basal cell marker CK5. However, distal α6 integrin$^+$ cells expressed CK5, but not Sca-1. Finally, α6 integrin appears to specifically stain CK5$^+$ cells, and not those cells with the CK8 *(23)*, observations that seem to support a linear differentiation mechanism. Additionally, the rat prostate epithelial line, NRP-152, has been demonstrated to differentiate from a basal phenotype toward a luminal, secretory phenotype under certain conditions *(53)*. Incidentally, Notch1 expression pattern was correlated to expression of basal markers p63 and CK14 *(77)*. Therefore, there is evidence to support the hypothesis that proximal basal cells are the precursors to other prostate cell types. However, this model does not address the origin of prostate neuroendocrine cells.

Alternatively, stem cells may differentiate via a branching pathway to generate progenitor cells for each lineage or basal cell and luminal/neuroendocrine lineages that separately undergo further maturation (Fig. 2) *(19, 58, 85)*. Both luminal and basal cells in the proximal region are able to retain BrdU label even after many cycles of androgen ablation and reintroduction *(36)*, suggesting that stem cells may not be limited to the basal layer. Seeming to contradict the branching differentiation model, p63-deficient mice were found to be completely unable to form prostatic buds *(86)*. The same group also found that the phenotype could be rescued by the injection of a p63 positive vector into embryonic stem cells, where chimeric mice formed prostatic buds exclusively of p63 positive cells *(87)*. However, another study found that p63 knockout mice could in fact regenerate prostate ductal tissue in kidney grafts. While prostate tissue lacked basal cells, it contained cells expressing normal luminal cell markers with secretory function. Additionally, neuroendocrine cells were present in these knockout mice *(88)*, suggesting that p63 is necessary for the development of basal cells, but that basal cells are not

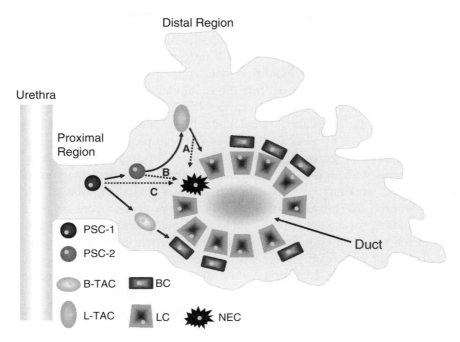

Fig. 2. The branching differentiation model of stem cell differentiation in the prostate. In this model the prostate stem cell (PSC-1) give rise to at least two different lineages; the luminal cell lineage, in which luminal transit amplifying cells (L-TAC) give rise to the more differentiated luminal cells; and the basal lineage, in which basal transit amplifying cells (B-TAC) give rise to more to differentiated basal cells (BC). Luminal cells surround the ducts into which they secrete various proteins. Neuroendocrine cells may differentiate from L-TAC (A), a stem/progenitor cell with a more restricted differentiation potential and common with that for luminal epithelium (PSC-2) (B), directly from PSC-1 (C) or from an independent precursor altogether *(see Color Plates)*.

necessary for the formation of luminal or neuroendocrine cells. Interestingly, double immunohisto-chemistry has shown that a small number of epithelial cells in the proximal region of the prostate coexpress synaptophysin and CK8 *(85)*; however, synaptophysin does not colocalize with CK5 *(89)* suggesting that neuroendocrine and luminal cells differentiate from a common precursor cell sub-population that is distinct from the precursors of basal cell population. This model, however, does not preclude a possibility that all three prostate epithelial lineages have a common precursor. In such a case, the commitment to basal cell differentiation would be expected to occur before that to luminal and neuroendocrine lineages. It also remains to be determined whether decision to differentiate into luminal and neuroendocrine cells takes place in stem cells with restricted differentiation potential or in transit-amplifying cells lacking capacity for long-term self-renewal.

SEARCHING FOR PROSTATE CANCER STEM CELLS: MODEL SYSTEMS AND PROSPECTS

Modeling Human Prostate Cancer in Mice

There is currently a strong interest on the genetic alterations that are frequently encountered in human prostate cancer in the design of the mouse models *(90, 91)*. The goal is to recapture the pathophysiologic characteristics of the human disease in a "natural" manner in immunocompetent mice to facilitate the exploration of the cellular and molecular mechanisms underlying prostate cancer as well as for the development or testing of new-targeted therapies. The strategies, however, are logical extensions of the earlier successful efforts to derive transgenic mouse models with prostate-specific expression of foreign genes, such as SV40 T antigens *(92–95)*. There is now ample evidence that specific genetic alterations in the mouse prostate epithelium can lead to the various stages of prostate carcinogenesis. For example, transgenic mouse models that represent activation of androgen receptor *(96)*, fibroblast growth factor 8, isoform b *(97)*, FGF receptor 1 *(98, 99)*, activated AKT *(100)*, or SKP2 *(101)* in the prostatic luminal epithelium, and those that address genome-wide knockout of a target gene, such as *Nkx3.1 (102)* or conditional prostate-specific gene inactivation of *Nkx3.1 (103)* or *RXRα(104)*, generally display a pattern of increasing degrees of phenotypic abnormalities, beginning with epithelial hyperplasia followed by presentations of preneoplastic lesions. Other types of modeling, like conditional homozygous disruption of the master tumor suppressor gene *Pten (105–107)*, overexpression of a strong proto-oncogene c-*Myc (108)*, or that of a mutant *AR (109)*, in the prostate epithelium lead to the development of invasive adenocarcinoma of the prostate. Evidence has been collected to show that in a *Pten* homozygous conditional deletion model, the primary cancer further progresses with micrometastases into lymph nodes and lung *(105, 110)*. Recently, the utility of the conditional *Pten* deletion model has been further improved by combining it with either a conditional luciferase or an enhanced green fluorescent protein reporter line *(89)*. In these models, the recombination mechanism that inactivates the *Pten* alleles also activates the reporter gene. In the luciferase reporter model, the growth of the primary cancer can be followed, noninvasively, by bioluminescence imaging. Surgical castration of tumor-bearing animals of this series leads to a progressive reduction of bioluminescence signal corresponding to tumor regression. Notably, the emergence of androgen depletion-independent cancer can also be detected using bioluminescence, when castrated animals are kept for further observations. Recurrence occurs at times varying from 7 to 28 weeks postcastration. Comparison of phenotypically distinct populations of epithelial cells in cancer tissues of these mice indicate that in addition to well-established hyperplasia of CK5-positive basal cell compartment *(78)*, *Pten* inactivation leads to the expansion of cells with neuroendocrine differentiation, marked by positive staining for synaptophysin. The hyperplasia of these differentiated cells increases after castration. This is similar to the appearance of the focal neuroendocrine phenotype in the recurrent human prostate carcinomas.

Considering that carcinogenesis is related to the accumulation of multiple genetic aberrations, it is likely to be better understood when a set of relevant genetic changes is present in a single model. In this regard, crosses between *Pten*[+/−] and *p27kip1*[+/−] mice were made, because low or absent expression of cyclin-dependent kinase inhibitor p27[KIP1] correlates with the poor prognosis of prostate cancer *(111)*, and PTEN controls p27[KIP1] through regulation of AKT kinase activity. Although *Pten*[+/−] mice display prostatic intraepithelial neoplasia (PIN) lesions, and *p27kip1*[+/−] display only mild hyperplasia, the double mutant mice exhibit multiple tumors in several different organs, including the prostate *(112)*. Loss of function of PTEN also seems to cooperate with NKX3.1 deficiency in mice. Increased incidence of high-grade PINs is detected in the *Nkx3.1*[−/−]*;Pten*[+/−] and *Nkx3.1*[+/−]*;Pten*[+/−] prostates, relative to *Nkx3.1*[+/+]*;Pten*[+/−] prostates *(113, 114)*. Furthermore, the majority of *Nkx3.1*[+/−]*;Pten*[+/−] mice have invasive prostatic adenocarcinoma with lymph node metastases, in less than 1 year of age *(115)*. Another example of synergy is noted when conditional *Pten* and *p53* deletions were combined. Although only PINs were found from conditional inactivation of the *p53* gene *(116)*, its combination with *Pten* deletions led to early onset of invasive cancer turning to lethality by 7 months of age *(117)*. It is suggested that the growth arrest induced by p53-dependent cellular senescence pathway under PTEN deficiency may be rescued by simultaneous loss of p53 function. A cooperativity of FGF8b overexpression and PTEN deficiency was expected based on the signaling pathways in which they are involved. Combinatorial modeling in mice, in fact shows that defects in FGF8b and PTEN expression, both of which are "natural" aberrations commonly found in human prostate cancer, can strongly cooperate in the induction of prostatic adenocarcinoma and its metastatic progression to regional lymph nodes *(118)*.

Since pathways mediated by p53 and Rb are frequently altered in aggressive human cancers, including prostate cancer, conditional inactivation of these genes in the prostate epithelium of the mouse was attempted *(116)*. While inactivation of either p53 or Rb leads to PIN, homozygous inactivation of both genes results in rapidly developing carcinomas showing both luminal epithelial and neuroendocrine differentiation. The resulting neoplasms are highly metastatic to sites such as the liver, the lung, and the regional lymph nodes, and resistant to androgen depletion from the early stage of development. Importantly, these tumors are marked with multiple gene expression signatures commonly found in human prostate carcinomas. In another model, the effect of the activation of the Wnt/β-catenin signaling pathway in the prostate epithelium was determined. As loss of APC is correlated with increased levels of β-catenin, a conditional *Apc* deletion in prostate epithelium was attempted *(119)*. Formation of adenocarcinoma in this model is fully penetrant and follows a consistent pattern of progression. Continued tumor growth, however, does not progress to metastasis in lymph nodes or other organs. Surgical castration of 6-week-old mice inhibits tumor formation, and castration of mice with more advanced tumors results in the partial regression of specific prostate glands. However, significant areas of carcinoma remain 2 months postcastration, suggesting that tumors induced by APC loss of function are capable of growth under conditions of androgen depletion. These and other related single gene or combinatorial gene mutant models available provide a diverse resource to identify and define the role of cancer stem cells in the genesis of prostate tumor and its progression.

Prospects

Although the generation of multiple different mouse models of prostate cancer presents opportunities to define the characteristics of prostate cancer stem/progenitor cells (a.k.a., tumor initiating or tumorigenic cells), most of the studies have only just begun. A few observations that have been reported to date, however, point to the optimism that novel information on the relationship between stem cell biology and malignant transformation could be forthcoming. For example, use of stage-by-stage evaluation of carcinogenesis in the combined p53 and Rb deficiency model *(116)*, demonstrates that malignant neoplasms arise from the proximal region of the prostate ducts, the compartment rich in prostate stem/progenitor cells *(85)*. Similar to the properties of normal mouse prostate stem cells, the cells of the earliest neoplastic lesions in this model express Sca-1 marker and are not sensitive to androgen withdrawal. Like the expression of both luminal and neuroendocrine differentiation markers in the carcinoma of this model, the early neoplastic cells also display such a coexpression pattern. While inactivation of *p53* and *Rb* also takes place in the lineage-committed transit amplifying and/or differentiated cells of distal regions of the prostatic ducts, the resulting early lesions in the distal region do not appear to progress to carcinoma. In contrast, the early mutant cells derived from either the proximal or distal region are capable of forming neoplasms in ectopic transplantation assays. These findings suggest that while p53 and Rb may be critical in the regulation of the prostate stem cell compartment, the transformation to aggressive cancer may secondarily depend on the context of the microenvironment in which the early lesions are formed.

Examples are also accumulating to suggest that the mechanisms of transformation of prostate cells with multiple stem/progenitor cell properties may be quite distinct based on the genes targeted for inactivation or activation in the models. Conditional deletion of the *Pten* tumor suppressor gene appears to lead to proliferation of p63-positive basal cells, and this expansion is concomitant with the expansion of Sca-1 positive cells. It is postulated that such an event is responsible for the selection of transformed transit amplifying/intermediate cells that progress to adenocarcinoma in the homozygous *Pten* deletion model *(78)*. Since both the *Pten* and *p53/Rb* tumor models are based on the same Cre-deletor mouse strain *PB-Cre4 (120)*, these early findings indicate that different genetic events may have unequal transforming effect on stem cells and their progeny, thereby leading to potential heterogeneity within the resulting transformed stem/progenitor units. For example, a transgenic line exists in which T-antigen expression is driven by the human fetal globin promoter, leading to the formation of prostate cancer with neuroendocrine differentiation. In this model, a subset of basal cells demonstrating expression of the viral oncogene are indicated to be the initiating cells that give rise to

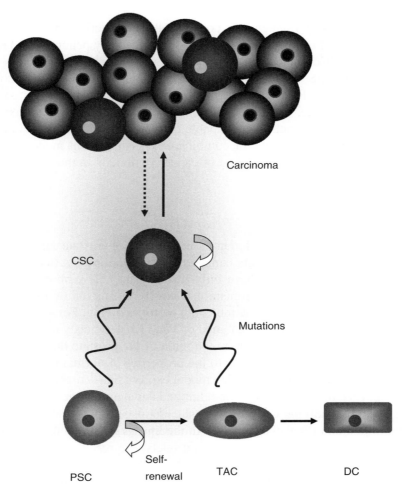

Fig. 3. Hypothetical origins of cancer stem/progenitor cells in a mouse model of prostate carcinoma. A prostate stem cell (PSC) undergoes genetic alterations (mutations) to give rise to cancer stem cell (CSC). An additional possibility is that more differentiated transit-amplifying cells (TAC) are targets for mutations, which lead to the acquisition of stem cell properties such as self-renewal and ability for multilineage differentiation. Differentiated cells (DC) probably do not typically contribute to tumor formation. The mutant series is denoted by red cytoplasm and the normal counterparts with blue cytoplasm. Neoplastic cells capable of only limited self-renewal are denoted in yellow cytoplasm. Theoretically, neoplastic cells of limited self-renewal may also acquire/reacquire stem cell properties (represented by the *dotted arrow*), thereby also giving rise to CSC.

the prostate cancer *(121)*. Genetic perturbations of prostate-regenerating cells from normal mouse prostates have indicated that discrete subpopulations may indeed serve as targets for initiation of prostate carcinogenesis. In another example, isolated prostate cells sorted for the Sca-1 cell surface marker and then transduced with activated *Akt1* gene result in the formation of preneoplastic lesions and foci of cancer in tissue grafting analysis *(29)*.

In each of the gene mutation-initiated cancer models, it is generally assumed that malignant transformation of the tissue stem cells due to the expression of a transgene or conditional regulation of one or more gene functions may be a primary necessary step in the oncogenic process. However, hypothetically mutations could accumulate in the cells of the transit amplifying cell compartment for their subsequent progression to cancer, and this notion remains to be tested. Another prevailing concept in prostate cancer is that antiprostate cancer hormonal therapies which target the bulk of the differentiated cells may be fairly ineffective against the cancer stem cell fraction that may be resistant to androgen blockade. This may explain why after initial control of the cancer by such therapy, the disease invariably recurs. Prostate cancer models that are initiated by Cre-mediated recombination within the epithelium and that present a pattern of progression, regression, and relapse similar to the human disease, such as the conditional homozygous *Pten* deletion model *(89, 105)*, are thus well suited to examine the important issue of the origin of the prostate adenocarcinoma-regenerating cells. For example, it is now possible to ask critically important questions such as: does castrate regressed cancer maintain stem/progenitor cells or does the pattern of genetic perturbations in the stem/progenitor cell compartment of the recurrent cancer vary from that of the primary cancer? It would also be important to know if certain differentiating/differentiated cancer cells may evolve or dedifferentiate to display the cancer stem cell properties when subjected to the stress of androgen deprived environment. It may be expected that there is significant heterogeneity in the cancer stem/progenitor compartment in terms of heterozygous and homozygous gene inactivations, and subsequent acquisition of a variable collection of temporal mutations all of which may differentially contribute to cell differentiation and tumor aggressiveness. A schematic diagram of this hypothetical scenario is presented in Fig. 3 to serve as a potential framework for exploration of the role of cancer stem cells in individual models and in identifying shared and overarching issues in general.

CONCLUSION

The extensive ability of the prostate to regenerate after numerous androgen ablation and reintroduction cycles is indicative of a reserve population of stem cells in the prostate. Stem cells have increasingly been demonstrated to exist in a specialized niche, and TGF-β, as well as several mitogens appear to be important regulators in the prostate niche. Investigators have used both cell culture and in vivo growth assays to analyze cells of various regions of the mouse prostate for their ability to reconstitute prostate tissue. Prostate epithelial cells of the proximal regions appear to have the most potential to do so. There is increasing evidence that cell markers such as Sca-1, BCL-2, prominin, and α6 integrin can be used to enrich for stem cells of the prostate. The traditional linear differentiation model has recently been challenged by a branching differentiation model where at least two types of progenitor cells may exist.

Several properties shared by both stem cells from the normal prostate and stem cell-like cells from the prostate tumor suggest that somatic stem cells or transit-amplifying cells that have acquired mutations to gain proliferation and oncogenic properties, or cancer cells that have reacquired stem cell properties, particularly the abilities for self-renewal and differentiation, may represent a renewable source for cancer persistence, growth or regrowth. Several autochthonous mouse models of prostate cancer are now available to critically examine these important issues. Particularly, models possessing the ability to follow progression, regression, and relapse of prostate cancer in living mice can serve as resources for isolation and characterization of enriched subpopulations of "stem cell-like," and more differentiated epithelial cells, as well as stromal cells at specific stages of growth or regrowth of the tumor. Phenotypic and biological evaluations of these cell systems singly and in combinations are likely to address the timely and important hypothesis that recurrent prostate cancer has an origin in cancer stem cells. However, it is also projected that like any neoplastic cells, prostate cancer stem cells are likely to be heterogeneous. In this regard, it may be overly simplistic to anticipate that the origin of prostate cancer stem cells could be assigned to a single cellular entity. Characterization of such heterogeneity and understanding its molecular and cellular mechanisms could pave a road toward development of individualized approaches toward treatment of prostate cancer.

NOTE ADDED IN PROOF

Recent study has identified CD117 (c-kit, stem cell factor receptor) as a new marker of adult mouse prostate stem cells (PSCs; Leong, K.G., Wang, B.E., Johnson, L., and Gao, W.Q. Nature *456*, 804–808, 2008). Long-term self-renewal capacity of CD117$^+$ PSCs was determined by serial isolation and transplantation in vivo. Furthermore, the authors have demonstrated that a single PSC defined by a Lin$^-$Sca-1$^+$CD133$^+$CD44$^+$CD117$^+$ phenotype and implanted under the renal capsule generates secretion-producing prostatic ducts consisting of basal, luminal and neuroendocrine cells.

ACKNOWLEDGMENTS

We would like to thank David Corney and Gohar Saribekyan for technical assistance. This work was supported by the National Institutes of Health to AYN (RO1 CA096823), to MGN (NIEHS Toxicology Training Grant), to PR-B (RO1 CA059705 and RO1 CA113392); by NYSTEM award to AYN; and by the California Institute of Regenerative Medicine Training Grant T1-00004 to C-PL.

REFERENCES

1. Hayward SW, Brody JR, Cunha GR. An edgewise look at basal epithelial cells: three-dimensional views of the rat prostate, mammary gland and salivary gland. Differentiation 1996;60(4):219–27.
2. Lee C, Sensibar JA, Dudek SM, Hiipakka RA, Liao ST. Prostatic ductal system in rats: regional variation in morphological and functional activities. Biol Reprod 1990;43(6):1079–86.
3. Sugimura Y, Cunha GR, Donjacour AA. Morphogenesis of ductal networks in the mouse prostate. Biol Reprod 1986;34(5):961–71.
4. Kasper S. Characterizing the prostate stem cell. J Urol 2007;178(2):375.
5. Guggenheim R, Bartsch G, Tannenbaum M, Rohr HP. Comparative scanning and transmission electron microscopy of the prostatic gland in different species (mouse, rat, dog, man). Scan Electron Microsc 1979(3):721–8.
6. Timms BG, Chandler JA, Sinowatz F. The ultrastructure of basal cells of rat and dog prostate. Cell Tissue Res 1976;173(4):543–54.
7. English HF, Santen RJ, Isaacs JT. Response of glandular versus basal rat ventral prostatic epithelial cells to androgen withdrawal and replacement. Prostate 1987;11(3):229–42.
8. English HF, Drago JR, Santen RJ. Cellular response to androgen depletion and repletion in the rat ventral prostate: autoradiography and morphometric analysis. Prostate 1985;7(1):41–51.
9. Kyprianou N, Isaacs JT. Activation of programmed cell death in the rat ventral prostate after castration. Endocrinology 1988;122(2):552–62.
10. Rouleau M, Leger J, Tenniswood M. Ductal heterogeneity of cytokeratins, gene expression, and cell death in the rat ventral prostate. Mol Endocrinol 1990;4(12):2003–13.
11. Hsing AY, Kadomatsu K, Bonham MJ, Danielpour D. Regulation of apoptosis induced by transforming growth factor-beta1 in nontumorigenic rat prostatic epithelial cell lines. Cancer Res 1996;56(22):5146–9.
12. Mahapokai W, Xue Y, van Garderen E, van Sluijs FJ, Mol JA, Schalken JA. Cell kinetics and differentiation after hormonal-induced prostatic hyperplasia in the dog. Prostate 2000;44(1):40–8.

13. Isaacs JT. Control of cell proliferation and cell death in normal and neoplastic prostate: a stem cell model. Benign prostatic hyperplasia Report No. INH 87-2881, Department of Health and Human Services, National Institutes of Health, Bethesda, MD, 1987;2:85–94.

14. Isaacs JT, Isaacs WB. Androgen receptor outwits prostate cancer drugs. Nat Med 2004;10(1):26–7.

15. Roy-Burman P, Tindall DJ, Robins DM, et al. Androgens and prostate cancer: are the descriptors valid? Cancer Biol Ther 2005;4(1):4–5.

16. Reya T, Morrison SJ, Clarke MF, Weissman IL. Stem cells, cancer, and cancer stem cells. Nature 2001;414(6859):105–11.

17. Feinberg AP, Ohlsson R, Henikoff S. The epigenetic progenitor origin of human cancer. Nat Rev Genet 2006;7(1):21–33.

18. Collins AT, Maitland NJ. Prostate cancer stem cells. Eur J Cancer 2006;42(9):1213–8.

19. Nikitin AY, Matoso A, Roy-Burman P. Prostate stem cells and cancer. Histol Histopathol 2007;22(9):1043–9.

20. Sharifi N, Kawasaki BT, Hurt EM, Farrar WL. Stem cells in prostate cancer: resolving the castrate-resistant conundrum and implications for hormonal therapy. Cancer Biol Ther 2006;5(8):901–6.

21. Dehm SM, Tindall DJ. Molecular regulation of androgen action in prostate cancer. J Cell Biochem 2006;99(2):333–44.

22. Sawicki JA, Rothman CJ. Evidence for stem cells in cultures of mouse prostate epithelial cells. Prostate 2002;50(1):46–53.

23. Lawson DA, Xin L, Lukacs RU, Cheng D, Witte ON. Isolation and functional characterization of murine prostate stem cells. Proc Natl Acad Sci USA 2007;104(1):181–6.

24. Shi X, Gipp J, Bushman W. Anchorage-independent culture maintains prostate stem cells. Dev Biol 2007;312(1):396–406.

25. Azuma M, Hirao A, Takubo K, Hamaguchi I, Kitamura T, Suda T. A quantitative matrigel assay for assessing repopulating capacity of prostate stem cells. Biochem Biophys Res Commun 2005;338(2):1164–70.

26. Cunha GR, Lung B. The possible influence of temporal factors in androgenic responsiveness of urogenital tissue recombinants from wild-type and androgen-insensitive (Tfm) mice. J Exp Zool 1978;205(2):181–93.

27. Xin L, Ide H, Kim Y, Dubey P, Witte ON. In vivo regeneration of murine prostate from dissociated cell populations of postnatal epithelia and urogenital sinus mesenchyme. Proc Natl Acad Sci USA 2003;100(Suppl 1):11896–903.

28. Burger PE, Xiong X, Coetzee S, et al. Sca-1 expression identifies stem cells in the proximal region of prostatic ducts with high capacity to reconstitute prostatic tissue. Proc Natl Acad Sci USA 2005;102(20):7180–5.

29. Xin L, Lawson DA, Witte ON. The Sca-1 cell surface marker enriches for a prostate-regenerating cell subpopulation that can initiate prostate tumorigenesis. Proc Natl Acad Sci USA 2005;102(19):6942–7.

30. Goto K, Salm SN, Coetzee S, et al. Proximal prostatic stem cells are programmed to regenerate a proximal-distal ductal axis. Stem Cells 2006;24(8):1859–68.

31. Lawson DA, Xin L, Lukacs R, Xu Q, Cheng D, Witte ON. Prostate stem cells and prostate cancer. Cold Spring Harb Symp Quant Biol 2005;70:187–96.

32. Salm SN, Burger PE, Coetzee S, Goto K, Moscatelli D, Wilson EL. TGF-{beta} maintains dormancy of prostatic stem cells in the proximal region of ducts. J Cell Biol 2005;170(1):81–90.

33. Sugimura Y, Cunha GR, Donjacour AA. Morphological and histological study of castration-induced degeneration and androgen-induced regeneration in the mouse prostate. Biol Reprod 1986;34(5):973–83.

34. Sugimura Y, Cunha GR, Donjacour AA, Bigsby RM, Brody JR. Whole-mount autoradiography study of DNA synthetic activity during postnatal development and androgen-induced regeneration in the mouse prostate. Biol Reprod 1986;34(5):985–95.

35. Kinbara H, Cunha GR, Boutin E, Hayashi N, Kawamura J. Evidence of stem cells in the adult prostatic epithelium based upon responsiveness to mesenchymal inductors. Prostate 1996;29(2):107–16.

36. Tsujimura A, Koikawa Y, Salm S, et al. Proximal location of mouse prostate epithelial stem cells: a model of prostatic homeostasis. J Cell Biol 2002;157(7):1257–65.

37. Cotsarelis G, Sun TT, Lavker RM. Label-retaining cells reside in the bulge area of pilosebaceous unit: implications for follicular stem cells, hair cycle, and skin carcinogenesis. Cell 1990;61(7):1329–37.

38. Zhang J, Niu C, Ye L, et al. Identification of the haematopoietic stem cell niche and control of the niche size. Nature 2003;425(6960):836–41.

39. Wright WE, Piatyszek MA, Rainey WE, Byrd W, Shay JW. Telomerase activity in human germline and embryonic tissues and cells. Dev Genet 1996;18(2):173–9.

40. Eisenhauer KM, Gerstein RM, Chiu CP, Conti M, Hsueh AJ. Telomerase activity in female and male rat germ cells undergoing meiosis and in early embryos. Biol Reprod 1997;56(5):1120–5.

41. Miura T, Katakura Y, Yamamoto K, et al. Neural stem cells lose telomerase activity upon differentiating into astrocytes. Cytotechnology 2004;36:137–44.

42. Sommerfeld HJ, Meeker AK, Posadas EM, Coffey DS. Frontiers in prostate cancer: telomeres and chaos. Cancer 1995;75:2027–37.

43. Banerjee PP, Banerjee S, Zirkin BR, Brown TR. Lobe-specific telomerase activity in the intact adult brown Norway rat prostate and its regional distribution within the prostatic ducts. Endocrinology 1998;139(2):513–9.

44. Sensibar JA, Griswold MD, Sylvester SR, et al. Prostatic ductal system in rats: regional variation in localization of an androgen-repressed gene product, sulfated glycoprotein-2. Endocrinology 1991;128(4):2091–102.

45. Whetton AD, Graham GJ. Homing and mobilization in the stem cell niche. Trends Cell Biol 1999;9(6):233–8.

46. Spradling A, Drummond-Barbosa D, Kai T. Stem cells find their niche. Nature 2001;414(6859):98–104.

47. Cashman JD, Eaves AC, Raines EW, Ross R, Eaves CJ. Mechanisms that regulate the cell cycle status of very primitive hematopoietic cells in long-term human marrow cultures. I. Stimulatory role of a variety of mesenchymal cell activators and inhibitory role of TGF-beta. Blood 1990;75(1):96–101.

48. Hatzfeld J, Li ML, Brown EL, et al. Release of early human hematopoietic progenitors from quiescence by antisense transforming growth factor beta 1 or Rb oligonucleotides. J Exp Med 1991;174(4):925–9.

49. Puolakkainen PA, Ranchalis JE, Gombotz WR, Hoffman AS, Mumper RJ, Twardzik DR. Novel delivery system for inducing quiescence in intestinal stem cells in rats by transforming growth factor beta 1. Gastroenterology 1994;107(5):1319–26.

50. Fortunel N, Hatzfeld J, Kisselev S, et al. Release from quiescence of primitive human hematopoietic stem/progenitor cells by blocking their cell-surface TGF-beta type II receptor in a short-term in vitro assay. Stem Cells 2000;18(2):102–11.

51. Fuchs E, Tumbar T, Guasch G. Socializing with the neighbors: stem cells and their niche. Cell 2004;116(6):769–78.

52. Kundu SD, Kim IY, Yang T, et al. Absence of proximal duct apoptosis in the ventral prostate of transgenic mice carrying the C3(1)-TGF-beta type II dominant negative receptor. Prostate 2000;43(2):118–24.

53. Danielpour D. Transdifferentiation of NRP-152 rat prostatic basal epithelial cells toward a luminal phenotype: regulation by glucocorticoid, insulin-like growth factor-I and transforming growth factor-beta. J Cell Sci 1999;112(Pt 2):169–79.

54. Nemeth JA, Lee C. Prostatic ductal system in rats: regional variation in stromal organization. Prostate 1996;28(2):124–8.

55. Nemeth JA, Sensibar JA, White RR, Zelner DJ, Kim IY, Lee C. Prostatic ductal system in rats: tissue-specific expression and regional variation in stromal distribution of transforming growth factor-beta 1. Prostate 1997;33(1):64–71.

56. Ilio KY, Sensibar JA, Lee C. Effect of TGF-beta 1, TGF-alpha, and EGF on cell proliferation and cell death in rat ventral prostatic epithelial cells in culture. J Androl 1995;16(6):482–90.

57. Long RM, Morrissey C, Fitzpatrick JM, Watson RW. Prostate epithelial cell differentiation and its relevance to the understanding of prostate cancer therapies. Clin Sci (Lond) 2005;108(1):1–11.

58. Xin L, Lukacs RU, Lawson DA, Cheng D, Witte ON. Self-renewal and multilineage differentiation in vitro from murine prostate stem cells. Stem Cells 2007;25(11):2760–9.

59. Spangrude GJ, Heimfeld S, Weissman IL. Purification and characterization of mouse hematopoietic stem cells. Science 1988;241(4861):58–62.

60. Montanaro F, Liadaki K, Volinski J, Flint A, Kunkel LM. Skeletal muscle engraftment potential of adult mouse skin side population cells. Proc Natl Acad Sci USA 2003;100(16):9336–41.

61. Falciatori I, Borsellino G, Haliassos N, et al. Identification and enrichment of spermatogonial stem cells displaying side-population phenotype in immature mouse testis. FASEB J 2004;18(2):376–8.

62. Matsuura K, Nagai T, Nishigaki N, et al. Adult cardiac Sca-1-positive cells differentiate into beating cardiomyocytes. J Biol Chem 2004;279(12):11384–91.

63. Tarone G, Hirsch E, Brancaccio M, et al. Integrin function and regulation in development. Int J Dev Biol 2000;44(6):725–31.

64. Shinohara T, Avarbock MR, Brinster RL. Beta1- and alpha6-integrin are surface markers on mouse spermatogonial stem cells. Proc Natl Acad Sci USA 1999;96(10):5504–9.

65. Tani H, Morris RJ, Kaur P. Enrichment for murine keratinocyte stem cells based on cell surface phenotype. Proc Natl Acad Sci USA 2000;97(20):10960–5.

66. Stingl J, Eirew P, Ricketson I, et al. Purification and unique properties of mammary epithelial stem cells. Nature 2006;439(7079):993–7.

67. Bhatt RI, Brown MD, Hart CA, et al. Novel method for the isolation and characterisation of the putative prostatic stem cell. Cytometry A 2003;54(2):89–99.

68. Hockenbery DM, Zutter M, Hickey W, Nahm M, Korsmeyer SJ. BCL2 protein is topographically restricted in tissues characterized by apoptotic cell death. Proc Natl Acad Sci USA 1991;88(16):6961–5.

69. Merritt AJ, Potten CS, Watson AJ, et al. Differential expression of bcl-2 in intestinal epithelia. Correlation with attenuation of apoptosis in colonic crypts and the incidence of colonic neoplasia. J Cell Sci 1995;108(Pt 6):2261–71.

70. Domen J, Weissman IL. Hematopoietic stem cells need two signals to prevent apoptosis; BCL-2 can provide one of these, Kitl/c-Kit signaling the other. J Exp Med 2000;192(12):1707–18.

71. Banerjee S, Banerjee PP, Zirkin BR, Brown TR. Regional expression of transforming growth factor-alpha in rat ventral prostate during postnatal development, after androgen ablation, and after androgen replacement. Endocrinology 1998;139(6):3005–13.

72. Bonkhoff H, Remberger K. Differentiation pathways and histogenetic aspects of normal and abnormal prostatic growth: a stem cell model. Prostate 1996;28(2):98–106.

73. Domen J, Cheshier SH, Weissman IL. The role of apoptosis in the regulation of hematopoietic stem cells: Overexpression of Bcl-2 increases both their number and repopulation potential. J Exp Med 2000;191(2):253–64.

74. Marzesco AM, Janich P, Wilsch-Brauninger M, et al. Release of extracellular membrane particles carrying the stem cell marker prominin-1 (CD133) from neural progenitors and other epithelial cells. J Cell Sci 2005;118(Pt 13):2849–58.

75. Florek M, Haase M, Marzesco AM, et al. Prominin-1/CD133, a neural and hematopoietic stem cell marker, is expressed in adult human differentiated cells and certain types of kidney cancer. Cell Tissue Res 2005;319(1):15–26.

76. Tsujimura A, Fujita K, Komori K, et al. Prostatic stem cell marker identified by cDNA microarray in mouse. J Urol 2007;178(2):686–91.

77. Wang XD, Shou J, Wong P, French DM, Gao WQ. Notch1-expressing cells are indispensable for prostatic branching morphogenesis during development and re-growth following castration and androgen replacement. J Biol Chem 2004;279(23):24733–44.

78. Wang S, Garcia AJ, Wu M, Lawson DA, Witte ON, Wu H. Pten deletion leads to the expansion of a prostatic stem/progenitor cell subpopulation and tumor initiation. Proc Natl Acad Sci USA 2006;103(5):1480–5.

79. Huss WJ, Gray DR, Greenberg NM, Mohler JL, Smith GJ. Breast cancer resistance protein-mediated efflux of androgen in putative benign and malignant prostate stem cells. Cancer Res 2005;65(15):6640–50.

80. Vander Borght S, Libbrecht L, Katoonizadeh A, et al. Breast cancer resistance protein (BCRP/ABCG2) is expressed by progenitor cells/reactive ductules and hepatocytes and its expression pattern is influenced by disease etiology and species type: possible functional consequences. J Histochem Cytochem 2006;54(9):1051–9.

81. Signoretti S, Loda M. Prostate stem cells: from development to cancer. Semin Cancer Biol 2007;17(3):219–24.

82. Al-Omari R, Shidaifat F, Dardaka M. Castration induced changes in dog prostate gland associated with diminished activin and activin receptor expression. Life Sci 2005;77(22):2752–9.

83. McDonnell TJ, Troncoso P, Brisbay SM, et al. Expression of the protooncogene bcl-2 in the prostate and its association with emergence of androgen-independent prostate cancer. Cancer Res 1992;52(24):6940–4.

84. Wang Y, Hayward S, Cao M, Thayer K, Cunha G. Cell differentiation lineage in the prostate. Differentiation 2001; 68(4–5):270–9.

85. Zhou Z, Flesken-Nikitin A, Nikitin AY. Prostate cancer associated with p53 and Rb deficiency arises from the stem/progenitor cell-enriched proximal region of prostatic ducts. Cancer Res 2007;67(12):5683–90.

86. Signoretti S, Waltregny D, Dilks J, et al. p63 is a prostate basal cell marker and is required for prostate development. Am J Pathol 2000;157(6):1769–75.

87. Signoretti S, Pires MM, Lindauer M, et al. p63 regulates commitment to the prostate cell lineage. Proc Natl Acad Sci USA 2005;102(32):11355–60.

88. Kurita T, Medina RT, Mills AA, Cunha GR. Role of p63 and basal cells in the prostate. Development 2004; 131(20):4955–64.

89. Liao CP, Zhong C, Saribekyan G, et al. Mouse models of prostate adenocarcinoma with the capacity to monitor spontaneous carcinogenesis by bioluminescence or fluorescence. Cancer Res 2007;67(15):7525–33.

90. Abate-Shen C, Shen MM. Mouse models of prostate carcinogenesis. Trends Genet 2002;18(5):S1–5.

91. Roy-Burman P, Wu H, Powell WC, Hagenkord J, Cohen MB. Genetically defined mouse models that mimic natural aspects of human prostate cancer development. Endocr Relat Cancer 2004;11(2):225–54.

92. Greenberg NM, DeMayo F, Finegold MJ, et al. Prostate cancer in a transgenic mouse. Proc Natl Acad Sci USA 1995;92(8):3439–43.

93. Gingrich JR, Barrios RJ, Kattan MW, Nahm HS, Finegold MJ, Greenberg NM. Androgen-independent prostate cancer progression in the TRAMP model. Cancer Res 1997;57(21):4687–91.

94. Kasper S, Sheppard PC, Yan Y, et al. Development, progression, and androgen-dependence of prostate tumors in probasin-large T antigen transgenic mice: a model for prostate cancer. Lab Invest 1998;78(3):319–33.

95. Masumori N, Thomas TZ, Chaurand P, et al. A probasin-large T antigen transgenic mouse line develops prostate adenocarcinoma and neuroendocrine carcinoma with metastatic potential. Cancer Res 2001;61(5):2239–49.

96. Stanbrough M, Leav I, Kwan PW, Bubley GJ, Balk SP. Prostatic intraepithelial neoplasia in mice expressing an androgen receptor transgene in prostate epithelium. Proc Natl Acad Sci USA 2001;98(19):10823–8.

97. Song Z, Wu X, Powell WC, et al. Fibroblast growth factor 8 isoform B overexpression in prostate epithelium: a new mouse model for prostatic intraepithelial neoplasia. Cancer Res 2002;62(17):5096–105.

98. Freeman KW, Gangula RD, Welm BE, et al. Conditional activation of fibroblast growth factor receptor (FGFR) 1, but not FGFR2, in prostate cancer cells leads to increased osteopontin induction, extracellular signal-regulated kinase activation, and in vivo proliferation. Cancer Res 2003;63(19):6237–43.

99. Jin C, McKeehan K, Guo W, et al. Cooperation between ectopic FGFR1 and depression of FGFR2 in induction of prostatic intraepithelial neoplasia in the mouse prostate. Cancer Res 2003;63(24):8784–90.

100. Majumder PK, Yeh JJ, George DJ, et al. Prostate intraepithelial neoplasia induced by prostate restricted Akt activation: the MPAKT model. Proc Natl Acad Sci USA 2003;100(13):7841–6.

101. Shim EH, Johnson L, Noh HL, et al. Expression of the F-box protein SKP2 induces hyperplasia, dysplasia, and low-grade carcinoma in the mouse prostate. Cancer Res 2003;63(7):1583–8.

102. Bhatia-Gaur R, Donjacour AA, Sciavolino PJ, et al. Roles for Nkx3.1 in prostate development and cancer. Genes Dev 1999;13(8):966–77.

103. Abdulkadir SA, Magee JA, Peters TJ, et al. Conditional loss of Nkx3.1 in adult mice induces prostatic intraepithelial neoplasia. Mol Cell Biol 2002;22(5):1495–503.

104. Huang J, Powell WC, Khodavirdi AC, et al. Prostatic intraepithelial neoplasia in mice with conditional disruption of the retinoid X receptor alpha allele in the prostate epithelium. Cancer Res 2002;62(16):4812–9.

105. Wang S, Gao J, Lei Q, et al. Prostate-specific deletion of the murine Pten tumor suppressor gene leads to metastatic prostate cancer. Cancer Cell 2003;4(3):209–21.

106. Trotman LC, Niki M, Dotan ZA, et al. Pten dose dictates cancer progression in the prostate. PLoS Biol 2003; 1(3):385–96.

107. Ma X, Ziel-van der Made AC, Autar B, et al. Targeted biallelic inactivation of Pten in the mouse prostate leads to prostate cancer accompanied by increased epithelial cell proliferation but not by reduced apoptosis. Cancer Res 2005; 65(13):5730–9.

108. Ellwood-Yen K, Graeber TG, Wongvipat J, et al. Myc-driven murine prostate cancer shares molecular features with human prostate tumors. Cancer Cell 2003;4(3):223–38.

109. Han G, Buchanan G, Ittmann M, et al. Mutation of the androgen receptor causes oncogenic transformation of the prostate. Proc Natl Acad Sci USA 2005;102(4):1151–6.

110. Khodavirdi AC, Song Z, Yang S, et al. Increased expression of osteopontin contributes to the progression of prostate cancer. Cancer Res 2006;66(2):883–8.

111. Macri E, Loda M. Role of p27 in prostate carcinogenesis. Cancer Metastasis Rev 1998;17(4):337–44.

112. Di Cristofano A, De Acetis M, Koff A, Cordon-Cardo C, Pandolfi PP. Pten and p27KIP1 cooperate in prostate cancer tumor suppression in the mouse. Nat Genet 2001;27(2):222–4.

113. Kim MJ, Cardiff RD, Desai N, et al. Cooperativity of Nkx3.1 and Pten loss of function in a mouse model of prostate carcinogenesis. Proc Natl Acad Sci USA 2002;99(5):2884–9.

114. Gary B, Azuero R, Mohanty GS, Bell WC, Eltoum IE, Abdulkadir SA. Interaction of Nkx3.1 and p27kip1 in prostate tumor initiation. Am J Pathol 2004;164(5):1607–14.

115. Abate-Shen C, Banach-Petrosky WA, Sun X, et al. Nkx3.1; Pten mutant mice develop invasive prostate adenocarcinoma and lymph node metastases. Cancer Res 2003;63(14):3886–90.

116. Zhou Z, Flesken-Nikitin A, Corney DC, et al. Synergy of p53 and Rb deficiency in a conditional mouse model for metastatic prostate cancer. Cancer Res 2006;66(16):7889–98.

117. Chen Z, Trotman LC, Shaffer D, et al. Crucial role of p53-dependent cellular senescence in suppression of Pten-deficient tumorigenesis. Nature 2005;436(7051):725–30.

118. Zhong C, Saribekyan G, Liao CP, Cohen MB, Roy-Burman P. Cooperation between FGF8b overexpression and PTEN deficiency in prostate tumorigenesis. Cancer Res 2006;66(4):2188–94.

119. Bruxvoort KJ, Charbonneau HM, Giambernardi TA, et al. Inactivation of Apc in the mouse prostate causes prostate carcinoma. Cancer Res 2007;67(6):2490–6.

120. Wu X, Wu J, Huang J, et al. Generation of a prostate epithelial cell-specific Cre transgenic mouse model for tissue-specific gene ablation. Mech Dev 2001;101(1–2):61–9.

121. Reiner T, de Las Pozas A, Parrondo R, Perez-Stable C. Progression of prostate cancer from a subset of p63-positive basal epithelial cells in FG/Tag transgenic mice. Mol Cancer Res 2007;5(11):1171–9.

17

Prostate Cancer Stem/Progenitor Cells

Sofia Honorio, Hangwen Li, and Dean G. Tang

ABSTRACT

The cancer stem cell (CSC) theory posits that only a small population of tumor cells within the tumor has the ability to reinitiate tumor development and is responsible for tumor homeostasis and progression. Tumor initiation is a defining property of putative CSCs, which have been reported in both blood malignancies and solid tumors. Here we provide evidence that both cultured prostate cancer cells and xenograft prostate tumors contain stem-like cells that can initiate serially transplantable tumors. We also present a hypothetical model of tumorigenic hierarchy of cancer cells in prostate tumors. Further studies on these important tumorigenic cells will help to understand prostate tumor biology and to develop novel diagnostic and prognostic markers and therapeutic agents.

Key Words: Prostate cancer, Cancer stem cells, Tumor progenitors, Clonal and clonogenic assays, Side population, Self-renewal, Transplantation sites, Sphere-formation assays

INTRODUCTION

Prostate cancer (PCa) is the most common noncutaneous malignant neoplasm in men in the Western world, accounts for the deaths of approximately 30,000 men per year in the United States, and constitutes the second leading cause of cancer-related deaths in American men *(1)*. Since PCa is a disease of aging men, the number of afflicted men is increasing rapidly as the population of males over the age of 50 grows worldwide. PCa is generally diagnosed through an elevated prostate-specific antigen (PSA) level or abnormal digital rectal exam *(2)*. PSA is a protein produced by normal epithelial cells of the prostate gland as well as PCa cells. It is present in small quantities in the serum of men without cancer, but is routinely elevated in the presence of PCa and in other benign prostate disorders such as infection, inflammation, and benign prostatic hyperplasia (BPH). Serum PSA as a screening tool sets the upper limit of normal at 4 ng/ml; levels above that point identify men who should be considered for prostate biopsy *(3)*. As a result of PSA screening, most cancers are now discovered while they are still localized to the gland, which makes metastatic disease at the time of diagnosis a relatively rare event.

From: *Cancer Drug Discovery and Development: Stem Cells and Cancer,*
Edited by: R.G. Bagley and B.A. Teicher, DOI: 10.1007/978-1-60327-933-8_17,
© Humana Press, a part of Springer Science + Business Media, LLC 2009

Localized disease is treated and often can be cured by surgery (prostatectomy) and radiation therapy (brachytherapy). The treatment of choice for advanced disease is androgen deprivation by either surgical or chemical castration *(2)*. While this approach leads to tumor regression in 70–80% of patients with advanced PCa, most patients eventually relapse with hormone-refractory metastatic PCa that remains incurable by current treatment regimens.

PCa generally develops slowly, sometimes over a period of 20–30 years *(3)*. Prostate carcinomas are multifocal (on average ≥5 cancer foci per patient) and highly heterogeneous. It is very common to find areas of cancer adjacent to prostatic intraepithelial neoplasia (PIN), considered to be the precursor lesions of PCa, and normal glands in human prostatectomy specimens. This degree of heterogeneity has resulted in the Gleason scoring/grading system *(4)*, in which the two most common histologic patterns are assigned a grade of 1–5 according to decreasing degree of differentiation (i.e., grade 1 corresponding to a well-differentiated histological pattern while grade 5 to a poorly differentiated pattern); these two grades are summed and reported as the total Gleason score, which serves as a prognostic indicator of clinical behavior *(5)*. Generally, PCa with a total Gleason score of 5–7 are considered to be intermediate grade/moderately differentiated and those with a score of 8–10 high grade/poorly differentiated.

CELLULAR ORGANIZATION OF THE PROSTATIC GLAND

The adult human prostate has three morphological zones: peripheral, transitional, and central. BPH occurs mainly in the transitional zone, while prostate carcinoma arises primarily in the peripheral zone. In contrast with the ductal-acinar histology of the human prostate, the rodent prostate gland consists of four distinct lobes: anterior, dorsal and lateral (collectively referred to as the dorsolateral lobe), and ventral. Although there is no clear analogy between the lobular structure of the rodent prostate and the zonal architecture of the human prostate, several studies claim that the dorsolateral lobe is most similar to the human peripheral zone *(6)*.

The prostate is a hormonally regulated glandular organ whose growth accelerates at sexual maturity due to androgen actions on both stroma and epithelial cells *(7)*. The prostatic glands contain two types of epithelial cells, i.e., the luminal secretory cells and the basal cells, and rare neuroendocrine (NE) cells (Fig. 1). External to the basal cells are also some transient (or reactive) "stromal" cell types whose identities remain unclear. These cells together form the pseudostratified prostatic glands. Basal cells form a layer of flattened cells along the basement membrane of each prostatic duct. Luminal cells form a layer of columnar shaped cells above the basal layer; they are the major cell type of the prostate and perform secretory function. NE cells often transverse both basal and luminal layers and secrete neuropeptides that support epithelial growth and viability. The prostatic epithelium is surrounded by a stromal component that includes fibroblasts, myofibroblasts, and smooth muscle cells that guide the growth and differentiation of the epithelium. Blood vessels, peripheral nerves and ganglia, and tissue infiltrating white blood cells are additional constituent cell elements of the normal adult human prostate.

The two epithelial cells express distinct markers (Fig. 1; Table 1) *(8–37)*. While luminal cells express the low molecular weight cytokeratins (CK) 8 and 18, androgen receptor (AR), PSA, prostatic acid phosphatase (PAP), CD57, and 15-lipoxygenase 2 (15-LOX2), basal cells express the high molecular weight CK5 and 14, CD44, Bcl-2, p63, telomerase, and GST-π. NE cells are androgen-independent cells and express chromogranin A, synaptophysin, and neuron-specific enolase (NSE). They also produce and secrete various neuropeptides such as serotonin, bombesin, calcitonin, neurotensin, and parathyroid hormone-related protein *(6)*.

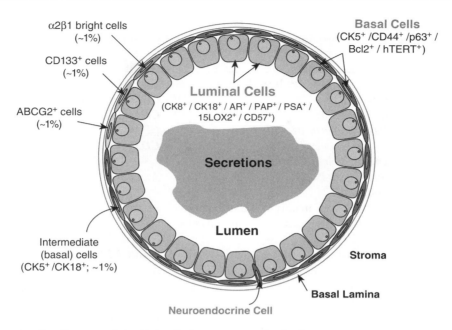

Fig. 1. Cartoon showing the general structure of a human prostatic gland.

NORMAL HUMAN PROSTATE STEM/PROGENITOR CELLS

The adult rodent prostate can undergo multiple rounds of castration-induced regression and testo-sterone-induced regeneration *(38)*: androgen withdrawal results in glandular involution due to apop-tosis of the terminally differentiated, androgen-dependent cells, while testosterone readministration restores the gland structure and its secretory function *(39)*, supposedly owing to the reconstitution of the luminal cell compartment by basal cells *(40)*. These data indicates that a population of stem cells (SCs), endowed with self-renewal and differentiation capacities, probably resides in the basal layer. This theory is further supported by findings that mice null for the basal cell marker p63 are born without prostate *(26)*. In the human prostate, several pieces of evidence suggest that the basal cell layer may contain stem-like cells. First, most (>80%) proliferating cells are found in this compartment *(41)*. Second, molecules important in maintaining SC self-renewal and proliferation (e.g., telomer-ase, p63), survival (Bcl-2), and detoxification (GST-π) preferentially localize in the basal layer (reviewed in *(37)*). Third, clonal analysis of dissociated adult human prostate epithelial cells reveals that only a small fraction (0.5–5%) of cells, all displaying basal cell characteristics, possess tremen-dous proliferative capacity *(42)*. Fourth, when recombined with rat urogenital sinus mesenchyme (rUGM) and implanted under the renal capsule, the basal-like prostate epithelial cells can, like their murine counterpart, generate glandular structures *(43)*. Finally, like other adult stem/progenitor cells, a small population of basal-like human prostate epithelial cells retains some developmental plasticity since, when cultured on mouse fibroblast feeder layers, they are able to "transdifferentiate" into neu-ronal/glial cells *(37)*.

Strictly speaking, a prostate SC should be a cell that has the ability to regenerate the whole prostatic gland, much like what has been demonstrated for murine mammary SCs *(44, 45)*. In this sense, the

Table 1
Representative marker expression in basal vs. luminal cells in human (and mouse) prostate[a]

	Basal cells	*Luminal cells*
Surface[b]	**ABCG2**(also BCRP; Brcp-1) *(8, 9)*	**CD57**(10)
	CD44(10)	**CD26**(Dipeptidyl peptidase I) (11)
	CD133(12, 13)	**CD13**(14)
	CD104 (integrin β4) (11, 15)	**CD10**(16)
	CD138 (syndecan) (15)	**CD38**(17)
	α2β1 integrin(18, 19)	
	Notch-1[c](20, 21)	**Jagged-1**[c]
	Her-2/neu(22)	
	Sca-1 (mouse); mainly in the proximal tubules also localized in luminal cells *(23, 24)*	
Cytoskeleton	**CK5/CK14**	**CK8/CK18**
Nuclear	**Sox9**(25); **p63** (26); **telomerase** (27, 28)	**AR**; **Nkx3.1**(29)
Cytosolic	**Bcl-2**(30)	**15-LOX2**(31, 32)
	GST-π(33)	**Probasin**(mouse) (34)
		PAP; **PSA**
		PSCA[d] (identifying TACs) *(35)*

Note: CD49a (integrin α1) is very specific for human prostate stromal cells, so are COL6A3, CD56, and CD90 (Thy-1) *(11)*. For mouse prostate, stromal, basal, luminal, and hematopoietic cells can be isolated by: CD34⁺, CD24⁺CD49f⁻, CD24⁺CD49f⁺, and CD45⁺ Ter119⁺ phenotype, respectively *(36)*.

[a] There are many differences between mouse and human prostates other than structural. For example, the basal cells in mouse prostate are only very scattered and do not form a continuous basal cell layer as in human. Mouse prostate epithelial cells express little PSA and no 15-LOX2, whereas probasin is unique to mouse prostate.

[b] The underlined surface molecules are homogeneously expressed in most basal or luminal cells while the rest surface markers are expressed in a subset of cells.

[c] Notch-1 is the receptor and Jagged-1 the ligand. These two markers have been identified from studies done in mouse prostate. It is not totally clear whether Jagged-1 is expressed only in the luminal cells.

[d] PSCA has been shown to be expressed in late intermediate epithelial cells that are still double positive for CK5/CK18.

true prostate SCs have not been identified. For this reason, prostatic cells with certain SC properties such as extended proliferative and anchorage-independent growth capacities and partial differentiation abilities (e.g., to form ductal or acinar structures in Matrigel or when mixed with rUGM and transplanted under the renal capsule) are often called prostate SCs, progenitor cells, or stem/progenitor cells *(37)*. Several candidate populations of NHP stem/progenitor cells have been reported. These include CK5 and CK18 double positive (CK5⁺/CK18⁺) intermediate cells, the side population (SP) cells and cells expressing the surface molecules CD44, ABCG2, integrin α2β1, or CD133 (reviewed in *(37)*). The *CK5⁺/CK18⁺ intermediate cell population* constitutes ~1% of the basal cells *(46)*. Since CK5 and CK18 are intracellular cytoskeletal proteins, the CK5⁺/CK18⁺ intermediate basal cells have not been prospectively purified and their putative stem/progenitor cell properties have not been directly tested. Putative prostatic SCs appear to be enriched in the *SP(47, 48)*, whose phenotype is mediated by multi-drug resistance family proteins such as MDR-1 and ABCG2 (reviewed in *(49)*). The SP in benign prostate constitutes 0.5–3% of epithelial cells and the SP cells cultured in Matrigel containing androgen have the ability to form acinus-like spheroids *(48)*. The majority of the SP cells are in the Go/G1 phase of the cell cycle *(47)*, a characteristic of SCs. The **ABCG2**-*expressing cells* in the benign prostate localize mainly in the basal layer *(8, 9)*, constitute <1% of total basal cell population, and share essentially the same transcriptome as the SP cells *(9)*. It has been proposed that the ABCG2$^+$ cells mark prostate SCs and that ABCG2 functions to efflux androgen to keep these cells under the undifferentiated state *(8)*. Interestingly, both SP and ABCG2$^+$ cells express genes indicative of a SC phenotype *(9)*. As of now, neither SP cells nor ABCG2$^+$ cells have been shown to have the ability to regenerate prostatic glands in vivo. **CD44** is expressed in nearly all basal cells in the human prostatic glands. Purified CD44$^+$ prostate basal cells, when cocultured with stromal cells in the presence of Matrigel and dihydrotestosterone (DHT), can produce PSA, presumably due to the differentiation of CD44$^+$ cells into luminal cells *(10)*. The *α2β1*^{hi}*cells* comprise 1–15% of the CD44$^+$ basal cell population and seem to possess higher in vitro colony-forming efficiency as well as the ability to generate prostatic-like acini when subcutaneously engrafted with stromal cells into the flanks of male, athymic nude mice *(19)*. Further characterization reveals that this proliferation and developmental potentials are preferentially harbored by the **CD133**-*expressing cells* within the CD44$^+$α2β1^{hi} population, which represent ~0.75% of the human prostate basal cells *(12)*. It has been proposed that the CD44$^+$α2β1^{hi}CD133$^+$ cells, constituting ~1% of the total epithelial cells, represent prostate SCs whereas CD44$^+$α2β1^{hi}CD133$^-$ cells represent the progenitor cells or transit amplifying cells *(12, 50)*. In support, the α2β1^{hi}CD133$^+$ cells are AR-negative while the α2β1^{hi}CD133$^-$ cells are AR-positive *(50)*. None of these purported prostate SCs have been demonstrated to regenerate the whole prostatic gland at the single cell level and the interrelationships among these reported prostate stem/progenitor cells are presently unclear.

STEM-LIKE CELLS IN TUMORS AND PCa STEM/PROGENITOR CELLS

Tumor development to a certain degree resembles and has been compared as "caricatures" of normal tissue histogenesis and organogenesis *(51)*. Indeed, most human tumors are heterogeneous in their cellular composition *(52–54)*. Although many posit that tumor cell heterogeneity is of a genetic basis associated with inherent high genomic instability in tumor cells, the heterogeneous cellular composition in tumors has also been hypothesized, early on, to be the consequence of abnormal tumor stem cell differentiation *(55)*. This latter postulate, called "cancer stem cell (CSC) hypothesis" was recently revived *(56)* mainly due to progresses made on studies of normal tissue stem cells. The CSC hypothesis has two central tenets – tumors are derived from transformation of normal stem cells or their progeny (i.e., progenitor or even differentiated cells) and every tumor contains a small population of stem-like cells that possess a unique ability to drive tumor formation and maintain tumor homeostasis *(56)*. In support of the first tenet, both CML (chronic myelogenous leukemia; *(57)*) and AML (acute myelogenous leukemia; *(58)*) appear to have arisen from the committed progenitor cells that have acquired self-renewing capabilities. In support of the second tenet, stem-like cells or CSCs that can initiate serially transplantable tumors in mice recapitulating the heterogeneous nature of patient tumors have been reported not only in leukemia but also in solid tumors including breast cancer, glioma, melanoma, colon and liver cancers, head and neck squamous cell carcinoma, and pancreatic cancer (Table 2) *(59–72)*.

Leukemic stem cells (LSCs), although constituting a minority (~0.1%) of the total cell population, are the only cells that can transfer the disease to NOD/SCID mice *(73)*. In the past 5 years, putative CSCs, or tumor-initiating cells, have been reported for many human solid tumors (Table 2). Several important principles have emerged from these studies. First, most CSCs have been identified using cell surface markers for the corresponding normal tissue stem/progenitor cells, suggesting that normal and cancer SCs share some phenotypic markers. Second, interestingly, although no markers may be truly SC-specific, CD44 and CD133 have been used to identify many types of CSCs. For example, CD44 has been used to enrich for breast, colon, pancreatic, liver, and head and neck CSCs, whereas CD133 for CSCs in lung and colon cancers and glioma (Table 2). Some other markers may be tumor specific, e.g., breast CSCs have a (CD44+)CD24⁻ phenotype *(59)* whereas pancreatic CSCs possess the (CD44+)CD24+ phenotype *(67)*. Third, in a particular tumor, CD44 and CD133 may identify distinct and/or overlapping populations of tumor stem/progenitor cells. For instance, both CD133 *(63–65)* and CD44 *(66)* have been utilized as the positive selection marker for colon CSCs. The same two markers have also been employed to independently select for pancreatic CSCs *(67, 68)*. In both cases, the interrelationship (inclusive, exclusive, or hierarchical) between the CD133 and CD44 selected CSCs remains unclear. These observations *(63–68)* emphasize the important point that the CSC population is likely heterogeneous, as elucidated in LSCs *(74)*, and also raise the possibility that combining CD44 and CD133 may enrich for more primitive CSCs. Fourth, CSCs are only operationally or functionally defined. Perhaps one of the most important criteria is that putative CSCs possess an enhanced ability to initiate serially transplantable tumors that phenotypically recapitulate patient tumor histology *(37, 75)*. In all of the above-mentioned CSC studies (Table 2), "naked" tumor cells were injected into the immunodeficient mice, implying that putative CSCs possess an intrinsic ability to establish a "niche" in a foreign microenvironment. Fifth, nevertheless, reconstitution of CSC activity and tumor development of human tumor cells in mice represents an extremely challenging task *(37, 76)* involving numerous variables associated with both tumors (availability, heterogeneity, stage/grade, size, quality, digestion/purification/implantation methods, etc.) and recipient mice (strains, degree of immune deficiency, pre-conditioning, injection/implantation sites, etc.). Consequently, different tumors have a wide variety of "empirical" details that cannot be interpreted readily and reconciled scientifically. For instance, although some tumorigenic subsets were implanted "orthotopically," many others were injected at ectopic sites, in particular, subcutaneously (s.c) or under the kidney capsule (Table 2). Sixth, as predicted, CSCs seem to be more resistant to antitumor therapeutics including chemotherapy and radiation *(68, 77–79)*. Of clinical significance, the abundance of CSCs significantly increases in breast cancer patients that have received prior therapies *(77)*.

The cellular origin of PCa is unknown. Because the majority of tumor cells in early PCa have a luminal cell phenotype expressing CK8, CK18, AR, and PSA, it has been proposed that PCa may arise from the transformation and dedifferentiation of luminal cells *(15, 26, 80–82)*. Nevertheless, some reports have identified intermediate cells coexpressing basal and luminal cell markers in PCa *(83)*. In addition, prostate stem cell antigen (PSCA), a putative marker of normal late-intermediate prostate cells, is also found to be upregulated in PCa *(35, 84)*. These data suggest that the disease might originate in an intermediate or transit-amplifying epithelial cell population. Furthermore, all PCa still contain a minor fraction of basal-like cells that express CD44, p63, ABCG2, or CD133, which identify normal prostate stem/progenitor cells. Therefore, it also remains possible that PCa might arise from normal prostate SCs.

Regardless of its origin, PCa seems to contain stem-like tumor cells, as evidenced by several observations. First, in long-term cultured PCa cells, only a small percentage of cells can establish serially passageable clones, colonies, or spheres *(37, 85)*. Second, for both long-term cultured and xenograft-derived PCa cells, generally a large number of cells needs be injected into the animals to reinitiate a tumor *(37, 49, 85–87)*, suggesting that PCa cells are not all equal in their tumor-initiating abilities. Third, PCa cells in culture, like keratinocytes, can form clones with distinct morphologies, i.e., holoclone, meroclone, and paraclone. Strikingly, only holoclones can be serially passaged and can initiate serially transplantable tumors *(85)*. Since <10% PCa cells can form holoclones *(37, 85)*, these observations again suggest that PCa cells are heterogeneous with respect to their tumor-initiating abilities and that only a small population of PCa cells have tumor-initiating ability.

Table 2
CSC studies in human solid tumors (2003–2008)

Tumor type	Samples	Marker	Mice	Transplantation	Results	Ref.
Breast cancer	9 (1 primary; 8 met.)	CD44$^+$ CD24$^{-/lo}$ESA$^+$ (FACS)	NOD/SCID mice pretreated with VP16	Mammary fat pad	>50-fold enrichment in tumorigenicity	(59)
Breast cancer	4 xenotransplants (from 2 primary; 2 met)	ALDH$^+$ (FACS)	NOD/SCID mice	Humanized mammary fat pad	500 ALDH$^+$ cells generate T; 20 ALDH$^+$ CD44$^+$ CD24$^-$Lin$^-$ cells generate T	(60)
Brain tumors	7 primary tumors	CD133$^+$ (MACS)	6–8 wk NOD/SCID	Intracranial injection	CD133$^+$ more tumorigenic	(61)
Prostate cancer	7 (4 primary, 1 benign, 2 LN mets)	CD44$^+$ α2β1^{hi}CD133$^+$ (MACS) purified from long-term cultured cells		*No tumor experiments*	Marker+ cells more clonogenic	(62)
Colon cancer	17 (6 primary, 10 liver and 1 retroperitoneal met.)	CD133$^+$ (double MACS)	8 wk NOD/SCID irradiated	Renal capsule	1 CSC/57,000 T cells; 1 CSC/262 CD133$^+$ cells	(63)
Colon cancer	19 primary (5 Dukes A)	CD133$^+$ (FACS or MACS)	SCID	Subcutaneous	3,000 CD133$^+$ cells generate T	(64)
Colon cancer	21 primary CRC	CD133$^+$	5–6 wk nude mice	Subcutaneous	2,500 CD133$^+$ cells generate T; 25 CD133$^+$-derived spheres generate T	(65)
Colon cancer	2 primary, 6 xenografts	EpCAMCD166$^+$ CD44$^+$ (FACS)	6–8 wk NOD/SCID	Subcutaneous	150 EpCAMCD166$^+$ CD44$^+$ cells generate T	(66)
Pancreatic cancer	10 (2 primary; 2 met.)	CD44$^+$CD24$^+$ESA$^+$	NOD/SCID	Subcutaneous + pancreas	>100-fold enrichment	(67)

(continued)

Table 2
(continued)

Tumor type	Samples	Marker	Mice	Transplantation	Results	Ref.
Pancreatic cancer	11 (6 met.); sorting for 7 L3.6pl metastatic line	CD133+ (MACS) CD133+ CXCR4+ (FACS)	8–12 wk nude mice	Pancreas	500 CD133+ cells generate T; the CD133+ CXCR4+ pop. mediates met.	(68)
Head & neck	25 primary (3 recurrences); 9 for sorting (4 primary + 5 xenografts)	CD44+ Lin−(FACS)	NOD/SCID & Rag2−/−	Subcutaneous	5,000 CD44+ Lin− cells generate T; only 13/25 HNSCC samples gave tumors	(69)
Melanoma	7 (1 primary; 4 LN & 2 visceral met.)	ABCB5+(MACS)	NOD/SCID	Subcutaneous	1 MMIC/1 million bulk T cells; primary xeno: 1 MMIC/160,000 ABCB5+cells; secondary xeno: 1 MMIC/120,000 ABCB5+cells	(70)
Lung cancer	19 (18 primary; 1 met.)	CD133+(FACS)	4 wk SCID or nude	Subcutaneous	10^4 CD133+ cells generate T	(71)
Liver cancer	28 primary (only 13 used)	CD45− CD90+ (MACS)	SCID	Intrahepatic	CD45− CD90+ more tumorigenic	(72)

The obvious challenge is to prospectively purify the stem-like cells out and further characterize their potential CSC properties. To this end, we have utilized three PCa xenograft models, i.e., Du145 (derived from brain metastasis), LAPC-4 (from a lymph node metastasis), and LAPC-9 (derived from a bony metastasis). Xenograft models have distinct advantages of being relatively genetically stable and providing a "renewable" source of specific populations of cells. Remarkably, these three xenograft tumors contain small populations of basal-like cells expressing ABCG2 *(49)*, CD44 *(86)*, and α2β1 *(87)*. We could also detect an SP, interestingly, only in LAPC-9 tumors *(49)*. Since normal prostate epithelial cells expressing these markers or showing the SP phenotype have been proposed as stem/progenitor cells (see above), we tested whether these marker-expressing cells in the xenograft tumors might have CSC properties. We prospectively purified these marker-expressing or the SP cells out from xenografts and compared their initiating abilities with the corresponding marker-negative or non-SP cells. We also studied the potential CSC properties of the matched populations. These studies have revealed that prostate tumor cells seem to be organized as a tumorigenic hierarchy (Fig. 2).

Several pieces of evidence provide support for this model (Fig. 2). First, most tumorigenicity resides in the relatively small population of CD44+ cells, which range from ~1–20% in xenograft tumors *(86, 87)*. In primary patient tumors, interestingly, the percentage of CD44+ cells seems to correlate with the Gleason grade, with Gleason grade 6–9 tumors having ~3, 9, 18, and 19% of CD44+ PCa cells (unpublished observations). Second, the CD44+ PCa cell population is still heterogeneous, encompassing tumor progenitor cells that are ABCG2+α2β1+ and relatively quiescent, slow-cycling CSCs that are CD44+ABCG2−α2β1−(Fig. 2). In support of this conjecture, all ABCG2+ cells and most (i.e., 70–80%) of the α2β1+ cells are included in the CD44+ cell population and overall the CD44+α2β1+ and LAPC-9 CD44+α2β1− cells have very similar tumorigenicities. In fact, the tumorigenicity of CD44+ (i.e., sorted using a single marker) cells is also indistinguishable from that of CD44+α2β1+ or CD44+α2β1− cells *(86, 87)*, suggesting that FACS sorting using either CD44 alone or CD44/α2β1 combination is purifying practically the same PCa cell population. Primary human tumors also reveal that ~75% of the α2β1+ cells are localized in the CD44+ PCa cell population.

Tumorigenic Hierarchy of PCa Cells in Xenograft Tumors

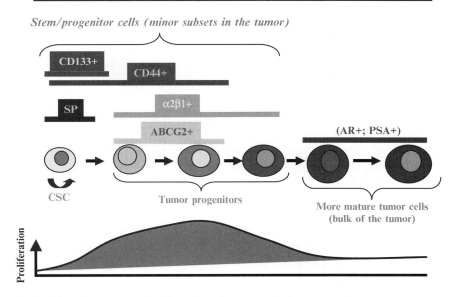

Fig. 2. Schematic depicting the tumorigenic hierarchy of tumor cells in xenograft tumors.

Third, the $\alpha2\beta1^+$ and $\alpha2\beta1^-$ cells are not significantly different in terms of their tumorigenicity, which can be explained by the fact that ~30% of the CD44$^+$ cells are localized in the $\alpha2\beta1^-$ cell population (87). In fact, the $\alpha2\beta1^-$ population appears to be slightly enriched in tumorigenic cells. For example, 100,000 of $\alpha2\beta1^-$Du145 cells orthotopically implanted in the DP can initiate tumor in four of the four injections whereas the same number of unfractionated Du145 cells cannot initiate any tumor development. Also, all tumors derived from the $\alpha2\beta1^-$ cells contain small numbers of $\alpha2\beta1^+$ cells. Remarkably, in tumors derived from high numbers (i.e., 100,000) of the LAPC4 $\alpha2\beta1^-$ or LAPC9 cells, more $\alpha2\beta1^+$ cells are observed than in unsorted tumors (87). All these observations support the hypothesis that $\alpha2\beta1^-$ population contains more primitive cells that can "regenerate" $\alpha2\beta1^+$ cells. Furthermore, when injected s.c, 100 LAPC-9 $\alpha2\beta1^-$ cells, like the unsorted cells, can initiate 50% tumor development whereas ten times more $\alpha2\beta1^+$ cells are required to achieve similar tumor take (87). These data suggest that the ~30% of the CD44$^+$ PCa cells that are $\alpha2\beta1^-$ might harbor primitive self-renewing CSCs (Fig. 2). Fourth, the CD44$^+\alpha2\beta1^-$ cells and CD44$^-\alpha2\beta1^+$ cells behave very similarly, in terms of their tumor-initiating abilities, to the $\alpha2\beta1^-$ and $\alpha2\beta1^+$ cells, respectively. Also, we have previously shown that 1,000 LAPC-9 CD44$^-$ cells injected s.c can initiate tumor development in five of the six injections (86), suggesting that there exist tumorigenic cells in the CD44$^-$ cell population. Also, 1,000 highly purified CD44$^-\alpha2\beta1^+$ cells initiate tumor development in nine of the ten implantations (87), suggesting that tumorigenic cells in CD44$^-$ population might all be $\alpha2\beta1^+$(i.e., having the CD44$^-\alpha2\beta1^+$ phenotype). These results emphasize the important concept that tumor progenitor cells, like the putative primitive CSCs, can be tumorigenic in regular tumor assays. Presumably, exhaustive serial tumor transplantation experiments can functionally distinguish putative CSCs from tumor progenitors. Fifth, in all xenograft models (DNp53-T, Du145, LAPC-4, and LAPC-9) as well as primary patient samples we have studied, the percentage of CD44$^+$ cells is always higher than that of $\alpha2\beta1$, supporting that CD44 marks both CSCs and tumor progenitors whereas $\alpha2\beta1$ expression identifies a subset of tumor progenitors (Fig. 2). Finally, since 100 LAPC9 SP cells can initiate tumor development whereas ≥1,000 CD44$^+$ cells are generally required to initiate tumor development, we hypothesize that the SP PCa cell population might contain more primitive CSCs than the CD44$^+$ cells (Fig. 2). In partial support, tumors initiated by the LAPC9 SP cells can be passaged for at least three generations (Fig. 3). Currently, the relationship between SP and CD44$^+$ cells remains unclear.

An obvious question pertains to the phenotypic properties of the putative CSCs in the CD44$^+$ PCa cell population (Fig. 2). The CD133$^+$ cells may represent good candidates as they have been reported to mark normal prostate SCs (12) and potential prostate CSCs with higher clonogenic potential (although tumorigenic potential has not been studied; (62)). We have also found that primary patient tumor samples contain 0.25–1.4% CD133$^+$ cells and that the CD133$^+$ PCa cells purified from LAPC-4 xenograft and HPCa13 patient tumors possess higher clonal and clonogenic potentials (Patrawala et al., unpublished observations). Studies are underway to characterize the in vivo tumorigenicity of CD44$^+$ CD133$^+$ PCa cells and to determine whether they may represent human prostate CSCs. Of particular interest, CD133 has recently been used as a marker to prospectively identify brain and colon tumor-initiating cells (Table 2), suggesting that this surface molecule, whose biological functions are yet to be elucidated, may represent more or less a "universal" normal SC and CSC marker. Another potential candidate population of primitive prostate CSCs might be in SP (Fig. 2). Since emerging evidence indicates that putative CSCs in solid tumors are more resistant to chemotherapeutic drugs and radiation and that CSCs might represent metastasis-mediating cells (68), identification and further characterization of prostate CSCs in patient tumors may lead to novel prognostic and therapeutic targets.

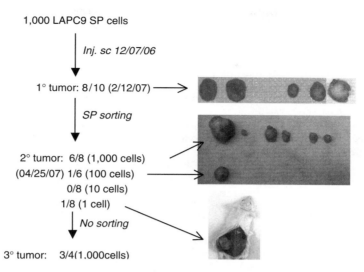

Fig. 3. The LAPC9 SP cell-initiated tumors can be serially passaged. 1,000 SP cells were acutely purified from the maintenance tumors *(49)* and injected s.c into the male NOD/SCID mice (on Dec. 7, 2006). The first-generation (1°) tumors, with an incidence of 8/10 (i.e., 8 tumors out of 10 injections), were further sorted for SP cells, which were used at different numbers in secondary tumor development. The secondary tumor cells, without further SP sorting, were used in tertiary tumor development (incidences and cell numbers indicated). Shown at the right are corresponding tumor images. Note the tumor derived from a single SP cell (right bottom).

ACKNOWLEDGMENTS

We thank Mr. Kent Claypool for assistance in FACS, Histology and Animal Facility Cores for technical assistance, and other members (past and present) of the Tang lab for discussion and support. This work was supported in part by grants from NIH (R01-AG023374, R01ES015888, and R21-ES015893–01A1), American Cancer Society (RSG MGO-105961), Department of Defense (W81XWH-07–1–0616 and PC073751), Prostate Cancer Foundation, and Elsa Pardee Foundation (D.G.T), and by two Center grants (CCSG-5 P30 CA166672 and ES07784). H. Li was supported in part by a predoctoral fellowship from DOD (W81XWH-07-1-0132).

BIBLIOGRAPHY

1. Jemal A, Siegel R, Ward E, Murray T, Xu J, Thun MJ. Cancer statistics, 2007. CA Cancer J Clin 2007;57:43–66.
2. National Comprehensive Cancer Network. 2007. NCCN Clinical Practice Guidelines in Oncology. Prostate cancer. v.2.2007. Available at: http://www.nccn.org/professionals/physician_gls/PDF/prostate.pdf.
3. Taichman RS, Loberg RD, Mehra R, Pienta KJ. The evolving biology and treatment of prostate cancer. J Clin Invest 2007;117:2351–61.
4. Gleason DF, Mellinger GT. Prediction of prognosis for prostatic adenocarcinoma by combined histological grading and clinical staging. J Urol 1974;111:58–64.
5. Bostwick DG, Foster CS. Predictive factors in prostate cancer: current concepts from the 1999 College of American Pathologists Conference on Solid Tumor Prognostic Factors and the 1999 World Health Organization Second International Consultation on Prostate Cancer. Semin Urol Oncol 1999;17:222–72.
6. Abate-Shen C, Shen MM. Molecular genetics of prostate cancer. Genes Dev 2000;14:2410–34.
7. Cunha GR, Harward SW, Wang YZ. Role of stroma in carcinogenesis of the prostate. Differentiation 2002;70:473–85.
8. Huss WJ, Gray DR, Greenberg NM, Mohler JL, Smith GJ. Breast cancer resistance protein-mediated efflux of androgen in putative benign and malignant prostate stem cells. Cancer Res 2005;65(15):6640–50.

9. Pascal LE, Oudes AJ, Petersen TW, Goo YA, Walashek LS, True LD, et al. Molecular and cellular characterization of ABCG2 in the prostate. BMC Urol 2007;7:6.

10. Liu AY, True LD, LaTray L, Nelson PS, Ellis WJ, Vessella RL, et al. Cell–cell interaction in prostate gene regulation and cyto-differentiation. Proc Natl Acad Sci USA 1997;94:10705–10.

11. Oudes AJ, Campbell DS, Sorensen CM, Walashek LS, True LD, Liu AY. Transcriptomes of human prostate cells. BMC Genomics 2006;7:92.

12. Richardson GD, Robson CN, Lang SH, Neal DE, Maitland NJ, Collins AT. CD133, a novel marker for human prostatic epithelial stem cells. J Cell Sci 2004;117:3539–45.

13. Miki J, Furusato B, Li H, Gu Y, Takahashi H, Egawa S, et al. Identification of putative stem cell markers, CD133 and CXCR4, in hTERT-immortalized primary nonmalignant and malignant tumor-derived human prostate epithelial cell lines and in prostate cancer specimens. Cancer Res 2007;67:3153–61.

14. Huang K, Takahara S, Kinouchi T, Takeyama M, Ishida T, Ueyama H, et al. Alanyl aminopeptidase from human seminal plasma: purification, characterization, and immunohistochemical localization in the male genital tract. J Biochem 1997;122:779–87.

15. Liu AY, True LD. Characterization of prostate cell types by CD cell surface molecules. Am J Pathol 2002;160:37–43.

16. Song J, Aumüller G, Xiao F, Wilhelm B, Albrecht M. Cell specific expression of CD10/neutral endopeptidase 24.11 gene in human prostatic tissue and cells. Prostate 2004;58:394–405.

17. Kramer G, Steiner G, Födinger D, Fiebiger E, Rappersberger C, Binder S, et al. High expression of a CD38-like molecule in normal prostatic epithelium and its differential loss in benign and malignant disease. J Urol 1995;154:1636–41.

18. Knox JD, Cress AE, Clark V, Manriquez L, Affinito KS, Dalkin BL, et al. Differential expression of extracellular matrix molecules and the alpha 6-integrins in the normal and neoplastic prostate. Am J Pathol 1994;145:167–74.

19. Collins AT, Habib FK, Maitland NJ, Neal DE. Identification and isolation of human prostate epithelial stem cells based on alpha(2)beta(1)-integrin expression. J Cell Sci 2001;114:3865–72.

20. Shou J, Ross S, Koeppen H, de Sauvage FJ, Gao WQ. Dynamics of notch expression during murine prostate development and tumorigenesis. Cancer Res 2001;61:7291–7.

21. Wang XD, Shou J, Wong P, French DM, Gao WQ. Notch1-expressing cells are indispensable for prostatic branching morphogenesis during development and re-growth following castration and androgen replacement. J Biol Chem 2004;279:24733–44.

22. Reiter RE, Sawyers CL. (2001). In: Chung LWK, Isaacs WB, Simons JW (eds). Prostate Cancer: Biology, Genetics, and the New Therapeutics. Humana Press: Totowa, NJ, 163–74.

23. Xin L, Lawson DA, Witte ON. The Sca-1 cell surface marker enriches for a prostate-regenerating cell subpopulation that can initiate prostate tumorigenesis. Proc Natl Acad Sci USA 2005;102:6942–7.

24. Burger PE, Xiong X, Coetzee S, Salm SN, Moscatelli D, Goto K, et al. Sca-1 expression identifies stem cells in the proximal region of prostatic ducts with high capacity to reconstitute prostatic tissue. Proc Natl Acad Sci USA 2005;102:7180–5.

25. Wang H, McKnight NC, Zhang T, Lu ML, Balk SP, Yuan X. SOX9 is expressed in normal prostate basal cells and regulates androgen receptor expression in prostate cancer cells. Cancer Res 2007;67:528–36.

26. Signoretti S, Waltregny D, Dilks J, Isaac B, Lin D, Garraway L, et al. p63 is a prostate basal cell marker and is required for prostate development. Am J Pathol 2000;157:1769–75.

27. Myers RB, Grizzle WE. Changes in biomarker expression in the development of prostatic adenocarcinoma. Biotech Histochem 1997;72:86–95.

28. Bui M, Reiter RE. Stem cell genes in androgen-independent prostate cancer. Cancer Mestastasis Rev 1999;17:391–9.

29. Ornstein DK, Cinquanta M, Weiler S, Duray PH, Emmert-Buck MR, Vocke CD, et al. Expression studies and mutational analysis of the androgen regulated homeobox gene NKX3.1 in benign and malignant prostate epithelium. J Urol 2001;165:1329–34.

30. McDonnell TJ, Troncoso P, Brisbay SM, Logothetis C, Chung LW, Hsieh JT, et al. Expression of the protooncogene bcl-2 in the prostate and its association with emergence of androgen-independent prostate cancer. Cancer Res 1992;52:6940–4.

31. Shappell SB, Boeglin WE, Olson SJ, Kasper S, Brash AR. 15-lipoxygenase-2 (15-LOX-2) is expressed in benign prostatic epithelium and reduced in prostate adenocarcinoma. Am J Pathol 1999;155:235–45.

32. Tang S, Bhatia B, Maldonado C, Yang P, Newman RA, Liu J, et al. Evidence that arachidonate 15-lipoxygenase 2 is a negative cell cycle regulator in normal prostate epithelial cells. J Biol Chem 2002;277:16189–201.

33. Cookson MS, Reuter VE, Linkov I, Fair WR. Glutathione S-transferase (GST-π) class expression by immunohistochemistry in benign and malignant prostate tissue. J Urol 1997;157:673–6.

34. Matuo Y, Nishi N, Muguruma Y, Yoshitake Y, Kurata N, Wada F. Localization of prostatic basic protein ("probasin") in the rat prostates by use of monoclonal antibody. Biochem Biophys Res Commun 1985;130:293–300.

35. Tran CP, Lin C, Yamashiro J, Reiter RE. Prostate stem cell antigen is a marker of late intermediate prostate epithelial cells. Mol Cancer Res 2002;1:113–21.

36. Lawson DA, Xin L, Lukacs RU, Cheng D, Witte ON. Isolation and functional characterization of murine prostate stem cells. Proc Natl Acad Sci USA 2007;104:181–6.

37. Tang DG, Patrawala L, Calhoun T, Bhatia B, Choy G, Schneider-Broussard R, et al. Prostate cancer stem/progenitor cells: identification, characterization, and implications. Mol Carcinog 2007;46:1–14.

38. Isaacs JT, Coffey DS. Etiology and disease process of benign prostatic hyperplasia. Prostate Suppl 1989;2:33–50.

39. English HF, Kyprianou N, Isaacs JT. Relationship between DNA fragmentation and apoptosis in the programmed cell death in the rat prostate following castration. Prostate 1989;15:233–50.

40. Bonkhoff H, Remberger K. Differentiation pathways and histogenetic aspects of normal and abnormal prostatic growth: a stem cell model. Prostate 1996;28:98–106.

41. Bonkhoff H, Stein U, Remberger K. The proliferative function of basal cells in the normal and hyperplastic human prostate. Prostate 1994;24:114–8.

42. Hudson DL, O'Hare M, Watt FM, Masters, JR. Proliferative heterogeneity in the human prostate: evidence for epithelial stem cells. Lab Invest 2000;80:1243–50.

43. Hayward SW, Haughney PC, Rosen MA, Greulich KM, Weier HU, Dahiya R, et al. Interactions between adult human prostatic epithelium and rat urogenital sinus mesenchyme in a tissue recombination model. Differentiation 1998; 63:131–40.

44. Shackleton M, Vaillant F, Simpson KJ, Stingl J, Smyth GK, Asselin-Labat ML, et al. Generation of a functional mammary gland from a single stem cell. Nature 2006;439:84–8.

45. Stingl J, Eirew P, Ricketson I, Shackleton M, Vaillant F, Choi D, et al. Purification and unique properties of mammary epithelial stem cells. Nature 2006;439:993–7.

46. van Leenders G, Dijkman H, Hulsbergen-van de Kaa C, Ruiter D, Schalken J. Demonstration of intermediate cells during human prostate epithelial differentiation in situ and in vitro using triple-staining confocal scanning microscopy. Lab Invest 2000;80:1251–8.

47. Bhatt RI, Brown MD, Hart CA, Gilmore P, Ramani VA, George NJ, et al. Novel method for the isolation and characterisation of the putative prostatic stem cell. Cytometry A 2003;54:89–99.

48. Brown MD, Gilmore PE, Hart CA, Samuel JD, Ramani VA, George NJ, et al. Characterization of benign and malignant prostate epithelial Hoechst 33342 side populations. Prostate 2007;67:1384–96.

49. Patrawala L, Calhoun T, Schneider-Broussard R, Zhou J, Claypool K, Tang DG. Side population is enriched in tumorigenic, stem-like cancer cells, whereas ABCG2+ and ABCG2 cancer cells are similarly tumorigenic. Cancer Res 2005;65:6207–19.

50. Heer R, Robson CN, Shenton BK, Leung HY. The role of androgen in determining differentiation and regulation of androgen receptor expression in the human prostatic epithelium transient amplifying population. J Cell Physiol 2007;212:572–8.

51. Sell S, Pierce GB. Maturation arrest of stem cell differentiation is a common pathway for the cellular origin of teratocarcinomas and epithelial cancers. Lab Invest 1994;70:6–22.

52. Dexter DL, Kowalski HM, Blazar BA, Fligiel Z, Vogel R, Heppner GH. Heterogeneity of tumor cells from a single mouse mammary tumor. Cancer Res 1978;38:3174–81.

53. Heppner GH. Tumor heterogeneity. Cancer Res 1984;44:2259–65.

54. Weiss L. Cancer cell heterogeneity. Cancer Metastasis Rev 2000;19:345–50.

55. Pierce GB. Neoplasms, differentiations and mutations. Am J Pathol 1974;77:103–18.

56. Reya T, Morrison SJ, Clarke MF, Weissman IL. Stem cells, cancer, and cancer stem cells. Nature 2001;414:105–11.

57. Jamieson CH, Ailles LE, Dylla SJ, Muijtjens M, Jones C, Zehnder JL, et al. Granulocyte-macrophage progenitors as candidate leukemic stem cells in blast-crisis CML. N Engl J Med 2004;351:657–67.

58. Krivtsov AV, Twomey D, Feng Z, Stubbs MC, Wang Y, Faber J, et al. Transformation from committed progenitor to leukaemia stem cell initiated by MLL-AF9. Nature 2006;442:818–22.

59. Al-Hajj M, Wicha MS, Benito-Hernandez A, Morrison SJ, Clarke MF. Prospective identification of tumorigenic breast cancer cells. Proc Natl Acad Sci USA 2003;100:3983–8.

60. Ginestier C, Hur MH, Charafe-Jauffret E, Monville F, Dutcher J, Brown M, et al. ALDH1 is a marker of normal and malignant human mammary stem cells and a predictor of poor clinical outcome. Cell Stem Cell 2007;1,555–67.

61. Singh SK, Hawkins C, Clarke ID, Squire JA, Bayani J, Hide T, et al. Identification of human brain tumour initiating cells. Nature 2004;432:396–401.

62. Collins AT, Berry PA, Hyde C, Stower MJ, Maitland NJ. Prospective identification of tumorigenic prostate cancer stem cells. Cancer Res 2005;65:10946–51.

63. O'Brien CA, Pollett A, Gallinger S, Dick JE. A human colon cancer cell capable of initiating tumour growth in immunodeficient mice. Nature 2007;445:106–10.

64. Ricci-Vitiani L, Lombardi DG, Pilozzi E, Biffoni M, Todaro M, Peschle C, et al. Identification and expansion of human colon-cancer-initiating cells. Nature 2007;445:111–5.

65. Todaro M, Alea MP, Di Stefano AB, Cammareri P, Vermeulen L, Iovino F, et al. Colon cancer stem cells dictate tumor growth and resist cell death by production of interleukin-4. Cell Stem Cell 2007;1:389–402.

66. Dalerba P, Dylla SJ, Park IK, Liu R, Wang X, Cho RW, et al. Phenotypic characterization of human colorectal cancer stem cells. Proc Natl Acad Sci USA 2007;104:10158–63.

67. Li C, Heidt DG, Dalerba P, Burant CF, Zhang L, Adsay V, et al. Identification of pancreatic cancer stem cells. Cancer Res 2007;67:1030–7.

68. Hermann PC, Huber SL, Herrler T, Aicher A, Ellwart JW, Guba M, et al. Distinct populations of cancer stem cells determine tumor growth and metastatic activity in human pancreatic cancer. Cell Stem Cell 2007;1:313–23.

69. Prince ME, Sivanandan R, Kaczorowski A, Wolf GT, Kaplan MJ, Dalerba P, et al. Identification of a subpopulation of cells with cancer stem cell properties in head and neck squamous cell carcinoma. Proc Natl Acad Sci USA 2007;104:973–8.

70. Schatton T, Murphy GF, Frank NY, Yamaura K, Waaga-Gasser AM, Gasser M, et al. Identification of cells initiating human melanomas. Nature 2008;451:345–9.

71. Eramo A, Lotti F, Sette G, Pilozzi E, Biffoni M, Di Virgilio A, et al. Identification and expansion of the tumorigenic lung cancer stem cell population. Cell Death Differ 2008;15:504–14.

72. Yang ZF, Ho DW, Ng MN, Lau CK, Yu WC, Ngai P, et al. Significance of CD90(+) cancer stem cells in human liver cancer. Cancer Cell 2008;13:153–66.
73. Lapidot T, Sirard C, Vormoor J, Murdoch B, Hoang T, Caceres-Cortes J, et al. A cell initiating human acute myeloid leukaemia after transplantation into SCID mice. Nature 1994;367:645–8.
74. Hope KJ, Jin L, Dick JE. Acute myeoloid leukemia originates from a hierarchy of leukemic stem cell classes that differ in self-renewal capacity. Nat Immunol 2004;5:738–43.
75. Clarke MF, Dick JE, Dirks PB, Eaves CJ, Jamieson CH, Jones DL, et al. Cancer stem cells – Perspectives on current status and future directions: AACR workshop on cancer stem cells. Cancer Res 2006;66:9339–44.
76. Hill RP. Identifying cancer stem cells in solid tumors: case not proven. Cancer Res 2006;66:1891–5.
77. Yu F, Yao H, Zhu P, Zhang X, Pan Q, Gong C, et al. let-7 regulates self renewal and tumorigenicity of breast cancer cells. Cell 2007:131:1109–23.
78. Bao S, Wu Q, McLendon RE, Hao Y, Shi Q, Hjelmeland AB, et al. Glioma stem cells promote radioresistance by preferential activation of the DNA damage response. Nature 2006;444:756–760.
79. Wang JCY. Evaluating therapeutic efficacy against cancer stem cells: New challenges posed by a new paradigm. Cell Stem Cell 2007;1:497–501.
80. Okada H, Tsubura A, Okamura A, Senzaki H, Naka Y, Komatz Y, et al. Keratin profiles in normal/hyperplastic prostates and prostate carcinoma. Virchows Arch A 1992;421:157–61.
81. De Marzo AM, Meeker AK, Epstein JI, Coffey DS. Prostate stem cell compartments: expression of the cell cycle inhibitor p27Kip1 in normal, hyperplastic, and neoplastic cells. Am J Pathol 1998;153:911–9.
82. Nagle RB, Ahmann FR, McDaniel KM, Paquin ML, Clark VA, Celniker A. Cytokeratin characterization of human prostatic carcinoma and its derived cell lines. Cancer Res 1987;47:281–6.
83. Verhagen AP, Ramaekers FC, Aalders TW, Schaafsma HE, Debruyne FM, Schalken JA. Colocalization of basal and luminal cell-type cytokeratins in human prostate cancer. Cancer Res 1992;52:6182–7.
84. Reiter RE, Gu Z, Watabe T, Thomas G, Szigeti K, Davis E, et al. Prostate stem cell antigen: a cell surface marker overexpressed in prostate cancer. Proc Natl Acad Sci USA 1998;95:1735–40.
85. Li H, Chen X, Calhoun-Davis T, Claypool K, Tang DG. PC3 human prostate carcinoma cell holoclones contain self-renewing tumor-initiating cells. Cancer Res 2008;68:1820–5.
86. Patrawala L, Calhoun T, Schneider-Broussard R, Li H, Bhatia B, Tang S, et al. Highly purified CD44+ prostate cancer cells from xenograft human tumors are enriched in tumorigenic and metastatic progenitor cells. Oncogene 2006;25:1696–708.
87. Patrawala L, Calhoun-Davis T, Schneider-Broussard R, Tang DG. Hierarchical organization of prostate cancer cells in xenograft tumors: the CD44+ α2β1+ cell population is enriched in tumor-initiating cells. Cancer Res 2007;67:6796–805.

18

Adult Prostate Epithelium Renewal, Stem Cells and Cancer

Chiara Grisanzio and Sabina Signoretti

ABSTRACT

Cancer is thought to develop from the neoplastic transformation of either stem cells that maintain the ability to self-renew or committed progenitor cells that undergo dedifferentiation and acquire stem cell characteristics. Thus, understanding prostate cell differentiation lineage during development as well as prostate epithelium renewal in adulthood represents a critical step in unraveling the mechanisms involved in prostate carcinogenesis. Recent advances in the field have started to clarify the hierarchical relationship between epithelial prostate cells. In addition, prostate cell populations with characteristics of stem cells have been identified. Further clarification of the processes that regulate normal prostate homeostasis is likely to shed additional light on the multistep process of prostate tumorigenesis.

Key Words: Adult, Prostate, Epithelium, Stem cells, Cancer, Development, Maintenance, Renewal

INTRODUCTION

Prostate cancer is the most frequent malignancy in men in the western world and the second leading cause of death from cancer in the United States *(1)*. Considerable effort is being placed in trying to clarify the molecular events underlying its development.

Normal tissue homeostasis is thought to depend on stem cell renewal and generation of committed progenitors that eventually give raise to differentiated cells. Similarly to other systems, cell proliferation and differentiation programs that regulate the renewal of the normal prostate epithelium are controlled by finely tuned mechanisms. Cancer occurs when such mechanisms are disrupted. Dysregulation of genes and pathways involved in the development, growth, and maintenance of normal prostate cells are likely to play a role in prostate carcinogenesis *(2–8)*.

It has become increasingly clear that the identification of the cell type(s) involved in neoplastic transformation is critical for unraveling the multistep process of tumorigenesis. In this respect, the characterization of stem cells of the normal prostate and their differentiation lineages is of great interest, as it will likely accelerate our understanding of the mechanisms underlying prostate cancer development and progression. In this chapter, we review the current knowledge on prostate stem cells and their possible involvement in normal epithelial homeostasis and cancer.

From: *Cancer Drug Discovery and Development: Stem Cells and Cancer,*
Edited by: R.G. Bagley and B.A. Teicher, DOI: 10.1007/978-1-60327-933-8_18,
© Humana Press, a part of Springer Science+Business Media, LLC 2009

THE ADULT PROSTATE GLAND

The prostate is an exocrine gland that surrounds the urethra at the base of the bladder and functions by producing proteins and ions that form the major fraction of the seminal fluid. Its presence has been described only in mammals and its function is dispensable for both survival and basal levels of fertility *(9)*. The human prostate gland is small during childhood, weighing around 2 g, and increases in size during puberty, reaching a weight of approximately 20 g in adulthood *(10)*. The normal adult prostate has a very slow growth rate. A daily renewal of about 1–2% of the cells is balanced by low rates of apoptotic cell death, resulting in a growth quiescent organ *(11–13)*. Accordingly, the weight of the gland remains fairly stable until the end of the third decade, when it tends to slowly increase due to a process of hyperplasia of both stromal and epithelial cells known as benign prostatic hyperplasia (BPH) *(14)*.

Several similarities and differences in the gross and microscopic anatomy of the human and murine prostate have been described. Classically, the developing human prostate has been divided into five lobes, namely the anterior, posterior, right and left lateral, and middle lobes. However, this anatomical arrangement is recognizable only in the embryo. The adult human prostate gland is instead subdivided into four biologically and anatomically different glandular regions defined as the peripheral, central, transitional, and periuretheral zones *(15)*. These four regions, which are tightly fused together within a common capsule and quite difficult to dissect, are differently involved in the development of pathological conditions. Of note, more than 80% of prostate cancers arise in the peripheral zone (PZ), which contains 70% of the prostate glandular elements *(16, 17)*.

On the other hand, the murine prostate consists of four easily distinguishable lobes: anterior, ventral, lateral, and dorsal. A mesothelial-lined capsule separates the lobes from one another *(18, 19)*. As opposed to the human prostate, the mouse gland is also characterized by the presence of very modest fibromuscular stroma surrounding the ducts *(20)*. Despite the differences, there is general agreement that the murine prostate represents a relevant and invaluable model for studying prostate development and carcinogenesis in humans *(21)*.

At microscopic examination, both the human and mouse glands consist of ducts lined by two layers of cells: a basal layer of low cuboidal cells surmounted by a luminal layer of columnar cells (i.e., secretory cells). Scattered neuroendocrine cells are localized on the basal layer, without extending to the lumina. In addition to the glandular part, the prostate gland contains a stromal component made of smooth muscle cells, fibroblasts, and myofibroblasts, as well as endothelial cells *(22–24)*.

The expression of molecular markers allows a clear differentiation among basal, secretory, and neuroendocrine cells. Secretory cells express prostate specific antigen (PSA), androgen receptor (AR), and low molecular weight cytokeratins (LMWCK) 8 and 18 *(25)*. The basal cell layer is characterized by the expression of high molecular weight cytokeratins (HMWCK) 5 and 14, as well as p63 *(25)*. In contrast to the secretory cells, basal cells express either low or undetectable AR levels. Neuroendocrine cells are rich in serotonin-containing granules, express chromogranin-A, and are negative for AR or PSA expression.

DEVELOPMENT OF THE PROSTATE

The prostate gland develops from the urogenital sinus (UGS), which is a midline structure that consists of an endodermally derived epithelial layer surrounded by a mesodermally derived mesenchymal layer. The prostate is initially formed by solid outgrowths of the UGS epithelium (i.e., prostatic buds) into the UGS mesenchyme *(12)*. As for many other glandular organs, epithelial-mesenchymal interactions are crucial for prostate formation *(18, 26)*.

The human gland starts developing during the third intrauterine month, reaching completion in the postnatal life, at sexual maturity *(15)*. Between the 11th and 14th weeks of postnatal life, the prostatic buds acquire a lumen and develop into tubulo-acinar glands. These structures remain small until puberty, when they increase in size and acquire cytological characteristics of the adult prostate due to the stimulation of high levels of androgens *(27)*. In mice, prostate organogenesis takes place through a similar process that starts at 17.5 days of gestation *(28, 29)*. Structural and cytological differentiation of the murine prostate occurs during the first 2–3 weeks after birth *(20, 30)*.

Considerable interest is focused on the identification of key molecules and pathways that regulate normal prostate formation and growth, due to their possible relevance to prostatic disease. Functional studies in animal models, tissues, or primary cells, have convincingly demonstrated that prostate development is under the control of several genes. Among these, p63, Sonic Hedgehog, Nkx3.1, and Notch-1 are of particular interest as they have been implicated in stem cell function and/or prostate carcinogenesis *(2–4)*.

p63

The p53-homolog p63 is highly expressed in normal prostate basal cells and is a clinically useful biomarker for the diagnosis of prostate cancer *(31, 32)*. Unlike p53, p63 plays a critical role in the regulation of epithelial cell development. p63-deficient (p63−/−) mice are born with severe developmental defects, i.e., striking craniofacial abnormalities, limb truncations, and agenesis of the epidermis and of the mammary, salivary, and lachrymal glands *(33, 34)*. Major abnormalities in the development of the urothelium are also observed *(34)*. The p63−/− mice die at day 1 because of maternal neglect and dehydration *(33, 34)*. Recent experimental evidence suggests that p63 is required for maintaining the proliferative potential of stem cells in epithelial tissues *(35)*.

Work from our group demonstrated that the UGS epithelium of p63−/− newborn mice fails to become stratified and is composed by a pseudostratified cell layer, in which cells with morphologic and phenotypic features of basal cells cannot be identified. Most importantly, prostate buds are not detectable at birth *(32)*. The agenesis of the early prostate in the p63−/− mice suggests that p63 is required for the formation of prostate stem cells that reside in the basal layer of the UGS epithelium. However, since the prostate undergoes significant postnatal development and p63−/− mice only survive a few hours after birth, the possibility that p63 deficiency simply causes a developmental delay in the prostate cannot be excluded. To study postnatal development of the p63-deficient prostate, both our group and others utilized renal grafting of the UGS *(36, 37)*. In these experiments, the UGS was isolated from p63−/− male embryos, implanted under the kidney capsule of recipient wild-type mice, and analyzed a few months after engrafting. Histological evaluation of the grafts showed the presence of glandular structures containing cells with molecular and histological characteristics of prostate secretory cells (i.e., positive for AR, CK8, and Nkx3.1 expression), while basal cells were completely absent. Surprisingly, the glands were also lined by mucus-secreting cells, which focally expressed markers of intestinal differentiation (e.g., Cdx-2). Interestingly, both the intestinal and prostate epithelia originate from the embryonic endoderm. However, in contrast to what is observed in the prostate, p63 is neither expressed in the intestine nor is it necessary for its development. Thus, our findings seem to suggest that p63 deficiency in the UGS endoderm prevents its full commitment to the prostate cell lineage and allows it to differentiate toward the p63-independent intestinal cell lineage.

Sonic Hedgehog

The hedgehog (Hh) family, originally identified in Drosophila, plays an important role in normal fetal development and tissue polarity *(38)*. Three family members have been identified in mammals:

Sonic Hedgehog (Shh), Desert Hedgehog (Dhh), and Indian Hedgehog (Ihh) *(39, 40)*. Several studies have demonstrated that Shh is critical for the development of several organs and structures, including the neural tube, gastrointestinal tract, pancreas, hair follicle, limbs, craniofacial bones, salivary glands, and lungs *(41–47)*. A recent study demonstrated that Shh and Dhh are both expressed in the epithelial compartment of the human developing prostate, suggesting their involvement in the regulation of human prostate organogenesis *(48)*. In mice, Shh is expressed in the epithelial cells of the UGS and specifically in the growing prostatic buds. The levels of expression decline after gestation and are scarcely detected during adulthood *(49–51)*. Antibody blockade of Hh in a renal grafting model inhibited prostate development and growth *(50)*, strongly suggesting that Shh plays a critical role in prostate development. Several studies have also shown that inhibition of Hh-signaling by cyclopamine has significant consequences on morphogenesis and differentiation of the prostate buds *(51–54)*. On the other hand, a study performed on Shh null mice demonstrated that the UGS of the mutant mice could form prostate buds in culture, and if transplanted under the renal capsule of a male host mouse, it could undergo budding and branching morphogenesis, resembling the normal prostate *(52)*. In this scenario, functional compensation by other members of the Hh signaling pathway has been proposed as a mechanism to overcome the absence of Shh. In support of this hypothesis, a recent study suggests that Ihh provides functional redundancy for Shh during prostate organogenesis *(55)*.

Moreover, Hh signaling has been implicated in the proliferation of stem/progenitor cells from various tissues/organs *(56–61)*. Further studies are needed to clarify whether the Hh pathway plays a role in prostate stem cell functions.

Nkx3.1

Nkx3.1 belongs to the NK-homeobox gene family, first identified in Drosophila *(62)*. The function of Nkx factors involves cell-type specification and organogenesis *(63)*. Murine Nkx3.1 is expressed in the male reproductive system *(64–67)*, as well as the dorsal aorta and the kidneys *(65)*.

In the genitourinary system, Nkx3.1 mRNA starts to be expressed in the lateral aspects of the UGS epithelium as early as 15.5 days of gestation, before prostate formation. In the early prostate, Nkx3.1 protein expression is detected in the whole epithelium but once the prostate ducts canalize, it becomes restricted to the secretory cell compartment *(3, 67)*. Targeted disruption of Nkx3.1 in the mouse results in defects in prostate ductal morphogenesis and in the production of secretory proteins *(67–69)*. In addition, Nkx3.1-deficient mice display prostatic epithelial hyperplasia and dysplasia that increases in severity with age. Several studies seem to support the hypothesis that Nkx.3.1 loss of function is implicated in prostate carcinogenesis *(3, 70)*.

Notch

The Notch signaling pathway is critical for cell-cell interaction, cell proliferation, and differentiation both during development and adult life *(71–73)*. To date four Notch genes have been described: Notch1, Notch2, Notch3, and Notch4. Of these, Notch1 has been shown to be expressed at high levels in the basal cells of the developing prostate *(4)*. Wang and colleagues generated a transgenic mouse line in which the Notch1-expressing cells could be selectively ablated by expressing the bacterial nitroreductase under the control of the Notch1 promoter. Results from this study demonstrated that Notch1-expressing cells are necessary for prostate branching morphogenesis during development and prostate cell regrowth following castration and androgen-induced regeneration *(74)*. These findings suggested that Notch1-expressing basal cells may represent the prostate progenitor/stem cells. In a more recent study, by using a conditional Notch1 gene deletion mouse model, the same group of investigators found that inactivation of Notch1 signaling resulted in prostatic alterations, including enhanced epithelial proliferation and impaired differentiation *(75)*. Taken together, these data strongly suggest that the Notch pathway plays an important role in regulating normal prostate epithelium growth and differentiation.

PROSTATE EPITHELIUM HOMEOSTASIS

The existence of a stem cell population within the prostate has been strongly supported by androgen cycling experiments from English and colleagues *(76)*. These studies have shown that castration of rodents causes prostate gland atrophy due to a process of apoptosis that mainly involves secretory cells. In response to androgen readministration, the gland regenerates and resumes its normal function. The authors suggested a hierarchical stem cell model of prostate cell maintenance according to which a basal stem cell layer generates transient amplifying cells that in turn develop into terminally differentiated secretory cells *(77)*.

Several findings support the hypothesis that secretory cells derive from progenitor basal cells. For example, a prostate cell line with a basaloid phenotype has been shown to generate cells that express secretory cell markers *(78, 79)*. Moreover, prostate epithelial cells with an intermediate phenotype between basal and secretory cells have been observed both with in vitro and in vivo experiments *(22, 80–86)*. Indeed, the prostate epithelium contains cells that express cytokeratins 5 and 8 but are negative for cytokeratin 14 expression *(84, 87)*. Such cells are thought to represent the transient amplifying cell population that is derived from basal stem cells and give rise to secretory cells. Interestingly, immunohistochemical analysis performed by Wang et al. have more recently shown that both human and mouse UGS epithelia are highly enriched for cells that express both secretory and basal cell markers *(85)*. On the basis of these observations, the authors have hypothesized that cells with intermediate characteristics represent prostate epithelial stem cells. Importantly, such cells have been sporadically identified also in the basal layer of the adult prostate, raising the possibility that they might represent the adult stem cells.

In line with the concept that stem cells are located in the basal cell compartment, other experiments have demonstrated that in both human and rodent prostate epithelia, basal cells display a higher proliferation rate than secretory cells *(88, 89)*. More specifically, the proliferation capacity of the basal cells has been shown to exceed that of the secretory cell compartment by a factor of seven *(88)*. It has also been proposed that a fraction of basal cells, capable of surviving in low androgen environments, is responsible for regenerating the androgen sensitive secretory prostate epithelium after castration and subsequent androgen administration *(22, 87, 90)*. Importantly, basal cells are characterized by the expression of bcl-2, a protein that is frequently upregulated in stem cells from other tissues *(84)*.

Significant progress in the understanding of the role of basal cells in several epithelial compartments has been achieved with the identification of the p63 gene and the discovery of its restricted expression in the basal layer of various epithelial organs *(31, 33, 34)*. Our group has previously demonstrated that, within the normal prostate epithelium, p63 is selectively expressed in the basal cells and is consistently absent in the secretory and neuroendocrine cells *(32)*. Double immunohistochemistry for p63 and HMWCK showed colocalization of the two antigens in the majority of basal cells. However, a small subset of p63-positive and HMWCK-negative cells was also observed, suggesting that the prostate basal cell compartment is functionally heterogeneous and might contain cells in different stages of differentiation. As already mentioned above, p63 was also found to be essential for normal prostate development. Specifically, by analyzing the genitourinary tract of the p63-deficient mice, we demonstrated that p63 is required for the formation of prostate buds and the development of prostate basal cells. In order to investigate the role of the basal cells as stem cells during normal prostate organogenesis, we subsequently constructed a novel mouse model based on the complementation of p63–/– embryos by normal embryonic stem (ES) cells *(36)*. In this model, the injection of normal (i.e., p63+/+) ES cells into p63–/– blastocysts generated chimeric mice with a morphologically normal prostate. In line with the finding that p63 is required for basal cell differentiation, the prostate of the chimeras contained entirely ES-cell-derived basal cells (Fig. 1a). Importantly, by assessing whether or not the secretory cells of the rescued prostate were also entirely derived from the injected ES cells, we were able to clarify the hierarchical relation between basal and secretory cells (Fig. 1b, c). Indeed, the observation that the whole epithelium was exclusively populated by cells that originated from the normal ES cells, in both the developing prostatic buds and the mature prostate, allowed us to conclude that secretory cells of the adult prostate derive from p63-positive progenitor/stem cells that constitute the prostate buds (Fig. 1d).

The finding that basal and secretory prostate cells are hierarchically related during development suggests that basal cells of the adult prostate might retain the capability to differentiate into secretory

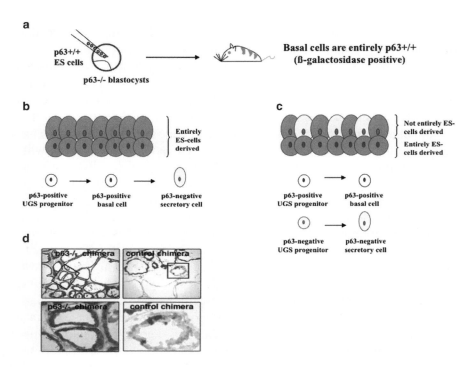

Fig. 1. p63-deficient blastocyst complementation. (**a**) Chimeric mice were created by injecting p63–/– blastocysts with p63+/+ ES cells constitutively expressing the β-galactosidase gene. As expected, the prostate of the rescued chimeras contained entirely ES-cell-derived basal cells. Insights on prostate cell lineages could be achieved by evaluating the relative contribution of the p63+/+ and p63–/– cells to the secretory cell compartment. (**b, c**). Models of epithelial development based on possible outcomes of blastocyst complementation experiments. In one scenario (**b**), both secretory cells and basal cells originate from the p63+/+ (β-galactosidase-positive) ES cells, indicating that the secretory cell compartment is derived from the p63-positive basal cell layer. In the alternative scenario (**c**), the secretory compartment is composed of both p63+/+ and p63–/– cells, implying that the basal and secretory cell compartments are not hierarchically related. (**d**) The results of our experiments show that only p63+/+ (β-galactosidase-positive) cells are present in the prostate epithelium (*left panels*) of rescued chimeras. In contrast, both β-galactosidase-positive and β-galactosidase-negative cells are detected in the prostate of control chimeras generated by injecting p63+/+ β-galactosidase-positive ES cells into p63+/+ blastocysts (*right panels*). Figure modified from Signoretti et al. *(36) (see Color Plates)*.

cells and thus function as adult stem cells. However, the role of basal cells in the maintenance of the adult prostate epithelium remains unclear and needs further investigation. It is generally believed that differentiated cells are postmitotic and are thus maintained by the proliferation of specialized progenitor/stem cells. Nevertheless, the concept that differentiated cells can be sustained by self-duplication is supported by recent findings in the endocrine pancreas. Two independent lineage tracing studies have surprisingly shown that the in vivo growth and regeneration of insulin-secreting beta-cells is based on self-renewal and does not involve specialized progenitor cells *(91, 92)*.

In the prostate, cell kinetic studies have unequivocally demonstrated that secretory cells are capable of proliferating in vivo *(76, 89, 93)*, raising the possibility that this cell compartment might be self-sustaining. Such analyses have also shown that upon androgen readministration after castration, a proliferative response is obtained mainly in the secretory cell compartment *(76, 93)*. In line with these findings, there is evidence that during rat prostate development the largest fraction of proliferating cells is contained within the secretory cell compartment *(89)*. Tsujimura and colleagues performed pulse-chase labeling experiments to identify label-retaining (slow cycling) cells within the prostate epithelium after castration-induced degeneration and androgen-induced regeneration of the mouse prostate *(94)*. In this study, the highest number of slow cycling cells was found within the proximal region of prostatic ducts. Epithelial cells isolated from the proximal ducts were also characterized by a greater in vitro proliferative capacity when compared to cells from the distal prostate region. Interestingly, label-retaining cells identified in vivo were present in both the basal and secretory layers. Although these findings can be explained by the presence of early transient amplifying cells within the secretory compartment, they seem to reinforce the concept that distinct basal and secretory progenitor/stem cells might exist. In accordance with the hypothesis that secretory cells are self-renewing and that progenitor/stem cells are proximally located, secretory cells of the proximal ducts have been shown to be less sensitive to androgen withdrawal after castration, whereas the intermediate and distal regions of the gland undergo rapid involution upon androgen deprivation *(28)*.

In summary, the way the prostate epithelium is renewed either in physiological conditions or after cell injury remains largely unknown. Further studies, including in vivo tracing of specific cell types and their progeny within the adult prostate will be invaluable in clarifying this important issue.

PROSTATE STEM CELL ASSAYS

Adult stem cells are defined by their capacity to self-renew and to generate terminally differentiated cells. There is evidence for adult stem cells in various organs, including bone marrow, blood vessels, peripheral blood, gastrointestinal tract, skeletal muscle, skin, breast, lung, and liver *(95–104)*.

The development of functional in vitro and in vivo assays to detect stem cell properties of a candidate cell population is a critical step in stem cell research. Recent advances in the development of cell culture systems have led to the optimization of in vitro procedures to test the self-renewal of prostate cell subpopulations by investigating known characteristics of stem cells, including colony-forming efficiency and ability to form spheroids.

Hudson et al. undertook a clonal analysis of cells isolated from freshly collected human prostate tissue. Primary cultures were grown at clonal density on a feeder layer of lethally irradiated NIH 3T3 cells, and two types of colonies were identified *(105)*. These colonies (named type I and II) were distinguished on the basis of their morphology, phenotype, and rate of growth. Specifically, Type I colonies were relatively small and irregular and contained a loose mixture of cells expressing both basal and secretory cell markers. In contrast, type II colonies were large, round, and homogeneous, and consisted almost exclusively of small undifferentiated and dividing cells with a basal cell phenotype. Type I colonies were approximately ten times more frequent than type II colonies and only about 1 in

200 of the plated cells was capable of forming a type II colony. Based on their results, the authors concluded that type II colonies may be the progeny of stem cells and the type I colonies derived from a more differentiated transit-amplifying population.

Lawson and collaborators recently utilized similar growth conditions to assess the colony-forming efficiency of murine epithelial prostate cells. Mixtures of prostate cells from transgenic animals expressing either green fluorescent protein (GFP) or red fluorescent protein from Discosoma (DsRed) were utilized to demonstrate that colonies were predominantly of clonal origin. When serial dilutions of prostate cells from wild-type mice were analyzed, the number of colonies grown at each dilution was proportional to the number of input cells. Moreover, the authors demonstrated that cells from castrated animals are at least fivefold enriched for colony-forming activity when compared with cells from intact animals. Taken together these data indicate that this colony-forming assay can be successfully utilized to test for prostate cell self-renewal capacities *(106)*.

Stem cells have the ability to proliferate in suspension culture, where they clonally generate spherical colonies (i.e., spheres). It has been shown that both mammary and neural cells can generate spheres when cultured on a nonadhesive substratum in serum-free medium supplemented with peptide growth factors. The stem cell properties of these cells was proved by serial passaging and differentiation along multiple lineages *(107–110)*. Work performed by Owen Witte's group recently demonstrated that murine prostate cells plated in vitro in laminin containing matrigel medium were able to grow and form prostate spheres *(106, 111)*. Of note, these spheres could be serially passaged individually or in bulk to generate daughter spheres with similar characteristics. The self-renewing ability was, however, limited, as only 1–2% of sphere cells formed new spheres upon replating. Nevertheless, prostate spheres spontaneously differentiated into basal and transit-amplifying cell types and could form glandular structures resembling murine prostate tissue in reconstitution experiments. In line with these findings, Shi et al. showed that the regenerative capacity of mouse prostate epithelial cells is rapidly lost when the cells are placed in monolayer culture but can be maintained by culture in anchorage-independent conditions *(112)*. Cells grown in spheres could be serially passaged and exhibited increased expression of putative stem cell markers as compared to cells grown in monolayer culture. Most importantly, passaged spheres were also capable of generating fully differentiated mouse prostate glands, when grafted in vivo. Overall, these data indicate that in vitro suspension culture systems might represent an important new tool for the study of prostate progenitor/stem cells.

Although in vitro assays are of paramount importance in assessing the self-renewal abilities of candidate stem cells, the gold standard for testing stem cell activity is represented by in vivo reconstitution experiments. For instance, bone marrow engraftment and cleared mammary gland fat pad transplantation methods have been classically utilized to study stem cells in the hematopoietic system and the breast, respectively. Cunha's group pioneered an in vivo prostate reconstitution assay in which prostate epithelial tissue fragments and embryonic urogenital sinus mesenchyme (UGM) coengrafted under the kidney capsule of recipient mice are able to regenerate prostate structures *(113)*. In vivo prostate reconstitution has been extensively utilized to study both normal prostate development and prostate carcinogenesis. More recently, this assay has been successfully modified to identify stem cells in the rodent prostate *(106, 114, 115)*. Specifically, Xin and colleagues were the first to utilize dissociated cell populations isolated from postnatal prostate epithelia and embryonic UGM *(115)*. This approach has proven invaluable in investigating the efficiency of candidate stem cell subpopulation in regenerating branching prostate glandular structures, within the subcapsular space of the kidney. Lynette Wilson's group recently employed serial in vivo prostate reconstitution experiments to study the regenerative potential of cells isolated from proximal ducts. Of note, primitive cells from the proximal prostatic region could be passaged through four generations of subrenal capsule grafts *(116)*.

An alternative in vivo method for assessing the repopulating capacity of prostate stem cells is based on subcutaneous engraftment of either matrigel or collagen containing a single-cell suspension from adult prostate cells *(117, 118)*. In this system, prostatic duct-like structures containing both basal and secretory cells can be observed in the gel a few weeks after transplantation. Interestingly, when a mixture with both EGFP-positive and negative prostate cells was transplanted, prostatic ducts consisted of either EGFP-positive or negative cells, suggesting that ducts were reconstituted from a single cell *(117)*.

ISOLATION OF PROSTATE STEM CELLS

In line with studies performed in the hematopoietic system where stem cells are isolated by means of specific antibodies recognizing surface antigens, several investigators have attempted to purify adult prostate cells with stem/progenitor characteristics by using cell surface markers *(114, 119, 120)*. However, none of the proposed markers appear to be specific for prostate stem cells *(121, 122)*.

Stem cell antigen 1 (Sca-1) is a cell surface protein of the Ly6 gene family, originally identified as an antigen upregulated on activated lymphocytes *(123)*. Sca-1 is the most common marker used to enrich adult murine hematopoietic stem cells and it is also utilized in combination with negative selection against mature markers for enrichment of stem and progenitor cells from a wide variety of murine tissues and organs *(123)*. Recently, Sca-1 expression was successfully utilized to isolate murine prostate cells with stem/progenitor cell-like features. Analysis of murine prostate tissue showed that Sca-1 is expressed in approximately 15% of prostatic cells and that a sixfold increase in Sca-1-positive cells occurs after castration *(114)*. Sca-1 is also expressed in the early stages of prostate organogenesis, suggesting that its expression could also identify prostate stem cells during development *(2)*. Importantly, engrafting experiments in immunodeficient recipient mice demonstrated that the Sca-1-positive cells display an in vivo proliferation capacity significantly higher than the Sca-1-negative cells *(114, 119)*. It has also been reported that the Sca-1-positive cells are more abundant in the proximal region of prostate ducts, where low-cycling putative progenitor cells have been shown to reside. In line with the hypothesis that the proximal ducts represent the prostate stem cell niche, Sca-1-positive cells isolated from this region were more effective in reconstituting prostate tissue when compared Sca-1-positive cells collected from the remaining areas of the gland *(119)*.

Immunohistochemical and flow cytometric analyses have demonstrated that CD49f (integrin $\alpha6$) expression could be utilized to discriminate prostate basal cells. By sorting the Sca-1$^+$CD49f$^+$ prostate cells, Lawson et al. showed that this population displayed higher colony forming activity as compared to the unfractionated cells *(106)*. Because non-epithelial cell lineages within the prostate also express CD49f and Sca-1, negative selection using hematopoietic (CD45, Ter119), and endothelial (CD31) lineage markers was performed to further enrich for prostate progenitor/stem cells. Importantly, sorting for cells with a CD45$^-$CD31$^-$Ter119$^-$Sca-1$^+$CD49f$^+$ antigenic profile resulted in a 60-fold enrichment for colony- and sphere-forming cells. Interestingly, these results indicated a similarity in cell surface profile between murine prostate and mammary gland stem cells and suggested that these markers may be conserved among epithelial stem cell populations *(101, 106)*.

CD44 is a transmembrane glycoprotein that functions as an extracellular matrix receptor involved in cell–cell interactions, cell adhesion, and migration in normal and tumor cells. It binds to hyaluronic acid and other ligands, including collagens, osteopontin, and matrix metalloproteases (MMPs) *(124)*. In prostatic glands, CD44 expression is observed mainly in basal cells but also in cytokeratin 14-negative, cytokeratin 19-positive intermediate cells *(125)*. Of note, Liu and coworkers showed that when the purified CD44-positive population is cocultured with stromal cells in the presence of dihydrotestosterone and matrigel, it is able to produce PSA, possibly reflecting its differentiation into secretory cells *(23)*. Thus, the CD44-positive cells seem to possess some characteristics of stem cells.

CD133, a human homolog of mouse prominin-1, is a five-transmembrane domain cell surface glyco-protein originally found on neuroepithelial stem cells in mice *(126)*. In humans, CD133 expression is restricted to undifferentiated cells that include endothelial progenitor cells *(127)*, hematopoietic stem cells *(128)*, fetal brain stem cells *(129)*, embryonic epithelium *(126, 130)*, and myogenic cells *(131)*. There is evidence that CD133 might also be a marker of prostate stem cells. CD133 is expressed in a small number of prostate epithelial cells with high in vitro proliferative potential. Immunofluorescence analysis indicated that such cells are localized in the basal cell compartment. The CD133-positive cells were also shown to coexpress high levels of integrin $\alpha2\beta1$, another putative prostate stem cell marker *(120)*. Finally, the CD133-positive cells displayed high colony-formation efficiency in vitro, and most importantly, were capable of reconstituting the prostate epithelium in vivo *(120)*.

A marker independent strategy to isolate putative stem cells from a variety of human and murine cell types relies on the ability of these cells to pump out the vital dye Hoechst 33342 through an active process that involves members of the ABC (ATP-Binding Cassette) transporter proteins *(132)*. Hoechst 33342 is a DNA-binding dye that binds preferentially to A-T rich regions of DNA. Goodell and colleagues were the first to identify a population of cells (called side population or SP) in the murine bone marrow that appeared particularly efficient in excluding the Hoechst dye *(133)*. Importantly, the SP cells were shown to have stem cell properties. There is now evidence that putative stem cells from solid tissues also possess this SP phenotype *(132)*. A side population recently isolated from primary prostate tissue accounted for approximately 1% of all epithelial cells. Interestingly, dual staining revealed that the SP fraction was highly enriched for basal integrin $\alpha2$-positive cells. Cell cycle analysis showed that the majority of SP cells were in either G0 or G1 *(134)*. Although, these features are consistent with a stem cell phenotype, further analyses are needed to characterize the prostate SP cells with respect to stem cells properties.

PROSTATE STEM CELLS AND CANCER

Prostate cancer is the sixth most common cancer in the world, and among men together with lung and colon cancer it is the most frequent form of malignancy *(135)*. In the last decades, the overall mortality from prostate cancer has been declining, due to significant advances in early detection and prevention. Nevertheless, the long-term survival of patients with metastatic disease has not changed significantly. Great hope lies in the development of new agents with higher specificity and decreased toxicity.

Cancer develops through the progressive acquisition of multiple genetic and epigenetic changes. There is increasing evidence that the molecular alterations required for cancer development might vary according to the differentiation stage of the cell that undergoes neoplastic transformation *(136, 137)*. An important implication of these novel findings is that the identification of the cell(s) of origin of prostate cancer is absolutely necessary for a full understanding of the molecular events leading to prostate cancer and the potential development of more effective therapies that specifically target such events.

The cell population that constitutes the majority of prostate cancers has secretory features and expresses low molecular weight cytokeratines, androgen receptor, and PSA. As a consequence, it has been classically assumed that prostate carcinoma originates from the malignant transformation of secretory cells *(138)*. However, several immunohistochemical studies have demonstrated that some prostate tumors, mainly in the androgen-independent stage, harbor a cell population coexpressing basal and secretory cells markers, suggesting that they might originate from a putative basal stem/

progenitor cell *(22, 80–86, 139)*. A recent study in a *Pten*-null murine model of prostate cancer appears to support such hypothesis *(140)*. Increased basal cell proliferation was, in fact, observed during the course of prostate tumor initiation and progression. *Pten* deletion in the basal cells also led to the expansion of cells expressing the Sca-1 and BCL-2 stem/progenitor markers. Thus, these findings suggest that prostate basal progenitor/stem cells might be the target of neoplastic transformation in this model.

There is increasing evidence that only a small subset of neoplastic cells with stem-like capacities [named cancer stem cells (CSCs) or cancer initiating cells] promote the maintenance and development of tumors *(141–143)*. Efforts aimed at isolating putative prostate CSCs from cultured prostate cancer cells, xenografts, and patient tumors are currently underway *(144)*. In hematologic malignancies, CSCs have been shown to derive from normal hematopoietic stem cells that undergo oncogene activation *(137)*. Alternatively, however, there is evidence that molecular alterations occurring in committed progenitor cells can cause them to become neoplastic through dedifferentiation and acquisition of self-renewal capacity *(136)*. As prostate carcinoma is a very heterogeneous disease and its cell(s) of origin remains unknown, it is possible to hypothesize that different subsets of prostate cancer derive from cell types that are in different stages of differentiation (Fig. 2). It is also tempting to speculate that the most aggressive form of prostate cancer, i.e., androgen-independent carcinoma, might develop from androgen-independent, basal stem cells.

CONCLUSIONS

Important advances have been made recently in the understanding of the processes underlying prostate cell development and differentiation. Prostate epithelial cell populations with characteristics of stem cells have been identified and their phenotype has already provided some insight in the cell of origin of prostate cancer. In addition, protein expression signatures identified in normal stem cells of various tissues are currently being utilized, singly and in combination, in the identification of putative

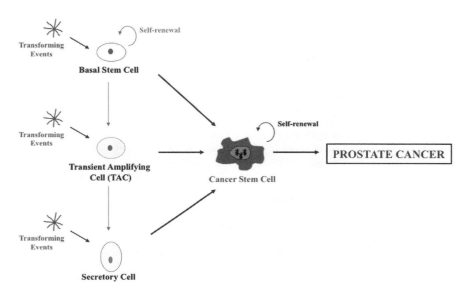

Fig. 2. Cell of origin of prostate cancer. In this proposed model, prostate cancer initiating/stem cells can originate from prostate epithelial cells that are at various stages of differentiation.

cancer stem cells. It must be stressed, however, that further clarification of the mechanisms regulating the homeostasis of the adult prostate epithelium is necessary for a complete understanding of the multi-step process of prostate tumorigenesis.

REFERENCES

1. Gronberg H. Prostate cancer epidemiology. Lancet 2003;361(9360):859–64.
2. Lawson DA, Xin L, Lukacs R, Xu Q, Cheng D, Witte ON. Prostate stem cells and prostate cancer. Cold Spring Harb Symp Quant Biol 2005;70:187–96.
3. Shen MM, Abate-Shen C. Roles of the Nkx3.1 homeobox gene in prostate organogenesis and carcinogenesis. Dev Dyn 2003;228(4):767–78.
4. Shou J, Ross S, Koeppen H, de Sauvage FJ, Gao WQ. Dynamics of notch expression during murine prostate development and tumorigenesis. Cancer Res 2001;61(19):7291–7.
5. Beachy PA, Karhadkar SS, Berman DM. Tissue repair and stem cell renewal in carcinogenesis. Nature 2004;432(7015):324–31.
6. Monk M, Holding C. Human embryonic genes re-expressed in cancer cells. Oncogene 2001;20(56):8085–91.
7. Reya T, Clevers H. Wnt signalling in stem cells and cancer. Nature 2005;434(7035):843–50.
8. Weng AP, Aster JC. Multiple niches for Notch in cancer: context is everything. Curr Opin Genet Dev 2004;14(1):48–54.
9. Abate-Shen C, Shen MM. Molecular genetics of prostate cancer. Genes Dev 2000;14(19):2410–34.
10. Hayward SW, Cunha GR. The prostate: development and physiology. Radiol Clin North Am 2000;38(1):1–14.
11. Isaacs JT, Furuya Y, Berges R. The role of androgen in the regulation of programmed cell death/apoptosis in normal and malignant prostatic tissue. Semin Cancer Biol 1994;5(5):391–400.
12. Closset J RE. Handbook of Cell Signaling, ch. Prostate; 2003.
13. Denmeade SR, Lin XS, Isaacs JT. Role of programmed (apoptotic) cell death during the progression and therapy for prostate cancer. Prostate 1996;28(4):251–65.
14. Walsh PC. Human benign prostatic hyperplasia: etiological considerations. Prog Clin Biol Res 1984;145:1–25.
15. Lowsley OS. Surgical pathology of the human prostate gland. Ann Surg 1918;68(4):399–415.
16. De Marzo AM, Meeker AK, Zha S, et al. Human prostate cancer precursors and pathobiology. Urology 2003;62(5 Suppl 1):55–62.
17. De Marzo AM, Coffey DS, Nelson WG. New concepts in tissue specificity for prostate cancer and benign prostatic hyperplasia. Urology 1999;53(3 Suppl 3a):29–39; discussion 42.
18. Cunha GR, Donjacour AA, Cooke PS, et al. The endocrinology and developmental biology of the prostate. Endocr Rev 1987;8(3):338–62.
19. McNeal JE. Normal and pathologic anatomy of prostate. Urology 1981;17(Suppl 3):11–6.
20. Marker PC, Donjacour AA, Dahiya R, Cunha GR. Hormonal, cellular, and molecular control of prostatic development. Dev Biol 2003;253(2):165–74.
21. Roy-Burman P, Wu H, Powell WC, Hagenkord J, Cohen MB. Genetically defined mouse models that mimic natural aspects of human prostate cancer development. Endocr Relat Cancer 2004;11(2):225–54.
22. Bonkhoff H, Remberger K. Differentiation pathways and histogenetic aspects of normal and abnormal prostatic growth: a stem cell model. Prostate 1996;28(2):98–106.
23. Liu AY, True LD, LaTray L, et al. Cell–cell interaction in prostate gene regulation and cytodifferentiation. Proc Natl Acad Sci USA 1997;94(20):10705–10.
24. Rizzo S, Attard G, Hudson DL. Prostate epithelial stem cells. Cell Prolif 2005;38(6):363–74.
25. Ware JL. Prostate cancer progression. Implications of histopathology. Am J Pathol 1994;145(5):983–93.
26. Wong YC, Wang XH, Ling MT. International Review of Cytology, ch. Prostate development and cytogenesis; 2003.
27. Kellokumpu-Lehtinen P, Santti R, Pelliniemi LJ. Correlation of early cytodifferentiation of the human fetal prostate and Leydig cells. Anat Rec 1980;196(3):263–73.
28. Sugimura Y, Cunha GR, Donjacour AA. Morphogenesis of ductal networks in the mouse prostate. Biol Reprod 1986;34(5):961–71.
29. Timms BG, Mohs TJ, Didio LJ. Ductal budding and branching patterns in the developing prostate. J Urol 1994;151(5):1427–32.
30. Barkley MS, Goldman BD. A quantitative study of serum testosterone, sex accessory organ growth, and the development of intermale aggression in the mouse. Horm Behav 1977;8(2):208–18.
31. Yang A, Kaghad M, Wang Y, et al. p63, a p53 homolog at 3q27–29, encodes multiple products with transactivating, death-inducing, and dominant-negative activities. Mol Cell 1998;2(3):305–16.
32. Signoretti S, Waltregny D, Dilks J, et al. p63 is a prostate basal cell marker and is required for prostate development. Am J Pathol 2000;157(6):1769–75.

33. Mills AA, Zheng B, Wang XJ, Vogel H, Roop DR, Bradley A. p63 is a p53 homologue required for limb and epidermal morphogenesis. Nature 1999;398(6729):708–13.

34. Yang A, Schweitzer R, Sun D, et al. p63 is essential for regenerative proliferation in limb, craniofacial and epithelial development. Nature 1999;398(6729):714–8.

35. Senoo M, Pinto F, Crum CP, McKeon F. p63 is essential for the proliferative potential of stem cells in stratified epithelia. Cell 2007;129(3):523–36.

36. Signoretti S, Pires MM, Lindauer M, et al. p63 regulates commitment to the prostate cell lineage. Proc Natl Acad Sci USA 2005;102(32):11355–60.

37. Kurita T, Medina RT, Mills AA, Cunha GR. Role of p63 and basal cells in the prostate. Development 2004;131(20):4955–64.

38. Ingham PW. Transducing Hedgehog: the story so far. EMBO J 1998;17(13):3505–11.

39. Weed M, Mundlos S, Olsen BR. The role of sonic hedgehog in vertebrate development. Matrix Biol 1997;16(2):53–8.

40. Ingham PW, McMahon AP. Hedgehog signaling in animal development: paradigms and principles. Genes Dev 2001;15(23):3059–87.

41. Ericson J, Muhr J, Placzek M, Lints T, Jessell TM, Edlund T. Sonic hedgehog induces the differentiation of ventral forebrain neurons: a common signal for ventral patterning within the neural tube. Cell 1995;81(5):747–56.

42. Fukuda K, Yasugi S. Versatile roles for sonic hedgehog in gut development. J Gastroenterol 2002;37(4):239–46.

43. Hebrok M, Kim SK, Melton DA. Notochord repression of endodermal Sonic hedgehog permits pancreas development. Genes Dev 1998;12(11):1705–13.

44. Niswander L, Jeffrey S, Martin GR, Tickle C. A positive feedback loop coordinates growth and patterning in the vertebrate limb. Nature 1994;371(6498):609–12.

45. Hu D, Helms JA. The role of sonic hedgehog in normal and abnormal craniofacial morphogenesis. Development 1999;126(21):4873–84.

46. Jaskoll T, Leo T, Witcher D, et al. Sonic hedgehog signaling plays an essential role during embryonic salivary gland epithelial branching morphogenesis. Dev Dyn 2004;229(4):722–32.

47. Pepicelli CV, Lewis PM, McMahon AP. Sonic hedgehog regulates branching morphogenesis in the mammalian lung. Curr Biol 1998;8(19):1083–6.

48. Zhu G, Zhau HE, He H, et al. Sonic and desert hedgehog signaling in human fetal prostate development. Prostate 2007;67(6):674–84.

49. Bitgood MJ, McMahon AP. Hedgehog and Bmp genes are coexpressed at many diverse sites of cell-cell interaction in the mouse embryo. Dev Biol 1995;172(1):126–38.

50. Podlasek CA, Barnett DH, Clemens JQ, Bak PM, Bushman W. Prostate development requires Sonic hedgehog expressed by the urogenital sinus epithelium. Dev Biol 1999;209(1):28–39.

51. Lamm ML, Catbagan WS, Laciak RJ, et al. Sonic hedgehog activates mesenchymal Gli1 expression during prostate ductal bud formation. Dev Biol 2002;249(2):349–66.

52. Berman DM, Desai N, Wang X, et al. Roles for Hedgehog signaling in androgen production and prostate ductal morphogenesis. Dev Biol 2004;267(2):387–98.

53. Freestone SH, Marker P, Grace OC, et al. Sonic hedgehog regulates prostatic growth and epithelial differentiation. Dev Biol 2003;264(2):352–62.

54. Wang BE, Shou J, Ross S, Koeppen H, De Sauvage FJ, Gao WQ. Inhibition of epithelial ductal branching in the prostate by sonic hedgehog is indirectly mediated by stromal cells. J Biol Chem 2003;278(20):18506–13.

55. Doles J, Cook C, Shi X, Valosky J, Lipinski R, Bushman W. Functional compensation in Hedgehog signaling during mouse prostate development. Dev Biol 2006;295(1):13–25.

56. Bhardwaj G, Murdoch B, Wu D, et al. Sonic hedgehog induces the proliferation of primitive human hematopoietic cells via BMP regulation. Nat Immunol 2001;2(2):172–80.

57. Lai K, Kaspar BK, Gage FH, Schaffer DV. Sonic hedgehog regulates adult neural progenitor proliferation in vitro and in vivo. Nat Neurosci 2003;6(1):21–7.

58. Machold R, Hayashi S, Rutlin M, et al. Sonic hedgehog is required for progenitor cell maintenance in telencephalic stem cell niches. Neuron 2003;39(6):937–50.

59. Zhang Y, Kalderon D. Hedgehog acts as a somatic stem cell factor in the Drosophila ovary. Nature 2001;410(6828):599–604.

60. Adolphe C, Narang M, Ellis T, Wicking C, Kaur P, Wainwright B. An in vivo comparative study of sonic, desert and Indian hedgehog reveals that hedgehog pathway activity regulates epidermal stem cell homeostasis. Development 2004;131(20):5009–19.

61. Rowitch DH, B SJ, Lee SM, Flax JD, Snyder EY, McMahon AP. Sonic hedgehog regulates proliferation and inhibits differentiation of CNS precursor cells. J Neurosci 1999;19(20):8954–65.

62. Kim Y, Nirenberg M. Drosophila NK-homeobox genes. Proc Natl Acad Sci USA 1989;86(20):7716–20.

63. Stanfel MN, Moses KA, Schwartz RJ, Zimmer WE. Regulation of organ development by the NKX-homeodomain factors: an NKX code. Cell Mol Biol (Noisy-le-grand) 2005;Suppl 51:OL785–99.

64. Bieberich CJ, Fujita K, He WW, Jay G. Prostate-specific and androgen-dependent expression of a novel homeobox gene. J Biol Chem 1996;271(50):31779–82.

65. Sciavolino PJ, Abrams EW, Yang L, Austenberg LP, Shen MM, Abate-Shen C. Tissue-specific expression of murine Nkx3.1 in the male urogenital system. Dev Dyn 1997;209(1):127–38.

66. Tanaka M, Lyons GE, Izumo S. Expression of the Nkx3.1 homobox gene during pre and postnatal development. Mech Dev 1999;85(1–2):179–82.
67. Bhatia-Gaur R, Donjacour AA, Sciavolino PJ, et al. Roles for Nkx3.1 in prostate development and cancer. Genes Dev 1999;13(8):966–77.
68. Schneider A, Brand T, Zweigerdt R, Arnold H. Targeted disruption of the Nkx3.1 gene in mice results in morphogenetic defects of minor salivary glands: parallels to glandular duct morphogenesis in prostate. Mech Dev 2000;95(1–2):163–74.
69. Tanaka M, Komuro I, Inagaki H, Jenkins NA, Copeland NG, Izumo S. Nkx3.1, a murine homolog of Drosophila bagpipe, regulates epithelial ductal branching and proliferation of the prostate and palatine glands. Dev Dyn 2000;219(2):248–60.
70. Abdulkadir SA. Mechanisms of prostate tumorigenesis: roles for transcription factors Nkx3.1 and Egr1. Ann N Y Acad Sci 2005;1059:33–40.
71. Artavanis-Tsakonas S, Rand MD, Lake RJ. Notch signaling: cell fate control and signal integration in development. Science 1999;284(5415):770–6.
72. Lai EC. Notch signaling: control of cell communication and cell fate. Development 2004;131(5):965–73.
73. Bray SJ. Notch signalling: a simple pathway becomes complex. Nat Rev Mol Cell Biol 2006;7(9):678–89.
74. Wang XD, Shou J, Wong P, French DM, Gao WQ. Notch1-expressing cells are indispensable for prostatic branching morphogenesis during development and re-growth following castration and androgen replacement. J Biol Chem 2004;279(23):24733–44.
75. Wang XD, Leow CC, Zha J, et al. Notch signaling is required for normal prostatic epithelial cell proliferation and differentiation. Dev Biol 2006;290(1):66–80.
76. English HF, Santen RJ, Isaacs JT. Response of glandular versus basal rat ventral prostatic epithelial cells to androgen withdrawal and replacement. Prostate 1987;11(3):229–42.
77. Isaacs JT, Coffey DS. Etiology and disease process of benign prostatic hyperplasia. Prostate 1989;Suppl 2:33–50.
78. Danielpour D. Transdifferentiation of NRP-152 rat prostatic basal epithelial cells toward a luminal phenotype: regulation by glucocorticoid, insulin-like growth factor-I and transforming growth factor-beta. J Cell Sci 1999;112(Pt 2):169–79.
79. Hayward SW, Haughney PC, Lopes ES, Danielpour D, Cunha GR. The rat prostatic epithelial cell line NRP-152 can differentiate in vivo in response to its stromal environment. Prostate 1999;39(3):205–12.
80. De Marzo AM, Meeker AK, Epstein JI, Coffey DS. Prostate stem cell compartments: expression of the cell cycle inhibitor p27Kip1 in normal, hyperplastic, and neoplastic cells. Am J Pathol 1998;153(3):911–9.
81. Hudson DL, Guy AT, Fry P, O'Hare MJ, Watt FM, Masters JR. Epithelial cell differentiation pathways in the human prostate: identification of intermediate phenotypes by keratin expression. J Histochem Cytochem 2001;49(2):271–8.
82. Peehl DM, Leung GK, Wong ST. Keratin expression: a measure of phenotypic modulation of human prostatic epithelial cells by growth inhibitory factors. Cell Tissue Res 1994;277(1):11–8.
83. Robinson EJ, Neal DE, Collins AT. Basal cells are progenitors of luminal cells in primary cultures of differentiating human prostatic epithelium. Prostate 1998;37(3):149–60.
84. Verhagen AP, Ramaekers FC, Aalders TW, Schaafsma HE, Debruyne FM, Schalken JA. Colocalization of basal and luminal cell-type cytokeratins in human prostate cancer. Cancer Res 1992;52(22):6182–7.
85. Wang Y, Hayward S, Cao M, Thayer K, Cunha G. Cell differentiation lineage in the prostate. Differentiation 2001;68(4–5):270–9.
86. Xue Y, Smedts F, Debruyne FM, de la Rosette JJ, Schalken JA. Identification of intermediate cell types by keratin expression in the developing human prostate. Prostate 1998;34(4):292–301.
87. Bonkhoff H. Role of the basal cells in premalignant changes of the human prostate: a stem cell concept for the development of prostate cancer. Eur Urol 1996;30(2):201–5.
88. Bonkhoff H, Stein U, Remberger K. The proliferative function of basal cells in the normal and hyperplastic human prostate. Prostate 1994;24(3):114–8.
89. Evans GS, Chandler JA. Cell proliferation studies in rat prostate. I. The proliferative role of basal and secretory epithelial cells during normal growth. Prostate 1987;10(2):163–78.
90. Bonkhoff H, Stein U, Remberger K. Multidirectional differentiation in the normal, hyperplastic, and neoplastic human prostate: simultaneous demonstration of cell-specific epithelial markers. Hum Pathol 1994;25(1):42–6.
91. Dor Y, Brown J, Martinez OI, Melton DA. Adult pancreatic beta-cells are formed by self-duplication rather than stem-cell differentiation. Nature 2004;429(6987):41–6.
92. Teta M, Rankin MM, Long SY, Stein GM, Kushner JA. Growth and regeneration of adult beta cells does not involve specialized progenitors. Dev Cell 2007;12(5):817–26.
93. Evans GS, Chandler JA. Cell proliferation studies in the rat prostate: II. The effects of castration and androgen-induced regeneration upon basal and secretory cell proliferation. Prostate 1987;11(4):339–51.
94. Tsujimura A, Koikawa Y, Salm S, et al. Proximal location of mouse prostate epithelial stem cells: a model of prostatic homeostasis. J Cell Biol 2002;157(7):1257–65.
95. Beltrami AP, Barlucchi L, Torella D, et al. Adult cardiac stem cells are multipotent and support myocardial regeneration. Cell 2003;114(6):763–76.
96. Collins CA, Olsen I, Zammit PS, et al. Stem cell function, self-renewal, and behavioral heterogeneity of cells from the adult muscle satellite cell niche. Cell 2005;122(2):289–301.

97. Herrera MB, Bruno S, Buttiglieri S, et al. Isolation and characterization of a stem cell population from adult human liver. Stem Cells 2006;24(12):2840–50.

98. Kim CF, Jackson EL, Woolfenden AE, et al. Identification of bronchioalveolar stem cells in normal lung and lung cancer. Cell 2005;121(6):823–35.

99. Merkle FT, Tramontin AD, Garcia-Verdugo JM, Alvarez-Buylla A. Radial glia give rise to adult neural stem cells in the subventricular zone. Proc Natl Acad Sci USA 2004;101(50):17528–32.

100. Oliver JA, Maarouf O, Cheema FH, Martens TP, Al-Awqati Q. The renal papilla is a niche for adult kidney stem cells. J Clin Invest 2004;114(6):795–804.

101. Stingl J, Eirew P, Ricketson I, et al. Purification and unique properties of mammary epithelial stem cells. Nature 2006;439(7079):993–7.

102. Till JE, Mc CE. A direct measurement of the radiation sensitivity of normal mouse bone marrow cells. Radiat Res 1961;14:213–22.

103. Tumbar T, Guasch G, Greco V, et al. Defining the epithelial stem cell niche in skin. Science 2004;303(5656):359–63.

104. Urbich C, Dimmeler S. Endothelial progenitor cells: characterization and role in vascular biology. Circ Res 2004;95(4):343–53.

105. Hudson DL, O'Hare M, Watt FM, Masters JR. Proliferative heterogeneity in the human prostate: evidence for epithelial stem cells. Lab Invest 2000;80(8):1243–50.

106. Lawson DA, Xin L, Lukacs RU, Cheng D, Witte ON. Isolation and functional characterization of murine prostate stem cells. Proc Natl Acad Sci USA 2007;104(1):181–6.

107. Reynolds BA, Weiss S. Clonal and population analyses demonstrate that an EGF-responsive mammalian embryonic CNS precursor is a stem cell. Dev Biol 1996;175(1):1–13.

108. Reynolds BA, Rietze RL. Neural stem cells and neurospheres – re-evaluating the relationship. Nat Methods 2005;2(5):333–6.

109. Dontu G, Abdallah WM, Foley JM, et al. In vitro propagation and transcriptional profiling of human mammary stem/progenitor cells. Genes Dev 2003;17(10):1253–70.

110. Dontu G, Jackson KW, McNicholas E, Kawamura MJ, Abdallah WM, Wicha MS. Role of Notch signaling in cell-fate determination of human mammary stem/progenitor cells. Breast Cancer Res 2004;6(6):R605–15.

111. Xin L, Lukacs RU, Lawson DA, Cheng D, Witte ON. Self-renewal and multilineage differentiation in vitro from murine prostate stem cells. Stem Cells 2007;25(11):2760–9.

112. Shi X, Gipp J, Bushman W. Anchorage-independent culture maintains prostate stem cells. Dev Biol 2007;312(1):396–406.

113. Cunha GR, Lung B. The possible influence of temporal factors in androgenic responsiveness of urogenital tissue recombinants from wild-type and androgen-insensitive (Tfm) mice. J Exp Zool 1978;205(2):181–93.

114. Xin L, Lawson DA, Witte ON. The Sca-1 cell surface marker enriches for a prostate-regenerating cell subpopulation that can initiate prostate tumorigenesis. Proc Natl Acad Sci USA 2005;102(19):6942–7.

115. Xin L, Ide H, Kim Y, Dubey P, Witte ON. In vivo regeneration of murine prostate from dissociated cell populations of postnatal epithelia and urogenital sinus mesenchyme. Proc Natl Acad Sci USA 2003;100(Suppl 1):11896–903.

116. Goto K, Salm SN, Coetzee S, et al. Proximal prostatic stem cells are programmed to regenerate a proximal–distal ductal axis. Stem Cells 2006;24(8):1859–68.

117. Azuma M, Hirao A, Takubo K, Hamaguchi I, Kitamura T, Suda T. A quantitative matrigel assay for assessing repopulating capacity of prostate stem cells. Biochem Biophys Res Commun 2005;338(2):1164–70.

118. Collins AT, Habib FK, Maitland NJ, Neal DE. Identification and isolation of human prostate epithelial stem cells based on alpha(2)beta(1)-integrin expression. J Cell Sci 2001;114(Pt 21):3865–72.

119. Burger PE, Xiong X, Coetzee S, et al. Sca-1 expression identifies stem cells in the proximal region of prostatic ducts with high capacity to reconstitute prostatic tissue. Proc Natl Acad Sci USA 2005;102(20):7180–5.

120. Richardson GD, Robson CN, Lang SH, Neal DE, Maitland NJ, Collins AT. CD133, a novel marker for human prostatic epithelial stem cells. J Cell Sci 2004;117(Pt 16):3539–45.

121. Liu H, Moy P, Kim S, et al. Monoclonal antibodies to the extracellular domain of prostate-specific membrane antigen also react with tumor vascular endothelium. Cancer Res 1997;57(17):3629–34.

122. Chang SS, Reuter VE, Heston WD, Bander NH, Grauer LS, Gaudin PB. Five different anti-prostate-specific membrane antigen (PSMA) antibodies confirm PSMA expression in tumor-associated neovasculature. Cancer Res 1999;59(13):3192–8.

123. Holmes C, Stanford WL. Concise review: stem cell antigen-1: expression, function, and enigma. Stem Cells 2007;25(6):1339–47.

124. Ponta H, Sherman L, Herrlich PA. CD44: from adhesion molecules to signalling regulators. Nat Rev Mol Cell Biol 2003;4(1):33–45.

125. Alam TN, O'Hare MJ, Laczko I, et al. Differential expression of CD44 during human prostate epithelial cell differentiation. J Histochem Cytochem 2004;52(8):1083–90.

126. Weigmann A, Corbeil D, Hellwig A, Huttner WB. Prominin, a novel microvilli-specific polytopic membrane protein of the apical surface of epithelial cells, is targeted to plasmalemmal protrusions of non-epithelial cells. Proc Natl Acad Sci USA 1997;94(23):12425–30.

127. Peichev M, Naiyer AJ, Pereira D, et al. Expression of VEGFR-2 and AC133 by circulating human CD34(+) cells identifies a population of functional endothelial precursors. Blood 2000;95(3):952–8.

128. Yin AH, Miraglia S, Zanjani ED, et al. AC133, a novel marker for human hematopoietic stem and progenitor cells. Blood 1997;90(12):5002–12.

129. Uchida N, Buck DW, He D, et al. Direct isolation of human central nervous system stem cells. Proc Natl Acad Sci USA 2000;97(26):14720–5.

130. Corbeil D, Roper K, Hellwig A, et al. The human AC133 hematopoietic stem cell antigen is also expressed in epithelial cells and targeted to plasma membrane protrusions. J Biol Chem 2000;275(8):5512–20.

131. Torrente Y, Belicchi M, Sampaolesi M, et al. Human circulating AC133(+) stem cells restore dystrophin expression and ameliorate function in dystrophic skeletal muscle. J Clin Invest 2004;114(2):182–95.

132. Challen GA, Little MH. A side order of stem cells: the SP phenotype. Stem Cells 2006;24(1):3–12.

133. Goodell MA, Brose K, Paradis G, Conner AS, Mulligan RC. Isolation and functional properties of murine hematopoietic stem cells that are replicating in vivo. J Exp Med 1996;183(4):1797–806.

134. Bhatt RI, Brown MD, Hart CA, et al. Novel method for the isolation and characterisation of the putative prostatic stem cell. Cytometry A 2003;54(2):89–99.

135. Jemal A, Siegel R, Ward E, Murray T, Xu J, Thun MJ. Cancer statistics, 2007. CA Cancer J Clin 2007;57(1):43–66.

136. Jamieson CH, Ailles LE, Dylla SJ, et al. Granulocyte-macrophage progenitors as candidate leukemic stem cells in blast-crisis CML. N Engl J Med 2004;351(7):657–67.

137. Daley GQ. Chronic myeloid leukemia: proving ground for cancer stem cells. Cell 2004;119(3):314–6.

138. De Marzo AM, Nelson WG, Meeker AK, Coffey DS. Stem cell features of benign and malignant prostate epithelial cells. J Urol 1998;160(6 Pt 2):2381–92.

139. Jones EG, Harper ME. Studies on the proliferation, secretory activities, and epidermal growth factor receptor expression in benign prostatic hyperplasia explant cultures. Prostate 1992;20(2):133–49.

140. Wang S, Garcia AJ, Wu M, Lawson DA, Witte ON, Wu H. Pten deletion leads to the expansion of a prostatic stem/progenitor cell subpopulation and tumor initiation. Proc Natl Acad Sci USA 2006;103(5):1480–5.

141. Pardal R, Clarke MF, Morrison SJ. Applying the principles of stem-cell biology to cancer. Nat Rev Cancer 2003;3(12):895–902.

142. Reya T, Morrison SJ, Clarke MF, Weissman IL. Stem cells, cancer, and cancer stem cells. Nature 2001;414(6859):105–11.

143. Tan BT, Park CY, Ailles LE, Weissman IL. The cancer stem cell hypothesis: a work in progress. Lab Invest 2006;86(12):1203–7.

144. Tang DG, Patrawala L, Calhoun T, et al. Prostate cancer stem/progenitor cells: identification, characterization, and implications. Mol Carcinog 2007;46(1):1–14.

19

Stem Cells, Angiogenesis, and Neurogenesis in Tumors

Judith A. Varner

ABSTRACT

Stem and progenitor cells promote repair of injured tissues by contributing to new blood vessel, muscle, and nerve formation. These same cells may contribute to tumor growth and spread by promoting new blood vessel growth and stimulating tumor invasiveness. Tumors can express factors that simultaneously induce both angiogenesis and neurogenesis, such as guidance receptors and ligands that regulate branching morphogenesis in neuronal and vascular systems. Vascular endothelial growth factor, brain-derived neurotrophic factor, Neuropilins, Semaphorins, Netrins, and Slit/Robos can promote branching morphogenesis of both neurons and blood vessels. Some of these factors can stimulate stem or progenitor cells to promote tumor angiogenesis and neurogenesis as well as tumor growth and spread. Innervation of tumors promotes cancer pain and can contribute to tumor spread along axons. An understanding of the mechanisms promoting development of neurons and blood vessels during tumor progression will assist in the development of new cancer therapies.

Key Words: Angiogenesis, Neurogenesis, Netrin, Semaphorin, VEGF, Neuropilin, Progenitor cell

INTRODUCTION

Neovascularization, the formation of blood vessels in embryonic and established tissues, plays important roles in development, inflammation, and wound repair. All cells require oxygen and nutrients for survival and are therefore located within the diffusion limit of oxygen of blood vessels or air. New blood vessels arise during embryogenesis by the differentiation of mesenchymal cells into endothelial cells and by the coalescence of these cells in structures with intact lumens. In older embryos and adult animals, blood vessels also arise from preexisting vessels by activation, proliferation, and migration of endothelial cells through a process named "angiogenesis" *(1)*. This process is characterized by sprouting of new capillaries from preexisting vessels; sprouting occurs when a "tip" cell migrates away from the preexisting vessels and other cells follow the path of this tip cell.

Specific growth factors, such as VEGF-A and bFGF, stimulate the proliferation, survival, and migration of quiescent endothelial cells in preexisting blood vessels. This stimulation results in the

From: *Cancer Drug Discovery and Development: Stem Cells and Cancer,*
Edited by: R.G. Bagley and B.A. Teicher, DOI: 10.1007/978-1-60327-933-8_19,
© Humana Press, a part of Springer Science + Business Media, LLC 2009

formation of new vessels during embryonic development and tumor growth (1). VEGF also promotes vasculogenesis, or the coalescence of new blood vessels from individual endothelial progenitor cells, that also occurs in tumors (2). VEGF and other factors such as SDF-1a can recruit circulating endothelial progenitor cells to tumors, where they can participate in new vessel growth. Additionally, myeloid lineage cells such as monocytes and macrophages are recruited by VEGF, SDF-1a, and other inflammatory factors and can modulate tumor angiogenesis and vasculogenesis (3).

A number of factors present in tumors promote the growth and guidance of both endothelium and neuronal cells, including vascular endothelial growth factor (VEGF) (4), basic fibroblast growth factor (bFGF) (5), neuropilins (6), netrins (7), semaphorins (8), slit/robo (9, 10), brain-derived neurotrophic factor (BDNF) (11), nerve growth factor (NGF) (12), and others. These factors have been shown to promote the development of both new blood vessels (angiogenesis) and nerves (neurogenesis). Circulating bone marrow-derived stem cells also contribute to both tumor neovascularization and neurogenesis (13).

Tumors express a number of neurotrophic factors that stimulate their own innervation (5, 6, 11, 12, 14). A key consequence of tumor innervation is cancer pain. Another consequence is tumor spread, or metastasis, along neural networks. Key neurotrophic factors such as nerve growth factor (NGF) (12), artemin (15), netrin (16, 17), BDNF (11), and even VEGF (14) play important roles in this process. For example, NGF promotes cancer pain; an anti-NGF function-blocking antibody suppresses skeletal pain induced by prostate tumor cells growing in bone (18). Tumor necrosis factor alpha, a key factor produced by most tumor cells, also stimulates neuropathic pain (19).

Neuronal innervation also promotes tumor spread along axons. A number of neurotrophic factors promote tumor invasion and metastasis. For example, netrin promotes mammary epithelial cell invasion and migration (16). Netrin-1 also promotes tumor cell survival through its receptor Deleted in Colon Carcinoma (17). Another neurotrophic factor, artemin, promotes pancreatic cancer cell invasion along pancreatic nerves (15). BDNF may also stimulate spread of tumors along nerves (11, 20, 21). Increased BDNF is observed in several tumors, including orthotopic hepatocellular carcinoma, multiple myeloma, and neuroblastoma, where it is a marker of a poor prognosis (20). This neurotrophic factor promotes migration and growth of multiple myeloma cells (21). It also activates TrkB, which stimulates VEGF expression in neuroblastoma cells (11). Thus, neurogenesis in tumors contributes significantly to cancer pathology.

SIMILARITIES BETWEEN TUMOR ANGIOGENESIS AND INNERVATION

Importantly, a number of similarities between the development of vascular networks and neural networks have been recently characterized. Both tissues form branching networks that are regulated by guidance factors and cytokines such as netrins (7), semaphorins (8, 22), plexins (23), neuropilins (6), and VEGF (14). Both can arise from nearby tissues or by the homing of circulating bone-marrow-derived stem cells. In some tissues, neuronal cells guide endothelial cells so that newly forming vessels coordinately track along recently migrated neuronal cells. This is especially clear in the developing retina in which astrocytes guide the newly migrating endothelial cells (23).

NEUROTROPHIC FACTORS THAT PROMOTE ANGIOGENESIS

A number of neurotrophic factors promote both neurogenesis and angiogenesis. These factors include NGF (12), BNDF (11), semaphorins (8),22), plexins (22), netrins (7), and neuropilins (6). Besides stimulating neurite outgrowth, NGF promotes angiogenesis in a quail chorioallantoic membrane model of angiogenesis *(12)*. Semaphorins and their receptors, the plexins and neuropilins, regulate guidance of neurons as well as guidance of new blood vessels *(22)*. The NGF receptor (tropomyosin related kinase – TrkA) has been shown to play a key role in angiogenesis *(2)*. VEGF has been shown to promote neuronal survival *(14)*. Semaphorin D provides a link between axon guidance and angiogenesis in tumors. It is expressed by invading cells of head and neck squamous cell carcinomas, breast carcinomas, prostate, and lung and stimulates endothelial cell migration as well as neurite outgrowth. Knockdown of Semaphorin D expression inhibits tumor vascularization *(24)*.

ANGIOGENIC FACTORS THAT PROMOTE NEURONAL OUTGROWTH

A number of clinical observations suggest that angiogenesis as well as angiogenic factors promote neurogenesis *(25)*. For example, brain injury due to seizures or cerebral ischemia stimulates angiogenesis, but it also stimulates neurogenesis *(26, 27)*. Neurogenesis is also observed in patients with Huntington's disease (HD) *(28)*, Alzheimer's *(29)*, and Parkinson's *(30)* and in animal models of HD, Alzheimer's, and Parkinson's disease *(29, 30)*. Angiogenic factors promote neurogenesis; when HD transgenic R6/2 mice and wild-type mice were treated by subcutaneous administration of bFGF, five-fold more proliferating cells were observed in the subventricular zone in HD mice than in wild-type mice. bFGF also induced the recruitment of new neurons from the subventricular zone into the neostriatum and cerebral cortex of HD mice and blocked cell death in primary striatal cultures *(5)*. VEGF also promotes neuronal survival. This key angiogenic factor promoted neuronal survival in a model of diabetic sensory neuropathy *(31)*. VEGF also protects neurons from hypoxia-induced apoptosis by activating Akt and ERK *(32)*. Reduced cerebrospinal fluid levels of VEGF have been implicated in the pathogenesis of amyotrophic lateral sclerosis (ALS), suggesting a possible role for *VEGF* gene delivery of VEGF suppressed motor neuron degeneration in a rat model of ALS *(33)*. Additionally, intracerebroventricular delivery of recombinant VEGF in a SOD1 (G93A) rat model of ALS delays onset of paralysis by 17 days, improves motor performance, and prolongs survival by 22 day *(34)*. Similar delivery of VEGF improves sensory and cognitive neural functions after focal cerebral ischemia *(35, 36)*. Additional factors that promote both neurogenesis and angiogenesis include sphingosine-1-phosophate. Mice lacking S-1-P receptor exhibited failure to close neural tube and defective embryonic angiogenesis *(37)*. Together these studies show that the regulation of angiogenesis and neurogenesis are closely intertwined.

BONE-MARROW-DERIVED STEM CELLS IN TUMORS

Bone-marrow-derived, CD34+ stem or progenitor cells have been shown to promote the repair of damaged tissues, offering promise for the treatment of hereditary and acquired human diseases. These cells differentiate into endothelial cells, hematopoietic cells, and, as reported in some studies into neurons, fibroblasts, and muscle *(2)*. CD34+ CD133+ progenitor cells participate in neovascularization by differentiating into endothelial cells *(38–40)*. Neovascularization stimulates healing of injured tissues, but also promotes tumor growth and inflammatory disease *(1)*. A number of studies indicate that bone-marrow-derived cells infiltrate tumors and directly participate in neovascularization *(38, 39, 41)*, giving rise to approximately 15% of the neovasculature *(41)*.

Other studies have shown that bone-marrow-derived cells of the myeloid lineage cell also home extensively to tumors and other neovascular or repairing tissues *(42)*. Macrophages express growth factors such as VEGF that stimulate angiogenesis *(43)*. Analyses of human sex-mismatched bone marrow transplantation patients provided evidence that endothelial cells do arise from bone marrow in humans. In one study, a small percentage of vasculature of sex mismatched transplant patients was derived from the transplanted bone marrow. When patients were analyzed on average 1 year after transplantation, 2% of all endothelial cells arose from the donor bone marrow *(44)*. In another study of human sex-mismatched bone marrow transplant recipients who later developed tumors, fluorescence in situ hybridization analysis showed that approximately 5% of endothelial cells infiltrating tumors were derived from bone-marrow *(45)*. Thus, experimental and clinical data confirm the existence of bone-marrow-derived endothelial progenitors.

Recent studies indicate that bone-marrow-derived stem cells also promote neurogenesis. Mesenchymal stem cells transfected with glial-derived neurotrophic factor promoted recovery from ischemia after cerebral artery occlusion *(46)*. Granulocyte colony stimulating factor and stem cell factor both promoted neurogenesis after focal cerebral artery occlusion in mice in part by mobilizing bone-marrow-derived stem cells into the brain where they appeared to differentiate into neuronal cells *(47)*. In additional studies, damaged skeletal muscle recovered function through synchronized vasculogenesis, myogenesis, and neurogenesis after transplantation of CD34+ CD45+ cells *(48)*. In one key study, CD34+ stem cells were used to promote neurogenesis after stroke in animal models. Surprisingly, rather than directly stimulating neurogenesis, CD34+ cells promoted angiogenesis, indirectly improving neuronal function *(49)*. Additional studies support a common lineage of precursors for endothelial cells, neuronal cells, and hematopoietic cells. The Zebrafish stem cell leukemia *(scl)* gene encodes a basic helix loop helix transcription factor that is essential for angiogenesis and hematopoietic cell specification in the zebrafish embryo. An upstream genomic DNA fragment containing the scl promoter was sufficient to drive expression of EGFP in endothelial cells, hematopoietic cells and in the brain and spinal cord, suggesting the existence of common precursor cells for these distinct cell types *(50)*.

Our lab has recently identified a molecular mechanism that promotes the homing and recruitment of bone-marrow-derived progenitor cells to remodeling tissues. We found that integrin α4β1 promotes the homing of circulating bone-marrow-derived progenitor cells to the α4β1 ligands, vascular cell adhesion molecule, and cellular fibronectin, which are expressed on neovasculature of tumors and other repairing tissues *(51)*. By regulating the homing of these cells, this integrin also promotes their participation in angiogenesis and tumor growth. In addition, our studies have shown that integrin α4β1 also promotes the homing of myeloid lineage cells to tumors *(43)*.

CONCLUSIONS

Tumors express growth factors that induce both angiogenesis and neurogenesis, leading to tumor growth, tumor invasion, and tumor pain. Tumors also recruit circulating bone-marrow-derived stem or progenitor cells, which can differentiate into endothelial cells or neuronal cells, thereby participating in cancer pathogenesis. Further investigation into the roles of stem cells in tumor innervation will assist in the development of new cancer therapies.

REFERENCES

1. Carmeliet P. Angiogenesis in life, disease and medicine. Nature 2005;428:932–936.
2. Garmy-Susini B, Varner J. Circulating endothelial progenitor cells. Br J Cancer 2005;93:855–858.
3. Schmid MC, Varner JA. Myeloid cell trafficking and tumor angiogenesis. Cancer Lett 2007;250:1–8.
4. Lazarovici P, Marcinkiewicz C, Lelkes PI. Cross talk between the cardiovascular and nervous systems: neurotrophic effects of vascular endothelial growth factor (VEGF) and angiogenic effects of nerve growth factor (NGF)-implications in drug development. Curr Pharm Des 2006;12:2609–2622.
5. Jin K, LaFevre-Bernt M, Sun Y, et al. FGF-2 promotes neurogenesis and neuroprotection and prolongs survival in a transgenic mouse model of Huntington's disease. Proc Natl Acad Sci USA 2005;102:18189–18194.
6. Ellis LM. The role of neuropilins in cancer. Mol Cancer Ther 2006;5:1099–1107.

7. Freitas C, Larrivee B, Eichman A. Netrins and Unc5 receptors in angiogenesis. Angiogenesis 2008;11:23–29.
8. Neufeld G, Kessler O. The semaphorins: versatile regulators of tumour progression and tumour angiogenesis. Nat Rev Cancer 2008;8:632–645.
9. Dickson BJ, Gilestro GF. Regulation of commissural axon pathfinding by slit and its Robo receptors. Annu Rev Cell Dev Biol 2006;22:651–675.
10. Jones CA, London NR, Chen H, et al. Robo4 stabilizes the vascular network by inhibiting pathologic angiogenesis and endothelial hyperpermeability. Nat Med 2008;14:448–453.
11. Nakamura K, Martin KC, Jackson JK, et al. Brain-derived neurotrophic factor activation of TrkB induces vascular endothelial growth factor expression via hypoxiainducible factor-1 alpha in neuroblastoma cells. Cancer Res 2006;66:4249–4255.
12. Lazarovici P, Gazit A, Staniszewska I, et al. Nerve growth factor (NGF) promotes angiogenesis in the quail chorioallantoic membrane. Endothelium 2006;13:51–59.
13. Wang L, Zhang Z, Wang Y, et al. Treatment of stroke with erythropoietin enhances neurogenesis and angiogenesis and improves neurological function in rats. Stroke 2004;35:1732–1737.
14. Lazarovici P, Marcinkiewicz C, Lelkes PI. Cross talk between the cardiovascular and nervous systems: neurotrophic effects of vascular endothelial growth factor (VEGF) and angiogenic effects of nerve growth factor (NGF)-implications in drug development. Curr Pharm Des 2006;12:2609–2622.
15. Ceyhan GO, Giese NA, Erkan M, et al. The neurotrophic factor artemin promotes pancreatic cancer invasion. Ann Surg 2006;244:274–281.
16. Strizzi L, Bianco C, Raafat A, et al. Netrin-1 regulates invasion and migration of mouse mammary epithelial cells overexpressing Cripto-1 in vitro and in vivo. J Cell Sci 2005;118:4633–4643.
17. Mehlen P, Furne C. Netrin-1: when a neuronal guidance cue turns out to be a regulator of tumorigenesis. Cell Mol Life Sci 2005;62:2599–2616.
18. Halvorson KG, Kubota K, Sevcik MA, et al. A blocking antibody to nerve growth factor attenuates skeletal pain induced by prostate tumor cells growing in bone. Cancer Res 2005;65:9426–9435.
19. Xu JT, Xin WJ, Zang Y, et al. The role of tumor necrosis factor-alpha in the neuropathic pain induced by Lumbar 5 ventral root transection in rat. Pain 2006;123:306–321.
20. Yang ZF, Ho DW, Lam CT, et al. Identification of brainderived neurotrophic factor as a novel functional protein in hepatocellular carcinoma. Cancer Res 2005;65:219–225.
21. Hu Y, Sun CY, Wang HF, et al. Brain-derived neurotrophic factor promotes growth and migration of multiple myeloma cells. Cancer Genet Cytogenet 2006;169:12–20.
22. Yazdani U, Terman JR. The semaphorins. Genome Biol 2006;7:211.
23. Gariano RF, Gardner TW. Retinal angiogenesis in development and disease. Nature 2005;438:960–966.
24. Basile JR, Castilho RM, Williams VP, et al. Semaphorin 4D provides a link between axon guidance processes and tumor-induced angiogenesis. Proc Natl Acad Sci USA 2006;103:9017–9022.
25. Greenberg DA, Jin K. From angiogenesis to neuropathology. Nature 2005;438:954–959.
26. Parent JM, Yu TW, Leibowitz RT, et al. Dentate granule cell neurogenesis is increased by seizures and contributes to aberrant network reorganization in the adult rat hippocampus. J Neurosci 1997;17:3727–3338.
27. Gu W, Brannstrom T, Wester P. Cortical neurogenesis in adult rats after reversible photothrombotic stroke. J Cereb Blood Flow Metab 2000;20:1166–1173.
28. Curtis MA, Penney EB, Pearson AG, et al. Increased cell proliferation and neurogenesis in the adult human Huntington's disease brain. Proc Natl Acad Sci USA 2003;100:9023–9027.
29. Jin K, Peel AL, Mao XO, et al. Increased hippocampal neurogenesis in Alzheimer's disease. Proc Natl Acad Sci USA 2004;101:343–347.
30. Wada K, Arai H, Takanashi M, et al. Expression levels of vascular endothelial growth factor and its receptors in Parkinson's disease. Neuroreport 2006;17:705–709.
31. Murakami T, Arai M, Sunada Y, et al. VEGF 164 gene transfer by electroporation improves diabetic sensory neuropathy in mice. J Gene Med 2006;8:773–781.
32. Zachary I. Neuroprotective role of vascular endothelial growth factor: signalling mechanisms, biological function, and therapeutic potential. Neurosignals 2005;14:207–221.
33. Devos D, Moreau C, Lassalle P, et al. Low levels of the vascular endothelial growth factor in CSF from early ALS patients. Neurology 2004;62:2127–2129.
34. Storkebaum E, Lambrechts D, Dewerchin M, et al. Treatment of motoneuron degeneration by intracerebroventricular delivery of VEGF in a rat model of ALS. Nat Neurosci 2005;8:85–92.
35. Wang Y, Galvan V, Gorostiza O, et al. Vascular endothelial growth factor improves recovery of sensorimotor and cognitive deficits after focal cerebral ischemia in the rat. Brain Res 2006;1115:186–193.
36. Jin K, Wang X, Xie L, et al. Evidence for stroke-induced neurogenesis in the human brain. Proc Natl Acad Sci USA 2006;103:13198–13202.
37. Mizugishi K, Yamashita T, Olivera A, et al. Essential role for sphingosine kinases in neural and vascular development. Mol Cell Biol 2005;25:11113–11121.
38. Asahara T, Murohara T, Sullivan A, et al. Isolation of putative progenitor endothelial cells for angiogenesis. Science 1997;275:964–67.

39. Hattori K, Dias S, Heissig B, et al. Vascular endothelial growth factor and angiopoietin-1 stimulate postnatal hematopoiesis by recruitment of vasculogenic and hematopoietic stem cells. J Exp Med 2001;193:1005–1014.
40. Lyden D, Hattori K, Dias S, et al. Impaired recruitment of bone-marrow-derived endothelial and hematopoietic precursor cells blocks tumor angiogenesis and growth. Nat Med 2001;7:1194–1201.
41. Ruzinova MB, Schoer RA, Gerald W, et al. Effect of angiogenesis inhibition by Id loss and the contribution of bone-marrow-derived endothelial cells in spontaneous murine tumors. Cancer Cell 2003;4:277–289.
42. Asahara T, Tomono T, Masuda H, et al. VEGF contributes to postnatal neovascularization by mobilizing bone marrow derived endothelial progenitor cells. EMBO J 1999;18:3964–3972.
43. Jin H, Su J, Garmy-Susini B, et al. Integrin alpha4beta1 promotes monocyte trafficking and angiogenesis in tumors. Cancer Res 2006;4:2146–2152.
44. Jiang S, Walker L, Afentoulis DA, et al. Transplanted human bone marrow contributes to vascular endothelium. Proc Natl Acad Sci USA 2004;101:16891–16896.
45. Peters BA, Diaz LA, Polyak K, et al. Contribution of bone marrow-derived endothelial cells to human tumor vasculature. Nat Med 2005;11:261–262.
46. Horita Y, Honmou O, Harada K, et al. Intravenous administration of glial cell line-derived neurotrophic factor gene-modified human mesenchymal stem cells protects against injury in a cerebral ischemia model in the adult rat. J Neurosci Res 2006;84:1495–1504.
47. Kawada H, Takizawa S, Takanashi T, et al. Administration of hematopoietic cytokines in the subacute phase after cerebral infarction is effective for functional recovery facilitating proliferation of intrinsic neural stem/progenitor cells and transition of bone marrow-derived neuronal cells. Circulation 2006;113:701–710.
48. Tamaki T, Uchiyama Y, Okada Y, et al. Functional recovery of damaged skeletal muscle through synchronized vasculogenesis, myogenesis, and neurogenesis by muscle-derived stem cells. Circulation 2005;112:2857–2866.
49. Taguchi A, Soma T, Tanaka H, et al. Administration of CD34+ cells after stroke enhances neurogenesis via angiogenesis in a mouse model. J Clin Invest 2004;114:330–338.
50. Jin H, Xu J, Qian F, et al. The 5 zebrafish scl promoter targets transcription to the brain, spinal cord, and hematopoietic and endothelial progenitors. Dev Dyn 2006;235:60–67.
51. Jin H, Aiyer A, Su J, et al. A homing mechanism for bone marrow-derived progenitor cell recruitment to the neovasculature. J Clin Invest 2006;3: 652–662.

V TARGETING CANCER STEM CELLS WITH THERAPY

20 Implications of Cancer Stem Cells for Cancer Therapy

Liang Cheng, Shaobo Zhang,
Darrell D. Davidson, Rodolfo Montironi,
and Antonio Lopez-Beltran

ABSTRACT

Our contemporary understanding of cancer biology is based on the stem cell hypothesis. This framework explains regression of premalignant lesions, radiation and drug resistant tumor cell subsets, relapse after complete therapeutic response, clonal similarity of metastatic implants and stromal requirements for cancer cultivation. The stem cell hypothesis also brings with it a new paradigm for cancer treatment. New therapies will increasingly target stem cell specific surface molecules, oncoproteins, regulation pathway elements, resistance mediators and stromal niche support factors. As our understanding of stem cell markers expands for various tumor subclasses, this knowledge of cancer stem cell biology and clinical significance will lead to more effective and safer treatments for human cancers.

Key Words: Cancer stem cell, pathway targeting, targeted therapy, personalized medicine, mesenchymal stem cell, stromal biology

INTRODUCTION

In the early 1990s, Lopidot et al. demonstrated that samples of human acute myeloid leukemia (AML) contain only a minority of cells with the capacity to engraft into nude mice *(1)*. Subsequently, Al-Hajii et al. reported the identification of cancer stem cells (CSC) from solid tumors *(2)*. They isolated a subpopulation of primary human breast cancer cells, with a high tumor forming ability in immunodeficient animal hosts *(2)*. The transplantable cells showed a distinct immunophenotype with high expression of CD44 and low or absent expression of CD24 (CD44+CD24−/low). Further evidence of a role for CSC in solid human tumors has also been observed in the neoplasms of brain, ovary, colon, prostate, pancreas, and other types of cancers *(3, 4)*.

A modern cancer model suggests that cancer is formed through clonal expansion of one or a few CSC *(5)*. CSC represents 1–4% of the viable cell population in a malignant neoplasm. These cells

From: *Cancer Drug Discovery and Development: Stem Cells and Cancer,*
Edited by: R.G. Bagley and B.A. Teicher, DOI: 10.1007/978-1-60327-933-8_20,
© Humana Press, a part of Springer Science+Business Media, LLC 2009

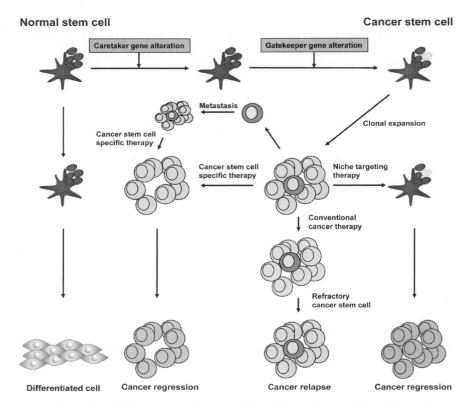

Fig. 1. Cancer stem cells are the cellular source of cancer cells and have characteristics of somatic stem cells. Normal stem cells renew themselves under the support of specialized microenvironment (niche) and differentiate into differentiated tissue cells (*left panel*). When genetic alterations involving caretaker and gatekeeper genes accumulate in the stem cell, a cancer stem cell may form (*upper right*). Subsequently, the cancer stem cells form a cancer through clonal expansion. The overall cellular population of a cancer consists of 1–4% cancer stem cells and 97–99% differentiated cancer cells. Only cancer stem cells are tumorigenic and form metastases. Conventional cancer therapy kills differentiated cancer cells but refractory cancer stem cells remain due to chemotherapy and radiation resistance. Cancer relapse occurs because of clonal expansion of surviving cancer stem cells. However, when cancer stem cell specific therapy is applied, the cancer stem cells are depleted and the differentiated cancer cells will die soon thereafter. Another option for therapy is to target the cancer stem cell microenvironment, niche. When the niche is interrupted the cancer stem cell cannot undergo self-renewal or clonal expansion (*see Color Plates*).

proliferate through asymmetric differentiation and can diversify into heterogeneous cancer cell lineages (*3, 6*). Each cancer stem cell and its progeny possess a unique set of genetic, epigenetic, and phenotypic features (*7*). These unique features provide an opportunity for stem cell therapy. (Fig. 1) Moreover, when tumors arise from CSC or progenitor cells, a specific microenvironment, niche, is essential for cancer formation. Mutations of stromal cells or somatic cell assistance to CSC in the niche may be necessary to promote cancer development and progression.

CSC AND PRECANCEROUS LESIONS: CLINICAL IMPLICATIONS

The three step carcinogenesis model, including dysplasia, in-situ carcinoma, and invasive carcinoma, has been well recognized and accepted (*5*). However, the notion that stem cells may be required for early precancerous lesions is still being debated. A recent study proposed that precancerous lesions are derived from precancerous stem cells (PSC), which have the potential for either benign or malignant differentiation *(8)*. CSCs may originate from a stem or progenitor cell through a precancerous stage, during which stem cells are hierarchically disturbed in their genetic program of self-renewal by environmental insults *(6, 9)*. But a criticism of this hypothesis is that it contradicts the clonal evolution theory of carcinogenesis. Supporters of the precancerous stem cell theory reply that clonal evolution is actually an aspect of CSC development from PSC. The dysregulated premalignant stem cells accumulate genetic changes until the malignant phenotype evolves. PSC have revealed evolutionary pathways involving progressive transformation of CSC cell phenotype, degree of differentiation, and stage of initiation or progression. Therefore, PSC are stem cells that may either remain noncancerous or progress to malignancy, depending on subsequent environmental influences.

PSC have biological features of both normal stem cells and of CSC regardless of their origin. A study indicated that Bmi1 was clearly overexpressed across a broad spectrum of gastrointestinal cancers, and the expression of Bmi1 increased in a manner that reflected the pathologic malignant features of precancerous colonic tissues (low-grade dysplasia, 13%; high-grade dysplasia, 83%; cancer, 90%) *(10)*. p16 was also strongly expressed in high-grade dysplasia, but not in cancers. p16 promoter methylation was detected only in some Bmi1-positive neoplastic cells *(10)*. Study results also indicated that in the tumor developed from PSC, most blood vessels were derived from PSC *(11)*. Some PSC constitutively expressed vasculogenic receptor VEGFR-2, which can be up-regulated by hypoxia and angiogenesis-promoting cytokines *(11)*. Anti-angiogenesis therapy may effect the progression of precancerous lesions to a cancer.

Accumulation of genetic alterations in PSC as they acquire increasingly malignant features is consistent with the multistep mutation process in classic carcinogenesis. Thus, the precancerous stem cell hypothesis covers the spectrum of developmental stages observed clinically in cancer. Precancerous lesion therapy is a part of cancer stem cell therapy.

CSC AND MESENCHYMAL STEM CELLS

CSC are the cells that can sustain unlimited cancer growth. The majority of cells in a growing cancer are committed cells that pass through dividing and differentiating stages but are destined to die. CSC, but then, always produces at least one daughter cell with unrestricted proliferation capacity. Nevertheless, CSC can form a cancer only within a specific microenvironment, niche, which includes unrelated mesenchymal stem cells. Mesenchymal stem cells are pluripotent progenitor cells that contribute to the maintenance and regeneration of a variety of supporting tissues *(12)*. These nonmalignant cells support and modulate the CSC in various ways. Actively growing cancer cells also recruit mesenchymal stem cells through the release of various endocrine and paracrine signals. Without the supporting niche, CSC fails to proliferate or produce progenitor cells to differentiate into a growing cancer. Thus, mesenchymal stem cells in the niche represent another potential target for cancer therapy.

RADIATION AND DRUG RESISTANCE OF CSC

Most current therapies against cancer target differentiated cancer cells. CSC is relatively resistant to conventional chemotherapy and radiotherapy *(3)*. There are several molecular mechanisms that may account for CSC therapy resistance. Many CSC are noncycling G_0 cells, and would not be susceptible to cell cycle specific chemotherapy agents. ATP-binding cassette proteins (ABC transporter), known to efflux chemotherapy drugs, are often overexpressed in CSC *(13)*. Other mechanisms of CSC resistance to chemotherapy include quiescence, increased expression of antiapoptotic proteins, and multidrug resistance molecules. CSC is also relatively radio-resistant because of increased tolerance to radiation induced DNA damage and enhanced DNA repair activity. Therapy resistance in the small CSC population of tumors accounts for most cancer relapse and posttherapy metastasis *(14, 15)*.

CSC AND CANCER RELAPSE

Cancer relapse occurs in many cases after the tumor has been grossly eradicated by surgical removal, chemotherapy, or radiation therapy. Relapse may now be attributed to incomplete CSC elimination *(16)*. Recent developments indicate that most current therapies eliminate differentiated cells, which are more sensitive to therapy than CSC. However, a small number of therapy resistant CSC remain or escape after ablation of the differentiated primary tumor cells. Proliferation and clonal expansion of these fugitive CSC results in establishment of new settlements wherever the surviving cells find a favorable niche (Fig. 1).

CSC AND CANCER METASTASIS

CSC are not only responsible for tumorigenesis, but also account for tumor metastasis *(17)*. Nevertheless, only a subset of CSC in a tumor has the ability to metastasize. The CSC model explains why metastases from a tumor with highly heterogeneous subpopulations all have striking similarities of morphology, gene expression profile, and molecular alterations *(18)*. This phenomenon of metastasis similarity contradicts the traditional cancer model that assumes origination and selection of metastasizing cells randomly. Metastases, according to the traditional model, would form subclones of the polygenetic and polyphenotypic primary cancer.

Cancer metastasis requires the "seeding" and successful colonization of specialized CSC at distant sites. The success of these exploits is determined by the microenvironment (Niche) and by molecules the niche cells provide. These molecules form a complex network of cellular interactions that facilitate both induction of a premetastasis niche by the primary tumor and formation of a nurturing microenvironment for migrating CSC *(19)*. Kaplan *(20)* et al. demonstrated that bone marrow-derived benign hematopoietic progenitor cells home to tumor-specific premetastatic sites and form cellular clusters before the arrival of tumor cells. Specific microenvironment, thus, appears to be a major regulator not only of tumor formation but also of cancer metastasis. Thus niche target therapy is an important option for cancer therapy (Fig. 1).

CSC AND PROGNOSIS

Current data about the relationship between CSC and prognosis indicate that the clinical behavior of a cancer is largely dependent on the characteristics of its CSC population. Distant metastasis correlates with the presence of $CD44^+/CD24^{-/low}$ stem cells in breast cancer. Zeppernick *(21)* et al. reported that $CD133^+$ glioma CSC are significant predictors of both progression-free survival and of overall survival, independent of tumor grade, extent of resection, or patient age. Since it is still difficult to detect individual CSC directly, some investigators have demonstrated that aggregate CSC associated gene expression may predict clinical outcome. Therefore, abundance of CSC generally correlates with unfavorable outcome and could be considered an independent risk factor for tumor recurrence and progression.

THERAPEUTICS TARGETING CSC

The CSC model has opened new opportunities for cancer therapy. Traditional cancer therapies are effective against differentiated, self-limiting transit-amplifying cancer cells. The transit-amplifying cells targeted by conventional therapy are the asymmetrically descended progeny of CSC without self-renewal capacity, yet forming a much larger branch with elevated but confined proliferation capacity. These differentiated cells typically have less active DNA repair systems and greater sensitivity to chemotherapy and radiotherapy than CSC. Therapy that targets CSC aims to deplete the CSC pool. CSC targeting therapy could be achieved through CSC surface molecule binding, oncoprotein inhibition, CSC regulation pathway disruption, and frustration of CSC therapy resistance machinery. There is no shortage of targets for CSC-directed treatments. However, an ideal CSC targeting agent must discriminate CSC from normal stem cells. Also functional assay techniques for CSC to monitor the effectiveness of targeted treatment are critical for the CSC targeting therapy *(22)*.

The historical hurdle of traditional therapy eliminating malignant, but not normal cells, are in no way circumvented by CSC targeting therapy. The latter approach, however, confers the additional benefits of potentially deleting the last malignant cell, targeting the precancerous pool of cells, eliminating cells resistant to conventional chemotherapy or radiotherapy, and aiming at the cells most likely to metastasize.

SURFACE MOLECULE TARGETING THERAPY

Since stem cells divide asymmetrically and the expression profiles of stem cells are strongly influenced by the microenvironment, it has been difficult to identify markers common to all stem cells. At this time little is known regarding the phenotype of CSC from various tissues and organs. Confirming CSC specific markers is confounded by the fact that stem cells represent only a small fraction of the total tumor cell population. Some of the CSC markers are shared by CSC from different tissues, whereas others are restricted to a specific tissue *(23)*. It is well known that CSC share many stem cell markers with their normal counterparts, which may not be suitable for target of therapy. Devising therapies specifically against CSC without harming normal stem cells is still a major challenge for CSC targeting therapy *(24)*. Although there are many phenotypic similarities between normal stem cells and CSC, subtle differences have been identified. Tissue-specific and cancer-specific stem cell markers provide the potential for more precise CSC targeting therapy and for functional assays to determine the efficacy of CSC therapy.

CSC surface antigen targeting is achieved by designing molecules to recognize a specific cell surface antigen and attach a toxin to the CSC plasma lemma. Ideally, this process would only recognize CSC while sparing normal cells and tissues. Humanized monoclonal antibodies against CSC surface antigens conjugated with cytotoxic agents or radio isotopes have been tested *(25)*. A highly potent cytotoxic drug, calicheamicin, has been conjugated to anti-CD33 antibody to produce *gemtuzumab ozogamicin*. This drug has been in clinical use in AML patients since 2000. Although CD33 has not been identified as a specific marker of stem cells, it is recognized as a marker of multipotent hematopoietic cells. Its precise biologic role, however, remains enigmatic. *Rituximab*, an anti-CD20 antibody targeting B-cell differentiation, has shown response of approximately half of the patients with minor toxicity in patients with refractory indolent B-cell lymphoma. *Alemtuzumab* (Campath-1H, anti-CD52), a complement and ADCC activating molecule, has shown encouraging results in chronic lymphocytic leukemia (CLL) and T-cell lymphoma. Response rates around one-third are found in patients with refractory CLL, although significant toxicity is observed. Moreover, anti-CD33 and anti-CD45 antibodies have been used to deliver radiation directly to leukemic cells. ^{131}I-tagged anti-CD45 antibodies target leukocyte membrane bound phosphatase. This compound has been studied in combination with standard therapy regimens in patients receiving bone marrow transplantation for leukemia. Beta emissions from ^{131}I damage nearby cells, including stem cells, whereas gamma decay products escape from the human body unimpeded. These studies have shown promising results in patients with recurrent AML and refractory myelodysplastic syndrome, apparently by eliminating therapy resistant cells from intractable cancers *(26)*.

ONCOPROTEIN TARGETING THERAPY

Oncogenic proteins play an important role in the initiation and progression of malignancies. Oncoproteins expressed by CSC, such as HER2/neu, ras, kit, bcr/abl, MLL, MOZ, and PML/RAR have also been investigated as therapy targets *(27–31)*. Many of these oncoproteins are involved in the self-renewal pathways of CSC. Recently, a tyrosine kinase inhibitor, *lapatinib*, reduced CD 44$^+$/CD 24$^{-/low}$ CSC in primary breast cancer.

Imatinib inhibits the *kit*-like constitutively expressed tyrosine kinase of the *bcr-abl* fusion protein (p210$^{bcr-abl}$) that is seen in CML. *Imatinib* is highly effective against bcr-abl positive chronic myeloid leukemia (CML). A recent model of *imatinib* therapy for CML suggests that long term remission is more likely if therapy is initiated early in the course of the disease or if there is a high degree of niche competition between CML and normal stem cells *(32)*. Under these circumstances, the CSC population is low and conditions promoting CSC survival by symmetric division are eliminated. Recent studies have indicated a more complicated CSC model. Some tumors may contain a heterogeneous population of CSC with varied phenotype *(33, 34)*. This type of tumor may require a combination of CSC targeting drugs to eliminate the complex CSC pool.

STEM CELL REGULATION PATHWAY TARGETING

Signal molecules of CSC regulation pathways, or downstream signal molecules, such as *Bmi-1, Notch, Wnt*, and *Sonic Hedgehog*, are also potential targets for CSC directed therapy. Such an approach may be less specific than conventional cancer therapies, but it covers more upstream pathways and targets more CSC subclones than other approaches. Some small molecule stem cell pathway inhibitors exhibit CSC specificity and spare the regulatory pathways of normal stem cells. It was recently reported that proteasome inhibitors down regulate NF-κB in AML stem cells but not in normal stem cells. Cyclopamine, a naturally occurring alkaloid, inhibits the G-protein coupled receptor smoothened (SMO), consequently inhibiting the growth of NIH 3T3 cells transfected with an *SmoA1* expression construct *(35)*. Cyclopamine also eliminated PC-3 and DU-145 xenografts in mice after 21 days of treatment. In both in vitro and in vivo experiments, scientists have blocked the Hedgehog signaling system with cyclopamine or purmorphamine to induce cell death of CSC. Other small molecules have shown efficacy against Wnt and NF-kB stem cell pathways *(36)*.

DRUG AND RADIATION RESISTANCE INHIBITORS

CSC has properties that allow them to survive through chemotherapy and radiation therapy. However, the mechanisms by which CSC evade or become resistant to targeted therapy are still largely unknown *(37)*. Chemotherapy resistance is largely attributed to CSC effluxing of the chemotherapeutic agents by drug transporter proteins, especially the ATP-binding cassette (ABC) transporter *(38)*. The radiation resistance properties of CSC are due to increased tolerance to DNA damage by ionizing particles and enhanced DNA repair activity. Combined use of standard chemotherapy drugs and ABC drug transporter inhibitors achieves a more efficient killing of CSC than the standard drugs alone *(39, 40)*. There are highly specific inhibitors of ABC drug transporter already used clinically and in development. CSC is also rendered less resistant to radiation therapy if inhibitors of two of the check point kinases, Chk1 and Chk2, are added to the treatment protocol *(41)*.

MESENCHYMAL STEM CELLS AND ANTI-NICHE CSC THERAPY

Mesenchymal stem cells and vascular stem cells are also emerging as new cancer therapy targets. Growth and metastasis of cancers depend upon a favorable microenvironment for proliferation and on formation of neo-vessels for nourishment *(42, 43)*. Vascular stem cells derived from bone marrow play an important role in tumor angiogenesis. Cancer cells release factors to attract vascular stem cells, to induce them to proliferate, and to cause neovessel incorporation into the developing tumor vasculature. Vascular stem cells, therefore, have become an important new target for anti-angiogenesis cancer treatment. Pathologists observed in the 1940s that cells of the aggressive brain tumor, glioblastoma multiform, migrate into normal brain around blood vessels (perivascular satellitosis) *(42)*. It was postulated that it is not tumor cells that invade and attract nourishing vessels, but stimulated vascular primordial cells that encroach and extend the glioma stem cell niche. Support for this concept is found in the clinically established principle that glioblastoma invasiveness is proportional to vascular endothelial growth factor (VEGF) secretion, and that the anti-angiogenesis agents, *bevicizumab* and *thalidomide*, potentiate other anti-glioma therapies.

Recent research in stem cell biology suggests that CSC tumorigenesis is governed by cells from the tumor cell niche. This microenvironment contains not only tumor stem cells, associated vascular bed and other mesenchyme-derived cells, but also extracellular matrix proteins and structures. Normal stem cells are highly responsive to basement membrane, spindle orientation, membrane adhesion molecules, growth factors, extracellular matrix integrin ligands, and to a host of paracrine signaling molecules. It is reasonable to assume that CSC retain some of these niche-dependent properties of normal stem cells *(44)*. Asymmetric division of CSC determines that some of the daughter cells are always retained within the niche, while others leave the niche to proliferate further, differentiate and eventually die. Therefore, CSC targeting therapy may benefit from anti-niche agents to compromise the microenvironment of the self-renewing, immortal branch of CSC.

Since stem cells divide asymmetrically and the expression profiles of stem cells are strongly influenced by the microenvironment, it has been difficult to identify markers common to all stem cells. At this time little is known regarding the phenotype of CSC from various tissues and organs. Confirming CSC specific markers is confounded by the fact that stem cells represent only a small fraction of the total tumor cell population. Some of the CSC markers are shared by CSC from different tissues, whereas others are restricted to a specific tissue *(23)*. Although there are many phenotypic similarities between normal stem cells and CSC, subtle differences have been identified. Tissue-specific and cancer-specific stem cell markers provide the potential for more precise CSC targeting therapy and for functional assays to determine the efficacy of CSC therapy.

CONCLUSIONS

Our contemporary understanding of cancer biology is based on the stem cell hypothesis. This framework explains regression of premalignant lesions, radiation, and drug resistant tumor cell subsets, relapse after complete therapeutic response, clonal similarity of metastatic implants, and stromal requirements for cancer cultivation. The stem cell hypothesis also brings with it a new paradigm for cancer treatment. New therapies will increasingly target stem cell-specific surface molecules, oncoproteins, regulation pathway elements, resistance mediators, and stromal niche support factors. As our understanding of stem cell markers expands for various tumor subclasses, this knowledge of cancer stem cell biology and clinical significance will lead to new, more effective, and safer treatments.

REFERENCES

1. Lapidot T, Sirard C, Vormoor J, et al.: A cell initiating human acute myeloid leukaemia after transplantation into SCID mice. Nature 367:645–8, 1994
2. Al-Hajj M, Wicha MS, Benito-Hernandez A, et al.: Prospective identification of tumorigenic breast cancer cells. Proc Natl Acad Sci USA 100:3983–8, 2003
3. Jordan CT, Guzman ML, Noble M: Cancer stem cells. N Engl J Med 355:1253–61, 2006
4. Pan CX, Zhu W, Cheng L: Implications of cancer stem cells in the treatment of cancer. Future Oncol 2:723–31, 2006
5. Cheng L, Zhang D: Molecular Genetic Pathology. Totowa, NJ, Humana Press, 2008
6. Reya T, Morrison SJ, Clarke MF, et al.: Stem cells, cancer, and cancer stem cells. Nature 404:105–11, 2001
7. Jordan CT, Guzman ML: Mechanisms controlling pathogenesis and survival of leukemic stem cells. Oncogene 23:7178–87, 2004
8. Gao JX: Cancer stem cells: the lessons from pre-cancerous stem cells. J Cell Mol Med 12:67–96, 2008

9. Houghton J, Stoicov C, Nomura S, et al.: Gastric cancer originating from bone marrow-derived cells. Science 306:1568–71, 2004
10. Tateishi K, Ohta M, Kanai F, et al.: Dysregulated expression of stem cell factor Bmi1 in precancerous lesions of the gastrointestinal tract. Clin Cancer Res 12:6960–6, 2006
11. Shen R, Ye Y, Chen L, et al.: Precancerous stem cells can serve as tumor vasculogenic progenitors. PLoS ONE 3:e1652, 2008
12. Prindull G, Zipori D: Environmental guidance of normal and tumor cell plasticity: epithelial mesenchymal transitions as a paradigm. Blood 103:2892–9, 2004
13. Chapuy B, Koch R, Radunski U, et al.: Intracellular ABC transporter A3 confers multidrug resistance in leukemia cells by lysosomal drug sequestration. Leukemia 22:1576–86, 2008
14. Tang C, Ang BT, Pervaiz S: Cancer stem cell: target for anti-cancer therapy. FASEB J 21:3777–85, 2007
15. Maitland NJ, Collins AT: Prostate cancer stem cells: a new target for therapy. J Clin Oncol 26:2862–70, 2008
16. Blagosklonny MV: Why therapeutic response may not prolong the life of a cancer patient: selection for oncogenic resistance. Cell Cycle 4:1693–8, 2005
17. Wicha MS: Cancer stem cells and metastasis: lethal seeds. Clin Cancer Res 12:5606–7, 2006
18. Lang JE, Hall CS, Singh B, et al.: Significance of micrometastasis in bone marrow and blood of operable breast cancer patients: research tool or clinical application? Expert Rev Anticancer Ther 7:1463–72, 2007
19. Steeg PS: Tumor metastasis: mechanistic insights and clinical challenges. Nat Med 12:895–904, 2006
20. Kaplan RN, Psaila B, Lyden D: Niche-to-niche migration of bone-marrow-derived cells. Trends Mol Med 13:72–81, 2007
21. Zeppernick F, Ahmadi R, Campos B, et al.: Stem cell marker CD133 affects clinical outcome in glioma patients. Clin Cancer Res 14:123–9, 2008
22. Kvinlaug BT, Huntly BJ: Targeting cancer stem cells. Expert Opin Ther Targets 11:915–27, 2007
23. Ailles LE, Weissman IL: Cancer stem cells in solid tumors. Curr Opin Biotechnol 18:460–6, 2007
24. Lichtman MA: Differentiation versus maturation of neoplastic hematopoietic cells: an important distinction. Blood Cells Mol Dis 27:649–52, 2001
25. Bernstein ID: Monoclonal antibodies to the myeloid stem cells: therapeutic implications of CMA-676, a humanized anti-CD33 antibody calicheamicin conjugate. Leukemia 14:474–5, 2000
26. Pagel JM, Appelbaum FR, Eary JF, et al.: 131I-anti-CD45 antibody plus busulfan and cyclophosphamide before allogeneic hematopoietic cell transplantation for treatment of acute myeloid leukemia in first remission. Blood 107:2184–91, 2006
27. Hu Y, Swerdlow S, Duffy TM, et al.: Targeting multiple kinase pathways in leukemic progenitors and stem cells is essential for improved treatment of Ph+ leukemia in mice. Proc Natl Acad Sci USA 103:16870–5, 2006
28. McCubrey JA, Steelman LS, Abrams SL, et al.: Targeting survival cascades induced by activation of Ras/Raf/MEK/ERK, PI3K/PTEN/Akt/mTOR and Jak/STAT pathways for effective leukemia therapy. Leukemia 22:708–22, 2008
29. Zhou H, Kim YS, Peletier A, et al.: Effects of the EGFR/HER2 kinase inhibitor GW572016 on EGFR- and HER2-overexpressing breast cancer cell line proliferation, radiosensitization, and resistance. Int J Radiat Oncol Biol Phys 58:344–52, 2004
30. Druker BJ, Tamura S, Buchdunger E, et al.: Effects of a selective inhibitor of the Abl tyrosine kinase on the growth of Bcr-Abl positive cells. Nat Med 2:561–6, 1996
31. Druker BJ, Sawyers CL, Kantarjian H, et al.: Activity of a specific inhibitor of the BCR-ABL tyrosine kinase in the blast crisis of chronic myeloid leukemia and acute lymphoblastic leukemia with the Philadelphia chromosome. N Engl J Med 344:1038–42, 2001
32. Kim PS, Lee PP, Levy D: Dynamics and potential impact of the immune response to chronic myelogenous leukemia. PLoS Comput Biol 4:e1000095, 2008
33. Stingl J, Caldas C: Molecular heterogeneity of breast carcinomas and the cancer stem cell hypothesis. Nat Rev Cancer 7:791–9, 2007
34. Schulenburg A, Ulrich-Pur H, Thurnher D, et al.: Neoplastic stem cells: a novel therapeutic target in clinical oncology. Cancer 107:2512–20, 2006
35. Chen JK, Taipale J, Young KE, et al.: Small molecule modulation of Smoothened activity. Proc Natl Acad Sci USA 99:14071–6, 2002
36. Schugar RC, Robbins PD, Deasy BM: Small molecules in stem cell self-renewal and differentiation. Gene Ther 15:126–35, 2008
37. Rapp UR, Ceteci F, Schreck R: Oncogene-induced plasticity and cancer stem cells. Cell Cycle 7:45–51, 2008
38. Goodell MA, Brose K, Paradis G, et al.: Isolation and functional properties of murine hematopoietic stem cells that are replicating in vivo. J Exp Med 183:1797–806, 1996
39. Kakarala M, Wicha MS: Cancer stem cells: implications for cancer treatment and prevention. Cancer J 13:271–5, 2007
40. Dean M, Fojo T, Bates S: Tumour stem cells and drug resistance. Nat Rev Cancer 5:275–84, 2005
41. Bao S, Wu Q, McLendon RE, et al.: Glioma stem cells promote radioresistance by preferential activation of the DNA damage response. Nature 444:756–60, 2006
42. Gilbertson RJ, Rich JN: Making a tumour's bed: glioblastoma stem cells and the vascular niche. Nat Rev Cancer 7:733–6, 2007
43. Yang ZJ, Wechsler-Reya RJ: Hit 'em where they live: targeting the cancer stem cell niche. Cancer Cell 11:3–5, 2007
44. Fuchs E, Tumbar T, Guasch G: Socializing with the neighbors: stem cells and their niche. Cell 116:769–78, 2004

21

Targeting Leukemic Stem Cells

Angelika M. Burger

ABSTRACT

The stem cell concept and asymmetric cell division are best understood in the hematopoietic system. Hematopoietic malignancies resemble many of the known normal mature hematopoietic lineages that originate from stem cells. Leukemias in particular, were shown to arise from leukemic stem cells. General characteristics of stem cells such as self-renewal, self-protection and proliferative quiescence clearly point toward the need for targeting leukemia stem cells in order to improve cure rates and to prevent relapse of this disease. However, leukemia stem cells share many stemness factors with hematopoietic stem cells, and owing to the inherent heterogeneity of leukemias, each subtype might have distinct stem cells. The successful targeting of leukemia stem cells will therefore require the careful consideration of these issues. This chapter gives an overview over leukemia stem cells and highlights pathways and disease specific markers that provide therapeutic targets. Agents that are under development or approved for cancer treatment and could target leukemia stem cells, are also reviewed.

Key Words: ALDH1, Disulfiram, Side population, BCRP, Pgp, Telomerase, Telomeres, Arsenic trioxide, BCR-ABL, Imatinib, CD34, CD38, Clonogenic assay

BACKGROUND

Adult human stem cells are best characterized in the hematopoietic system. At least eight distinct lineages of mature blood cells are known that replenish continuously throughout adult life. Owing to that fact, the existence of a rare subpopulation of cells with self-renewal capacity, termed hematopoietic stem cells (HSCs), from which all hematopoietic cells are derived, has been recognized *(1)*.

The hematopoietic system is hierarchically organized; a long-term HSC divides asymmetrically into a long-term HSC and a short-term HSC, which in turn facilitates cell expansion by generating multipotent progenitor cells lacking self-renewal. Multipotent progenitors differentiate into lymphoid progenitors, granulocyte/macrophage progenitors, megakaryocyte/erythroid progenitors, mast cell and basophile progenitors, as well as macrophage and dendritic cell progenitors. The resulting mature blood cell lineages comprise B and T cells, red blood cells, monocytic, granulocytic and basophilic myeloid cells, and megakaryocytes *(1, 2)*.

From: *Cancer Drug Discovery and Development: Stem Cells and Cancer,*
Edited by: R.G. Bagley and B.A. Teicher DOI: 10.1007/978-1-60327-933-8_21,
© Humana Press, a part of Springer Science+Business Media, LLC 2009

Hematopoietic malignancies resemble various normal, mature cell types of the hematopoietic system and their origin. In particular, leukemia has been shown to arise from leukemic stem cells (LSC), which can differentiate into multiple types of leukemia, dependent on which developmental and signaling pathways become dysregulated. Acute lymphoblastic leukemia (ALL) is characterized by an upregulation of Hedgehog and Notch signaling, and acute myeloid leukemia (AML) is governed by self-renewal pathways, or chronic myelogenous leukemia (CML) by the BCR-ABL kinase signaling pathway (2, 3).

HEMATOPOIETIC AND LEUKEMIC STEM CELLS: COMMONALITIES AND DIFFERENCES

The origin of leukemic stem cells is still not clearly defined. Existing experimental evidence suggests that LSCs can arise from HSCs, but also progenitor cells such as common myeloid progenitors or granulocytes/macrophage progenitors after introducing certain transforming leukemia fusion proteins such as MOZ-TIF2, the mixed lineage leukemia (MLL) oncogenic fusion proteins MLL-ENL, or MLL-Af9 (4–6). The close relationship between HSCs and LSCs has been demonstrated by genomic profiling of cell populations enriched for HSCs and LSCs (7). Gal and coworkers found that 34 out of the 148 genes that were at least twofold up regulated in LSCs compared with the LSC-depleted bulk cell fractions were also typical to normal HSCs. The latter include, e.g., *MLL* gene and Jagged 2, a ligand of the Notch extracellular domain, which is important in the Notch-developmental signaling pathway (7). In addition, 104 out of the 261 genes that were down regulated in LSC compared with LSC-depleted bulk cells showed a similar behavior in normal HSC. For example, myeloid cell nuclear differentiation antigen and the HSC and LSC maturation marker CD38, whose level of surface expression was shown to decrease during differentiation, were under expressed (7). Overall, 34% of the modulated genes in that study were shared by both LSC and HSC and the degree of similarity is high (7). Another common characteristic of HSCs and LSCs is the positivity for the cell–cell adhesion factor CD34 and the lack of the maturation marker CD38, which are both cell surface antigens and facilitate the isolation of HSCs and LSCs by cell sorting methods such as fluorescence activated cell sorting (FACS) (8–10). It has been shown that both, CD34+/CD38– HSC and LSC are capable of self-renewal and can either repopulate bone marrow or the leukemia from which they originate at a low dilution of cells (1–100) in nonobese diabetic mice with severe combined immunodeficiency disease (NOD/SCID) (10). However, immunophenotyping has revealed that the use of additional cell surface markers such as CD90[-], CD117[-], and CD123[+] can help to distinguish between HSC and LSC. The latter three antigens are not expressed in HSCs, but by LSCs of acute myeloid leukemia (9). Another characteristic common to HSCs, LSCs, and stem cells in general is the capability to grow colonies in a semi solid matrix such as soft agar or methylcellulose (Fig. 1) (12, 13). As shown in Fig. 1 for AML, APL, and CML cell lines in the soft agar clonogenic assay, 3–6% of a bulk tumor cell mass can grow anchorage independent, suggesting the presence of multipotent leukemic stem cells and/or progenitor cells. The colony forming ability of leukemia cells is, however, highly dependent on the number of bulk cells that were seeded per well (Fig. 1). Optimal colony formation was seen at a density of 5,000 cells/well, while less than 2,000 cells or more than 10,000 cells per well appeared to permit colony formation, perhaps because of unfavorable environmental conditions (Fig. 1).

LEUKEMIC STEM CELL TYPES

Malignant stem cells with proven self-renewal and disease repopulation abilities have been identified in acute myelogenous leukemia (AML) and subtypes thereof such as acute promyelocytic leukemia (APL), chronic myeloid leukemia (CML), and some types of acute lymphoblastic leukemia (ALL)

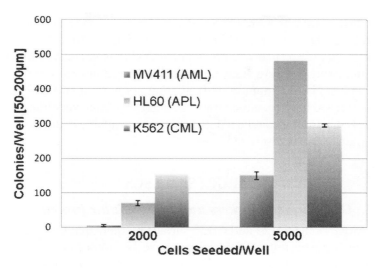

Fig. 1. Clonogenicity of leukemia cells. Soft agar colony formation of leukemia cell lines seeded at a density of 2,000 and 5,000 cells per well in a 24-well plate, respectively. The modified two layer soft agar technique was used as described by us before *(11)*. Colony growth was monitored and after 7–10 days in culture 100 μL of the vital dye iodonitro tetrazolium blue (2 mg/mL) were added per well and the cells incubated with that dye over night. Viable colonies (stained purple) of a size between 50 and 200 μm were counted the next day with an automated colony analyzer (Microbiology International). Twelve wells were analyzed per cell density for each cell line and the experiment repeated three more times. Mean values for a representative experiment ± standard deviation are shown. MV411 is an acute myelogenous leukemia (AML, *dark blue*) cell line, HL60 is an acute promyelocytic leukemia (APL, *light blue*), and K562 is chronic myelogenous leukemia (CML, *green*) cell line.

Table 1
Leukemia cell lines and CD34/CD38 expression

Surface marker	MV411 AML (%)	KG1a AML (%)	HL60 APL (%)	K562 CML (%)
CD34+	0.13	90.54	0.42	0.1
CD38+	70.67	0.07	0.42	0.07
CD38–	29.33	99.83	99.58	99.93

(2, 10, 14–16). AML, APL, CML, and ALL leukemic stem cells are all known to be CD34$^+$/CD38$^-$. As shown for representative leukemia cell lines in Table 1, the bulk mass of cells contains mostly only a very small fraction of CD34+/CD38– cells (<1%) consistent with the stem cell hypothesis that only a rare number of cells is capable of self-renewal and to differentiate into any mature cell type of the tumor of origin (Table 1) *(10, 14, 16)*. However, KG1a, a very aggressive AML cell line with minimally or undifferentiated features, high P-glycoprotein expression, high bcl-2/bax ratio, an unfavorable karyotype, frequent internal tandem duplications, and mutations in the key hematopoietic cytokines Flt-3 (receptor for Flt-ligand), c-kit (receptor for stem cell factor) and fms (receptor for M-CSF) has over 90% of CD34-positive and CD38-negative cells (Table 1) *(17)*. This could point toward a selection of stem-like or pluripotent cells in KG1a in an in vitro culture environment and that KG1a would be a good line for studying AML stem cell directed treatments. But then, the large population of CD34+/CD38– cells also demonstrates that in vitro cultures of cancer cells may not reflect the patient situation and that other cell types than pluripotent cells might express CD34+/CD38–.

Among leukemia, AML stem cells (AMLSCs) are best characterized and additional surface markers such as CD90−, CD117−, CD123+, or CD33+ have been identified *(9, 18, 19)*. Although CD33 is found on all AML cells including mature cells, when CD33 was ablated and CD34+/CD33− cells of patients were grown in colony-forming assays, the resulting colonies were polyclonal and normal in origin, suggesting that CD33 is important in AMLSCs but not normal HSCs *(19)*. Hence, CD123 and CD33 are epitopes that can and have been used for targeting. Despite the very limited information relating to differences between LSCs from distinct leukemia subtypes, available evidence suggests that subtype-specific stem cell markers exist as discussed later.

TARGETS IN LSCS

Cell Surface Markers and Intracellular Proteins

AML Markers: In AML, both CD123 and CD33 surface markers that have been found to be disease specific, not to be expressed on normal HSCs, and have been exploited for specifically targeting toxins to leukemic cells *(18–20)*. CD123, also known as IL3, has been conjugated with a diphtheria protein by fusing human interleukin-3 (IL3) to a truncated form of diphtheria toxin (DT) with a $(G_4S)_2$ linker (L). Exposure of mononuclear cells to 680 pm DTLIL3 for 48 h in culture reduced the number of cells capable of forming colonies in semisolid medium (colony-forming units leukemia) ≥ 10-fold in 4/11 (36%) patients with myeloid acute phase chronic myeloid leukemia (CML) and 3/9 (33%) patients with acute myeloid leukemia (AML). Normal myeloid progenitors (colony-forming unit granulocyte–macrophage) from five different donors treated and assayed under identical conditions showed intermediate sensitivity with three to fivefold reductions in colonies. The sensitivity to DTLIL3 of leukemic progenitors from a number of acute phase CML patients suggests that this agent could have therapeutic potential for some patients with this disease *(18)*.

CD33 is another cell surface molecule that can be used to direct toxins to AMLSCs. It has been shown that AML cells capable of initiating tumors in NOD/SCID mice express CD33. In fact, the CD33-calicheamicin immunoconjugate gemtuzumab ozogamicin (Mylotarg) has been FDA approved for clinical use in AML (Table 2) and should be tested for AMLSC specific activity *(19, 20)*.

Table 2
Leukemia stem cell targets and targeted treatments

Leukemia subtype	Stem cell target	Targeted treatment	Reference
AML (APL)	CD123	DTLIL3	*(18)*
	CD33	Mylotarg	*(19, 20)*
	C-kit/SCF	SCF mab	*(17)*
	Pgp	Cyclosporin A, Zosquidar	*(21, 22)*
	Telomeres/telomerase	ATO, GRN136L	*(23, 24)*
	Differentiation	ATRA	*(25, 26)*
	Sonic Hedgehog	GDC-0449	*(27)*
CML	BCR-ABL	Imatinib + G-CSF, SKI-606	*(28, 29)*
	ALDH1	Disulfiram	*(30, 31)*
ALL (T-ALL)	Notch 1	MK-0752	*(32)*
	DLL4	Soluble DLL4, DLL4 mab	*(33, 34)*

AML, acute myelogenous leukemia; APL, acute promyelocytic leukemia; SCF, stem cell factor; mab, monoclonal antibody; Pgp, P-glycoprotein; ATO, arsenic trioxide; ATRA, all-*trans*-retinoic acid; G-CSF, granulocyte-colony stimulating factor; ALDH1, aldehyde dehydrogenase 1; DLL4, delta-like 4

Stem cell factor (SCF) and its receptor c-kit regulate the proliferation, survival, and differentiation of normal and malignant hematopoietic stem cells and germ cells. It has recently been shown that anti-SCF antibodies can significantly enhance the low dose cytarabine and daunorubicine-induced bcl-2 reduction in drug resistant CD34+ AML cells, suggesting that targeting c-kit signaling has anti-AMLSC activity. For example in the extremely resistant KG1a CD34+ AML cells, enhancing activity of anti-SCF on low dose chemotherapy-induced apoptosis and necrosis went up from 26.7 ± 0.6 to $64.6 \pm 1.0\%$ and from 59.8 ± 3.1 to $80.1 \pm 7.9\%$, respectively ($p < 0.01$) *(17)* (Table 2).

CML Markers: In chronic myelogenous leukemia (CML), the formation of the BCR-ABL fusion gene and expression of the p210(BCR-ABL) kinase is a hallmark of the disease and the most important molecular target *(35)*. It has recently been found that quiescent CML stem cells are resistant to the BCR-ABL inhibitor imatinib, because this drug can only eliminate cycling cells *(28)*. Thus, the failure of imatinib to eradicate CML stem cells leads eventually to disease relapse. Interestingly, exposure of CD34+ CML cells to granulocyte-colony stimulating factor (G-CSF) in vitro drives long-term, quiescent stem cells out of their niche (a specialized environment) into a short-term cycling stage in which they can be targeted by imatinib. Treating CML patients with imatinib that incorporates G-CSF exposure shows great promise for obtaining improved responses and perhaps more durable remissions in vivo *(28)*.

In addition to imatinib, SKI-606, a potent new BCR-ABL and Src kinase inhibitor without anti-PDGF or c-Kit activity, has been reported to effectively inhibit CD34+ CML stem and progenitor cells, but compared with imatinib, SKI-606 had relatively little effect on normal progenitors *(29)* (Table 2). The effectiveness of BCR-ABL inhibitors against CML stem and progenitor cells indicates that CML, which is a disease with a causative single gene defect, can be traced back to CML stem cells, and those cancer stem cells need to be targeted to achieve curative outcomes.

Aldehyde dehydrogenase 1 (ALDH1): The aldehyde dehydrogenase (ALDH) family of enzymes comprises more than 15 members; in particular the ALDH1 isoform mediates the synthesis of intracellular all-*trans*-retinoic acid that is required for the growth of normal stem cells in the hematopoietic system and other tissues *(36, 37)*. The role of ALDH is not limited to retinoic acid metabolism, as it is also involved in the detoxification of a variety of compounds such as ethanol and the chemotherapeutic drug cyclophosphamide, thus implicating the enzyme into anticancer drug resistance. Furthermore, high expression of ALDH appears to be a marker for stem cells from many tissues and has been identified as a cancer stem cell associated gene in breast cancer, AML, and CML *(30, 37–41)*. Methodology to detect and isolate viable cells by ALDH1 activity using a fluorescent-labeled aldehyde substrate (Aldefluor) is available as shown by us for the CML cell line K562 (Fig. 2a) *(37, 38)*. Within some AML samples, a high ALDH1 activity has been shown to identify patients' CD34$^+$/CD38$^-$ leukemic stem cells. In leukemic stem cells exhibiting extremely high ALDH1 activity, the enzyme may have important implications for resistance to chemotherapy *(30)*. Interestingly, agents that can inhibit ALDH1 exist, one being approved for the treatment of alcoholism, namely disulfiram (Antabus). The latter has shown antitumor activity in in vitro and in vivo models of breast cancer *(31)*. We have tested whether disulfiram can abolish the ALDH1+ subpopulation in K562 CML cells. Figure 2c demonstrates depletion of the stem cell fraction (in R1) following treatment of K562 cells (containing a relatively high percentage of progenitor cells) with disulfiram. Owing to its ALDH+ cell inhibitory potency, disulfiram should be investigated in clinical trials as a potential LSC targeting drug.

Drug efflux pumps: A common property of normal and leukemic stem cells is the expression of high levels of ATP-binding cassette (ABC) transporters, in particular the drug efflux pumps P-glycoprotein (Pgp/ABCB1) and BCRP (breast cancer resistance protein, ABCG2) *(42, 43)*.

ABC transporters provide a mechanism of self-protection in HSCs, and they are involved in multi-drug resistance of leukemia (AML and ALL) to a wide variety of the clinically used cytotoxic agents

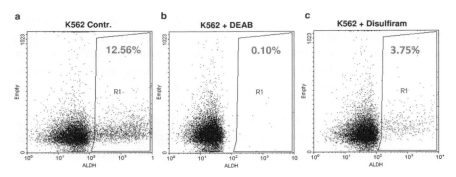

Fig. 2. ALDH1 expression in leukemia cells. The CML cell line K562 is known to express ALDH1 activity. To detect ALDH1, we used the Aldefluor assay kit (StemCell Technologies, Vancouver, CA) and followed the manufacturer's instructions. The assay is based on the principle that ALDH1 can convert uncharged ALDH-substrate, BAAA (BODIPY – aminoacetaldehyde) into a negatively charged reaction product BAA (BODIPY – aminoacetate), which is retained inside cells expressing high levels of ALDH, causing them become brightly fluorescent. (**a**) K562 cells stained with Aldefluor have a fluo escent cell population of 12.56%. (**b**) Negative control; K562 cells stained with Aldefluor in the presence of the known ALDH1 inhibitor diethylaminobenzaldehyde (DEAB, 15 μM, supplied with kit). DEAB blocks the ALDH+ population (0.1% = background). (**c**) Effects of disulfiram on the ALDH+ leukemic stem cell population in K562 cells. Disulfiram (15 μM) was added to K562 cells together with Aldefluor and instead of DEAB. Disulfiram was able to reduce the number of ALDH+ cells more than three times. Data were analyzed by fluorescence activated cell sorting (FACS) using a BD LSR I four-laser flow cytometer (BD Biosciences, San Jose, CA), channel 1 (FL1).

such as daunorubicine, vincristine, vinblastine, methotrexate, or mitoxantrone *(43)*. Furthermore, the ABC transporters Pgp and BCRP define a distinct fraction of cells termed the side population (SP). The SP is composed approximately 0.1% of all cells in bone marrow (BM) from mice, and is detected by flow activated cell sorting (FACS) with a characteristic appearance in the left lower quadrant of the readouts based on its capability to efflux the vital dye Hoechst 33342, which is a substrate of the transporters *(44)*. In mouse BM, the SP was found to be enriched at least 1,000-fold for in vivo BM reconstitution activity in lethally irradiated animals, thus suggesting that the ABC transporter+ cell fraction has stem cell properties *(44)*. SP cells were also detected in leukemia such as T-ALL. The latter implies that ABC transporter expressing leukemia cells are either derived from leukemia stem cells that survive drug treatment or are stem cells *(45)*. Therefore, ABC transporters represent LSC drug targets and existing Pgp or BCRP inhibitors should be exploited for their potential to inhibit LSCs.

Pgp-inhibitors have been studied in leukemia patients as drug resistance modifiers. The Pgp inhibitor cyclosporine A was found to enhance clinical outcomes in combination with standard cytotoxic chemotherapy in poor risk patients with AML (Table 2) *(21)*. However, subsequent clinical studies with a second generation, more specific Pgp inhibitor, valspodar (PSC-833), failed to show benefit *(46)*. A third molecule of this class of drugs, namely zosquidar, is currently in clinical trials in leukemia in combination with standard cytotoxic agents *(22)*. BCRP inhibitors will likely be more selective and effective, but are still in preclinical development (Table 2).

Self-Renewal

Telomerase: Self-renewal is the key characteristic of any stem cell, normal, or cancerous. It essentially means that such cells can differentiate in any cell type of a tissue including themselves. This requires the expression of a set of "stemness" genes that promote immortality. Telomerase is a ribonucleo-protein enzyme complex composed of the human telomerase reverse transcriptase (hTERT), the human telomerase RNA component (hTERC), and dyskerin *(47)*. Its biological function is to synthesize telomeric repeats onto chromosomal ends, thereby preventing telomere erosion and eventual loss of coding DNA sequences with each cell division. Cells that lack the capability to activate telomerase undergo successive telomere shortening and have a finite lifespan, whereas cells that possess telomerase activity such as stem cells or cancer cells can maintain their telomeres and are immortal *(47, 48)*. Although stem cells possess in general a limitless proliferative capacity and long telomeres, telomerase appears differentially expressed in quiescent long-term (LT) HSCs and short-term (ST) cycling HSCs. LT-HSCs are unable to prevent telomere shortening upon serial transplantation, because of low levels of telomerase expression. In short term-HSCs or more committed progenitors cells however, telomerase activity is high and indicates actively cycling cells *(49, 50)*. These data are consistent with recent findings in genetically-engineered mouse models in which over expression of TERT was shown to promote the mobilization of "quiescent" epidermal stem cells out of their niches, leading to stem cell proliferation in vitro and excessive hair growth in vivo *(51, 52)*.

In human hematopoietic stem cells and leukemic stem cells, telomere lengths were comparatively analyzed. It was found that telomeres in LSCs isolated from CML patients were significantly shorter than in HSCs, and that telomerase activity in LSCs was high *(49)*. In line with these observations, we have analyzed telomere length in three AML cell lines (MV411, KG1a, MOLM14) and the acute lymphoblastic the human T cell line MOLT-4 (Fig. 3) and found that both AML cell lines for which we know the CD34/CD38 status (Table 1: MV411 and KG1a) have relatively short telomeres of 2.5 and 1.5 Kb, respectively (Fig. 3, lanes 2 and 5). Importantly, the KG1a line, which has >90% of CD34+ cells, has critically short telomeres of 1.5 Kb. In contrast, the acute lymphoblastic human T cell line MOLT-4 has relatively long telomeres (8 Kb, Fig. 3, lane 3).

The reported differential in telomere length and telomerase activity between HSCs and LSCs and the very short telomeres seen in a highly CD34-positive AML cell line by us (Fig. 3) opens avenues for exploiting telomere and telomerase-directed treatments as stem cell therapeutics *(23)*.

Drugs with telomerase modulating properties that have been already approved for use in patients or are in clinical trials in leukemia include the telomere binding/poisoning agent arsenic trioxide (ATO, approved for APL), the hTERC antisense oligonucleotide GRN163L (in phase I in chronic lymphocytic leukemia), and hTERT vaccines (in chronic lymphocytic leukemia, Table 2) *(23, 24)*.

Differentiating Agents: Another approach to interfere with leukemia stem cells self-renewal capacity is to force them into differentiation. An example for the effectiveness of differentiating agents as a strategy to eliminate cancer stem cells is retinoic acid. All-*trans* retinoic acid (ATRA) has been used with great success in combination chemotherapy in acute promyelocytic leukemia (APL), a disease with a cure rate of more than 70% *(25)*; the high cure rate of APL suggests that cancer stem cells are successfully eliminated by treatment.

Intriguingly, it was demonstrated that when the telomere poison arsenic trioxide (ATO) was combined with ATRA, the cure in patients with APL further improved *(25, 26)*. In a study that combined ATRA and ATO vs. ATRA plus chemotherapy in untreated APL patients, the rate of complete remissions increased to 89% *(26)*.

Developmental Pathways

Developmental pathways control cell fate during embryogenesis and organogenesis and comprise Notch, Wnt, and Hedgehog signaling *(53)*. These pathways are often shared between HSC and LSC. It has been suggested that leukemogenesis associated with pathway activation may result from mis-specification of cells towards stem-cell or stem cell-like fates *(53, 54)*.

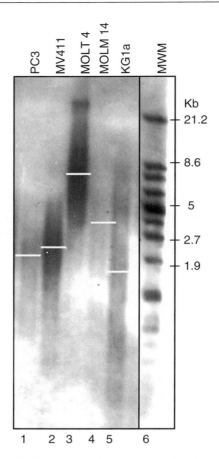

Fig. 3. Telomere length in leukemia cells. The mean telomere restriction fragment length (TRF) was analyzed in 5 cell lines, the PC3 prostate cancer cell line with known mean TRF length of 2.5 kb *(lane 1)* as positive control, and the three AML cell lines MV411 *(lane 2)*, MLOM14 *(lane 4)*, and KG1a *(lane 5)*, as well as the T cell leukemia line MOLT4 *(lane 3)*. *Lane 6* depicts a molecular weight marker. To detect the TRF length of leukemia cells, genomic DNA was isolated using a Qiagen DNeasy plant mini kit (Qiagen, Valencia, CA) and 2 μg each digested with *Hinf*I and *Rsa*I, then loaded onto a 0.8% agarose gel, separated at low voltage (50 V) and transferred to a nylon membrane (GE Healthcare). Southern blotting was performed using the TeloTAGG Telomere Length Assay Kit (Roche) and developed as described by us in *(24)*. Mean TRF lengths are indicated by a *white line*.

The **Notch** signaling pathway in particular regulates cell specification and differentiation *(54)*. Four Notch transmembrane heterodimeric receptors (Notch 1–4) and several ligands are known. The ligands Jagged 1, 2 and Delta 1–4 (DLL1 to 4) can initiate Notch signaling by releasing the intracellular domain of the receptor (Notch-IC) through proteolytic cleavage involving α-secretase and γ-secretase. Notch-IC then enters the nucleus and induces the transcription of Notch-responsive genes *(33, 54)*. In leukemia, Notch signaling plays a crucial role in T-ALL. Fifty % of human T-ALLs from all major molecular oncogenic subtypes exhibit activating Notch 1 mutations *(55)*. Furthermore, experiments using genetically-engineered mice showed that the interaction between the Notch ligand DLL4 and Notch 1 provide key signals for the development of T-cells and T-ALL *(56)*. BM, spleen, lymph nodes, and peripheral blood of Dll4- overexpressing mice contained predominantly CD4+CD8+ T cells and virtually lacked B cells. The Dll4-mice developed a lethal phenotype of a T cell lympho-proliferative disease that progressed to transplantable monoclonal T cell leukemia and scattered to multiple organs *(56)*. Knockout DLL4 mice revealed that DLL4 is specific and critical for normal vascular development and proper arterial formation in mice and appears to be the cognate Notch 1 ligand in vascular development *(33)*. The Notch 1 and DLL4 data suggest that they represent promising anti-leukemia targets.

In fact, several Notch inhibitors are in preclinical and clinical development for the treatment of cancer, including MK-0752, a γ-secretase inhibitor that is in phase I studies in patients with T-ALL and other leukemias (Table 2)*(32)*. Most recently fully humanized antibodies against DLL4 (Regeneron Pharmaceuticals, Inc., Tarrytown, NY) and a soluble form of DLL4 (D4ECD-Fc) are being developed as anticancer therapies and are currently in advanced preclinical studies *(33, 34)*.

The other developmental pathway that provides a therapeutic target in leukemia is the Sonic Hedgehog (Shh) signaling pathway. A recent analysis of bone marrow smears of patients with hematological malignancies has revealed that Shh, a ligand of Ptc, which is the gene encoding the Shh receptor, and Gli1, which is a downstream effector of Ptc, are differentially expressed in leukemia *(57)*. APL had the highest frequency of positive staining both for Shh and Gli1 (100%). Forty-five percent of all AML were also positive for Shh and Gli1. In contrast, all AML and CML cases were negative for both Shh and Gli1 *(57)*. GDC-0449, a potent systemic inhibitor of Shh signal transduction is currently in phase I clinical trials in patients with refractory solid tumors. Initial results of the first in human trial are very exciting in hat no dose-limiting toxicities were seen and dramatic responses occurred in basal cell carcinoma associated with a down-regulation of Gli1 in skin biopsies *(27)*. The APL and AML Shh and Gli1 expression data suggest that GDC-0449 or other Shh inhibitors that are currently in preclinical development should also be investigated for clinical efficacy in these leukemias *(27)*.

CONCLUSIONS AND FUTURE PERSPECTIVES

The idea of the existence of leukemia-initiating/leukemic stem cells has been introduced many decades ago, and it has been clear that these cells play an important role in disease relapse and therapy resistance. However, a molecular understanding of the pathways that govern LSC function and fate was lacking until recently. The pioneering work of John Dick's laboratory in Toronto has provided us with the means of isolating LSCs and HSCs and to test their critical self-renewal property in the NOD/SCID mouse repopulation model. This, together with emerging knowledge in developmental and self-renewal pathways has led to the identification of several targets that are differentially regulated by HSCs and LSCs and could be exploited for the development of LSC-directed anticancer drugs. They are summarized in Table 2. In addition, drugs already exist that are either approved or in advanced clinical development, and can be used to inhibit LSC targets. For a successful use of these agents as LSC treatments, the current clinical practice of how trials are designed needs to be revisited. Standard cytotoxic agents are used with the intent to kill the bulk tumor mass, and thus their effect is assessed in terms of tumor shrinkage. Drugs directed toward LSCs will require the use of novel study endpoints and surrogate markers and will need to be combined with agents that target mature, differentiated leukemic cells to reduce a patient's tumor burden. It is hoped that when tumor burden is low, subsequent, chronically administered LSC-directed treatments will prevent repopulation of tumor mass with resistant cells that arise from LSCs. The selective eradication of leukemia over hematopoietic stem cells will be absolutely necessary to ultimately achieve cures and improve leukemia outcomes. Whether this will be possible or whether side effects associated with the depletion of normal tissue stem cells will occur due to the high degree of similarity between HSCs and LSCs remains to be seen. Nevertheless, LSC targeting agents offer great promise and it could be argued the success of ATRA/ATO combinations in curing APL provides proof that the concept works (see Table 2). If drug combinations that include LSC targeting can be found for each of the disease subtypes, the natural history of leukemias and their prognosis could greatly be altered in the near future.

ACKNOWLEDGMENTS

This work was supported by the Maryland Cancer Research Fund and in part by CA127258-01. I wish to thank Dr. Dean Mann and the University of Maryland, School of Medicine Flow Cytometry Core Facility for assistance with generating the FACS data.

REFERENCES

1. Metcalf D, Nicola NA, Robb L. Differentiation commitment in normal hematopoiesis and leukemic transformation. J Cell Physiol 1997;173:131–4.
2. Chumsri S, Matsui W, Burger AM. Therapeutic implications of leukemic stem cell pathways. Clin Cancer Res 2007;13:6549–54.
3. Wang JCY, Dick JE. Cancer stem cells: Lessons from leukemia. Trends Cell Biol 2005;15:494–501.
4. Stubbs MC, Armstrong SA. Therapeutic implications of leukemia stem cell development. Clin Cancer Res 2007;13:3439–42.
5. Huntly BJ, Shigematsu H, Deguchi K, et al. MOZ-TIF2, but not BCR-ABL, confers properties of leukemic stem cells to committed murine hematopoietic progenitors. Cancer Cell 2004;6:587–96.
6. Krivtsov AV, Twomey D, Feng Z, et al. Transformation from committed progenitor to leukaemia stem cell initiated by MLL-AF9. Nature 2006;442:818–22.
7. Gal H, Amariglio N, Trakhtenbrot L, et al. Gene expression profiles of AML derived stem cells; similarity to hematopoietic stem cells. Leukemia 2006;20:2147–54.
8. Gilliland DG, Jordan CT, Felix CA. The molecular basis of leukemia. Hematology Am Soc Hematol Educ Program 2004:80–97
9. Hope KJ, Jin L, Dick JE. Human acute myeloid leukemia stem cells. Arch Med Res 2003;34:507–14.
10. Bonnet D, Dick JE. Human acute myeloid leukemia is organized as a hierarchy that originates from a primitive hematopoietic cell. Nat Med 1997;3:730–7.
11. Fiebig HH, Maier A, Burger AM. Clonogenic assay with established human tumor xenografts: correlation of *in vitro* to *in vivo* activity as a basis for anticancer drug discovery. Eur J Cancer 2004;40:802–20.
12. Dicke KA, Tindle SE, Davis FM, et al. Leukemic cell colony formation in soft agar by bone marrow cells and peripheral blood cells from untreated acute leukemia patients. Exp Hematol 1983;11:341–50.
13. Allieri MA, Douay L, Deloux J et al. The role of methylcellulose on colony growth of human myeloid leukemic progenitors (AML-CFU). Exp-Hematol 1990;18:911–5.
14. Holyoake TL, Jiang X, Drummond MW, et al. Elucidating critical mechanisms of deregulated stem cell turnover in the chronic phase of chronic myeloid leukemia. Leukemia 2002;16:549–58.
15. Guzman ML, Jordan CT. Considerations for targeting malignant stem cells in leukemia. Cancer Control 2004;11:97–104.
16. George AA, Franklin J, Kerkof K, et al. Detection of leukemic cells in the CD34(+)CD38(-) bone marrow progenitor population in children with acute lymphoblastic leukemia. Blood 2001;97:3925–30.
17. Lu C, Hassan HT. Human stem cell factor-antibody [anti-SCF] enhances chemotherapy cytoxicity in human CD34+ resistant myeloid leukaemia cells. Leuk Res 2006;30:296–302.
18. Frankel AE, McCubrey JA, Miller MS, et al. Diphtheria toxin fused to human interleukin-3 is toxic to blasts from patients with myeloid leukemias. Leukemia 2000;14:576–85.
19. Bernstein ID. Monoclonal antibodies to the myeloid stem cells: therapeutic implications of CMA-676, a humanized anti-CD33 antibody calicheamicin conjugate. Leukemia 2000;14:474–5.
20. Sievers EL, Larson RA, Stadtmauer EA, et al. Efficacy and safety of gemtuzumab ozogamicin in patients with CD33-positive acute myeloid leukemia in first relapse. J Clin Oncol 2001;19:3244–54.
21. List AF, Kopecky KJ, Willman CL, et al. Benefit of cyclosporine modulation of drug resistance in patients with poor-risk acute myeloid leukemia: a Southwest Oncology Group study. Blood 2001;98:3212–20.
22. Fracasso PM, Goldstein LJ, de Alwis DP, et al. Phase I study of docetaxel in combination with the P-glycoprotein inhibitor, zosuquidar, in resistant malignancies. Clin Cancer Res 2004;10:7220–8.
23. Phatak P, Burger AM. Telomerase and its potential for therapeutic intervention. Br J Pharmacol 2007;152:1003–11.
24. Phatak P, Dai F, Butler M, et al. KML001 Cytotoxic activity is associated with its binding to telomeric sequences and telomere erosion in prostate cancer cells. Clin Cancer Res 2008;14:4593–602.
25. Douer D. Advances in the treatment of relapsed acute promyelocytic leukemia. Acta Haematol 2002;107:1–17.
26. Estey E, Garcia-Manero G, Ferrajoli A, et al. Use of all-trans retinoic acid plus arsenic trioxide as an alternative to chemotherapy in untreated acute promyelocytic leukemia. Blood 2006;107:3469–73.

27. LoRusso PM, Rudin CM, Borad MJ. A first-in-human, first-in-class, phase (ph) I study of systemic Hedgehog (Hh) pathway antagonist, GDC-0449, in patients (pts) with advanced solid tumors. J Clin Oncol 2008;26:3516.

28. Jørgensen HG, Copland M, Allan EK, et al. Intermittent exposure of primitive quiescent chronic myeloid leukemia cells to granulocyte-colony stimulating factor in vitro promotes their elimination by imatinib mesylate. Clin Cancer Res 2006;12:626–33.

29. Konig H, Holyoake TL, Bhatia R. Effective and selective inhibition of chronic myeloid leukemia primitive hematopoietic progenitors by the dual Src/Abl kinase inhibitor SKI-606. Blood 2008;111:2329–38.

30. Pearce DJ, Taussig D, Simpson C, et al. Characterization of cells with a high aldehyde dehydrogenase activity from cord blood and acute myeloid leukemia samples. Stem Cells 2005;23:752–60.

31. Chen D, Cui QC, Yan H, et al. Disulfiram, a clinically used anti-alcoholism drug and copper-binding agent, induces apoptotic cell death in breast cancer cultures and xenografts via inhibition of the proteasome activity. Cancer Res 2006;66:10425–33.

32. Deangelo DJ, Stone RM, Silverman LB, et al. A phase I clinical trial of the notch inhibitor MK-0752 in patients with T-cell acute lymphoblastic leukemia/lymphoma (T-ALL) and other leukemias. J Clin Oncol 2006;24 (18S):6585.

33. Turston G, Noguera-Troise I, Yancopoulos GD. The Delta paradox: DLL4 blockade leads to more tumour vessels but less tumour growth. *Nat Rev Cancer* 2007;7:327–31.

34. Li JL, Sainson RC, Shi W, et al. Delta-like 4 Notch ligand regulates tumor angiogenesis, improves tumor vascular function, and promotes tumor growth in vivo. Cancer Res 2007;67:11244–53.

35. Jiang X, Saw KM, Eaves A, et al. Instability of BCR-ABL gene in primary and cultured chronic myeloid leukemia stem cells. J Natl Cancer Inst 2007;99:680–93.

36. Lee MO, Manthey CL, Sladek NE. Identification of mouse liver aldehyde dehydrogenases that catalyze the oxidation of retinaldehyde to retinoic acid. Biochem Pharmacol 1991;42:1279–85.

37. Jones RJ, Matsui W. Cancer Stem Cells: From Bench to Bedside. Biol Blood Marrow Transplant 2007;13:47–52.

38. Jones RJ, Barber JP, Vala MS, et al. Assessment of aldehyde dehydrogenase in viable cells. *Blood* 1995;85:2742–6.

39. Corti S, Locatelli F, Papadimitriou D, et al. Identification of a primitive brain-derived neural stem cell population based on aldehyde dehydrogenase activity. Stem Cells 2006;24:975–85.

40. Ginestier C, Hur MH, Charafe-Jauffret E, et al. ALDH1 Is a marker of normal and malignant human mammary stem cells and a predictor of poor clinical outcome. Cancer Stem Cell 2007;1:555–67.

41. Graham SM, Vass JK, Holyoake TL, et al. Transcriptional analysis of quiescent and proliferating CD34+ human hemopoietic cells from normal and chronic myeloid leukemia sources. Stem Cells 2007;25:3111–20.

42. Plasschaert SL, Van Der Kolk DM, De Bont ES, et al. Breast cancer resistance protein (BCRP) in acute leukemia. Leuk Lymphoma 2004;45:649–54.

43. Steinbach D, Legrand O. ABC transporters and drug resistance in leukemia: was P-gp nothing but the first head of the Hydra? Leukemia 2007;21:1172–6.

44. Goodell MA, Brose K, Paradis G, et al: Isolation and functional properties of murine hematopoietic stem cells that are replicating in vivo. J Exp Med 1996;183:1797–806.

45. Kayo H, Yamazaki H, Nishida H, et al. Stem cell properties and the side population cells as a target for interferon-alpha in adult T-cell leukemia/lymphoma. Biochem Biophys Res Commun 2007;364:808–14.

46. Baer MR, George SL, Dodge RK, et al. Phase 3 study of the multidrug resistance modulator PSC-833 in previously untreated patients 60 years of age and older with acute myeloid leukemia: Cancer and Leukemia Group B Study 9720. Blood 2003;100:1224–32.

47. Cohen SB, Graham ME, Lovrecz GO, et al. Protein composition of catalytically active human telomerase from immortal cells. Science 2007;315:1850–3.

48. Blasco MA. Telomeres and human disease: ageing, cancer and beyond. Nat Rev Genet 2005; 6: 611–622.

49. Brummendorf TH, Balabanov S. Telomere length dynamics in normal hematopoiesis and in disease states characterized by increased stem cell turnover. Leukemia 2006;20:1706–16.

50. Hiyama E, Hiyama K. Telomere and telomerase in stem cells. Br J Cancer 2007;96:1020–4.

51. Sarin KY, Cheung P, Gilison D, et al. Conditional telomerase induction causes proliferation of hair follicle stem cells. Nature 2005;436:1048–52.

52. Flores I, Cayuela ML, Blasco MA. Effects of telomerase and telomere length on epidermal stem cell behavior. Science 2005;309:1253–6.

53. Taipale J, Beachy PA. The Hedgehog and Wnt signalling pathways in cancer. Nature 2001;411:349–354.

54. Artavanis-Tsakonas S, Rand MD, Lake RJ. Notch signaling: cell fate control and signal integration in development. Science 1999;284:770–6.

55. Weng AP, Ferrando AA, Lee W, et al. Activating mutations of NOTCH1 in human T cell acute lymphoblastic leukemia. Science 2004;306:269–71.

56. Yan XQ, Sarmiento U, Sun Y, et al. A novel Notch ligand, Dll4, induces T-cell leukemia/lymphoma when overexpressed in mice by retroviral-mediated gene transfer. Blood 2001;98:3793–9.

57. Bai, LY, Chiu, CF, Lin CW, et al. Differential expression of Sonic hedgehog and Gli1 in hematological malignancies. Leukemia 2008;22:226–8.

22

Targeting Brain Cancer Stem Cells in the Clinic

Gentao Liu, Keith L. Black, and John S. Yu

ABSTRACT

Malignant gliomas (MG) include glioblastoma multiforme (GBM), the most frequent and aggressive of primary brain tumors (Holland, Proc Natl Acad Sci USA 97:6242–6244, 2000). The standard of care for GBM, including surgery followed by radiotherapy and chemotherapy with temozolomide, is associated with a median overall survival of 14.6 months following diagnosis (Reardon et al., J Clin Oncol 24:1253–1265, 2006). The identification of brain cancer stem cells has led to a great opportunity to exploit stem cell mechanisms to inhibit brain tumor initiation, progression, and invasion. Brain cancer stem cells – also called tumor initiating cells or tumor propagating cells - share features with normal neural stem cells but do not necessarily originate from stem cells. Although most cancers have only a small fraction of cancer stem cells, these tumor cells have been shown in laboratory studies to contribute to therapeutic resistance, formation of new blood vessels to supply the tumor and tumor invasion. The presence of this population of cells can explain the recurrence of some brain tumors after chemotherapy, radiation therapy, and other current treatments. In fact, a few of these cells is enough to give rise to a new recurrent tumor. Viewing cancer through the prism of the cancer stem cell hypothesis may fundamentally transform brain cancer therapeutics and translate into improved prognosis of brain tumor patients through a novel means for testing of new strategies for treating brain tumors that focus on the eradication of the cancer stem cells. In animal models, dendritic cell immunotherapy and novel drugs that target stem cell pathways active in brain tumors have been efficacious against cancer stem cells suggesting that anti-cancer stem cell therapies may improve brain tumor therapy. In this chapter, we will discuss the approaches to isolate cancer stem cells and test the therapeutic resistance of cancer stem cells. We will then focus on the implications of cancer stem cells in the clinic, such as the effect of cancer stem cells in prognosis. Finally, we will explore several new strategies to target cancer stem cells.

Key Words: Glioma, Brain tumor-initiating cells, Brain tumor propagating cells, Neurospheres, Tumorospheres, Glioblastoma, Dendritic cell vaccine, Side population, CD133

IDENTIFICATION AND ISOLATION OF BRAIN CANCER STEM CELLS

To be considered as brain cancer stem cells, cells must display the following characteristics (3). (a) they must generate clonally derived cells forming neurospheres, (b) they must self-renew and proliferate, (c) they must be able to differentiate and express markers typical of brain cells (i.e., markers for astrocytes,

From: *Cancer Drug Discovery and Development: Stem Cells and Cancer,*
Edited by: R.G. Bagley and B.A. Teicher, DOI: 10.1007/978-1-60327-933-8_22,
© Humana Press, a part of Springer Science+Business Media, LLC 2009

oligodendrocytes, and neurons), and (d) they must be able to recapitulate their original human tumors after in vivo transplantation in immunodeficient animal models. We and several other groups have identified human brain cancer stem cells based on the formation of neurospheres, a cell culture phenotype associated with neural stem cells *(4)*, as a relevant phenotype *(5–11)*. The significance of the neurosphere phenotype is supported by the success of tumor-derived neurospheres to self-renew, and differentiate to multiple lineages (neural, astrocytic, and oligodendroglial) and recapitulate the complexity of primary GBM in immunocompromised rodents with as few as 100 cells *(11)*.

Similar to the results reported by Kondo et al. on a rat GBM cell line C6 *(12, 13)*, we have successfully isolated cancer stem-like cells defined as tumorospheres from the commercial cell line, 9L, which are cultured under differentiating conditions for years using conditions appropriate for neural stem cell expansion. This observation implies that even after years of passaging, this glioma cell line may retain the capacity to display a stem-like phenotype. These neurosphere cells are able to differentiate after the withdrawal of growth factors and give rise to a progeny of cells expressing markers of astrocytic and neuronal lineage markers. However, concerns have been raised about the true reflection of "stemness" with the generation of neurospheres which may contain cells that coalesce to form similar structures *(14)*. In addition, the culturing of tumor cells until the formation of neurospheres precludes the direct comparison of cancer stem cells with non-stem cell populations.

The ideal approach to isolate cancer stem cells should be through the use of cell surface markers. The cell surface marker CD133 (Prominin 1) is expressed by embryonic neural stem cells *(4, 15)* and has been used to select for brain cancer stem cells *(5, 6, 16)*.

In 2003, Dirks and collaborators *(6)* reported the identification and purification of cancer stem cells from human brain tumors on the basis of cells expressing the neural stem cell surface antigen, CD133. The authors demonstrated that the CD133+ cells can differentiate in vitro into tumor cells that phenotypically resemble the patient's tumor. The cancer stem cells represent a fraction of the total cells comprising the tumor, identified by CD133 expression. The authors were able to confirm the stem cell activity of CD133+ tumor cells by plating cancer stem cells at limiting dilutions and by demonstrating that the self-renewal capacity of tumor cells was only present in the CD133+ fraction and not in the CD133– fraction. The CD133+ population also displayed proliferative capacity, which is not present in the CD133– fraction.

Furthermore, the same group reported that only CD133+ cells are able to generate tumors after grafting in mice brain and that these tumors resemble the patient's original tumor *(5)*. Injection of only 100 CD133+ cells into NOD-SCID mice brain led to the growth of a tumor that could also be serially transplanted and that is histologically identical to the tumor of the patient from whom these cells were derived. In contrast, the injection of 1×10^5 CD133– cells does not generate tumor growth *(5)*.

However, other reports suggest that cells without CD133 expression may generate brain tumors *(17–19)*. Another group has found that the IQGAP1 scaffold protein regulates neural stem cells and is a marker for amplifying cancer cells in glioblastomas *(20, 21)*.

Cancer stem cells could also be identified from the side population (SP) using flow cytometry as stem cells which exclude Hoechst blue dye. The 72-kDa breast cancer resistance protein (BRCP) is a member of the subfamily G of the human ATP-binding cassette transporter superfamily, designated also as ABCG2 *(22, 23)*. Overexpression of BRCP is associated with high levels of resistance to a variety of anticancer agents, including anthracyclines, mitoxantrone, and camphothecins by enhancing drug efflux *(22, 24)*. Zhou and collaborators *(25)* demonstrated that ABCG2 is expressed in stem cells from a wide variety of sources. They found that the expression of ABCG2 is strictly correlated with the SP of cells from different sources (murine bone marrow, skeletal muscle, and cultured embryonic stem cells). The SP is defined as the population of cells able to efflux the Hoechst 33342 dye and is rich of highly repopulating cells *(26)*. The SP was demonstrated first in hematopoietic stem cells of different species and also in murine skeletal muscle and neurospheres derived from embryonic mice. The SP was also found in various cancer cell lines including C6 rat glioma, MCF7 breast cancer, B104 neuroblastoma, and HeLa adenocarcinoma cell lines *(12)*. There are about 0.4% SP cells in glioma C6, this small percentage of cells can be cultured and can give rise to both SP and non-SP cells, including neurons and glia. The SP cells are also highly tumorigenic in immune-deficient mice *(12, 27)*. This suggests that even if these cells constitute only a very small percentage of the population, the SP cells contain not only tumor stem cells that proliferate, but also cells that can differentiate.

The persistence of SP cells in cancer cell lines cultured in serum-containing medium for decades suggests that SP may be a general source of cancer stem cells. However, the SP cells have been also shown to be very heterogeneous. In fact, the SP detected in cancer stem cells contained a wide variety of cells, some of which express ABCG2.

The diversity of markers that may be used to define cancer stem cells may be due to patient-to-patient differences in cancer stem cells or a lack of absolute marker fingerprints. It is clear that the expression of a cancer stem cell marker is not sufficient to claim a cancer stem cell phenotype. The precise methodologies employed for isolation of cancer stem cells (even for the same marker) and in functional assays may be dramatically different between laboratory groups, limiting the ability to generalize conclusions regarding the cell biology of the derived populations. Thus, every lab performing cancer stem cell studies must confirm critical cancer stem cell functional assays to permit comparisons across studies.

CANCER STEM CELLS IN THERAPEUTIC RESISTANCE

Cancer stem cells are likely to share many of the properties of normal stem cells that provide for a long lifespan, including relative quiescence, resistance to drugs and toxins through the expression of several ABC transporters, an active DNA-repair capacity, and resistance to apoptosis. Several groups, including our laboratory, have demonstrated that brain tumor stem cells or cells expressing stem cell markers from multiple cancer types exhibit resistance to conventional cancer therapies.

We demonstrated that CD133+ cancer stem cells express higher levels of BCRP and MGMT mRNA, as well as higher mRNA levels of genes that inhibit apoptosis. Furthermore, CD133+ cells were significantly resistant to chemotherapeutic agents including temozolomide, carboplatin, paclitaxel (Taxol), and etoposide (VP16) compared to autologous CD133– cells *(28)*. Our study provided evidence that CD133+ cancer stem cells display chemoresistance. This resistance is probably conferred in the CD133+ cell by higher expression of on BCRP and MGMT, as well as antiapoptosis proteins and inhibitors of apoptosis protein families *(28)*. Salmaggi and colleagues also found that multidrug resistance-associated proteins 1 and 3 as well as other molecules conferring multidrug resistance were higher in the selected populations of cancer stem-like cells defined as tumorospheres that were obtained from human glioblastoma when compared with primary adherent cells derived from the same tumor *(29)*. In addition to resistance to chemotherapy, brain cancer stem cells are also resistant to the effects of ionizing radiation with proficient capacity to repair DNA damage due to preferential activation of the DNA damage checkpoint response *(16)*. Additional studies from other groups investigating brain tumor stem cell models confirmed that cells expressing cancer stem cell markers are resistant to radiation *(30)*.

Cancer stem cells share another property with normal stem cells: they are able to migrate to different areas of the brain. Cancers stem cells are capable of migrating and hiding themselves in the "safe corner" of the brain to escape removal by surgery, chemotherapy, and radiation therapy. The invading cells, having migrated several millimeters or even centimeters from the main focus of the tumor, return to cycle phase under the control of some as yet unknown microenvironmental cue to form a recurrent tumor adjacent to the original site of presentation. Clinical and experimental data demonstrate that glioma cell migration is a complex combination of multiple molecular processes, including the alteration of tumor cell adhesion to a modified extracellular matrix, the secretion of proteases by the cells, and modifications to the actin cytoskeleton. Intracellular signaling pathways involved in the acquisition of resistance to apoptosis by migrating glioma cells include PI3K, Akt, mTOR, NF-kappaB, the Rho family of small GTPases, and autophagy (programmed cell death type II) *(31)*. However, high expression of chemokine receptors, such as CXCR4, are probably one of the most important mechanisms related to cancer stem cells migration *(28, 29, 32)*.

Clinically it is observed that tumors respond to chemotherapies and radiation therapy only to recur with renewed resilience and aggression. Although chemotherapy kills most of the cells in a tumor, chemoresistant cancer stem cells may be left behind, which then recur. Therefore, recurrent brain tumors contain greater numbers of brain tumor stem cells that are also selected for greater resistance to therapy. Hence, the lethality of high grade brain tumors as well as the virulence of recurrent tumors might be better explained *(33)*.

CANCER STEM CELLS IN PROGNOSIS

Current prognosis (and thus clinical management) of brain tumor patients utilizes patient characteristics (age, performance status, etc.) and tumor characteristics (histology, grade, extent of resection and presence of metastasis in some tumor types). Prognosis for GBM patients remains dismal although we have showed that levels of CD8(+) recent thymic emigrants (RTEs) accounted for the prognostic power of age on clinical outcome in GBM patients *(34, 35)*. To date, molecular testing has only modestly contributed to patient management *(36–38)* as these markers are imperfect and require refinement as the status of the direct molecular target for any therapy does not solely determine the outcome of treatment. Recently, several studies employed genomic signatures to predict patient prognosis and response to therapy. Glinsky et al. *(39)* investigated 11 stemness-related gene signatures in several independent therapy-outcome sets of clinical samples obtained from 1,153 cancer patients diagnosed with 11 different types of cancer, including 5 epithelial malignancies (prostate, breast, lung, ovarian, and bladder cancers) and 5 nonepithelial malignancies (lymphoma, mesothelioma, medulloblastoma, glioma, and acute myeloid leukemia). Kaplan-Meier analysis demonstrated that a stem cell-like expression profile of the 11-gene signature in primary tumors is a consistent powerful predictor of a short interval to disease recurrence, distant metastasis, and death after therapy in cancer patients diagnosed with 11 distinct types of cancer *(39)*. More recently, Liu et al. also found that a cancer stem gene expression profile derived from breast cancers did predict patient survival *(40)*. We also demonstrated that CD133 expression was significantly higher in recurrent GBM tissue obtained from five patients as compared to their respective newly diagnosed tumors *(28)*. Furthermore, based on the analysis of CD133 expression in a series of 95 gliomas of various grade and histology by immunohistochemistry on cryostat sections and multivariate survival analysis *(41)*, Zeppernick et al. found that both the proportion of CD133+ cells and their topological organization in clusters were significant ($P < 0.001$) prognostic factors for adverse progression-free survival and overall survival independent of tumor grade, extent of resection, or patient age. Furthermore, proportion of CD133+ cells was an independent risk factor for tumor regrowth and time to malignant progression in WHO grade 2 and 3 tumors *(41)*. These studies indicated that prognostic models may be strengthened if cancer stem cell populations are directly characterized. Cancer markers like CA-125 have been developed to follow the course of patients in response to therapy and predict recurrence. Many of these markers are expressed by the more differentiated cancer cell compartments *(42, 43)*. Characterizing cancer stem cells at diagnosis and during treatment may yield novel cancer markers that more closely predict the clinical course of cancer patients.

DIFFERENTIATION THERAPY

If the malignant cells of cancers are initiated by cancer stem cells, then it should be possible to treat cancers by inducing differentiation of the stem cells, i.e., differentiation therapy *(44)*. If tumor cells can be forced to differentiate and to cease proliferation, then their malignant potential will be controlled. Although a number of agents have been studied over the years *(45)*, the most thoroughly examined and clinically tested as a differentiating agent is retinoic acid (RA, Vitamin A), in particular all-trans-retinoic acid (ATRA) *(46, 47)*.

Currently about 90% of newly diagnosed patients with acute promyelocytic leukemia (APL) achieve complete remission and over 70% are cured by ATRA therapy *(48)* with or without concomitant chemotherapy with methotrexate and cytarabine *(49)*. The clinical presentation of APL is frequently associated with hemorrhage and low platelet counts due to the decreased ability of the bone marrow to produce platelets. Poor prognostic factors include older age, elevated white blood cell count, low platelets, and CD56 expression *(50)*. The overall survival rate is greatly increased by ATRA vs. chemotherapy remission. Maintenance therapy with ATRA with low-dose chemotherapy may be useful. Despite overall success in treating APL with retinoids, relapse with the development of acquired resistance to retinoid induced maturation is not uncommon and is responsible for treatment failure *(48)*. The mechanism of resistance to RA therapy is not well understood. It may be due to increased ATRA metabolism, increased expression of the RA binding proteins, P-gylcoprotein expression, or mutations in the ligand binding domain of RAR-α. Due to severe side effects of ATRA treatment, dosing schedules are critical to the success of treatment. Treatment with other differentiating-inducing agents, cytotoxic or chromatin remodeling agents, as well as receptor-selective and modified retinoids may overcome this resistance *(48)*. Cytotoxic treatment with arsenic trioxide is the treatment of choice for refractory ATRA resistance *(49, 50)*. In addition, resistance can be overcome to some extent by combining histone deacetylase inhibitors, such as sodium butyrate, with RA. This treatment facilitates RA-induced gene transcription and induction of apoptosis, but has little effect on granulocytic differentiation of the promyelocytic leukemia cells *(51)*.

Early-stage mouse embryonic stem cells could also be differentiated into neural cells by ATRA in vitro *(52)*. ATRA can greatly increase the percentage of neurons in the course of inducing the human embryonic neural stem cells to differentiate by downregulation of Notch1 expression *(53)*. ATRA can accelerate differentiation of NSCs into neuron-likes cells and upregulate the expression of RAR-beta mRNA in neonatal rat striatal neural stem cells *(54)*. In C6 rat glioma cells, ATRA stimulates the differentiation toward oligodendrocytic cells *(55)*.These studies raised the possibility of using ATRA to induce differentiation of brain cancer stem cells as a therapy.

TARGETING SIGNAL TRANSDUCTION PATHWAYS OF CANCER STEM CELLS

The signals that determine which daughter cell of an adult stem cell remains a stem cell, and which begins the process of determination, may also be the signals that control the growth and differentiation of cancer stem cells *(46)*. Key signaling pathways that regulate neural stem cell fate and differentiation – Olig2, sonic hedgehog, Notch, BMI-1, bone morphogenic proteins (BMPs), maternal embryonic leucine zipper kinase (MELK), etc. – may contribute to brain tumor malignancy through regulation of proliferation, apoptosis, and angiogenesis of brain tumor stem cells. Hemmati and collaborators *(9)* demonstrated that normal and tumor-derived spheres express *bmi-1*, even after mitogen withdrawal from the medium. *Bmi-1* has been demonstrated to be important for self-renewal of both leukemic *(56)* and normal hematopoietic stem cells *(57)*. The presence and the persistent expression of *bmi-1* in tumor cells could indicate a greater capacity of these cells to self-renew.

The first generation of anticancer stem cell therapies has focused on signal transduction pathways that regulate cell differentiation: Notch, BMP, hedgehog, etc. *(58–61)*. Growth factor pathways may function in stem cell maintenance [e.g., epidermal growth factor (EGF) and basic fibroblast growth factor (bFGF)] *(10)* and the relationship with the cancer stem cell niche may be targeted *(62, 63)*. Bao et al. recently demonstrated that brain tumor stem cells generate highly vascular tumors through the secretion of high levels of vascular endothelial growth factor (VEGF) *(64)*. This finding is important as VEGF is a validated therapeutic target in glioma therapy *(65–67)*.

A cautionary note may be struck with potential toxicities to normal stem cells. The role of neural stem cells remains to be defined but neural stem cells are clearly important in the pediatric population. Therefore, antistem cell therapies may display significant therapeutic indices. Target identification studies may identify novel molecular cancer stem cell targets that are differentially expressed or regulated relative to normal stem cells.

TARGETING CANCER STEM CELLS USING ACTIVE IMMUNOTHERAPY

The presence and high expression of ABC transporter proteins, antiapoptosis proteins, and DNA repair checkpoint proteins in cancer stem cells could explain why common therapies and, in particular, chemotherapy and radiation are not enough to eradicate the tumor. Because normal neural stem cells do not express major histocompatibility (MHC) antigens which are necessary for recognition by T cells, neural stem cells would not be susceptible to T cell killing. Cancer stem cells, on the other hand, express high levels of MHC antigens. Therefore, active immunotherapy in which a vaccination strategy is used to induce a T cell response specifically against cancer stem cells may be an effective means of exploiting this therapeutic window. Hence, immunotherapy with dendritic cell vaccination opens a new way to target infiltrating cancer stem cells.

Dendritic cells (DCs) are antigen-presenting cells that stimulate the naïve immune system and play a role in maintaining self-tolerance *(68)*. Through the expression of high levels of MHC class I and class II molecules, adhesion and costimulatory molecules (CD40, CD45, CD80, and CD86), and stimulatory cytokines (IL-12, IL-15, and IL-18) DCs lead to an efficient priming of cytotoxic T cells and CD4+ T helper cells, thus inducing a specific and therapeutic immune response *(69)*. In fact, cytotoxic T cells are believed to be the main cells involved in tumor rejection because these cells can recognize antigens loaded onto MHC class I molecules, while CD4+ T cells are activated after MHC class II-restricted presentation of exogenous antigens by DC. It was also reported that DCs can prime CD8+ T cell-mediated response against exogenous tumor antigens *(70)*. DCs can be generated in culture both from peripheral blood CD14+ monocytic precursors and from proliferating CD34+ progenitor cells by the addition of cytokines, including IL-4, GM-CSF, TNF-alpha, c-kit, and Flt-3 ligand *(69)*.

In vaccination studies, DCs have been loaded in culture with different tumor-derived substrates, including specific tumor-associated peptides, tumor RNA and cDNA, tumor cell lysate, or apoptotic tumor cells *(69)*. Many animal studies and clinical trials based on DC immunotherapy have been reported to successfully improve and prolong the survival of tumor-bearing experimental animals or patients *(71–76)*. The use of a dendritic cell (DC) vaccine in patients with newly diagnosed high grade glioma was described in a phase I study by Yu and colleagues *(77)*. Following surgical resection and external-beam radiotherapy, nine patients were given a series of three DC vaccinations using DCs cultured from patients' peripheral blood mononuclear cells (PBMC) pulsed ex vivo with autologous tumor cell-surface peptide isolated by means of acid elution. Each DC vaccination was given intradermally every other week over a 6-week period. Four of the nine patients who had radiological evidence of disease progression underwent repeat surgery after receiving the third vaccination. Two of the four patients who underwent re-resection had robust infiltration of CD8+ and CD45RO+

T cells which was not apparent in the tumor specimen resected prior to DC trial entry. Comparison of long-term survival data between the study group and matched controls demonstrated an increase in median survival of 455 days vs. 257 days for the control group, conferring some survival benefit after DC vaccination.

Given the promising results and absence of observed destructive autoimmune response in the Phase I study, Yu and colleagues pursued an additonal phase I trial using tumor lysate as an antigen source *(78)*. Fourteen patients with recurrent *(12)* and newly diagnosed *(2)* malignant glioma including anaplastic astrocytoma and glioblastoma multiforme were given three vaccinations with autologous DC pulsed with autologous tumor-lysate every other week over a 6-week period. As part of a HLA-restricted tetramer staining assay, it was established in four out of nine patients, that there was one or more tumor-associated antigen (TAA)-specific cytotoxic T-lymphocyte (CTL) clones against melanoma antigen-encoding gene-1, gp100 and human epidermal growth factor receptor (HER)-2. DC vaccination offers a significant survival benefit as evidenced by an increase in median survival of 133 weeks for the study group vs. 30 weeks for the control group.

In another phase I study by Liau and colleagues, 12 patients with glioblastoma multiforme (7 newly diagnosed, 5 recurrent) were enrolled into a dose-escalation study and treated with 1, 5, or 10 million autologous dendritic cells pulsed with acid-eluted autologous tumor peptides *(79)*. They found that the DC vaccinations were well tolerated with no major adverse events or autoimmune reactions. Using conventional CTL assays, six patients were found to have peripheral tumor-specific CTL activity postvaccination where they did not have peripheral CTL activity prior to vaccination. They also found that those who developed systemic antitumor cytotoxicity had longer survival time compared to those patients who did not. All of the patients who had stable/minimal residual disease at baseline generated a positive CTL response (100%) whereas those with active progressive disease at baseline did not produce statistically significant cell-mediated CTL responses (0%) suggesting that those with active tumor progression/recurrence may have an impaired ability to mount an effective cellular antitumor immune response *(79)*.

More recently, Pellegatta and colleagues have found that DC targeting of mouse glioma GL261 neurospheres (GL261-NS) provides more efficient protection against GL261 tumors than targeting of GL261 adherent cells(GL261-AC) *(80)*. We generated very similar results using 9L rat glioma model (unpublished data). Thus, these results demonstrated that CTLs generated by vaccinations with DC pulsed with tumor lysate derived form cancer stem cells could efficiently deplete the tumor of its hierarchically highest and most relevant population: CSCs. Pellegatta also found that GL261-NS, but not GL261-AC, express high levels of MHC class II and costimulatory molecules, CD80 and CD86. Normal neurospheres, on the other hand, express MHC II molecules but are weakly immunogenic because of the low expression levels of costimulatory molecules *(81)*. Therefore, it seems that GL261-NS have a peculiar set of expression of molecules highly relevant for immune recognition. To translate these observations to the clinical setting, we need to assess how representative the GL261 model is of human glioma. If the glioblastoma neurosphere subpopulation enriches for tumor-initiating cells and displays higher immunogenicity as in the GL261 model, this approach may warrant clinical investigation. GBM cells from relatively small amounts of tumor tissue could be amplified in vitro as neurospheres and used for treating the relapse, usually taking place 6 months or more after the first surgery.

SOX2 was regarded as a critical gene for self-renewal in both normal neural stem cells and brain cancer stem cells. SOX2 were tested for the activation of glioma-reactive CD8+ cytotoxic T lymphocytes (CTLs). Specific CTLs were raised against the HLA-A0201-restricted SOX2-derived peptide (TLMKKDKYTL) and were capable of lysing glioma cells *(82)*. Furthermore, detection of anti-SOX2 T cells predicts favorable clinical outcome in patients with asymptomatic plasma proliferative disorders *(83)*.The abundant and glioma-restricted overexpression of SOX2 and the generation of SOX2-specific and tumor-reactive CTLs may implicate this antigen as a target for T cell-based immunotherapy of brain cancer stem cells. SOX2 was highly expressed on cancer stem cells as compared to their differentiated cells in glioblastoma cells *(28)*. Harnessing immunity to antigens expressed by tumor progenitor cells may be critical for prevention and therapy of human cancer *(83)*.

The challenge with vaccination strategies is to break tolerance so that the patient's immune system will recognize cancer cells. The success of vaccines depends on the identification of appropriate tumor antigens, establishment of effective immunization strategies, and their ability to circumvent inhibitory immune mechanisms. On the other hand, several aspects of DC vaccine need to be optimized, including the protocol of DC generation, DC subtype, dose and timing interval of vaccination, route of administration, approaches of antigen loading, and especially, DC maturation *(84)*. Future vaccination therapies may be directly driven toward CSCs lysates or specific tumor antigens of CSCs to improve and ameliorate the DC vaccine efficacy (mostly evaluated as overall survival) *(3)*. In this case, the activated immune system can directly and specifically attack tumor stem cells.

In addition, the effects of immunotherapy depend on the development of antigen-specific memory CD8+ T cells that can express cytokines and kill antigen-bearing cells when they encounter the tumor. The induction of specific CD8-mediated antitumor immunity by DC vaccine involves the following six steps: antigen threshold, antigen presentation, T cell response, T cell traffic, target destruction, and generation of memory. Each of these steps could be significantly impacted by chemotherapy *(85)*. Cytotoxic chemotherapy can be integrated with tumor vaccines using unique doses and schedules to break down the barriers to cancer immunotherapy, releasing the full potential of the antitumor immune response to eradicate disease. The development of new protocols by combining chemotherapy with immunotherapy to achieve therapeutic synergy will be applicable to many cancer types *(86)*. Furthermore, synergistic effects of DC immunotherapy followed by chemotherapy have also been observed. Sensitization of malignant glioma to chemotherapy through dendritic cell vaccination provides a novel strategy to overcome the immune escape of cancer cells by immunoediting *(84, 87)*.

TARGETING CANCER STEM CELLS WITH PASSIVE IMMUNOTHERAPY

Other modalities are being adapted toward brain tumor stem cell ablation, particularly antibody therapy (passive immunotherapy). Krause et al. found that CD44 is specifically required on leukemic cells that initiate CML. Antibody to CD44 attenuates induction of CML-like leukemia in recipients *(88)*. Further, Jin et al. reported a therapeutic approach using an activating monoclonal antibody directed to the adhesion molecule CD44. In vivo administration of this antibody to nonobese diabetic-severe combined immune-deficient mice transplanted with human AML markedly reduced leukemic repopulation. Absence of leukemia in serially transplanted mice demonstrated that AML LSCs are directly targeted *(63)*. Developing antibody targeting solid cancer stem cells is attracting attention and financial investment from small biotech companies to pharmaceutical giants. GlaxoSmithKline (GSK) and OncoMed Pharmaceuticals (OncoMed) recently announced a worldwide strategic alliance to discover, develop, and market novel antibody therapeutics to target cancer stem cells. OncoMed has established a diverse pipeline of monoclonal antibodies to target multiple pathways important in the activity of cancer stem cells. The alliance with GSK includes OncoMed's lead antibody product candidate, OMP-21M18.

SUMMARY

The FDA has required improved survival as the endpoint for approval of most cancer therapies. Surrogate endpoints, such as radiographic tumor response, are attractive for clinical trials, but tumor response (i.e., shrinkage of tumor) may not correlate with survival. Non-stem tumor cells account for the bulk of the tumor and may display preferential sensitivity to some cancer therapies while cancer stem cells may represent restricted subsets of tumor populations but contribute to tumor progression and recurrence – and thus, tumor lethality. Obviously, brain tumor stem cells must be addressed for therapeutic success but cancer stem cells may present special challenges and opportunities. We may be entering a new phase in cancer research based on the cancer stem cell paradigm in which the ability of oncologists to provide improved prognosis and therapy may be at hand.

In conclusion, while more studies are necessary to better understand the biology and the behavior of tumor stem-like cells, it is evident that these cells will represent a new target for future tumor therapies.

REFERENCES

1. Holland, E. C. Glioblastoma multiforme: the terminator. Proc Natl Acad Sci USA, 97: 6242–6244, 2000.
2. Reardon, D. A., Rich, J. N., Friedman, H. S., and Bigner, D. D. Recent advances in the treatment of malignant astrocytoma. J Clin Oncol, 24: 1253–1265, 2006.
3. Tunici, P., Irvin, D., Liu, G., Yuan, X., Zhaohui, Z., Ng, H., and Yu, J. S Brain tumor stem cells: new targets for clinical treatments?. Neurosurg Focus, 20: E27, 2006.
4. Uchida, N., Buck, D. W., He, D., Reitsma, M. J., Masek, M., Phan, T. V., Tsukamoto, A. S., Gage, F. H., and Weissman, I. L. Direct isolation of human central nervous system stem cells. Proc Natl Acad Sci USA, 97: 14720–14725, 2000.
5. Singh, S. K., Hawkins, C., Clarke, I. D., Squire, J. A., Bayani, J., Hide, T., Henkelman, R. M., Cusimano, M. D., and Dirks, P. B. Identification of human brain tumour initiating cells. Nature, 432: 396–401, 2004.
6. Singh, S. K., Clarke, I. D., Terasaki, M., Bonn, V. E., Hawkins, C., Squire, J., and Dirks, P. B. Identification of a cancer stem cell in human brain tumors. Cancer Res, 63: 5821–5828, 2003.
7. Galli, R., Binda, E., Orfanelli, U., Cipelletti, B., Gritti, A., De Vitis, S., Fiocco, R., Foroni, C., Dimeco, F., and Vescovi, A. Isolation and characterization of tumorigenic, stem-like neural precursors from human glioblastoma. Cancer Res, 64: 7011–7021, 2004.
8. Ignatova, T. N., Kukekov, V. G., Laywell, E. D., Suslov, O. N., Vrionis, F. D., and Steindler, D. A. Human cortical glial tumors contain neural stem-like cells expressing astroglial and neuronal markers in vitro. Glia, 39: 193–206, 2002.
9. Hemmati, H. D., Nakano, I., Lazareff, J. A., Masterman-Smith, M., Geschwind, D. H., Bronner-Fraser, M., and Kornblum, H. I. Cancerous stem cells can arise from pediatric brain tumors. Proc Natl Acad Sci USA, 100: 15178–15183, 2003.
10. Lee, J., Kotliarova, S., Kotliarov, Y., Li, A., Su, Q., Donin, N. M., Pastorino, S., Purow, B. W., Christopher, N., Zhang, W., Park, J. K., and Fine, H. A. Tumor stem cells derived from glioblastomas cultured in bFGF and EGF more closely mirror the phenotype and genotype of primary tumors than do serum-cultured cell lines. Cancer Cell, 9: 391–403, 2006.
11. Yuan, X., Curtin, J., Xiong, Y., Liu, G., Waschsmann-Hogiu, S., Farkas, D. L., Black, K. L., and Yu, J. S. Isolation of cancer stem cells from adult glioblastoma multiforme. Oncogene, 23: 9392–9400, 2004.
12. Kondo, T., Setoguchi, T., and Taga, T. Persistence of a small subpopulation of cancer stem-like cells in the C6 glioma cell line. Proc Natl Acad Sci USA, 101: 781–786, 2004.
13. Ghods, A. J., Irvin, D., Liu, G., Yuan, X., Abdulkadir, I. R., Tunici, P., Konda, B., Wachsmann-Hogiu, S., Black, K. L., and Yu, J. S. Spheres isolated from 9L gliosarcoma rat cell line possess chemoresistant and aggressive cancer stem-like cells. Stem Cells, 25: 1645–1653, 2007.
14. Singec, I., Knoth, R., Meyer, R. P., Maciaczyk, J., Volk, B., Nikkhah, G., Frotscher, M., and Snyder, E. Y. Defining the actual sensitivity and specificity of the neurosphere assay in stem cell biology. Nat Methods, 3: 801–806, 2006.
15. Pfenninger, C. V., Roschupkina, T., Hertwig, F., Kottwitz, D., Englund, E., Bengzon, J., Jacobsen, S. E., and Nuber, U. A. CD133 is not present on neurogenic astrocytes in the adult subventricular zone, but on embryonic neural stem cells, ependymal cells, and glioblastoma cells. Cancer Res, 67: 5727–5736, 2007.
16. Bao, S., Wu, Q., McLendon, R. E., Hao, Y., Shi, Q., Hjelmeland, A. B., Dewhirst, M. W., Bigner, D. D., and Rich, J. N. Glioma stem cells promote radioresistance by preferential activation of the DNA damage response. Nature, 444: 756–760, 2006.
17. Beier, D., Hau, P., Proescholdt, M., Lohmeier, A., Wischhusen, J., Oefner, P. J., Aigner, L., Brawanski, A., Bogdahn, U., and Beier, C. P. CD133(+) and CD133(−) glioblastoma-derived cancer stem cells show differential growth characteristics and molecular profiles. Cancer Res, 67: 4010–4015, 2007.

18. Zheng, X., Shen, G., Yang, X., and Liu, W. Most C6 cells are cancer stem cells: evidence from clonal and population analyses. Cancer Res, 67: 3691–3697, 2007.

19. Wang, J., Sakariassen, P. O., Tsinkalovsky, O., Immervoll, H., Boe, S. O., Svendsen, A., Prestegarden, L., Rosland, G., Thorsen, F., Stuhr, L., Molven, A., Bjerkvig, R., and Enger, P. O. CD133 negative glioma cells form tumors in nude rats and give rise to CD133 positive cells. Int J Cancer, 122: 761–768, 2008.

20. Balenci, L., Saoudi, Y., Grunwald, D., Deloulme, J. C., Bouron, A., Bernards, A., and Baudier, J. IQGAP1 regulates adult neural progenitors in vivo and vascular endothelial growth factor-triggered neural progenitor migration in vitro. J Neurosci, 27: 4716–4724, 2007.

21. Balenci, L., Clarke, I. D., Dirks, P. B., Assard, N., Ducray, F., Jouvet, A., Belin, M. F., Honnorat, J., and Baudier, J. IQGAP1 protein specifies amplifying cancer cells in glioblastoma multiforme. Cancer Res, 66: 9074–9082, 2006.

22. Doyle, L. A. and Ross, D. D. Multidrug resistance mediated by the breast cancer resistance protein BCRP (ABCG2). Oncogene, 22: 7340–7358, 2003.

23. Ejendal, K. F. and Hrycyna, C. A. Multidrug resistance and cancer: the role of the human ABC transporter ABCG2. Curr Protein Pept Sci, 3: 503–511, 2002.

24. Mao, Q. and Unadkat, J. D. Role of the breast cancer resistance protein (ABCG2) in drug transport. AAPS J, 7: E118–133, 2005.

25. Zhou, S., Schuetz, J. D., Bunting, K. D., Colapietro, A. M., Sampath, J., Morris, J. J., Lagutina, I., Grosveld, G. C., Osawa, M., Nakauchi, H., and Sorrentino, B. P. The ABC transporter Bcrp1/ABCG2 is expressed in a wide variety of stem cells and is a molecular determinant of the side-population phenotype. Nat Med, 7: 1028–1034, 2001.

26. Kim, M. and Morshead, C. M. Distinct populations of forebrain neural stem and progenitor cells can be isolated using side-population analysis. J Neurosci, 23: 10703–10709, 2003.

27. Setoguchi, T., Taga, T., and Kondo, T. Cancer stem cells persist in many cancer cell lines. Cell Cycle, 3: 414–415, 2004.

28. Liu, G., Yuan, X., Zeng, Z., Tunici, P., Ng, H., Abdulkadir, I. R., Lu, L., Irvin, D., Black, K. L., and Yu, J. S. Analysis of gene expression and chemoresistance of CD133+ cancer stem cells in glioblastoma. Mol Cancer, 5: 67, 2006.

29. Salmaggi, A., Boiardi, A., Gelati, M., Russo, A., Calatozzolo, C., Ciusani, E., Sciacca, F. L., Ottolina, A., Parati, E. A., La Porta, C., Alessandri, G., Marras, C., Croci, D., and De Rossi, M. Glioblastoma-derived tumorospheres identify a population of tumor stem-like cells with angiogenic potential and enhanced multidrug resistance phenotype. Glia, 54: 850–860, 2006.

30. Blazek, E. R., Foutch, J. L., and Maki, G. Daoy medulloblastoma cells that express CD133 are radioresistant relative to CD133− cells, and the CD133+ sector is enlarged by hypoxia. Int J Radiat Oncol Biol Phys, 67: 1–5, 2007.

31. Lefranc, F., Brotchi, J., and Kiss, R. Possible future issues in the treatment of glioblastomas: special emphasis on cell migration and the resistance of migrating glioblastoma cells to apoptosis. J Clin Oncol, 23: 2411–2422, 2005.

32. Dirks, P. B. Glioma migration: clues from the biology of neural progenitor cells and embryonic CNS cell migration. J Neurooncol, 53: 203–212, 2001.

33. Bolteus, A. J., Berens, M. E., and Pilkington, G. J. Migration and invasion in brain neoplasms. Curr Neurol Neurosci Rep, 1: 225–232, 2001.

34. Reavey-Cantwell, J. F., Haroun, R. I., Zahurak, M., Clatterbuck, R. E., Parker, R. J., Mehta, R., Fruehauf, J. P., and Brem, H. The prognostic value of tumor markers in patients with glioblastoma multiforme: analysis of 32 patients and review of the literature. J Neurooncol, 55: 195–204, 2001.

35. Wheeler, C. J., Black, K. L., Liu, G., Ying, H., Yu, J. S., Zhang, W., and Lee, P. K. Thymic CD8+ T cell production strongly influences tumor antigen recognition and age-dependent glioma mortality. J Immunol, 171: 4927–4933, 2003.

36. Mischel, P. S. and Cloughesy, T. Using molecular information to guide brain tumor therapy. Nat Clin Pract Neurol, 2: 232–233, 2006.

37. Louis, D. N. Molecular pathology of malignant gliomas. Annu Rev Pathol, 1: 97–117, 2006.

38. Furnari, F. B., Fenton, T., Bachoo, R. M., Mukasa, A., Stommel, J. M., Stegh, A., Hahn, W. C., Ligon, K. L., Louis, D. N., Brennan, C., Chin, L., DePinho, R. A., and Cavenee, W. K. Malignant astrocytic glioma: genetics, biology, and paths to treatment. Genes Dev, 21: 2683–2710, 2007.

39. Glinsky, G. V., Berezovska, O., and Glinskii, A. B. Microarray analysis identifies a death-from-cancer signature predicting therapy failure in patients with multiple types of cancer. J Clin Invest, 115: 1503–1521, 2005.

40. Liu, R., Wang, X., Chen, G. Y., Dalerba, P., Gurney, A., Hoey, T., Sherlock, G., Lewicki, J., Shedden, K., and Clarke, M. F. The prognostic role of a gene signature from tumorigenic breast-cancer cells. N Engl J Med, 356: 217–226, 2007.

41. Zeppernick, F., Ahmadi, R., Campos, B., Dictus, C., Helmke, B. M., Becker, N., Lichter, P., Unterberg, A., Radlwimmer, B., and Herold-Mende, C. C. Stem cell marker CD133 affects clinical outcome in glioma patients. Clin Cancer Res, 14: 123–129, 2008.

42. Markmann, S., Gerber, B., and Briese, V. Prognostic value of Ca 125 levels during primary therapy. Anticancer Res, 27: 1837–1839, 2007.

43. Bairey, O., Blickstein, D., Stark, P., Prokocimer, M., Nativ, H. M., Kirgner, I., and Shaklai, M. Serum CA 125 as a prognostic factor in non-Hodgkin's lymphoma. Leuk Lymphoma, 44: 1733–1738, 2003.

44. Rowley, J. D. The role of chromosome translocations in leukemogenesis. Semin Hematol, 36: 59–72, 1999.

45. Schmidt, C. A. and Przybylski, G. K What can we learn from leukemia as for the process of lineage commitment in hematopoiesis?. Int Rev Immunol, 20: 107–115, 2001.

46. Sell, S. Cancer stem cells and differentiation therapy. Tumour Biol, 27: 59–70, 2006.

47. Sell, S. Leukemia: stem cells, maturation arrest, and differentiation therapy. Stem Cell Rev, 1: 197–205, 2005.

48. Sell, S. Stem cell origin of cancer and differentiation therapy. Crit Rev Oncol Hematol, 51: 1–28, 2004.
49. Gerl, A., Clemm, C., Schmeller, N., Hentrich, M., Lamerz, R., and Wilmanns, W. Late relapse of germ cell tumors after cisplatin-based chemotherapy. Ann Oncol, 8: 41–47, 1997.
50. Chou, T. C., Motzer, R. J., Tong, Y., and Bosl, G. J. Computerized quantitation of synergism and antagonism of taxol, topotecan, and cisplatin against human teratocarcinoma cell growth: a rational approach to clinical protocol design. J Natl Cancer Inst, 86: 1517–1524, 1994.
51. Zhong, S., Salomoni, P., and Pandolfi, P. P. The transcriptional role of PML and the nuclear body. Nat Cell Biol, 2: E85–90, 2000.
52. Guo, X., Ying, W., Wan, J., Hu, Z., Qian, X., Zhang, H., and He, F. Proteomic characterization of early-stage differentiation of mouse embryonic stem cells into neural cells induced by all-trans retinoic acid in vitro. Electrophoresis, 22: 3067–3075, 2001.
53. Wang, F., Li, S. T., Huang, Q., and Lan, Q. Expression of Notch1 gene in the differentiation of the human embryonic neural stem cells to neurons. Xi Bao Yu Fen Zi Mian Yi Xue Za Zhi, 20: 769–772, 2004.
54. Deng, H., Zou, F., and Luo, H. J. Differentiation of neonatal rat striatal neural stem cells induced by all-trans retinoic acid. Di Yi Jun Yi Da Xue Xue Bao, 25: 1357–1360, 1374, 2005.
55. Bianchi, M. G., Gazzola, G. C., Tognazzi, L., and Bussolati, O. C6 glioma cells differentiated by retinoic acid overexpress the glutamate transporter excitatory amino acid carrier 1 (EAAC1). Neuroscience, 151: 1042–1052, 2008.
56. Lessard, J. and Sauvageau, G. Bmi-1 determines the proliferative capacity of normal and leukaemic stem cells. Nature, 423: 255–260, 2003.
57. Park, I. K., Qian, D., Kiel, M., Becker, M. W., Pihalja, M., Weissman, I. L., Morrison, S. J., and Clarke, M. F. Bmi-1 is required for maintenance of adult self-renewing haematopoietic stem cells. Nature, 423: 302–305, 2003.
58. Clement, V., Sanchez, P., de Tribolet, N., Radovanovic, I., and Ruiz i Altaba, A. HEDGEHOG-GLI1 signaling regulates human glioma growth, cancer stem cell self-renewal, and tumorigenicity. Curr Biol, 17: 165–172, 2007.
59. Bar, E. E., Chaudhry, A., Lin, A., Fan, X., Schreck, K., Matsui, W., Piccirillo, S., Vescovi, A. L., DiMeco, F., Olivi, A., and Eberhart, C. G. Cyclopamine-mediated hedgehog pathway inhibition depletes stem-like cancer cells in glioblastoma. Stem Cells, 25: 2524–2533, 2007.
60. Fan, X., Matsui, W., Khaki, L., Stearns, D., Chun, J., Li, Y. M., and Eberhart, C. G. Notch pathway inhibition depletes stem-like cells and blocks engraftment in embryonal brain tumors. Cancer Res, 66: 7445–7452, 2006.
61. Piccirillo, S. G., Reynolds, B. A., Zanetti, N., Lamorte, G., Binda, E., Broggi, G., Brem, H., Olivi, A., Dimeco, F., and Vescovi, A. L. Bone morphogenetic proteins inhibit the tumorigenic potential of human brain tumour-initiating cells. Nature, 444: 761–765, 2006.
62. Calabrese, C., Poppleton, H., Kocak, M., Hogg, T. L., Fuller, C., Hamner, B., Oh, E. Y., Gaber, M. W., Finklestein, D., Allen, M., Frank, A., Bayazitov, I. T., Zakharenko, S. S., Gajjar, A., Davidoff, A., and Gilbertson, R. J. A perivascular niche for brain tumor stem cells. Cancer Cell, 11: 69–82, 2007.
63. Jin, L., Hope, K. J., Zhai, Q., Smadja-Joffe, F., and Dick, J. E. Targeting of CD44 eradicates human acute myeloid leukemic stem cells. Nat Med, 12: 1167–1174, 2006.
64. Bao, S., Wu, Q., Sathornsumetee, S., Hao, Y., Li, Z., Hjelmeland, A. B., Shi, Q., McLendon, R. E., Bigner, D. D., and Rich, J. N. Stem cell-like glioma cells promote tumor angiogenesis through vascular endothelial growth factor. Cancer Res, 66: 7843–7848, 2006.
65. Vredenburgh, J. J., Desjardins, A., Herndon, J. E., 2nd, Marcello, J., Reardon, D. A., Quinn, J. A., Rich, J. N., Sathornsumetee, S., Gururangan, S., Sampson, J., Wagner, M., Bailey, L., Bigner, D. D., Friedman, A. H., and Friedman, H. S. Bevacizumab plus irinotecan in recurrent glioblastoma multiforme. J Clin Oncol, 25: 4722–4729, 2007.
66. Vredenburgh, J. J., Desjardins, A., Herndon, J. E., 2nd, Dowell, J. M., Reardon, D. A., Quinn, J. A., Rich, J. N., Sathornsumetee, S., Gururangan, S., Wagner, M., Bigner, D. D., Friedman, A. H., and Friedman, H. S. Phase II trial of bevacizumab and irinotecan in recurrent malignant glioma. Clin Cancer Res, 13: 1253–1259, 2007.
67. Batchelor, T. T., Sorensen, A. G., di Tomaso, E., Zhang, W. T., Duda, D. G., Cohen, K. S., Kozak, K. R., Cahill, D. P., Chen, P. J., Zhu, M., Ancukiewicz, M., Mrugala, M. M., Plotkin, S., Drappatz, J., Louis, D. N., Ivy, P., Scadden, D. T., Benner, T., Loeffler, J. S., Wen, P. Y., and Jain, R. K. AZD2171, a pan-VEGF receptor tyrosine kinase inhibitor, normalizes tumor vasculature and alleviates edema in glioblastoma patients. Cancer Cell, 11: 83–95, 2007.
68. Steinman, R. M., Turley, S., Mellman, I., and Inaba, K. The induction of tolerance by dendritic cells that have captured apoptotic cells. J Exp Med, 191: 411–416, 2000.
69. Soling, A. and Rainov, N. G. Dendritic cell therapy of primary brain tumors. Mol Med, 7: 659–667, 2001.
70. Hoffmann, T. K., Meidenbauer, N., Dworacki, G., Kanaya, H., and Whiteside, T. L. Generation of tumor-specific T-lymphocytes by cross-priming with human dendritic cells ingesting apoptotic tumor cells. Cancer Res, 60: 3542–3549, 2000.
71. Ashley, D. M., Faiola, B., Nair, S., Hale, L. P., Bigner, D. D., and Gilboa, E. Bone marrow-generated dendritic cells pulsed with tumor extracts or tumor RNA induce antitumor immunity against central nervous system tumors. J Exp Med, 186: 1177–1182, 1997.
72. Heimberger, A. B., Crotty, L. E., Archer, G. E., McLendon, R. E., Friedman, A., Dranoff, G., Bigner, D. D., and Sampson, J. H. Bone marrow-derived dendritic cells pulsed with tumor homogenate induce immunity against syngeneic intracerebral glioma. J Neuroimmunol, 103: 16–25, 2000.
73. Liau, L. M., Black, K. L., Prins, R. M., Sykes, S. N., DiPatre, P. L., Cloughesy, T. F., Becker, D. P., and Bronstein, J. M. Treatment of intracranial gliomas with bone marrow-derived dendritic cells pulsed with tumor antigens. J Neurosurg, 90: 1115–1124, 1999.

74. Ni, H. T., Spellman, S. R., Jean, W. C., Hall, W. A., and Low, W. C. Immunization with dendritic cells pulsed with tumor extract increases survival of mice bearing intracranial gliomas. J Neurooncol, 51: 1–9, 2001.

75. Okada, H., Tahara, H., Shurin, M. R., Attanucci, J., Giezeman-Smits, K. M., Fellows, W. K., Lotze, M. T., Chambers, W. H., and Bozik, M. E. Bone marrow-derived dendritic cells pulsed with a tumor-specific peptide elicit effective anti-tumor immunity against intracranial neoplasms. Int J Cancer, 78: 196–201, 1998.

76. Yamanaka, R., Zullo, S. A., Tanaka, R., Blaese, M., and Xanthopoulos, K. G. Enhancement of antitumor immune response in glioma models in mice by genetically modified dendritic cells pulsed with Semliki forest virus-mediated complementary DNA. J Neurosurg, 94: 474–481, 2001.

77. Fong, L., Hou, Y., Rivas, A., Benike, C., Yuen, A., Fisher, G. A., Davis, M. M., and Engleman, E. G. Altered peptide ligand vaccination with Flt3 ligand expanded dendritic cells for tumor immunotherapy. Proc Natl Acad Sci USA, 98: 8809–8814, 2001.

78. Yu, J. S., Liu, G., Ying, H., Yong, W. H., Black, K. L., and Wheeler, C. J. Vaccination with tumor lysate-pulsed dendritic cells elicits antigen-specific, cytotoxic T-cells in patients with malignant glioma. Cancer Res, 64: 4973–4979, 2004.

79. Liau, L. M., Prins, R. M., Kiertscher, S. M., Odesa, S. K., Kremen, T. J., Giovannone, A. J., Lin, J. W., Chute, D. J., Mischel, P. S., Cloughesy, T. F., and Roth, M. D. Dendritic cell vaccination in glioblastoma patients induces systemic and intracranial T-cell responses modulated by the local central nervous system tumor microenvironment. Clin Cancer Res, 11: 5515–5525, 2005.

80. Pellegatta, S., Poliani, P. L., Corno, D., Menghi, F., Ghielmetti, F., Suarez-Merino, B., Caldera, V., Nava, S., Ravanini, M., Facchetti, F., Bruzzone, M. G., and Finocchiaro, G. Neurospheres enriched in cancer stem-like cells are highly effective in eliciting a dendritic cell-mediated immune response against malignant gliomas. Cancer Res, 66: 10247–10252, 2006.

81. Odeberg, J., Piao, J. H., Samuelsson, E. B., Falci, S., and Akesson, E. Low immunogenicity of in vitro-expanded human neural cells despite high MHC expression. J Neuroimmunol, 161: 1–11, 2005.

82. Schmitz, M., Temme, A., Senner, V., Ebner, R., Schwind, S., Stevanovic, S., Wehner, R., Schackert, G., Schackert, H. K., Fussel, M., Bachmann, M., Rieber, E. P., and Weigle, B. Identification of SOX2 as a novel glioma-associated antigen and potential target for T cell-based immunotherapy. Br J Cancer, 96: 1293–1301, 2007.

83. Spisek, R., Kukreja, A., Chen, L. C., Matthews, P., Mazumder, A., Vesole, D., Jagannath, S., Zebroski, H. A., Simpson, A. J., Ritter, G., Durie, B., Crowley, J., Shaughnessy, J. D., Jr., Scanlan, M. J., Gure, A. O., Barlogie, B., and Dhodapkar, M. V. Frequent and specific immunity to the embryonal stem cell-associated antigen SOX2 in patients with monoclonal gammopathy. J Exp Med, 204: 831–840, 2007.

84. Liu, G., Black, K. L., and Yu, J. S. Sensitization of malignant glioma to chemotherapy through dendritic cell vaccination. Expert Rev Vaccines, 5: 233–247, 2006.

85. Lake, R. A. and Robinson, B. W. Immunotherapy and chemotherapy - a practical partnership. Nat Rev Cancer, 5: 397–405, 2005.

86. Emens, L. A. and Jaffee, E. M. Leveraging the activity of tumor vaccines with cytotoxic chemotherapy. Cancer Res, 65: 8059–8064, 2005.

87. Dunn, G. P., Bruce, A. T., Ikeda, H., Old, L. J., and Schreiber, R. D. Cancer immunoediting: from immunosurveillance to tumor escape. Nat Immunol, 3: 991–998, 2002.

88. Krause, D. S., Lazarides, K., von Andrian, U. H., and Van Etten, R. A. Requirement for CD44 in homing and engraftment of BCR-ABL-expressing leukemic stem cells. Nat Med, 12: 1175–1180, 2006.

23

Critical Roles of Tumorigenic and Migrating Cancer Stem/Progenitor Cells in Cancer Progression and their Therapeutic Implications

Murielle Mimeault and Surinder K. Batra

ABSTRACT

Recent progress in cancer stem/progenitor cell research has revealed that these poorly differentiated, multipotent, and malignant cells may provide critical functions for tumor formation, metastases, resistance to current clinical therapies, and disease relapse. More specifically, the malignant transformation of tissue-resident adult stem/progenitor cells into tumorigenic and migrating cancer stem/progenitor cells during cancer progression, and more particularly the acquisition of a migratory phenotype during epithelial–mesenchymal transition (EMT) program, may lead to more aggressive and metastatic cancer subtypes. The EMT process is generally associated with changes in the local microenvironment, niche of cancer stem/progenitor cells, cell–cell detachment, and remodeling stromal components including the activation of host stromal cells, myofibroblasts, and immune cells. These molecular events may result in the activation of a complex network of oncogenic signaling pathways in cancer stem/progenitor cells and their differentiated progenies, initiating autocrine and paracrine manners by diverse growth factors, cytokines, and extracellular matrix components during cancer progression. The stimulation of these tumorigenic cascades may contribute to the sustained growth, survival, migration, invasion, and treatment resistance of cancer stem/progenitor cells. On the basis of these observations, it appears that the molecular targeting of tumorigenic and migrating cancer stem/progenitor cells may represent a new promising therapeutic strategy that may be exploited to improve the current therapies against aggressive, metastatic, recurrent, and lethal cancers.

Key Words: Cancer stem/progenitor cells, Stromal microenvironment, Epithelial–mesenchymal transition, Tumor growth, Invasion, Metastasis, Targeting therapies

INTRODUCTION

Recent advances in the field of stem cell research have provided a growing body of experimental evidence that most solid tumors may arise from the malignant transformation of tissue-resident adult stem cells into tumorigenic and migrating cancer stem/progenitor cells *(1–21)*. More specifically, the genetic alterations in adult stem cells and changes in their specialized local microenvironment, niche, and stroma occurring during aging or pathological conditions such as inflammatory atrophies and

From: *Cancer Drug Discovery and Development: Stem Cells and Cancer,*
Edited by: R.G. Bagley and B.A. Teicher, DOI: 10.1007/978-1-60327-933-8_23,
© Humana Press, a part of Springer Science+Business Media, LLC 2009

fibrosis associated with intense tissue injuries may notably lead to cancer initiation (1–23). Moreover, the accumulation of genetic and/or epigenetic alterations in tumorigenic cancer stem/progenitor cells concomitant with a stromal remodeling during cancer progression may result in their acquisition a more malignant behavior (5, 8, 11–20, 24–29). Importantly, the epithelial–mesenchymal transition (EMT) phenomenon, which occurs during embryonic development and wound healing, is also reactivated during the progression from numerous aggressive cancers into locally invasive forms (5, 8, 30–37). Among these aggressive cancers, there are brain, skin, prostate, mammary, hepatic, gastrointestinal, pancreatic, and colorectal carcinomas. More particularly, the EMT program implicates the morphogenetic changes in polarized cancer cells concomitant with a deregulation of cell–cell adhesion junctions that lead to a loss of the epithelial phenotype and the acquisition of mesenchymal properties conferring an enhanced motility and invasive ability to cancer cells (18, 19, 30, 31, 37–46). This is generally due to a sustained activation of diverse oncogenic cascades in the cancer cells during the progression from premalignant lesions into locally invasive cancers (3, 5, 8, 11–19, 30–32, 38, 47–67). Hence, the acquisition of a migratory phenotype by tumorigenic cancer stem/progenitor cells during the EMT process may lead to their invasion, dissemination, and formation of aggressive and metastatic cancers at distant sites.

The cancer progression is also associated with up-regulated expression and sustained activation of diverse tumorigenic cascades activated by diverse growth factors and cytokines in cancer stem/progenitor cells and the release of soluble factors by host stromal cells that may provide them with a more aggressive behavior (5, 8, 11–20, 24–29, 31). These oncogenic events may promote a transition from localized cancers into invasive and metastatic disease stages. The tumorigenic and migrating cancer stem/progenitor cells, which are endowed with a self-renewal potential, aberrant multilineage differentiation capacity, and migratory ability, can provide critical roles in tumor formation and metastases at distant tissues/organs by giving rise to the bulk mass of cancer cells (Fig. 1). Moreover, the stromal activated cells and tissue-resident endothelial progenitor cells (EPCs) and mesenchymal stem cells (MSCs) or the recruitment of bone marrow-derived cells such as circulating EPCs and hematopoietic stem cells (HSCs) at the primary neoplasms or premetastatic sites may also promote their malignant transformation or tumoral angiogenesis process (11–20, 68–72). Hence, all of these molecular and cellular changes may contribute to the multiple steps leading to carcinogenesis and metastases.

On the basis of this new cancer stem/progenitor cell concept of carcinogenesis, it is likely that the intratumoral heterogeneity or differences between cancer subtypes may be due, a least in part, to the occurrence of different genetic/epigenetic alterations, which lead to the generation of distinct tumorigenic and/or migrating cancer stem/progenitor cells during cancer initiation and progression (1, 5, 8, 9, 11–19, 25, 60, 67, 73–100). Moreover, the resistance of tumorigenic and migrating cancer stem/progenitor cells to current therapies and their persistence at primary or secondary neoplasms after treatment initiation may also explain, at least in part, the recurrence of aggressive and metastatic cancers (9–20, 29, 101–103). Therefore, these new concepts have important repercussions on basic and clinical research and must be considered to improve the diagnostic and prognostic methods as well as the therapeutic strategies to treat the aggressive and recurrent cancers. Particularly, the molecular targeting of tumorigenic and migrating cancer stem/progenitor cells appears to be essential for eradicating these cancer-initiating cells that can contribute to tumor growth, metastases, and disease relapse. We review here numerous recent lines of evidence supporting the critical roles of tumorigenic and migrating cancer stem/progenitor cells in tumor formation, metastases, treatment resistance, and disease recurrence. We also discuss the implications of new concepts on cancer stem/progenitor cells for the development of novel therapeutic strategies based on their molecular targeting to improve the current clinical therapies. The information should help develop novel therapeutic strategies that could be translated into curative treatments for the patients diagnosed with locally advanced cancers at high risk of relapse as well as metastatic and recurrent cancers.

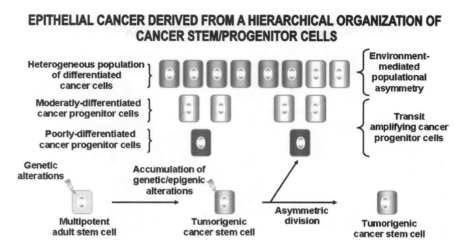

Fig. 1. New concept on epithelial cancer formation derived from the malignant transformation of adult stem cells into tumorigenic cancer stem/progenitor cells. This scheme shows the malignant transformation of adult stem cells into tumorigenic cancer stem cells (CSCs), which may be induced through the genetic and/or epigenetic alterations. More specifically, an asymmetric division of a CSC that gives rise to one CSC daughter and one poorly-differentiated cancer progenitor cell termed early transit-amplifying (TA)/intermediate cancer progenitor cell is indicated. Moreover, the possibility that early poorly-differentiated TA cells, which possess a high proliferative potential, may in turn, generate the moderately-differentiated cancer progenitor cells and subsequently the bulk mass of well-differentiated cancer cells is also illustrated. This hierarchical model of carcinogenesis also implicates that the changes in the local environmental of early and late TA cancer progenitor cells during the amplification process and their migration at distant sites from niche may influence the phenotype of their further and terminally differentiated progenies, and thereby contribute to the populational asymmetry and cellular diversity characterizing cancer subtype *(see Color Plates)*.

FUNCTIONS OF TUMORIGENIC AND MIGRATING CANCER STEM/ PROGENITOR CELLS IN CANCER PROGRESSION AND METASTASES

The establishment of the molecular events responsible of the tumor initiation and progression into locally invasive and metastatic cancers is of immense interest in basic cancer research. This should lead to the development of new effective diagnostic and prognostic methods and clinical therapeutic options against the aggressive, recurrent, and lethal cancers. Several recent lines of evidence have revealed that the accumulation of genetic and/or epigenetic alterations in the multipotent adult stem cells and/or their early progenies may contribute to their malignant transformation during cancer initiation and progression (Fig. 1) *(1–21)*. In support with this, a small subpopulation of cancer cells expressing the stem cell-like markers such as CD133, CD44, CD90, Oct-3/4, and/or ATP-binding cassette (ABC) multidrug transporters has been isolated from primary and/or secondary neoplasms from patients with skin, lung, liver, brain, gastrointestinal, pancreatic, prostatic, breast, and ovarian cancers and well-established cancer cell lines *(1, 11–21, 24, 25, 74, 77, 104–121)*. These tumorigenic cancer stem/progenitor cells (also designated as cancer-initiating cells or tumor-initiating cells), which are endowed with unique self-renewal ability and tumorigenic potential, were able to give rise through an asymmetric division to a hierarchical lineage of more differentiated cancer cell types in vitro and in vivo (Fig. 1) *(4, 21, 24, 25, 74, 77, 104–110, 112)*. Furthermore, the acquisition of a migratory phenotype by tumorigenic cancer stem/progenitor cells may also promote their invasion, thereby lead to more aggressive and metastatic cancer subtypes (Fig. 2).

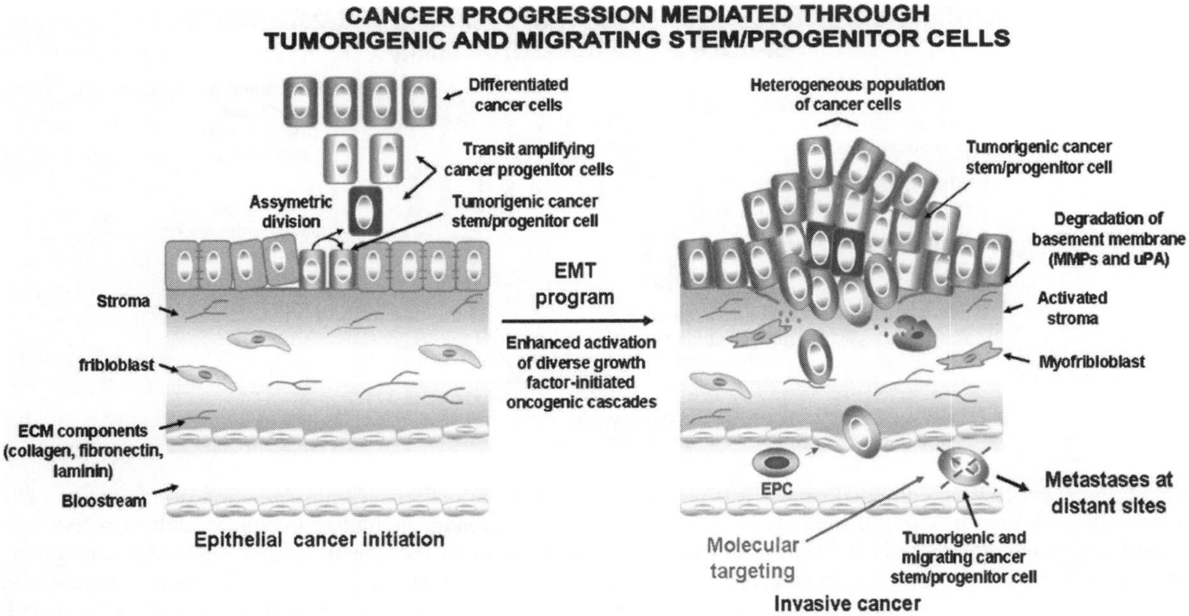

Fig. 2. Cellular events associated with the initiation and progression of epithelial cancer mediated through tumorigenic and migrating cancer stem/progenitor cells. The asymmetric division of cancer stem cells localized in the basal compartment into transit-amplifying cancer progenitor cells that, in turn, may regenerate the further differentiated cancer cells is illustrated. The oncogenic transformation of tumorigenic stem/progenitor cells into migrating cancer progenitor cells, which may be induced by the sustained activation of distinct growth factor signaling cascades during the epithelial-mesenchymal transition (EMT) program is also shown. The invasion of tumorigenic and migrating cancer stem/progenitor cells in the bloodstream, which may lead to their dissemination at distant sites and metastases, is also indicated. This model of carcinogenesis supports the therapeutic interest of targeting tumorigenic and migrating cancer stem/progenitor cells to counteract the cancer progression and metastases at distant sites. *ECM* extracellular matrix, *MMPs* matrix metalloproteinases, and *uPA* urokinase type-plasminogene activator *(see Color Plates)*.

Significant advancements have led to the identification of specific oncogenic products that are often implicated in the malignant transformation of adult stem/progenitor cells or precancerous stem cells (pre-CSCs) into tumorigenic and migrating cancer stem/progenitor cells during cancer initiation and progression to the invasive and metastatic stages. The occurrence of some genetic abnormalities leading to an aberrant expression and/or activation of a complex network of oncogenic signaling elements [MYC, nuclear factor- κB "NF-κB", phosphatidylinositol 3'-kinase "PI_3K"/Akt, Bcl-2 and/ or survivin] in adult stem/progenitor cells may notably result in cancer initiation *(10–20, 29, 58, 102, 103, 122–127)*. Moreover, the down-regulation or inactivation of tumor suppressor gene products [p53, phosphatase and tensin homolog deleted on chromosome ten "PTEN" and/or retinoblastoma "Rb"] in adult stem/progenitor cells may also promote the tumor formation. Additionally, the stimulation of numerous tumorigenic signaling cascades initiated by hormones and/or distinct growth factors, cytokines, and their cognate receptors in tumorigenic cancer stem/progenitor cells and/or their early progenies may also contribute to their sustained growth, survival, invasion, and/or metastatic spread during cancer progression, treatment resistance, and disease relapse *(1, 2, 5, 7, 10–20, 58, 102, 103, 126–129)*. Particularly, the acquisition of a mesenchymal phenotype and enhanced motile and invasive abilities by tumorigenic cancer stem/progenitor cells during the EMT process may lead to their invasion from the primary neoplasm and metastatic spread to distant sites, and thereby contribute to the disease recurrence. In this matter, we describe the molecular events that are often associated with the EMT process during the early and late stages of cancer progression from organ-confined tumors into aggressive, invasive, and metastatic disease stages. The emphasis is on the critical functions assumed by several growth factors, cytokines, and integrins as well as the changes in stromal components for inducing a more complete EMT program in cancer stem/progenitor cells.

Molecular Events Associated with the EMT Process, Invasion, and Metastasis of Cancer Stem/Progenitor Cells and Their Progenies

The EMT phenomenon, which occurs during embryonic development, throughout adult life, and in some pathological conditions such as tissue injuries and cancers, is an important process *(5, 8, 22, 23, 30–32)*. The EMT process generally progresses along multiple steps that usually result in the changes of morphology and an enhanced migratory ability of cells. Certain molecular events that are frequently associated with the induction of the EMT program in embryonic stem cells (ESCs) are also reactivated in adult stem cells during their malignant transformation. In particular, recent studies have shown that the induction of the differentiation of the pluripotent mouse, monkey, and human ESCs in a monolayer culture was accompanied by an up-regulated expression and/or activity of gelatinase (matrix metalloproteinases, MMP-2 and MMP-9), metastasis-associated 5T4 oncofetal antigen, vimentin, and E-cadherin transcriptional repressor molecules (snail and slug proteins) *(33–36)*. These cellular events ultimately resulted in an E- to N-cadherin switch, altered actin cytoskeleton arrangement, and a loss of cell–cell contact concomitant with the acquisition of a mesenchymal phenotype and an enhanced motility of differentiating human ESCs *(33, 35, 36)*. Similarly, during carcinogenesis, the occurrence of EMT events may contribute to the malignant transformation of tissue-resident adult stem/progenitor cells into tumorigenic and migrating cancer stem/progenitor cells during the transition from premalignant lesions into locally invasive cancers and disseminated diseases (Fig. 2) *(11–20)*. More specifically, in the early stages of carcinogenesis, a disorganization of intercellular junctional complexes including adherens-, tight-, gap-, and/or desmosomal junctions may occur during the EMT process (Fig. 2) *(11–20, 30–32, 38, 47, 48, 130–136)*. This event may result in a disruption of intercellular adhesion and cell–cell dissociation, thereby leading to the detachment of cancer cells including cancer stem/progenitor cells from the tumor mass. Moreover, the EMT process may also result in a reduction of expression levels and/or redistribution of other junctional component types that acquire an intracellular or extracellular localization *(18, 19, 137)*. In regard with this, the EMT program is also accompanied by the activation of mechanisms that are involved in the cell detachment-induced apoptotic death (anoikis) *(18)*. In fact, a positive selection occurs during which certain cancer cell subpopulations and adjacent normal epithelial cells can trigger apoptotic death, while other tumor cells, including the cancer stem/progenitor cells or their early progenies possessing the oncogenic phenotype advantages, can survive *(8, 18, 19, 31, 48)*. For instance, the normal basal epithelial cells in the primary neoplasms, including prostate and breast carcinomas, are gradually destroyed during the transition from low-, intermediate- and high-grade intraepithelial neoplasms into well-established invasive cancers *(138, 139)*. Hence, all of these molecular events may lead to a loss of polarity and changes in the structural shape as well as the acquisition of a more malignant behavior by a subpopulation of tumorigenic cancer stem/progenitor cells due to a disorganization of cell–cell interactions and actin cytoskeleton rearrangement. Particularly, the acquisition of a migratory fibroblastoid phenotype by the cancer cells, which is generally accompanied by the expression of mesenchymal markers such as vimentin and a switch from E-cadherin to N-cadherin expression, may promote their invasion in activated stroma (Fig. 2) *(18, 19, 30, 31, 38–43)*.

In general, a gain of migratory and invasive capabilities by tumor cells, including cancer stem/progenitor cells and their further differentiated progenies, at the invasive front appears to represent a critical step in the transition from preinvasive primary neoplasms into locally invasive and metastatic cancers. In support with this, it has been observed that a loss of E-cadherin concomitant with the up-regulation of N-cadherin in tumor cells may lead to abrogation of cell–cell contacts and an increased mobility of tumor cells in some invasive cancer types such as colorectal, pancreatic, breast, prostate, bladder, thyroid, and squamous cell carcinomas *(18, 19, 37, 44–46)*. The E-cadherin to N-cadherin switch may be mediated via an inhibition of expression of E-cadherin expression by binding a transcriptional repressor such as snail and slug to E-cadherin gene promoter. Moreover, the activation of growth factor receptors such as EGFR and hepatocyte growth factor (Met) receptor may also lead to a proteolytic degradation or internalization of cell surface E-cadherin proteins *(18, 19, 37, 140, 141)*. In support with a critical role provided by E-cadherin as a repressor of cancer cell invasion, it has been observed that the overexpression of the wild-type E-cadherin protein in tumor epithelial cells may reverse their mesenchymal phenotype and invasive ability. Although the progression of some epithelial cancers is often associated with a loss of E-cadherin function and the achievement of a complete EMT process, certain cancer subtypes may also occur in its absence or after a partial EMT program or implicate other molecular mechanisms *(8, 18, 19, 25, 142, 143)*. For example, it has been observed that the EMT process occurred during tumor progression in HRas and Myc-induced mammary carcinomas as inferred by the expression of mesenchymal cell markers, while the EMT events were not detected in neoplasms arising in transgenic mice for erbB2 and Wnt-1 *(144)*. More intriguingly, the up-regulated expression of a small mucin-like transmembrane glycoprotein, podoplanin in the invasive front of human cancers, also induced tumor cell migration and invasion in cancer cells without the up-regulation of EMT-associated mesenchymal markers and the E- to N-cadherin switch *(142)*. Together these observations suggest that a partial or complete EMT program is not a necessary prerequisite to invasion and metastases in all types of cancer. Also, other alternative pathways may contribute to cancer cell invasion as well.

Other molecular and cellular events that may occur during the EMT program include an enhanced expression and/or activation of stromal matrix components such as collagen, fibrinogen, and laminin as well as extracellular matrix metalloproteinases (MMPs) and urokinase-type plasminogen activator (uPA) system *(18, 19, 31, 39–43, 48, 145–148)*. These molecular events may lead to a degradation of the basement membrane and altered adhesion of tumor cells to ECM components, thereby promoting cancer cell invasion in the reactive stroma. In this regard, we describe the implication of diverse autocrine and paracrine loops stimulated by distinct growth factors, cytokines, and integrins in tumor cells, activated fibroblasts, and infiltrating inflammatory cells that may contribute to the sustained growth and survival of cancer stem/progenitor cells and their differentiated progenies during cancer progression. These survival factors may also reciprocally collaborate to induce a fuller EMT program and the invasion process in diverse cancer types *(5, 8, 32, 48, 149)*.

Interplay of Some Growth Factors for Inducing a More Complete EMT Program

The progression from premalignant epithelial lesions into locally invasive cancers and disseminated diseases generally involves the stimulation of diverse oncogenic pathways induced by multiple growth factors, cytokines, and integrins in tumorigenic cancer stem/progenitor cells and host stromal cells that contribute to their malignant transformation during the EMT program (Fig. 2) *(5, 8, 11–14, 16–19, 32, 48, 52–56, 62, 67, 149)*. The up-regulated expression and sustained activation of diverse developmental cascades in cancer stem/progenitor cells and their progenies, which are involved in the stringent control of self-renewal and differentiation of adult stem cells, may give them a more malignant behavior *(3, 5, 8, 11–19, 30–32, 38, 47–67).* Among these deregulated pathways, there are epidermal growth factor (EGF)-EGFR system, hedgehog, Wnt/β-catenin, fibroblast growth factor (FGF)/FGFR, transforming growth factor-β (TGF-β)/TGF-βR, and/or stromal cell-derived growth factor-1 (SDF-1)/CXCR4 pathways. These potent morphogens may cooperate to induce the molecular events associated with a complete EMT program, including the disruption of the cell–cell adhesion contacts and tumor cell dissociation as well as the alterations in epithelial cell shape and an increase of motile ability and invasiveness of tumorigenic cancer stem/progenitor cells *(5, 8, 11–14, 16–19, 30, 31, 38, 47–56, 67, 133, 134, 149–153).* Particularly, these growth factors may induce an increase of the expression of transcriptional repressors of E-cadherin expression (snail, slug, and/or twist) and a subset of mesenchymal genes (vimentin, fibronectin, and N-cadherin) in certain tumorigenic cancer stem/progenitor cells and their progenies during the EMT process *(11–14, 16–19, 31, 39–43, 48, 51, 67, 146–148, 150, 154–156).* Moreover, these growth factors may also stimulate the production of enzymes such as MMPs and uPa system that are involved in degradation of basement membrane and breakdown of cell–cell and cell–ECM interactions. Changes in the expression of these gene products may lead to the abrogation of cell–cell contacts and contribute to the sustained growth, survival, and/ or a gain of motile ability of tumorigenic and migrating cancer stem/progenitor cells and their progenies, which is necessary for their invasion in adjacent reactive stroma. For instance, the activation of receptor tyrosine kinases (RTKs), such as EGFR, Met receptor, platelet-derived growth factor receptor (PDGFR), and Src tyrosine kinase may bring out the adherens junctions, including catenin-E-cadherin complexes by tyrosine phosphorylation of catenin components, and thereby induce the cytoskeletal rearrangements controlling cell polarity and locomotion *(18, 19, 137, 157).* Furthermore, the stimulation of RTKs through autocrine and paracrine loops and integrins by ECM components may also lead to the activation of diverse signal transduction effectors. Among them, there are Src, mitogen-activated protein kinase (MAPK), PI_3K/Akt, NF-κB, small GTPases of the Rho family (Rac1, Cdc42 and RhoA), and/or phospholipase C-γ (PLC-γ) *(8, 11–19, 31, 39–43, 47, 58, 67, 130, 137, 157–163).* In turn, these signaling elements can induce a reorganization of the actin cytoskeleton and changes in cell adhesion that leads to morphogenic changes associated with the migration and invasion of cancer cells, including cancer stem/progenitor cells.

Molecular Events in Reactive Tumor Stroma Associated with the EMT Program

Cancer progression is also accompanied by an extensive tumor stromal remodeling of the extracellular matrix (ECM) components and changes in the gene expression pattern in the tumor-associated activated myofibroblasts and/or stellate cells during the EMT process *(11–19, 23, 32, 67–72, 136).* Moreover, the recruitment of circulating EPCs and immune cells such as macrophages into tumor stroma may also occur during the EMT process. Particularly, tumor stromal cells secrete a variety of soluble growth factors and cytokines such as EGF, insulin-like growth factor (IGF), hepatocyte growth factor (HGF), and TGF-β as well as MMPs and uPA in reactive stroma, which may promote the molecular events associated with the malignant transformation of cancer stem/progenitor cells during the EMT process (Fig. 2) *(5, 11–14, 16–19, 22, 32, 47, 48, 67, 146–149).* For instance, the persistent induction of the stromal fibroblasts into activated myofibroblasts may cause fibrosis characterized by an excess production and deposition of extracellular matrix components in the stroma. This molecular event may lead to the secretion of diverse angiogenic factors and proinflammatory factors by myofibroblasts that may stimulate the tumor neovascularization process in a paracrine manner and cancer cell proliferation and invasion into reactive stroma (Fig. 2) *(22, 23).*

Hence, the integration of these distinct internal and external signals may provide tumorigenic and migrating stem/progenitor cells with the ability to evade from primary neoplasms, spread via the

lymphatic vessels and systemic circulation at near lymph nodes and form metastases at distant tissues/
organs (Fig. 2). Particularly, the acquisition of migratory phenotype by tumorigenic cancer stem/
progenitor cells during the EMT program has been associated with the occurrence of highly aggressive and invasive cancer subtypes that may progress to metastatic and recurrent disease states *(8, 18, 19)*.
In respect with this, we are reporting accumulating lines of evidence supporting the implication of
tumorigenic and migrating cancer progenitor cells in the formation of different aggressive and metastatic cancer subtypes, treatment resistance, and disease relapse. Of particular therapeutic interest, we
also describe novel cancer therapeutic strategies based on the molecular targeting of the oncogenic
signaling elements that are often deregulated in tumorigenic and migrating cancer stem/progenitor
cells during the transition from premalignant lesions into aggressive and invasive forms.

NEW CONCEPT ON HETEROGENEITY OF CANCERS DERIVED FROM DISTINCT TUMORIGENIC AND MIGRATING CANCER STEM/PROGENITOR CELLS

Numerous investigations revealed that the occurrence of different malignant transforming events in
adult stem/progenitor cells during cancer initiation as well as the accumulation of distinct genetic/
epigenetic alterations in cancer stem/progenitor cells along cancer progression may lead to the
development of different cancer subtypes with distinct levels of differentiation and invasiveness *(1, 5,
8, 9, 11–19, 25, 60, 67, 73–100)*. For instance, the expression of mesenchymal genes and the
acquisition of a migratory phenotype by poorly or moderately-differentiated tumorigenic cancer stem/
progenitor cells during the EMT program may result in the formation of highly invasive cancer
subtypes characterized by a poorly to moderately-differentiated state *(18, 19, 98–100)*. In contrast, the
tumorigenic cancer stem/progenitor cells that do not undertake the EMT transition could rather give
rise to weakly invasive cancer subtypes *(18)*. In support with this model, at least five subtypes of
breast cancer have been identified based on the gene expression signatures and classified as basal-like
(CK5/6$^+$, estrogen receptor "ERα^-", progesterone receptor "PR$^-$", erbB2$^{-/low}$, EGFR$^+$, vimentin$^+$ and
KIT$^+$); erbB2/HER2$^+$ overexpressing (ERα^- and PR$^-$); luminal A (ERα^+ and/or PR$^+$ and erbB2$^-$);
luminal B (ERα^+ and/or PR$^+$ and erbB2$^+$) and normal-like cancer subtype (high expression of normal
epithelium genes and low expression of luminal epithelial gene products) *(73, 98–100, 164–170)*.
Among these cancer subtypes, the ERα-negative basal-like breast cancer and erbB2-overexpressing
breast cancer are aggressive cancer forms that are associated with a poor prognosis of survival with
current clinical therapies relative to other breast cancer subtypes *(164, 166–168, 171, 172)*. In regard
with this, it has been reported that the targeted expression of stabilized β-catenin in the basal
myoepithelial cells of mouse mammary epithelium resulted in an enhanced proliferation of basal-type
cell-like progenitors possessing an abnormal differentiation potential, whose oncogenic event led to
the development of invasive basal-type carcinomas *(78)*. Moreover, it has also been noted that the
ERα-negative breast cancer cells, which did not express the metastasis-associated gene 3 (MTA3) that
inhibits snail transcriptional activity, may express a lower level of E-cadherin, and therefore possess
a higher migratory capacity than the ERα-positive breast cancer cells *(173)*. In this same pathway, an
increased expression of NF-kB in ERα-negative breast cancer cells may also lead to EMT induction
throughout the stimulation of transcription RelB and enhanced expression of the antiapoptotic protein
Bcl-2 *(174)*. The primary glioblastoma multiforms, which represent a heterogeneous population of
cancer cells, may also arise from the malignant transformation of neural stem cells (NSCs) that
acquire the mesenchymal properties like mesenchymal stem cells and give rise to further differentiated
progenies *(8, 24, 25)*. In fact, these aggressive glioblastomas, which are frequently accompanied by
the overexpression of EGFR, seem to progress rapidly without evidence of a transitory step of lower-grade

tumor. On the opposite end, the secondary or progressive glioblastoma multiforms, which are often characterized by the mutations in the *p53* suppressor gene, appear to derive from low-grade tumors that did not show the changes in the gene expression pattern that are usually associated with the EMT program *(8)*.

In addition, the changes in the local microenvironment of tumorigenic cancer stem/progenitor cells resulting in the expression of a different subset of oncogenic gene products may also be responsible, at least in part, for the intratumoral heterogeneity. This line of thought is well-supported by the observations that have indicated that certain invasive cancer types such as mammary, ovarian, prostatic, pancreatic, gastric, colorectal, and squamous cell carcinomas may harbor an intratumoral heterogeneity *(5, 8, 18, 21, 25, 94)*. Particularly, certain tumors show distinct proliferating and differentiating regions, including a preferential localization of migrating cancer stem/progenitor cells at the invasive front (Fig. 2). As a matter of fact, the data from immunohistochemical analyses of pancreatic adenocarcinoma specimens from patients have revealed the presence of two different subpopulations of pancreatic cancer stem/progenitor cells, including tumorigenic $CD133^+$ cells and migrating $CD133^+$/$CXCR4^+$ localized in the bulk mass and invasive front of pancreatic tumor, respectively *(21)*. Hence, this suggests that the migrating $CD133^+$/$CXCR4^+$ cells may correspond to a more malignant cell subpopulation than tumorigenic $CD133^+$ cells, which may have acquired a migratory phenotype during the EMT program, and may thereby be involved in invasion and metastases to distant sites. Consistently, it has been observed that the depletion of $CD133^+$/$CXCR4^+$ migrating cancer stem/progenitor cells effectively abrogated the metastatic capacity of pancreatic tumors without altering their tumorigenic potential *(21)*.

In light of these observations, it appears that distinct aggressive and invasive cancer subtypes may originate from different tumorigenic and migrating cancer stem/progenitor cells expressing a specific oncogenic gene profile, and thereby may require different therapeutic strategies. In respect with this, we describe the recent accumulating data obtained on the analyses of the gene expression profiles specific to this very small subpopulation of cancer cells that have indicated the major implication of tumorigenic and migrating cancer stem/progenitor cells in resistance to current clinical treatments. We also reviewed novel therapeutic approaches based on the molecular targeting of the signaling elements deregulated in these tumor-initiating cells.

Characterization of the Differently-Expressed Gene Profiles of Cancer Stem/Progenitor Cells

Since the gene expression analyses on the total mass of the mixed cancer cell population may principally reflect the phenotype of the major population of differentiated and nontumorigenic cancer cells, new analyses of gene expression pattern restricted to tumorigenic and/or migrating cancer stem/progenitor cells must be consider to identify a molecular signature *(11, 18, 19, 26, 28, 75, 101, 175–182)*. This information could be used to identify new potential diagnostic, predictors and prognostic indicators and drug targets. In respect with this, the data from a recent comparative microarray analysis between the differently expressed genes observed for $CD44^+CD24^{-/low}$ tumorigenic breast cancer stem/progenitor cells relative to that of normal breast epithelium have indicated that a 186-gene, designated as invasiveness gene signature (IGS), may be associated with the overall survival and metastasis-free survival of patients with breast cancer *(183)*. Among the genes expressed in this very little population of tumor-initiating cells, there are the gene products associated with the NF-κB and MAPK pathways, and epigenetic control of gene expression *(183)*. The results from another study have also revealed that the TGF-β pathway may be specifically activated in $CD44^+$ breast cancer cells suggesting that this cellular subpopulation could be targeted by using the specific inhibitor of TGF-β signaling *(184)*. Additionally, CD133-positive cells, which expressed higher mRNA levels of a multidrug efflux pump, brain cancer resistance protein (BCRP1/ABCG2) and antiapoptotic products were also more resistant to chemotherapeutic agents such as temozolomide, carboplatin, etoposide, and paclitaxel when compared with the CD133 cell fraction *(26)*. Importantly, the CD133 stem cell surface marker was also expressed at higher levels in recurrent GBM tissue obtained from five patients relative to their respective newly diagnosed tumors. Altogether, these studies suggest that a very small population of cancer stem/progenitor cells may express higher level of survival factors, and thereby be more resistant than their differentiated progenies to current therapies *(26)*. Hence, this supports the clinical interest of using newly identified biomarkers expressed by tumorigenic cancer stem/progenitor cells as prognostic indicators and molecular targets to eradicate these tumor-initiating cells that can provide critical roles in treatment resistance and disease relapse.

NOVEL THERAPIES AGAINST AGGRESSIVE AND RECURRENT CANCERS

The development of invasive, metastatic, and recurrent cancers represents one of the major causes of cancer-related deaths *(11–20, 29, 58, 67, 185–189)*. Therefore, the molecular targeting of oncogenic products underlying cancer progression into locally invasive and metastatic disease stages offers great promise for developing new therapeutic options against aggressive cancers *(11–14, 16–20, 67, 85, 155, 177)*. Since recent studies revealed that only a small population of tumorigenic and/or migrating cancer stem/progenitor cells possesses a high potential to drive tumor growth and invasion from primary neoplasm and metastases at distant sites, the molecular targeting of deregulated signaling elements in these tumor-initiating cells must then be considered *(11–14, 16–20, 67, 155, 180, 190, 191)*. In support with this, recent experimental lines of evidence have indeed indicated that the cancer stem/progenitor cells, which express high levels of anti-apoptotic factors, ABC multidrug efflux pumps and enhanced DNA repair mechanisms, could be more resistant than their differentiated progenies to radiation, hormonal, and/or chemotherapeutic treatments *(3, 8, 11–20, 26–28, 75, 101–103, 106, 115, 125, 180–182, 192, 193)*. We review here the new therapeutic strategies to eradicate the tumorigenic and migrating cancer stem/progenitor cells, and thereby improve the current therapies against aggressive, invasive, and metastatic cancers.

Molecular Targeting of Tumorigenic and Migrating Cancer Stem/Progenitor Cells

Recent important advancements have been made in the development of new therapeutic strategies aiming to eradicate the tumorigenic and migrating cancer stem/progenitor cells and their further differentiated progenies *(2, 3, 5, 8, 10–14, 16–20, 26, 29, 67, 76, 102, 103, 124, 194–196)*. Particularly, the molecular targeting of the deregulated signaling elements that mediate the transforming events occurring in tumorigenic and migrating cancer stem/progenitor cells and their local microenvironment during cancer progression, and more particularly during the EMT process, represents new promising therapeutic strategies to improve the current clinical therapies against the most locally aggressive, invasive, metastatic, and recurrent cancers *(5, 11–14, 16–20, 48, 67, 129, 151, 152, 155, 197–201)*. Among the potential targets often deregulated in tumor-initiating cells, there are signaling elements involved in the stringent control of self-renewal and differentiation of adult stem cells including hedgehog, polycomb gene Bmi-1, EGFR, Wnt/β-catenin, FGF/FGFR, SCF-1/CXCR4, TGF-β/TGF-βR, and/or integrin cascades *(3, 8, 9, 11–20, 51, 64, 67, 102, 128, 155, 174, 202–205)*. It has been observed that the blockade of these tumorigenic pathways by using specific inhibitor or antagonists, monoclonal antibody (mAb), or antisense oligonucleotides (As) led to a growth inhibition, apoptotic cell death, and/or a reduction of invasiveness or metastatic spread of tumor-initiating cells and their progenies in vitro or in animal models in vivo (Table 1; Fig. 3) *(3, 11–14, 16, 17, 62, 64, 102, 128,*

Table 1
New molecular targeting strategies by using specific inhibitory agents of deregulated signaling, elements involved in sustained growth, survival, invasion, and/or drug resistance of cancer stem/progenitor cells and their differentiated progenies

Targeted deregulated element	Name of inhibitory agent
EGFR family member inhibitor	
Anti-EGFR (erbB1) antibody	mAb-C225, IMC-C225, EKB-569
Anti-EGF antibody	ABX-EGF
Anti-EGFR, EGF, or TGF- toxin	425(scFv)-ETA, DAB389EGF, TP40
EGFR-TKI	Gefitinib, eriotinib, AG1478,
Anti-erbB2 antibody	Trastuzumab
EGFR-erbB2-TKI	PKI-166, TAK165, GW572017 (lapatinib)
erbB1/erbB2/erbB3/erbB4-TKI	CI1033
Other growth factor signaling inhibitor	
Hedgehog	SMO inhibitor (cyclopamine), anti-SHH antibody
Wnt/β-catenin	Anti-Wnt antibody, WIF-1
Notch	Y-secretase inhibitor DAPT, GSI-18
PDGFR/KIT/ABL-TKI	Imatinib mesylate (STI571)
SDF-1/CXCR4	Anti-SDF-1 or anti-CXCR4 antibody, CXCR4 antagonist (TC14012, TN14003, or AMD3100)
TGF-β/TGF-βR	Anti-TGF-β or TGF-βR antibody, TGF-βR kinase inhibitor (SD-093 and SD-208)
VEGF	Anti-VEGF antibody
VEGFR	Anti-VEGFR antibody, SU5416
ECM component/integrin	Anti-integrin antibody
Intracellular signaling inhibitor	
Telomerase	Telomerase template antagonist
MYC	As-MYC
Bcl-2	ABT-737
PI$_3$K	LY294002, rapamycin, CCI-779
NF-κB	IκBα inhibitor, sulfasalazine, bortezomib (PS-341)
Cripto-1 oncofetal gene product	Anti-Cripto antibody
Tenascin-C	Anti-tenacin C antibody
COX-2	NS-398, etodolax, celecoxib, rofecoxib
Drug transporter inhibitor	
ABC multidrug efflux transporter	
MDR1/ABCB1/P-gp	MS-209, gefitinib, CI1033, tamoxifen, cyclopamine
MRP1/ABCC1	MS-209
ABCG2/BCRP	Gefitinib, CI1033, tamoxifen derivatives, cyclopamine
Organic cation intracellular transporter Oct-1	Prazosin

ABC ATP-binding cassette, *As* antisense, *BCRP* brain cancer resistance protein, *CXCR* CXC-chemokine receptor, *COX* cyclooxygenase, *DAPTN*-[N-(3,5-difluorophenacetyl)-l-alanyl]-*S*-phenylglycine t-butyl ester, *ECM* extracellular matrix, *EGF* epidermal growth factor, *EGFR* epidermal growth factor receptor, *KIT* stem cell factor (SCF) receptor, *GSI-18* [11-*endo*]-*N*-(5,6,7,8,9,10-hexahydro-6,9-methanobenzo[a][8]annulen-11-yl-thiophene-2 sulfonamide, *IκBα* inhibitor of nuclear factor-κBα, *mAb* monoclonal antibody, *MDR1* multidrug resistance, 1, *MRP1* multidrug resistance-associated protein 1, *MRP2* multidrug resistance-associated protein 2, *NF-κB* nuclear factor-κB, *PDGFR* platelet-derived growth factor receptor, *P-gp* P-glycoprotein, *PI$_3$K* phosphatidylinositide-3' kinase, *SMO* smoothened, *TKI* tyrosine kinase inhibitor, *TGF* transforming growth factor, *VEGF* vascular epithelial growth factor, *VEGFR* vascular epithelial growth factor receptor, *WIF-1* Wingless inhibitory factor-1 and *Wnt* Wingless ligand

NOVEL CANCER THERAPY BY TARGETING DEREGULATED SIGNALING ELEMENTS IN TUMORIGENIC AND MIGRATING STEM/PROGENITOR CELLS

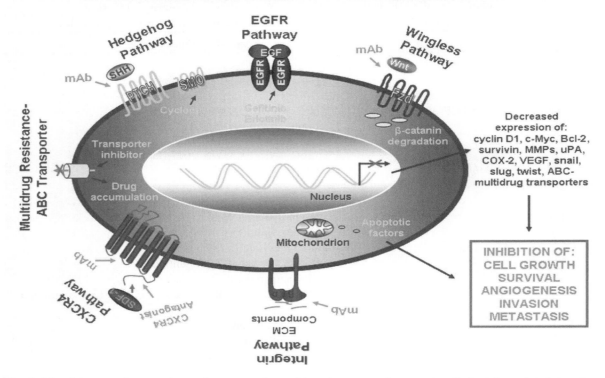

Fig. 3. Novel therapeutic strategies against aggressive and invasive cancers by targeting distinct deregulated signaling cascades in tumorigenic and migrating cancer progenitor cells. The inhibitory effects on the tumorigenic signaling cascades induced by using pharmacological agents such as the selective inhibitors of smoothened (SMO) hedgehog signaling element (cyclopamine) and epidermal growth factor receptor (EGFR) tyrosine kinase activity (gefitinib or erlotinib) are indicated. Moreover, the anti-carcinogenic effects induced by a CXC chemokine receptor 4 (CXCR4) antagonist or monoclonal antibody (mAb) directed against stromal cell-derived factor-1 (SDF-1), CXCR4, Wingless ligand (Wnt) or integrin are also indicated. Particularly, the anti-proliferative, anti-invasive and apoptotic effects induced by these pharmacological agents in cancer stem/progenitor cells through the down-regulation of the expression levels of numerous gene products are also indicated. In addition, the potent inhibitory effect mediated by a specific inhibitor of ATP-binding cassette (ABC)-multidrug transporter on drug efflux is also indicated. *COX-2* cyclooxygenase 2, *ECM* extracellular matrix, *EGF* epidermal growth factor, *Fzd* Frizzled receptor, *MMPs* matrix metalloproteinases, *PTCH* hedgehog-patched receptor, *uPA* urokinase type-plasminogene activator, and *VEGF* vascular endothelial growth factor *(see Color Plates)*.

174, 194, 195, 202–214). Particularly, the blockade of the SDF-1/CXCR4 axis, which provides a critical function for metastases by using a monoclonal antibody directed against SDF-1 or CXCR4 or selective CXCR4 antagonists, such as 14-mer peptide (TN14003) and AMD 3100, constitutes a promising strategy to counteract the migration of cancer stem/progenitor cells to distant sites and metastases (Fig. 3) *(11–14, 16–20, 67, 153, 200, 215–221).* Moreover, other potential molecular targets also include the cellular signaling effectors [telomerase, interleukin-4 (IL-4), Cripto-1, tenacin C, NF-κβ, PI_3K/Akt, Bcl-2, survivin and/or ABC multidrug efflux pump] that are frequently involved in sustained growth, enhanced survival, and invasion during the EMT process and/or drug resistance of cancer stem/progenitor cells and their progenies (Table 1) *(3, 11–14, 16–20, 67, 102, 128, 174, 202, 222, 223).* For instance, it has been observed that the molecular targeting of IL-4, whose cytokine may protect the tumorigenic CD133[+] cancer stem/progenitor cells from human colon carcinoma of apoptotic death, by using IL-4Rα antagonist or anti-IL-4 neutralizing antibody strongly sensitized these tumor-initiating cells to the antitumor effects induced by standard chemotherapeutic drugs *(224)*. In addition, the induction of the differentiation of cancer stem/progenitor cells by using agents such as retinoic acid and its synthetic analogues or histone deacetylase inhibitors, which induce the differentiation, growth arrest and/or apoptotic death of cancer cells, may also represent a promising therapeutic strategy *(2, 129, 225, 226)*.

Molecular Targeting of Local Microenvironment of Tumorigenic and Migrating Cancer Stem/Progenitor Cells

Since the local microenvironment of cancer stem/progenitor cells also plays an active role in cancer progression, efforts are being made to counteract cancer progression by targeting the host stromal cells. In particular, the targeting of the myofibroblasts and immune cells that support the malignant transformation of cancer stem/progenitor cells as well as the use of anti-angiogenic agents may also constitute an adjuvant treatment for counteracting cancer progression to metastatic and lethal disease states *(11–14, 16–20, 67, 68, 70, 153, 227–234)*. More specifically, the combined use of the cytotoxic agents targeting cancer stem/progenitor cells plus a selective inhibitor of the angiogenic process such as cyclooxygenase-1 or 2 (COX-1 or -2), NF-kB, and/or VEGF-VEFGR may constitute more potential strategies to prevent disease relapse (Table 1) *(235–247)*. As a matter of fact, it has been observed that the treatment of the mice-bearing orthotopic U87 glioma cell xenografts with an anti-VEGF monoclonal antibody, called bevacizumab, noticeably reduced the microvasculature density and tumor growth *(232)*. This anticarcinogenic effect was also accompanied by a decrease of the number of vessel-associated self-renewing CD133$^+$/nestin$^+$ tumor-initiating cells *(232)*.

CONCLUSIONS AND FUTURE RESEARCH

In few last years, major progress has been made in establishing the physiological functions provided by tissue-resident adult stem cells to maintain tissue homeostasis as well as the implication of their malignant counterpart, tumorigenic and migrating cancer stem/progenitor cells in tumor formation and metastases. Future investigations are still essential to more precisely to determine the genetic/epigenic alterations occurring in adult stem/progenitor cells and the changes in their intercellular interactions with neighboring cells constituting their niche during cancer initiation. Since the acquisition of a migratory phenotype and invasive ability by tumorigenic cancer stem/progenitor cells constitutes an important event in cancer progression from localized primary neoplasms into metastatic disease stages, it will be important to more precisely establish the molecular events underlying the EMT program in tumorigenic cancer stem/progenitor cells. These additional studies should lead to the identification of new biomarkers and oncogenic targets specific to tumorigenic and migrating cancer stem/progenitor cells. Hence, these new biomarkers could be exploited to develop new diagnostic and prognostic methods and preventive and therapeutic approaches for treating and even curing patients diagnosed with locally advanced, invasive, metastatic, and recurrent cancers, which remain incurable in the clinics with the current therapeutic options.

ACKNOWLEDGMENTS

The authors of this manuscript are supported by the grants from the U.S. Department of Defense (PC04502, OC04110) and the National Institutes of Health (CA78590, CA133774). We thank Ms. Kristi L. Berger for editing the manuscript.

REFERENCES

1. Al-Hajj M, Clarke MF. Self-renewal and solid tumor stem cells. Oncogene 2004;23:7274–82.
2. Sell S. Stem cell origin of cancer and differentiation therapy. Crit Rev Oncol Hematol 2004;51:1–28.
3. Beachy PA, Karhadkar SS, Berman DM. Tissue repair and stem cell renewal in carcinogenesis. Nature 2004;432:324–31.
4. Bapat SA, Mali AM, Koppikar CB, Kurrey NK. Stem and progenitor-like cells contribute to the aggressive behavior of human epithelial ovarian cancer. Cancer Res 2005;65:3025–9.
5. Brabletz T, Jung A, Spaderna S, Hlubek F, Kirchner T. Opinion: migrating cancer stem cells – an integrated concept of malignant tumour progression. Nat Rev Cancer 2005;5:744–9.
6. Li L, Neaves WB. Normal stem cells and cancer stem cells: the niche matters. Cancer Res 2006;66:4553–7.
7. Vescovi AL, Galli R, Reynolds BA. Brain tumour stem cells. Nat Rev Cancer 2006;6:425–36.
8. Tso CL, Shintaku P, Chen J et al. Primary glioblastomas express mesenchymal stem-like properties. Mol Cancer Res 2006;4: 607–19.
9. Liu S, Dontu G, Mantle ID et al. Hedgehog signaling and Bmi-1 regulate self-renewal of normal and malignant human mammary stem cells. Cancer Res 2006;66:6063–71.
10. Nicolis SK. Cancer stem cells and "stemness" genes in neuro-oncology. Neurobiol Dis 2007;25:217–29.
11. Mimeault M, Hauke R, Batra SK. Recent advances on the molecular mechanisms involved in drug-resistance of cancer cells and novel targeting therapies. Clin Pharmacol Ther 2008;83:673–91.
12. Mimeault M, Hauke R, Mehta PP, Batra SK. Recent advances on cancer stem/progenitor cell research: therapeutic implications for overcoming resistance to the most aggressive cancers. J Mol Cell Med 2007;11:981–1011.
13. Mimeault M, Hauke R, Batra SK. Stem cells – A revolution in therapeutics–Recent advances on the stem cell biology and their therapeutic applications in regenerative medicine and cancer therapies. Clin Pharmacol Ther 2007;82:252–64.
14. Mimeault M, Batra SK. Stem cell applications in disease research: Recent advances on stem cell and cancer stem cell biology and their therapeutic implications. In: Allen V. Faraday and Jonathon T. Dyer, eds. Progress in stem cell applications, NOVA Publisher 2008;57–98.
15. Mimeault M, Batra SK. Recent advances on multiple tumorigenic cascades involved in prostatic cancer progression and targeting therapies. Carcinogenesis 2006;27:1–22.
16. Mimeault M, Batra SK. Recent advances on the significance of stem cells in tissue regeneration and cancer therapies. Stem Cells 2006; 24:2319–45.
17. Mimeault M, Mehta PP, Hauke R, Batra SK. Functions of normal and malignant prostatic stem/progenitor cells in tissue regeneration and cancer progression and novel targeting therapies against advanced prostate cancers. Endocr Rev 2008;29:234–52.
18. Mimeault M, Batra SK. Interplay of distinct growth factors during epithelial-mesenchymal transition of cancer progenitor cells and molecular targeting as novel cancer therapies. Ann Oncol 2007;18:1605–19.
19. Mimeault M, Batra SK. Functions of tumorigenic and migrating cancer progenitor cells in cancer progression and metastasis and their therapeutic implications. Cancer Metastasis Rev 2007;26:203–14.
20. Mimeault M, Batra SK. Recent progress on tissue-resident adult stem cell biology and their therapeutic implications. Stem Cell Rev 2008;4:27–49.
21. Hermann PC, Huber SL, Herrler T et al. Distinct populations of cancer stem cells determine tumor growth and metastatic activity in human pancreatic cancer. Cell Stem Cells 2007;1:313–23.
22. Radisky ES, Radisky DC. Stromal induction of breast cancer: inflammation and invasion. Rev Endocr Metab Disord 2007;8: 279–287.
23. Kleeff J, Beckhove P, Esposito I et al. Pancreatic cancer microenvironment. Int J Cancer 2007;121:699–705.
24. Yuan X, Curtin J, Xiong Y et al. Isolation of cancer stem cells from adult glioblastoma multiforme. Oncogene 2004;23: 9392–400.
25. Galli R, Binda E, Orfanelli U et al. Isolation and characterization of tumorigenic, stem-like neural precursors from human glioblastoma. Cancer Res 2004;64:7011–21.
26. Liu G, Yuan X, Zeng Z et al. Analysis of gene expression and chemoresistance of CD133+ cancer stem cells in glioblastoma. Mol Cancer 2006;5:67.
27. Bao S, Wu Q, McLendon RE et al. Glioma stem cells promote radioresistance by preferential activation of the DNA damage response. Nature 2006;444:756–60.
28. Haraguchi N, Utsunomiya T, Inoue H et al. Characterization of a side population of cancer cells from human gastrointestinal system. Stem Cells 2006;24:506–13.
29. Sato M, Shames DS, Gazdar AF, Minna JD. A translational view of the molecular pathogenesis of lung cancer. J Thorac Oncol 2007;2:327–43.
30. Larue L, Bellacosa A. Epithelial-mesenchymal transition in development and cancer: role of phosphatidylinositol 3′ kinase/ AKT pathways. Oncogene 2005;24:7443–54.
31. Thiery JP. Epithelial-mesenchymal transitions in tumour progression. Nat Rev Cancer 2002;2:442–54.
32. Gotzmann J, Mikula M, Eger A et al. Molecular aspects of epithelial cell plasticity: implications for local tumor invasion and metastasis. Mutat Res 2004;566:9–20.
33. Eastham AM, Spencer H, Soncin F et al. Epithelial-mesenchymal transition events during human embryonic stem cell differentiation. Cancer Res 2007;67:11254–62.

34. Behr R, Heneweer C, Viebahn C, Denker HW, Thie M. Epithelial-mesenchymal transition in colonies of rhesus monkey embryonic stem cells: a model for processes involved in gastrulation. Stem Cells 2005;23:805–16.
35. Barrow KM, Ward CM, Rutter J, Ali S, Stern PL. Embryonic expression of murine 5T4 oncofoetal antigen is associated with morphogenetic events at implantation and in developing epithelia. Dev Dyn 2005;233:1535–45.
36. Ullmann U, In't VP, Gilles C et al. Epithelial-mesenchymal transition process in human embryonic stem cells cultured in feeder-free conditions. Mol Hum Reprod 2007;13:21–32.
37. Derycke LD, Bracke ME. N-cadherin in the spotlight of cell-cell adhesion, differentiation, embryogenesis, invasion and signalling. Int J Dev Biol 2004;48:463–76.
38. Lee JM, Dedhar S, Kalluri R, Thompson EW. The epithelial-mesenchymal transition: new insights in signaling, development, and disease. J Cell Biol 2006;172:973–81.
39. Grunert S, Jechlinger M, Beug H. Diverse cellular and molecular mechanisms contribute to epithelial plasticity and metastasis. Nat Rev Mol Cell Biol 2003;4:657–65.
40. Cavallaro U, Christofori G. Cell adhesion and signalling by cadherins and Ig-CAMs in cancer. Nat Rev Cancer 2004;4: 118–32.
41. Cavallaro U, Christofori G. Multitasking in tumor progression: signaling functions of cell adhesion molecules. Ann N Y Acad Sci 2004;1014:58–66.
42. Thiery JP. Epithelial-mesenchymal transitions in development and pathologies. Curr Opin Cell Biol 2003;15:740–6.
43. Sahai E, Marshall CJ. RHO-GTPases and cancer. Nat Rev Cancer 2002;2(2):133–142.
44. Seidel B, Braeg S, Adler G, Wedlich D, Menke A. E- and N-cadherin differ with respect to their associated p120ctn isoforms and their ability to suppress invasive growth in pancreatic cancer cells. Oncogene 2004;23:5532–42.
45. Bates RC, Mercurio AM. The epithelial-mesenchymal transition (EMT) and colorectal cancer progression. Cancer Biol Ther 2005;4:365–70.
46. Sarrio D, Perez-Mies B, Hardisson D et al. Cytoplasmic localization of p120ctn and E-cadherin loss characterize lobular breast carcinoma from preinvasive to metastatic lesions. Oncogene 2004;23:3272–83.
47. Savagner P. Leaving the neighborhood: molecular mechanisms involved during epithelial-mesenchymal transition. Bioessays 2001;23:912–23.
48. Bissell MJ, Radisky D. Putting tumours in context. Nat Rev Cancer 2001;1:46–54.
49. Huber MA, Kraut N, Beug H. Molecular requirements for epithelial-mesenchymal transition during tumor progression. Curr Opin Cell Biol 2005;17:548–58.
50. Zavadil J, Cermak L, Soto-Nieves N, Bottinger EP. Integration of TGF-beta/Smad and Jagged1/Notch signalling in epithelial-to-mesenchymal transition. EMBO J 2004;23:1155–65.
51. Katoh M, Katoh M. Cross-talk of WNT and FGF signaling pathways at GSK3beta to regulate beta-catenin and SNAIL signaling cascades. Cancer Biol Ther 2006;5:1059–64.
52. Davies M, Robinson M, Smith E, Huntley S, Prime S, Paterson I. Induction of an epithelial to mesenchymal transition in human immortal and malignant keratinocytes by TGF-beta1 involves MAPK, Smad and AP-1 signalling pathways. J Cell Biochem 2005;95:918–31.
53. Grande M, Franzen A, Karlsson JO, Ericson LE, Heldin NE, Nilsson M. Transforming growth factor-beta and epidermal growth factor synergistically stimulate epithelial to mesenchymal transition (EMT) through a MEK-dependent mechanism in primary cultured pig thyrocytes. J Cell Sci 2002;115:4227–36.
54. Bigelow RL, Jen EY, Delehedde M, Chari NS, McDonnell TJ. Sonic hedgehog induces epidermal growth factor dependent matrix infiltration in HaCaT keratinocytes. J Invest Dermatol 2005;124:457–65.
55. Kasper M, Schnidar H, Neill GW et al. Selective modulation of hedgehog/GLI target gene expression by epidermal growth factor signaling in human keratinocytes. Mol Cell Biol 2006;26:6283–98.
56. Oku N, Sasabe E, Ueta E, Yamamoto T, Osaki T. Tight junction protein claudin-1 enhances the invasive activity of oral squamous cell carcinoma cells by promoting cleavage of laminin-5 gamma2 chain via matrix metalloproteinase (MMP)-2 and membrane-type MMP-1. Cancer Res 2006;66:1–5257.
57. Hajra KM, Fearon ER. Cadherin and catenin alterations in human cancer. Genes Chromosomes Cancer 2002;34:255–68.
58. Mimeault M, Brand RE, Sasson AA, Batra SK. Recent advances on the molecular mechanisms involved in pancreatic cancer progression and therapies. Pancreas 2005;31:301–16.
59. Reya T, Clevers H. Wnt signalling in stem cells and cancer. Nature 2005;434:843–50.
60. Woodward WA, Chen MS, Behbod F, Rosen JM. On mammary stem cells. J Cell Sci 2005;118:3585–94.
61. Owens DM, Watt FM. Contribution of stem cells and differentiated cells to epidermal tumours. Nat Rev Cancer 2003;3: 444–51.
62. Mimeault M, Moore E, Moniaux N et al. Cytotoxic effects induced by a combination of cyclopamine and gefitinib, the selective hedgehog and epidermal growth factor receptor signaling inhibitors, in prostate cancer cells. Int J Cancer 2006; 118:1022–031.
63. Rao G, Pedone CA, Valle LD, Reiss K, Holland EC, Fults DW. Sonic hedgehog and insulin-like growth factor signaling synergize to induce medulloblastoma formation from nestin-expressing neural progenitors in mice. Oncogene 2004; 23:6156–62.
64. Derynck R, Akhurst RJ, Balmain A. TGF-beta signaling in tumor suppression and cancer progression. Nat Genet 2001; 29:117–29.

65. Jechlinger M, Sommer A, Moriggl R et al. Autocrine PDGFR signaling promotes mammary cancer metastasis. J metastasis. J metastasis. J Clin Invest 2006;116:1561–70.
66. Waerner T, Alacakaptan M, Tamir I et al. ILEI: a cytokine essential for EMT, tumor formation, and late events in metastasis in epithelial cells. Cancer Cell 2006;10:227–39.
67. Mimeault M, Batra SK. Targeting of cancer stem/progenitor cells plus stem cell-based therapies:an ultimate hope for treating and curing the aggressive and recurrent cancers. Panminerva Medica 2008;50:3–18.
68. Rafii S, Lyden D, Benezra R, Hattori K, Heissig B. Vascular and haematopoietic stem cells: novel targets for anti-angiogenesis therapy? Nat Rev Cancer 2002;2:826–35.
69. Orimo A, Weinberg RA. Stromal fibroblasts in cancer: A novel tumor-promoting cell type. Cell Cycle 2006;5:1597–601.
70. Ganss R. Tumor stroma fosters neovascularization by recruitment of progenitor cells into the tumor bed. J Cell Mol Med 2006;10:857–65.
71. Kaplan RN, Riba RD, Zacharoulis S et al. VEGFR1-positive haematopoietic bone marrow progenitors initiate the pre-metastatic niche. Nature 2005;438:820–7.
72. Bruno S, Bussolati B, Grange C et al. CD133+ renal progenitor cells contribute to tumor angiogenesis. Am J Pathol 2006;169:2223–35.
73. Sorlie T, Wang Y, Xiao C et al. Distinct molecular mechanisms underlying clinically relevant subtypes of breast cancer: gene expression analyses across three different platforms. BMC Genomics 2006;7:127.
74. Al-Hajj M, Wicha MS, ito-Hernandez A, Morrison SJ, Clarke MF. Prospective identification of tumorigenic breast cancer cells. Proc Natl Acad Sci USA 2003;100:3983–8.
75. Dontu G, El-Ashry D, Wicha MS. Breast cancer, stem/progenitor cells and the estrogen receptor. Trends Endocrinol Metab 2004;15:193–7.
76. Liu S, Dontu G, Wicha MS. Mammary stem cells, self-renewal pathways, and carcinogenesis. Breast Cancer Res 2005;7:86–95.
77. Ponti D, Costa A, Zaffaroni N et al. Isolation and *in vitro* propagation of tumorigenic breast cancer cells with stem/progenitor cell properties. Cancer Res 2005;65:5506–11.
78. Teuliere J, Faraldo MM, Deugnier MA et al. Targeted activation of beta-catenin signaling in basal mammary epithelial cells affects mammary development and leads to hyperplasia. Development 2005;132:267–77.
79. Clarke RB, Spence K, Anderson E, Howell A, Okano H, Potten CS. A putative human breast stem cell population is enriched for steroid receptor-positive cells. Dev Biol 2005;277:443–56.
80. Du Z, Podsypanina K, Huang S et al. Introduction of oncogenes into mammary glands in vivo with an avian retroviral vector initiates and promotes carcinogenesis in mouse models. Proc Natl Acad Sci USA 2006;103:17396–401.
81. Tang P, Wang X, Schiffhauer L et al. Expression patterns of ER-alpha, PR, HER-2/neu, and EGFR in different cell origin subtypes of high grade and non-high grade ductal carcinoma in situ. Ann Clin Lab Sci 2006;36:137–43.
82. Fodde R, Brabletz T. Wnt/beta-catenin signaling in cancer stemness and malignant behavior. Curr Opin Cell Biol 2007;19:150–8.
83. Moraes RC, Zhang X, Harrington N et al. Constitutive activation of smoothened (SMO) in mammary glands of transgenic mice leads to increased proliferation, altered differentiation and ductal dysplasia. Development 2007;134(6):1231–1242.
84. Chung LW, Baseman A, Assikis V, Zhau HE. Molecular insights into prostate cancer progression: the missing link of tumor microenvironment. J Urol 2005;173:10–20.
85. Langley RR, Fidler IJ. Tumor cell-organ microenvironment interactions in the pathogenesis of cancer metastasis. Endocr Rev 2007;28:297–321.
86. Carver BS, Pandolfi PP. Mouse modeling in oncologic preclinical and translational research. Clin Cancer Res 2006;12:5305–11.
87. Zhou Z, Flesken-Nikitin A, Nikitin AY. Prostate cancer associated with p53 and Rb deficiency arises from the stem/progenitor cell-enriched proximal region of prostatic ducts. Cancer Res 2007;67:5683–90.
88. Chen Z, Trotman LC, Shaffer D et al. Crucial role of p53-dependent cellular senescence in suppression of Pten-deficient tumorigenesis. Nature 2005;436:725–30.
89. Wang S, Gao J, Lei Q et al. Prostate-specific deletion of the murine Pten tumor suppressor gene leads to metastatic prostate cancer. Cancer Cell 2003;4:209–21.
90. Wang S, Garcia AJ, Wu M, Lawson DA, Witte ON, Wu H. Pten deletion leads to the expansion of a prostatic stem/progenitor cell subpopulation and tumor initiation. Proc Natl Acad Sci USA 2006;103:1480–5.
91. Bruxvoort KJ, Charbonneau HM, Giambernardi TA et al. Inactivation of Apc in the mouse prostate causes prostate carcinoma. Cancer Res 2007;67:2490–6.
92. Nikitin AY, Matoso A, Roy-Burman P. Prostate stem cells and cancer. Histol Histopathol 2007;22:1043–9.
93. Reiner T, de Las PA, Parrondo R, Perez-Stable C. Progression of prostate cancer from a subset of p63-positive basal epithelial cells in FG/Tag transgenic mice. Mol Cancer Res 2007;5:1171–9.
94. Kalluri R, Zeisberg M. Fibroblasts in cancer. Nat Rev Cancer 2006;6:392–401.
95. Laakso M, Tanner M, Nilsson J et al. Basoluminal carcinoma: a new biologically and prognostically distinct entity between basal and luminal breast cancer. Clin Cancer Res 2006;12:4185–91.
96. Simon R. Development and evaluation of therapeutically relevant predictive classifiers using gene expression profiling. J Natl Cancer Inst 2006;98:1169–71.

97. Leonard GD, Swain SM. Ductal carcinoma *in situ*, complexities and challenges. J Natl Cancer Inst 2004;96:906–20.

98. Buyse M, Loi S, van't VL et al. Validation and clinical utility of a 70-gene prognostic signature for women with node-negative breast cancer. J Natl Cancer Inst 2006;98:1183–92.

99. Anderson WF, Matsuno R. Breast cancer heterogeneity: a mixture of at least two main types? J Natl Cancer Inst 2006;98:948–51.

100. Asselin-Labat ML, Shackleton M, Stingl J et al. Steroid hormone receptor status of mouse mammary stem cells. J Natl Cancer Inst 2006;98:1011–4.

101. Hirschmann-Jax C, Foster AE, Wulf GG et al. A distinct "side population" of cells with high drug efflux capacity in human tumor cells. Proc Natl Acad Sci USA 2004;101:14228–33.

102. Dean M, Fojo T, Bates S. Tumour stem cells and drug resistance. Nat Rev Cancer 2005;5:275–84.

103. Milas L, Raju U, Liao Z, Ajani J. Targeting molecular determinants of tumor chemo-radioresistance. Semin Oncol 2005;32:S78–S81.

104. Hemmati HD, Nakano I, Lazareff JA et al. Cancerous stem cells can arise from pediatric brain tumors. Proc Natl Acad Sci USA 2003;100:15178–83.

105. Singh SK, Hawkins C, Clarke ID et al. Identification of human brain tumour initiating cells. Nature 2004;432:396–401.

106. Collins AT, Berry PA, Hyde C, Stower MJ, Maitland NJ. Prospective identification of tumorigenic prostate cancer stem cells. Cancer Res 2005;65:10946–51.

107. Patrawala L, Calhoun T, Schneider-Broussard R et al. Highly purified CD44+ prostate cancer cells from xenograft human tumors are enriched in tumorigenic and metastatic progenitor cells. Oncogene 2006;25:1696–708.

108. Li C, Heidt DG, Dalerba P et al. Identification of pancreatic cancer stem cells. Cancer Res 2007;67:1030–7.

109. Ricci-Vitiani L, Lombardi DG, Pilozzi E et al. Identification and expansion of human colon-cancer-initiating cells. Nature 2007;445:111–5.

110. Prince ME, Sivanandan R, Kaczorowski A et al. Identification of a subpopulation of cells with cancer stem cell properties in head and neck squamous cell carcinoma. Proc Natl Acad Sci USA 2007;104:973–8.

111. Taylor MD, Poppleton H, Fuller C et al. Radial glia cells are candidate stem cells of ependymoma. Cancer Cell 2005;8:323–35.

112. Fang D, Nguyen TK, Leishear K et al. A tumorigenic subpopulation with stem cell properties in melanomas. Cancer Res 2005;65:9328–37.

113. Patrawala L, Calhoun T, Schneider-Broussard R, Zhou J, Claypool K, Tang DG. Side population is enriched in tumorigenic, stem-like cancer cells, whereas ABCG2+ and ABCG2- cancer cells are similarly tumorigenic. Cancer Res 2005;65:6207–19.

114. Tai MH, Chang CC, Kiupel M, Webster JD, Olson LK, Trosko JE. Oct4 expression in adult human stem cells: evidence in support of the stem cell theory of carcinogenesis. Carcinogenesis 2005;26:495–502.

115. Ho MM, Ng AV, Lam S, Hung JY. Side population in human lung cancer cell lines and tumors is enriched with stem-like cancer cells. Cancer Res 2007;67:4827–33.

116. Hadnagy A, Gaboury L, Beaulieu R, Balicki D. SP analysis may be used to identify cancer stem cell populations. Exp Cell Res 2006;312:3701–10.

117. Klein WM, Wu BP, Zhao S, Wu H, Klein-Szanto AJ, Tahan SR. Increased expression of stem cell markers in malignant melanoma. Mod Pathol 2007;20:102–7.

118. Immervoll H, Hoem D, Sakariassen PO, Steffensen OJ, Molven A. Expression of the "stem cell marker" CD133 in pancreas and pancreatic ductal adenocarcinomas. BMC Cancer 2008;8:48.

119. Wright MH, Calcagno AM, Salcido CD, Carlson MD, Ambudkar SV, Varticovski L. Brca1 breast tumors contain distinct CD44+/CD24- and CD133+ cells with cancer stem cell characteristics. Breast Cancer Res 2008;10:R10.

120. Eramo A, Lotti F, Sette G et al. Identification and expansion of the tumorigenic lung cancer stem cell population. Cell Death Differ 2008;15:504–14.

121. Yang ZF, Ho DW, Ng MN et al. Significance of CD90(+) cancer stem cells in human liver cancer. Cancer Cell 2008;13:153–66.

122. Gao JX. Cancer stem cells: the lessons from precancerous stem cells. J Cell Mol Med 2008;12:67–96.

123. Blanco-Aparicio C, Renner O, Leal JF, Carnero A. PTEN, more than the AKT pathway. Carcinogenesis 2007;28:1379–86.

124. Fuster JJ, Sanz-Gonzalez SM, Moll UM, Andres V. Classic and novel roles of p53: prospects for anticancer therapy. Trends Mol Med 2007;13:192–9.

125. de Jonge-Peeters SD, Kuipers F, de Vries EG, Vellenga E. ABC transporter expression in hematopoietic stem cells and the role in AML drug resistance. Crit Rev Oncol Hematol 2007;62:214–26.

126. Mimeault M, Pommery N, Henichart JP. New advances on prostate carcinogenesis and therapies: involvement of EGF-EGFR transduction system. Growth Factors 2003;21:1–14.

127. Mimeault M, Bonenfant D, Batra SK. New advances on the functions of epidermal growth factor receptor and ceramides in skin cell differentiation, disorders and cancers. Skin Pharmacol Physiol 2004;17:153–66.

128. Chen BY, Liu JY, Chang HH et al. Hedgehog is involved in prostate basal cell hyperplasia formation and its progressing towards tumorigenesis. Biochem Biophys Res Commun 2007;357:1084–9.

129. Massard C, Deutsch E, Soria JC. Tumour stem cell-targeted treatment: elimination or differentiation. Ann Oncol 2006;17:1620–4.

130. Edme N, Downward J, Thiery JP, Boyer B. Ras induces NBT-II epithelial cell scattering through the coordinate activities of Rac and MAPK pathways. J Cell Sci 2002;115:2591–601.

131. Yin T, Getsios S, Caldelari R et al. Mechanisms of plakoglobin-dependent adhesion: desmosome-specific functions in assembly and regulation by epidermal growth factor receptor. J Biol Chem 2005;280:40355–63.

132. Lorch JH, Klessner J, Park JK et al. Epidermal growth factor receptor inhibition promotes desmosome assembly and strengthens intercellular adhesion in squamous cell carcinoma cells. J Biol Chem 2004;279:37191–200.

133. Vandewalle C, Comijn J, De CB et al. SIP1/ZEB2 induces EMT by repressing genes of different epithelial cell-cell junctions. Nucleic Acids Res 2005;33:6566–78.

134. De Craene B, Gilbert B, Stove C, Bruyneel E, van RF, Berx G. The transcription factor snail induces tumor cell invasion through modulation of the epithelial cell differentiation program. Cancer Res 2005;65:6237–44.

135. Trosko JE, Tai MH. Adult stem cell theory of the multi-stage, multi-mechanism theory of carcinogenesis: role of inflammation on the promotion of initiated stem cells. Contrib Microbiol 2006;13:45–65.

136. Kopfstein L, Christofori G. Metastasis: cell-autonomous mechanisms versus contributions by the tumor microenvironment. Cell Mol Life Sci 2006;63:449–68.

137. Cozzolino M, Stagni V, Spinardi L et al. p120 Catenin is required for growth factor-dependent cell motility and scattering in epithelial cells. Mol Biol Cell 2003;14:1964–77.

138. Man YG, Sang QX. The significance of focal myoepithelial cell layer disruptions in human breast tumor invasion: a paradigm shift from the "protease-centered" hypothesis. Exp Cell Res 2004;301:103–18.

139. Hildenbrand R, Arens N. Protein and mRNA expression of uPAR and PAI-1 in myoepithelial cells of early breast cancer lesions and normal breast tissue. Br J Cancer 2004;91:564–71.

140. Nieto MA. The snail superfamily of zinc-finger transcription factors. Nat Rev Mol Cell Biol 2002;3:155–66.

141. Barrallo-Gimeno A, Nieto MA. The Snail genes as inducers of cell movement and survival: implications in development and cancer. Development 2005;132:3151–61.

142. Wicki A, Lehembre F, Wick N, Hantusch B, Kerjaschki D, Christofori G. Tumor invasion in the absence of epithelial-mesenchymal transition: podoplanin-mediated remodeling of the actin cytoskeleton. Cancer Cell 2006;9:261–72.

143. Christiansen JJ, Rajasekaran AK. Reassessing epithelial to mesenchymal transition as a prerequisite for carcinoma invasion and metastasis. Cancer Res 2006;66:8319–26.

144. Mikaelian I, Blades N, Churchill GA et al. Proteotypic classification of spontaneous and transgenic mammary neoplasms. Breast Cancer Res 2004;6:R668–79.

145. Polette M, Nawrocki-Raby B, Gilles C, Clavel C, Birembaut P. Tumour invasion and matrix metalloproteinases. Crit Rev Oncol Hematol 2004;49:179–86.

146. Radisky DC, Bissell MJ. Matrix metalloproteinase-induced genomic instability. Curr Opin Genet Dev 2006; 16:45–50.

147. Bergers G, Coussens LM. Extrinsic regulators of epithelial tumor progression: metalloproteinases. Curr Opin Genet Dev 2000;10:120–7.

148. Reiss K, Ludwig A, Saftig P. Breaking up the tie: Disintegrin-like metalloproteinases as regulators of cell migration in inflammation and invasion. Pharmacol Ther 2006;111:985–1006.

149. Yang J, Mani SA, Weinberg RA. Exploring a new twist on tumor metastasis. Cancer Res 2006;66:4549–52.

150. Lo HW, Hsu SC, Xia W et al. Epidermal growth factor receptor cooperates with signal transducer and activator of transcription 3 to induce epithelial-mesenchymal transition in cancer cells via up-regulation of TWIST gene expression. Cancer Res 2007;67:9066–76.

151. Kajita M, McClinic KN, Wade PA. Aberrant expression of the transcription factors snail and slug alters the response to genotoxic stress. Mol Cell Biol 2004;24:7559–66.

152. Vega S, Morales AV, Ocana OH, Valdes F, Fabregat I, Nieto MA. Snail blocks the cell cycle and confers resistance to cell death. Genes Dev 2004;18:1131–43.

153. Onoue T, Uchida D, Begum NM, Tomizuka Y, Yoshida H, Sato M. Epithelial-mesenchymal transition induced by the stromal cell-derived factor-1/CXCR4 system in oral squamous cell carcinoma cells. Int J Oncol 2006;29:1133–8.

154. Kang Y, Massague J. Epithelial-mesenchymal transitions: twist in development and metastasis. Cell 2004;118:277–9.

155. Croker AK, Allan AL. Cancer Stem Cells: Implications for the progression and treatment of metastatic disease. J Cell Mol Med 2007.

156. Ii M, Yamamoto H, Adachi Y, Maruyama Y, Shinomura Y. Role of matrix metalloproteinase-7 (matrilysin) in human cancer invasion, apoptosis, growth, and angiogenesis. Exp Biol Med (Maywood) 2006;231:20–27.

157. Liu H, Radisky DC, Wang F, Bissell MJ. Polarity and proliferation are controlled by distinct signaling pathways downstream of PI3-kinase in breast epithelial tumor cells. J Cell Biol 2004;164:603–12.

158. Festuccia C, Angelucci A, Gravina GL et al. Epidermal growth factor modulates prostate cancer cell invasiveness regulating urokinase-type plasminogen activator activity. EGF-receptor inhibition may prevent tumor cell dissemination. Thromb Haemost 2005;93:964–75.

159. Shelton JG, Steelman LS, Abrams SL et al. The epidermal growth factor receptor gene family as a target for therapeutic intervention in numerous cancers: what's genetics got to do with it? Expert Opin Ther Targets 2005;9:1009–30.

160. Miravet S, Piedra J, Castano J et al. Tyrosine phosphorylation of plakoglobin causes contrary effects on its association with desmosomes and adherens junction components and modulates beta-catenin-mediated transcription. Mol Cell Biol 2003;23:7391–402.

161. Ahmed N, Maines-Bandiera S, Quinn MA, Unger WG, Dedhar S, Auersperg N. Molecular pathways regulating EGF-induced epithelio-mesenchymal transition in human ovarian surface epithelium. Am J Physiol Cell Physiol 2006;290:C1532–42.

162. Cattan N, Rochet N, Mazeau C et al. Establishment of two new human bladder carcinoma cell lines, CAL 29 and CAL 185. Comparative study of cell scattering and epithelial to mesenchyme transition induced by growth factors. Br J Cancer 2001;85:1412–7.

163. Lu Z, Ghosh S, Wang Z, Hunter T. Downregulation of caveolin-1 function by EGF leads to the loss of E-cadherin, increased transcriptional activity of beta-catenin, and enhanced tumor cell invasion. Cancer Cell 2003;4:499–515.

164. Nielsen TO, Hsu FD, Jensen K et al. Immunohistochemical and clinical characterization of the basal-like subtype of invasive breast carcinoma. Clin Cancer Res 2004;10:5367–74.

165. Birnbaum D, Bertucci F, Ginestier C, Tagett R, Jacquemier J, Charafe-Jauffret E. Basal and luminal breast cancers: basic or luminous? (review). Int J Oncol 2004;25:249–58.

166. Livasy CA, Karaca G, Nanda R et al. Phenotypic evaluation of the basal-like subtype of invasive breast carcinoma. Mod Pathol 2006;19:264–71.

167. Carey LA, Perou CM, Livasy CA et al. Race, breast cancer subtypes, and survival in the Carolina Breast Cancer Study. JAMA 2006;295:2492–502.

168. Jumppanen M, Gruvberger-Saal S, Kauraniemi P et al. Basal-like phenotype is not associated with patient survival in estrogen receptor negative breast cancers. Breast Cancer Res 2007;9:R16.

169. Lacroix M. Significance, detection and markers of disseminated breast cancer cells. Endocr Relat Cancer 2006;13:1033–067.

170. Calza S, Hall P, Auer G et al. Intrinsic molecular signature of breast cancer in a population-based cohort of 412 patients. Breast Cancer Res 2006;8:R34.

171. Potemski P, Kusinska R, Watala C, Pluciennik E, Bednarek AK, Kordek R. Prognostic relevance of basal cytokeratin expression in operable breast cancer. Oncology 2005;69:478–85.

172. Rakha EA, El-Sayed ME, Green AR, Lee AH, Robertson JF, Ellis IO. Prognostic markers in triple-negative breast cancer. Cancer 2007;109:25–32.

173. Fujita N, Jaye DL, Kajita M, Geigerman C, Moreno CS, Wade PA. MTA3, a Mi-2/NuRD complex subunit, regulates an invasive growth pathway in breast cancer. Cell 2003;113:207–19.

174. Wang X, Belguise K, Kersual N et al. Oestrogen signalling inhibits invasive phenotype by repressing RelB and its target BCL2. Nat Cell Biol 2007;9:470–8.

175. Hu M, Polyak K. Serial analysis of gene expression. Nat Protoc 2006;1:1743–60.

176. Porter D, Yao J, Polyak K. SAGE and related approaches for cancer target identification. Drug Discov Today 2006;11:110–8.

177. Nguyen DX, Massague J. Genetic determinants of cancer metastasis. Nat Rev Genet 2007;8:341–52.

178. Price ND, Foltz G, Madan A, Hood L, Tian Q. Systems Biology and Cancer Stem Cells. J Cell Mol Med 2007.

179. Yang ZF, Ngai P, Ho DW et al. Identification of local and circulating cancer stem cells in human liver cancer. Hepatology 2008;47:919–28.

180. Eramo A, Ricci-Vitiani L, Zeuner A et al. Chemotherapy resistance of glioblastoma stem cells. Cell Death Differ 2006;13:1238–41.

181. Salmaggi A, Boiardi A, Gelati M et al. Glioblastoma-derived tumorospheres identify a population of tumor stem-like cells with angiogenic potential and enhanced multidrug resistance phenotype. Glia 2006;54:850–60.

182. Frank NY, Margaryan A, Huang Y et al. ABCB5-mediated doxorubicin transport and chemoresistance in human malignant melanoma. Cancer Res 2005;65:4320–33.

183. Liu R, Wang X, Chen GY et al. The prognostic role of a gene signature from tumorigenic breast-cancer cells. N Engl J Med 2007;356:217–26.

184. Shipitsin M, Campbell LL, Argani P et al. Molecular definition of breast tumor heterogeneity. Cancer Cell 2007;11:259–73.

185. Goldman J, Gordon M. Why do chronic myelogenous leukemia stem cells survive allogeneic stem cell transplantation or imatinib: does it really matter? Leuk Lymphoma 2006;47:1–7.

186. Copland M, Jorgensen HG, Holyoake TL. Evolving molecular therapy for chronic myeloid leukaemia–are we on target? Hematology 2005;10:349–59.

187. Copland M, Hamilton A, Elrick LJ et al. Dasatinib (BMS-354825) targets an earlier progenitor population than imatinib in primary CML but does not eliminate the quiescent fraction. Blood 2006;107:4532–9.

188. Mauro MJ. Defining and managing imatinib resistance. Hematology Am Soc Hematol Educ Program 2006;219–25.

189. Jemal A, Siegel R, Ward E, Murray T, Xu J, Thun MJ. Cancer statistics, 2007. CA Cancer J Clin 2007;57:43–66.

190. Knizetova P, Darling JL, Bartek J. Vascular endothelial growth factor in astroglioma stem cell biology and response to therapy. J Cell Mol Med 2008;12:111–25.

191. Kang MK, Kang SK. Tumorigenesis of chemotherapeutic drug-resistant cancer stem-like cells in brain glioma. Stem Cells Dev 2007;16:837–47.

192. Chen MS, Woodward WA, Behbod F et al. Wnt/beta-catenin mediates radiation resistance of Sca1+ progenitors in an immortalized mammary gland cell line. J Cell Sci 2007;120:468–77.

193. Kurbel S. Selective reduction of estrogen receptor (ER) positive breast cancer occurrence by estrogen receptor modulators supports etiological distinction between ER positive and ER negative breast cancers. Med Hypotheses 2005;64:1182–7.

194. Fan X, Matsui W, Khaki L et al. Notch pathway inhibition depletes stem-like cells and blocks engraftment in embryonal brain tumors. Cancer Res 2006;66:7445–52.

195. Karhadkar SS, Bova GS, Abdallah N et al. Hedgehog signalling in prostate regeneration, neoplasia and metastasis. Nature 2004;431:707–12.

196. Gray-Schopfer V, Wellbrock C, Marais R. Melanoma biology and new targeted therapy. Nature 2007;445:851–7.

197. Jung A, Schrauder M, Oswald U et al. The invasion front of human colorectal adenocarcinomas shows co-localization of nuclear beta-catenin, cyclin D1, and p16INK4A and is a region of low proliferation. Am J Pathol 2001; 159:1613–7.

198. Rintoul RC, Sethi T. Extracellular matrix regulation of drug resistance in small-cell lung cancer. Clin Sci (Lond) 2002;102:417–24.

199. Warshamana-Greene GS, Litz J, Buchdunger E, Hofmann F, Garcia-Echeverria C, Krystal GW. The insulin-like growth factor-I (IGF-I) receptor kinase inhibitor NVP-ADW742, in combination with STI571, delineates a spectrum of dependence of small cell lung cancer on IGF-I and stem cell factor signaling. Mol Cancer Ther 2004;3:527–35.

200. Kucia M, Reca R, Miekus K et al. Trafficking of normal stem cells and metastasis of cancer stem cells involve similar mechanisms: pivotal role of the SDF-1-CXCR4 axis. Stem Cells 2005;23:879–94.

201. Warshamana-Greene GS, Litz J, Buchdunger E, Garcia-Echeverria C, Hofmann F, Krystal GW. The insulin-like growth factor-I receptor kinase inhibitor, NVP-ADW742, sensitizes small cell lung cancer cell lines to the effects of chemotherapy. Clin Cancer Res 2005;11:1563–71.

202. Feldmann G, Dhara S, Fendrich V et al. Blockade of hedgehog signaling inhibits pancreatic cancer invasion and metastases: a new paradigm for combination therapy in solid cancers. Cancer Res 2007;67:2187–96.

203. Biswas S, Criswell TL, Wang SE, Arteaga CL. Inhibition of transforming growth factor-beta signaling in human cancer: targeting a tumor suppressor network as a therapeutic strategy. Clin Cancer Res 2006;12:4142–6.

204. Bierie B, Moses HL. Tumour microenvironment: TGFbeta: the molecular Jekyll and Hyde of cancer. Nat Rev Cancer 2006;6:506–20.

205. Park CC, Zhang H, Pallavicini M et al. Beta1 integrin inhibitory antibody induces apoptosis of breast cancer cells, inhibits growth, and distinguishes malignant from normal phenotype in three dimensional cultures and *in vivo*. Cancer Res 2006;66:1526–35.

206. Mimeault M, Johansson SL, Venkatraman G et al. Combined targeting of epidermal growth factor receptor and hedgehog signaling by gefitinib and cyclopamine cooperatively improves the cytotoxic effects of docetaxel on metastatic prostate cancer cells. Mol Cancer Ther 2007;6:967–78.

207. Mimeault M, Venkatraman G, Johansson SL et al. Novel combination therapy against metastatic and androgen-independent prostate cancer by using gefitinib, tamoxifen and etoposide. Int etoposide. Int etoposide. Int J Cancer 2007;120(1):160–169.

208. Mimeault M, Mehta PP, Hauke R et al. Improvement of cytotoxic effects of mitoxantrone on hormone-refractory metastatic prostate cancer cells by co-targeting epidermal growth factor receptor and hedgehog signaling cascades. Growth Factors 2007;25:400–16.

209. Chen JS, Pardo FS, Wang-Rodriguez J et al. EGFR regulates the side population in head and neck squamous cell carcinoma. Laryngoscope 2006;116:401–6.

210. Peacock CD, Wang Q, Gesell GS et al. Hedgehog signaling maintains a tumor stem cell compartment in multiple myeloma. Proc Natl Acad Sci USA 2007;104:4048–53.

211. Sims-Mourtada J, Izzo JG, Ajani J, Chao KS. Sonic Hedgehog promotes multiple drug resistance by regulation of drug transport. Oncogene 2007;26:5674–9.

212. Clement V, Sanchez P, de Tribolet N, Radovanovic I, Altaba A. HEDGEHOG-GLI1 signaling regulates human glioma growth, cancer stem cell self-renewal, and tumorigenicity. Curr Biol 2007;17:165–72.

213. Galmozzi E, Facchetti F, La Porta CA. Cancer stem cells and therapeutic perspectives. Curr Med Chem 2006; 13:603–7.

214. Wang J, Guo LP, Chen LZ, Zeng YX, Lu SH. Identification of cancer stem cell-like side population cells in human nasopharyngeal carcinoma cell line. Cancer Res 2007;67:3716–24.

215. Kang H, Watkins G, Douglas-Jones A, Mansel RE, Jiang WG. The elevated level of CXCR4 is correlated with nodal metastasis of human breast cancer. Breast 2005;14:360–7.

216. Rubin JB, Kung AL, Klein RS et al. A small-molecule antagonist of CXCR4 inhibits intracranial growth of primary brain tumors. Proc Natl Acad Sci USA 2003;100:13513–8.

217. Liang Z, Wu T, Lou H et al. Inhibition of breast cancer metastasis by selective synthetic polypeptide against CXCR4. Cancer Res 2004;64:4302–8.

218. Kulbe H, Levinson NR, Balkwill F, Wilson JL. The chemokine network in cancer–much more than directing cell movement. Int J Dev Biol 2004;48:489–96.

219. Balkwill F. Cancer and the chemokine network. Nat Rev Cancer 2004;4:540–50.

220. Hart CA, Brown M, Bagley S, Sharrard M, Clarke NW. Invasive characteristics of human prostatic epithelial cells: understanding the metastatic process. Br J Cancer 2005;92:503–12.

221. Engl T, Relja B, Marian D et al. CXCR4 chemokine receptor mediates prostate tumor cell adhesion through alpha5 and beta3 integrins. Neoplasia 2006;8:290–301.

222. Strizzi L, Bianco C, Normanno N, Salomon D. Cripto-1: a multifunctional modulator during embryogenesis and oncogenesis. Oncogene 2005;24:5731–41.

223. Hu XF, Xing PX. Cripto as a target for cancer immunotherapy. Expert Opin Ther Targets 2005;9:383–94.

224. Todaro M, Mileidys Perez Alea MP, Di Stefano AB et al. Colon cancer stem cells dictate tumor growth and resist cell death by production of interleukin-4. Cell Stem Cells 2007;1:389–402.

225. Sano T, Kagawa M, Okuno M et al. Prevention of rat hepatocarcinogenesis by acyclic retinoid is accompanied by reduction in emergence of both TGF-alpha-expressing oval-like cells and activated hepatic stellate cells. Nutr Cancer 2005;51:197–206.

226. Perabo FG, Muller SC. New agents for treatment of advanced transitional cell carcinoma. Ann Oncol 2007;18:1118.

227. Davidoff AM, Ng CY, Brown P et al. Bone marrow-derived cells contribute to tumor neovasculature and, when modified to express an angiogenesis inhibitor, can restrict tumor growth in mice. Clin Cancer Res 2001;7: 2870–9.

228. Rafii S, Lyden D. Contribution of hematopoietic and vascular progenitor cells to the neoangiogenic niche. Am Assoc Res Edu Book 2006;181–5.

229. Byrne AM, Bouchier-Hayes DJ, Harmey JH. Angiogenic and cell survival functions of vascular endothelial growth factor (VEGF). J Cell Mol Med 2005;9:777–94.

230. Moreira IS, Fernandes PA, Ramos MJ. Vascular endothelial growth factor (VEGF) inhibition–a critical review. Anticancer Agents Med Chem 2007;7:223–45.

231. Rosell R, Cecere F, Cognetti F et al. Future directions in the second-line treatment of non-small cell lung cancer. Semin Oncol 2006;33:S45–51.

232. Calabrese C, Poppleton H, Kocak M et al. A perivascular niche for brain tumor stem cells. Cancer Cell 2007; 11:69–82.

233. Folkins C, Man S, Xu P, Shaked Y, Hicklin DJ, Kerbel RS. Anticancer therapies combining antiangiogenic and tumor cell cytotoxic effects reduce the tumor stem-like cell fraction in glioma xenograft tumors. Cancer Res 2007; 67:3560–4.

234. Yang ZJ, Wechsler-Reya RJ. Hit 'em where they live: targeting the cancer stem cell niche. Cancer Cell 2007;11:3–5.

235. Sun SY, Hail N, Jr., Lotan R. Apoptosis as a novel target for cancer chemoprevention. J Natl Cancer Inst 2004; 96:662–72.

236. Miller JC, Sorensen AG. Imaging biomarkers predictive of disease/therapy outcome: ischemic stroke and drug development. Prog Drug Res 2005;62:319–56.

237. Arora A, Scholar EM. Role of tyrosine kinase inhibitors in cancer therapy. J Pharmacol Exp Ther 2005;315:971–9.

238. Zhong H, Bowen JP. Antiangiogenesis drug design: multiple pathways targeting tumor vasculature. Curr Med Chem 2006;13:849–62.

239. Meric JB, Rottey S, Olaussen K et al. Cyclooxygenase-2 as a target for anticancer drug development. Crit Rev Oncol Hematol 2006;59:51–64.

240. Aggarwal BB, Shishodia S, Sandur SK, Pandey MK, Sethi G. Inflammation and cancer: How hot is the link? Biochem Pharmacol 2006;72:1605–21.

241. Kobayashi H, Lin PC. Antiangiogenic and radiotherapy for cancer treatment. Histol Histopathol 2006;21:1125–34.

242. Grosch S, Maier TJ, Schiffmann S, Geisslinger G. Cyclooxygenase-2 (COX-2)-independent anticarcinogenic effects of selective COX-2 inhibitors. J Natl Cancer Inst 2006;98:736–47.

243. Cairns R, Papandreou I, Denko N. Overcoming physiologic barriers to cancer treatment by molecularly targeting the tumor microenvironment. Mol Cancer Res 2006;4:61–70.

244. Lu H, Ouyang W, Huang C. Inflammation, a Key Event in Cancer Development. Mol Cancer Res 2006;4:221–33.

245. Lyden D, Hattori K, Dias S et al. Impaired recruitment of bone-marrow-derived endothelial and hematopoietic precursor cells blocks tumor angiogenesis and growth. Nat Med 2001;7:1194–201.

246. Vosseler S, Mirancea N, Bohlen P, Mueller MM, Fusenig NE. Angiogenesis inhibition by vascular endothelial growth factor receptor-2 blockade reduces stromal matrix metalloproteinase expression, normalizes stromal tissue, and reverts epithelial tumor phenotype in surface heterotransplants. Cancer Res 2005;65:1294–305.

247. van Beijnum J, Dings RP, van der LE et al. Gene expression of tumor angiogenesis dissected; specific targeting of colon cancer angiogenic vasculature. Blood 2006;108:2339–48.

24

Therapeutic Index and the Cancer Stem Cell Paradigm

Vera S. Donnenberg and Albert D. Donnenberg

ABSTRACT

The therapeutic index of antineoplastic therapies has traditionally been driven by the concepts of maximally tolerated dose and treatment response. When the tumor is viewed as homogeneous with respect to response, and response is defined by tumor regression, there are many effective antineoplastic regimens. However, the persistent problem of cancer recurrence in the face of apparently successful therapy, and the recognition that tumors are at least as heterogeneous as normal tissue, necessitates a reevaluation of the concept of therapeutic index from the standpoint of the most therapy resistant cells within the tumor vs. the maximal disruption that critical tissues can withstand. The cancer stem cell paradigm helps explain some of the heterogeneity within tumors and posits that therapy resistance originates with the strategies by which normal tissue stem cells protect themselves from toxic insults. The recognition that at any given time, self-renewing (tumorigenic) tumor cells are protected by mechanisms, such as multiple drug resistance (MDR) transporters, detoxifying enzymes, a resting state, and niche effects, ensures that a proportion of tumor cells will have toxicity profiles similar to normal tissue stem cells. The problem of therapeutic index is compounded by the fact that clonogenic cancer cells have merely to survive and reactivate to perpetuate the neoplasm, whereas vital organ functions cannot be compromised for long without lethal consequences. In this chapter, we review the evolving concepts of therapeutic index, maximal tolerated dose, and tumor heterogeneity in the context of the cancer stem cell paradigm. Primary clinical isolates are used to provide examples of heterogeneity within the tumorigenic compartment, within cells that resist therapy, and within cells protected by MDR transporters.

Key Words: Cancer stem cells, Multiple drug resistance transporters (MDR), Therapeutic index, Maximal tolerated dose, Lung cancer, Breast cancer, Flow cytometry, CD90, CD117, CD133, Side population (SP), Minimal residual disease (MRD)

INTRODUCTION

Complete Response Defined: According to the NCI Dictionary of Cancer Terms, a complete response (also called a complete remission) is *"the disappearance of all signs of cancer in response to treatment. This does not always mean the cancer has been cured."* This practical definition has proven useful for evaluating and comparing therapeutic regimens. However, it has wreaked havoc with the notion of therapeutic index, in the sense in which it is used in nononcologic applications.

From: *Cancer Drug Discovery and Development: Stem Cells and Cancer,*
Edited by: R.G. Bagley and B.A. Teicher, DOI: 10.1007/978-1-60327-933-8_24,
© Humana Press, a part of Springer Science+Business Media, LLC 2009

Therapeutic index is conventionally defined as the Lethal Dose$_{50}$ divided by the Effective Dose$_{50}$, and by the effectiveness criterion of *Complete Response*, the antineoplastic armamentarium is filled with agents and regimens with high therapeutic indices. The cancer stem cell paradigm provides a useful way to frame a hypothesis explaining why these therapies have largely proven inefficacious in the long run.

Therapeutic Index and Acute Dose Limiting Toxicity: Defining the therapeutic index of anti-cancer agents as the ratio of the toxicity to tumor vs. normal tissue regeneration and maintenance is not a new idea. The pioneers of bone marrow transplantation, E. Donnall Thomas *(1)*, George W. Santos *(2)*, and George Mathé *(3)* capitalized on the observation that bone marrow rescue after radio-chemotherapy permitted significant dose intensification, implicitly recognizing that cancer therapy must balance tumor kill against normal tissue repair. To this day, the majority of preparative regimens used in hematopoietic stem cell transplantation are myeloablative, meaning that they destroy the regenerative capacity of bone marrow. The earliest studies of radiation sensitivity revealed that hematopoietic stem cells are among the most sensitive in the body *(4)*. It is the differential sensitivity of hematopoietic vs. other tissue stem cells that makes dose intensive therapy followed by hematopoietic stem cell rescue possible. The dose limiting toxicity in the setting of hematopoietic stem cell transplantation is defined by the thresholds of irreversible skin, gut, and liver damage.

In the setting of autologous stem cell rescue after high dose therapy, the best risk acute myelocytic leukemia (AML) patients have an 81% probability of 12-year disease-free survival *(5)*, indicating that the most resistant leukemia cells are more sensitive to conventional therapeutic agents than nonhematopoietic tissue stem cells.

In epithelial and other nonhematopoietic tumors, there is no analogous strategy to rescue tissue irreversibly damaged by therapy. Further, therapeutic index pits retention of vital organ function against mere survival of clonogenic tumor cells. This concept is illustrated in Fig. 1, in which the most therapy resistant cells within a tumor are shown as being somewhat more sensitive to a hypothetical

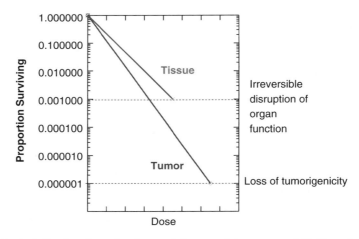

Fig. 1. Therapeutic Index is defined as the ratio of normal tissue toxicity to tumor kill. Hypothetical antineoplastic dose response curves are given for normal tissue stem cells (Tissue), and the most therapy resistant cells within an epithelial tumor (Tumor). The *dashed lines* indicate 3 and 6 logs of kill. Making the conservative assumptions that: (1) The most resistant cells within a tumor are at least as therapy-sensitive as tissue stem cells (here they are shown as slightly more sensitive), (2) normal tissue function will be irreversibly disrupted at a dose that destroys 99.9% of stem cells (*dashed line*), (3) tumor eradication requires at least 6 logs of kill of the most resistant cell, it follows that there can be no dose of a nonselective agent, which spares normal tissue function and eradicates tumor.

therapy than the corresponding tissue stem cells. Even so, organ function is depicted as irreversibly disrupted when 99.9% of the tissue stem cells have been killed, whereas loss of tumorigenicity hypothetically requires 6 logs of kill of the most therapy resistant cells.

The Temporal Component of Therapeutic Index: A damaged organ such as liver, skin, or gut has a finite amount of time to regenerate function before life threatening complications ensue. In contrast, surviving tumor cells have the patient's lifetime in which to reestablish whatever genetic, epigenetic, or niche effects are required for reactivation of their invasive phenotype. Dingli and Michor took bone marrow toxicity into account in their model of the kinetics of tumor reactivation after cessation of therapy, concluding that successful therapy requires the eradication of stem-like cells within the tumor *(6)*. It is worth noting that patients receiving dose-intensive therapy and allogeneic hematopoietic stem cell rescue occasionally have spontaneous autologous bone marrow recovery *(7)*. It is only the intensive supportive care (including the allograft) following transplant that permitted the bone marrow to recover from what would have been a lethal bone marrow insult. This emphasizes the point that the maximal tolerated dose is exceeded when the function of a vital organ is disrupted for a critical time period, and this does not necessarily require the death of every last stem cell.

Maximum tolerated dose: Conventionally, dose limiting toxicity is considered in an acute setting as the highest dose of anti-neoplastic therapy that can be tolerated before vital organ function is seriously compromised. Maximally tolerated drug doses, alone and in combination, are defined in phase I clinical trials, and regimens are specifically designed to minimize such acute toxicities. The principle of combining therapeutic agents in a way that maximizes the delivered dose of each agent and avoids synergistic toxicities has been termed summation dose intensity *(8)*. However, this approach does not take into account long-term effects of anti-neoplastic regimens on the capacity for organ maintenance and regeneration, functions mediated by tissue stem cells and their progeny. Long-term manifestations such as cardiotoxicity may take years to manifest, as demonstrated by long-term studies of causes of death in long-term survivors of pediatric cancers *(9)*. In general, therapy related adverse events are difficult to capture *(10)*, difficult to relate to specific interventions, and more difficult still to ascribe to specific mechanisms, such as compromise of the tissue stem cell compartment.

Regenerative Responses to Anti-Neoplastic Therapy and Cancer Relapse: Another factor that may influence the therapeutic index of anti-neoplastic therapy is the possibility that therapy induced damage, and the tissue repair that ensues, may create a more favorable environment for survival of persistent tumor cells. Inflammation shares a number of central mediators and pathways with tumor growth and invasiveness *(11)*. In particular, the proinflammatory cytokine IL-18 has been proposed to play a role in cancer metastasis and angiogenesis *(12)*.

Progenitor vs. Stem Cell Toxicity: Examining the difference between myelosuppressive and myeloablative chemotherapeutic regimens highlights the important distinction between progenitor and stem cell toxicity. Many antineoplastic agents are myelosuppressive at conventional doses. The attendant cytopenias are transient and red cell, granulocyte, and platelet counts rebound upon cessation of therapy. In these scenarios, anemia occurs not because of toxicity to mature anucleate erythrocytes, but because the mitotically active erythroid progenitors are selectively targeted. Recovery from these symptoms is mediated by more primitive hematopoietic stem cells, which give rise to erythroid progenitors on demand. In contrast, myeloablative therapy overcomes the mechanisms that protect hematopoietic stem cells, resulting in irreversible bone marrow aplasia, requiring stem cell rescue. It is worth reinforcing that irreversible hematopoietic stem cell toxicity occurs at doses that only transiently damage skin and gut. Progenitor toxicity is also dramatically demonstrated in the case of chemotherapy induced alopecia, which occurs with many agents that only transiently affect the bone marrow. Alopecia results from toxicity to hair follicle progenitor cells

(13), but their stem cells, which have been well characterized and reside in a niche within the follicle bulge *(14)*, are highly protected and regenerate the progenitor population upon discontinuation of therapy.

Taken together, the therapeutic index of anticancer agents must consider the differential toxicity to the most sensitive of the normal tissue stem cells vs. the most resistant clonogenic tumor cells, as well as the temporal constraints on normal tissue regeneration. Normal tissue must not be damaged such that vital functions are acutely disrupted, or can their regenerative capacity be irreversibly compromised in the longer term. In contrast, tumor recurrence requires only persistence of clonogenic cells, and if they persist in a dormant state, appropriate conditions for their reactivation. Tumor dormancy is well documented but poorly understood. It has been attributed to a variety of niche effects including maintenance of G0/G1state, protection from immune surveillance, as well as expression of multiple drug resistance transporters *(15)*. Activation from the dormant state may accordingly result from changes in the niche, including signals associated with normal tissue repair.

TUMOR HETEROGENEITY AND THE IDENTIFICATION OF TUMOR STEM CELL SUBSETS

Although it is clear that in many epithelial cancers, the majority of tumor cells are not tumorigenic, Kern and Shibata's analysis of the literature *(16)* suggests more than one, and perhaps many distinct tumorigenic subpopulations coexist within a tumor. According to these authors, this dilemma may result from markers used to define the subpopulations, where some markers, such as CD44 *(17–19)*, are "promiscuously expressed outside the definable stem populations," whereas others are "too restricted, failing to mark all of the stem-like cells" (e.g., side population, CD133) so that cells outside the stem cell fraction are also tumorigenic *(20–23)*.

Our own experience leads us to believe that *tumorigenicity* (as opposed to therapy resistance) and tumor *stemness* have little in common, save the requirement for self-renewal. In an experiment in which we provisionally defined tumor stem cells isolated from breast cancer malignant effusions as CD45– CD44+ CD90+ ABCG2+ with small resting morphology (low forward and side light scatter), and tumor progenitor cells as CD45– CD44+ CD90+ ABCG2– with complex light scatter comparable to the bulk of the tumor, we found that both subsets were tumorigenic and serially transplantable *(24)*. Further, we were surprised to find that tumors derived from the high light scatter ABCG2– "progenitor" fraction gave rise to substantial numbers of low light scatter CD90+ ABCG2+ resting tumor "stem" cells (Fig. 2). In fact, CD45–/CD44+/ABCG2+ cells were more numerous in the tumor xenograft (4%) than in the original pleural effusion (1.5%).

Although this may have been due to "contamination" of the progenitor fraction with "stem" cells, we find this unlikely, since the progenitor cells were 228-fold more numerous than the stem cells and very well separated in multiparameter space. The more likely interpretation is that there is a bidirectional relationship between tumor "stem" and "progenitor" cells that is contrary to a rigid hierarchal model of normal tissue differentiation, but consistent with more recent observations that conditionally differentiated cells in normal airway *(25)*, liver *(26)*, and pancreas *(27)* can assume a self-renewing phenotype after injury.

Taken together, it seems unlikely that any one phenotypically defined subset will encompass all tumorigenic cells to the exclusion of all nontumorigenic cells in all tumors. Phenotype, defined by a handful of markers, is a moving target among genetically unstable cells of unpredictable plasticity. This by no means excludes the possibility that functionally important proteins, such as adherence/signaling molecules (CD44, CXCR4, CD90), growth factor receptors (CD117), and other stem/pro-

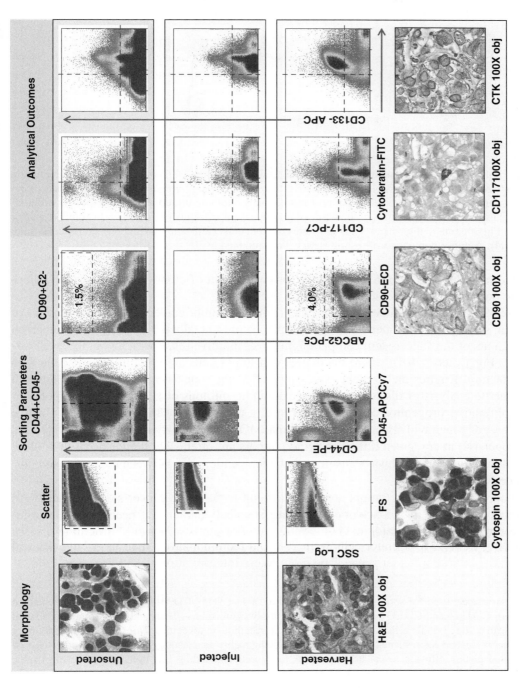

Fig. 2. Implantation of high light scatter/CD45−/CD44+/CD90+/ABCG2− cells sorted from a breast cancer pleural effusion gives rise to a heterogeneous tumor. 13,200 sorted cells were admixed with 10,000 heavily irradiated (10,000 cGy) CD45− tumor cells suspended in matrigel. The cells were injected subcutaneously into the mammary fatpad of NOD/SCID mice. Tumor was harvested 204 days after injection, disaggregated, and stained for flow cytometry. Immunohistochemical staining for human specific CD90, CD117, and pancytokeratin was performed on the tumor xenograft. *First row*, Unsorted freshly isolated pleural effusion (*left to right*): A Wright-Giemsa stained cytocentrifuge preparation immediately prior to sorting; gating on forward vs. side light scatter and CD45 vs. CD44. ABCG2+ cells (dashed box) comprised 1.5% of CD45−/CD44+ cells. Analytical outcomes within the light scatter, CD45−/CD44+ gate: Distinct patterns of the stem/progenitor markers CD117 and CD133 vs. the epithelial differentiation marker cytokeratin are seen. *Second row*, Injected (sorted) tumor cells (*left to right*): Logical gating

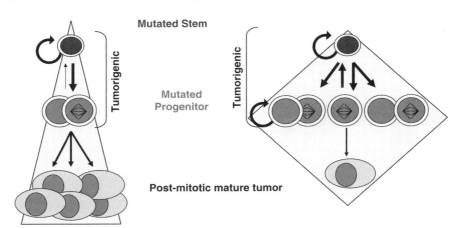

Fig. 3. Maturation profiles of low grade and high grade tumors. Low grade tumors (*left panel*) follow a differentiation pathway more closely related to normal regenerating tissue. Resting self-renewing (*circular arrow*) stem cells are rare, proliferating progenitor cells are more prevalent, but post mitotic cells retaining discernable tissue specific differentiation markers and some histological features of the tissue of origin make up the bulk of the tumor. In contrast, a large proportion of cells in high grade malignancies share attributes of stem cells (self-renewal) and progenitor cells (high proliferative potential). A minor population of resting stem cells is retained.

genitor associated markers (CD133) may be useful for enrichment of clonogenic tumor cells, diagnostic/prognostic purposes, or drug discovery.

Histologic Tumor Grade and Therapeutic Index: Depending on tumor grade, architectural features of the tissue of origin, such as ducts in adenocarcinomas, may be present, albeit in a disorganized manner. Current interpretations of the cancer stem cell paradigm make intuitive sense with low grade, well differentiated tumors Fig. 3, left panel), where the majority of tumor cells are nontumorigenic cells with discernable architectural features and protein expression reflecting their tissue of origin *(28)*. In such cases, flow cytometric analysis of dissociated tumor examining millions of cells reveals a minor subpopulation of proliferating progenitor cells and, rarer still, a population of stem cell marker positive resting cells, a subset of which will also express constitutive MDR and detoxifying enzyme activity (e.g., aldehyde dehydrogenase) at any given time. Low grade tumors are often slow growing, but their close relation to normal differentiation pathways ensures a low therapeutic index between the tumor and normal tissue stem cells.

High grade, poorly differentiated tumors are more difficult to fit to the cancer stem cell paradigm (Fig. 3, right panel). In fact, the abundance of cells bearing stem cell markers has been used as an argument against the cancer stem cell paradigm *(16)*. The tissue of origin is sometimes difficult to discern and the majority of cells express both the proliferative capacity of progenitor cells and the self-renewal

---

Fig. 2. (continued) parameters used for sorting (high light scatter, CD44+/CD45–/CD90+). The sorted cells contained distinct populations of CD117+ and CD133+ cells and were uniformly cytokeratin+. These data are from an analytical tube run in parallel with sorting (viable cells cannot be stained for intracellular cytokeratin). *Third row*, Xenograft tumor (*left to right*): A hematoxylin and eosin stained paraffin section showing highly anaplastic cells; superimposed gates used for sorting the original pleural effusion reveal heterogeneous light scatter including low light scatter (resting) cells, CD44- cells and ABCG2+ (4%) cells not present in the sorted injected fraction. The tumor xenograft has rare CD117+ cells, and virtually all cytokeratin dim cells are CD133+. Fourth row, Tumor xenograft histology (*left to right*): A cytocentrifuge preparation of disaggregated tumor xenograft cells immediately prior to staining. Immunohistochemical staining of tumor xenograft paraffin sections confirm abundant expression of CD90, rare isolated CD117+ cells and abundant cytokeratin staining.

of the stem cell. Whether these proliferating cells retain or have acquired the self-protective mechanisms of the tissue stem cell will determine whether there is a low therapeutic index (as in many poorly differentiated carcinomas) or high therapeutic index (as some high grade lymphomas).

Tumor Heterogeneity, Intrinsic Drug Resistance, and Selection: Cancer is ultimately a disease of dysregulation of proliferation, differentiation, and programmed cell death, resulting from initial mutations and proceeding to epigenetic changes, genetic instability and selection of favorable clones for outgrowth. The common threads are the multiple pathways leading to growth dysregulation and metastasis. The tissue characteristics and heterogeneity that tumors express during their evolution from a local primary lesion to a lethal disseminated mass consist of traits that are essential for the invasive, growth-dysregulated phenotype, those that are merely helpful, and those which are passenger traits, secondary to these genetic and epigenetic changes. Superimposed on the natural history of the temporal and spatial evolution of the tumor is therapy-driven selection imposed directly on the tumor, and indirectly by alteration of its supporting niche. As occurs in the initial selective process for growth independence, selection for traits conferring therapy resistance in the face of genetic and epigenetic instability may be accompanied by the expression of traits irrelevant to the pathologic process. Taken together, we are faced with enormous phenotypic heterogeneity, both within tumors and between patients. Without specific loss and gain of function studies, one can only speculate on the significance of a particular trait, such as the expression of a particular stem/progenitor or differentiation marker.

The most important contribution of the cancer stem cell paradigm is the recognition that traits retained from normal tissue stem cells or acquired as the result of mutation guarantee that a proportion of tumor cells will be intrinsically at least as therapy resistant as their normal tissue counterparts. The selective pressure of chemotherapy may further promote the outgrowth of cells with improved resistance, but the key factors initially mediating therapy resistance are: *(1)* intrinsic expression of MDR transporters identical to that of the native tissue; *(2)* intrinsic activity of detoxifying enzymes (aldehyde dehydrogenase) indistinguishable to that of normal tissue stem cells; (3) a resting state, which renders cells resistant to agents dependent on DNA synthesis or high metabolic activity; (4) lack of differentiation markers such as receptors (ER/PR, EGFR, VEGFR) and tissue specific signaling proteins (tyrosine kinase), which constitute targets of therapy in more mature tumor cells; and (5) resistance to apoptosis mediated by interaction of surface receptors in the tumor niche.

In normal tissues self-renewal and self-protection by the mechanisms outlined above coexist in tissue stem cell. It should be stressed that this is not necessarily the case in tumors, which have been likened to caricatures of the process of tissues renewal *(29)*. It is trivially true that the tumorgenicity of a particular cell within a tumor requires self-renewal, in the sense that some daughter cells must retain the proliferative potential of the parent. However, if tumor *stemness* is to be used in a meaningful and useful way, it must also refer to those protective properties, which permit a subset of tumorigenic cells to survive therapy. This complicates a neat division between tumor cells into stem and nonstem, since protective traits, such as MDR transporter activity are only conditionally active, with ABCG2− tumor cells giving rise to ABCG2+ cells (Fig. 2) and vice versa in the absence of drug selection.

MULTIPLE DRUG RESISTANCE TRANSPORTERS
AND CANCER STEM CELLS: TWO EXAMPLES

MDR Transporter Activity is not Limited to Cells Expressing Stem/Progenitor Markers in Newly Diagnosed Untreated NSC Lung Cancer. The ability to cotransport R123 and Ho33342 has been proposed as a marker for the most primitive hematopoietic stem cells *(30)*. We hypothesize that the most drug resistant tumor cells share this activity. Primary tumors are heterogeneous with respect to expression of tissue differentiation and stem/progenitor markers. To assess the association of MDR transporter activity with differentiation, we stained a freshly isolated therapy naïve disaggregated lung tumor with the stem/progenitor marker CD90, the epithelial differentiation marker EpCAM, and simultaneously measured transport of the ABCB1 and ABCG2 substrate dyes rhodamine 123 (R123) and Hoechst 33342 (Ho). CD90 is expressed on thymocytes and primitive bone marrow progenitor cells but is also present on stem/progenitor cells in a variety of nonhematopoietic tissues. This GPI anchored glycoprotein is involved in integrin-mediated cell–cell and cell–matrix interactions *(31)* and is thought to regulate survival/apoptosis. EpCAM (CD326), an epithelial-specific adhesion molecule involved in cell environment interactions, is prominently expressed in many epithelial carcinomas. Anti-CD45 was used to eliminate hematopoietic cells, and propidium iodide (PI) was used to exclude dye permeant (dead) cells.

In this particular tumor, CD90 was the most prevalent of the stem/progenitor markers (48% of nonhematopoietic cells), with CD117+ cells representing 4.8% and CD133+ cells comprising 4.5% (not shown). Figure 4 shows MDR activity as a function of CD90 and EpCAM expression. The

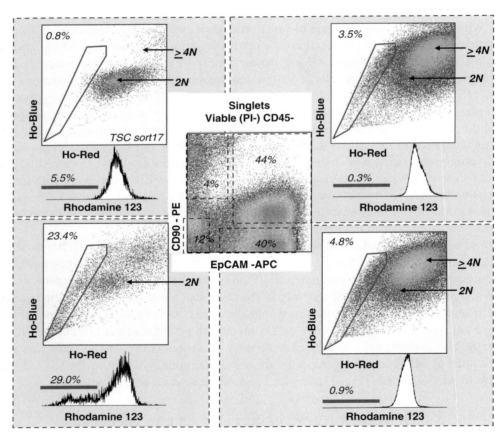

Fig. 4. Multiple drug resistance transporter activity is not limited to cells expressing stem/progenitor markers in newly diagnosed untreated nonsmall cell lung cancer. The central histogram shows four populations based on the expression of the epithelial differentiation marker EpCAM, and the stem/progenitor marker CD90 within nonhematopoietic tumor cells. Adjacent to each corner of the central histogram are a two-parameter histogram showing Hoechst 33342 fluorescence, and a one-parameter histogram showing rhodamine 123 fluorescence within each EpCAM/CD90 subpopulation.

EpCAM− CD90− population (12%) had the greatest transport of both Ho (23.4%) and R123 (29%). The epithelial stem candidate (here CD90+/EpCAM− because of relative insensitivity to APC detection, cf. Figs. 6 and 7) has virtually no Ho transporter activity and little R123 transport, whereas the epithelial progenitor (EpCAM+/CD90+) and mature populations (EpCAM+/CD90−) have a small subpopulation (3.5–4.8%), which transport Ho but not R123. The other interesting feature that these data reveal is that in cells without MDR activity, Ho can be used to estimate DNA content. The EpCAM negative and dim populations are largely diploid (2N, G0/G1), whereas endothelial progenitor and mature cells have greater DNA content (≥4N, aneuploid or cycling).

Figure 5 shows the light scatter properties of the nonhematopoietic cells, which transport both Ho and R123 (color evented red). Low light scatter cells (small cells of simple morphology) comprise only 3.1% of the total nonhematopoietic tumor population, but small cells increase in frequency with MDR transporter activity: 10.9% of the Ho transporting cells are small, compared with 33.3% of R123 transporting cells, and 68.6% of cells which cotransport both dyes. The majority of cotransporting cells (57.3%) are the least differentiated cells within the tumor (EpCAM−/CD90−), followed by EpCAM+/CD90− (mature cells, 32.1%), and EpCAM−/CD90+ (stem candidate, 8.5%).

It is uncertain whether EpCAM−/MDR+ cells are resting tumor cells or normal tissue progenitor cells recruited into the tumor, although their predominantly resting diploid state suggests the former (Fig. 4). The EpCAM negative or dim CD90+ epithelial stem cell candidate, also a resting diploid cell, was devoid of constitutive Ho transporting activity, whereas progenitor and mature tumor populations had moderate Ho transport capacity and minimal R123 transport. R123 is thought to be transported chiefly by ABCB1 (P-glycoprotein) (32), whereas ablation of Ho transport requires knockout of both ABCB1 and ABCG2 (33). Taken together, this example of a newly diagnosed untreated epithelial malignancy indicates the difficulties in defining stem and progenitor cells (and even distinguishing between bona fide tumor cells and reactive cells) within a very heterogeneous tumor on the basis of MDR activity. It also illustrates that significant MDR activity preexists in lung tumors before the initiation of therapy. The bottom line, as far as therapeutic index is concerned, is not which cells

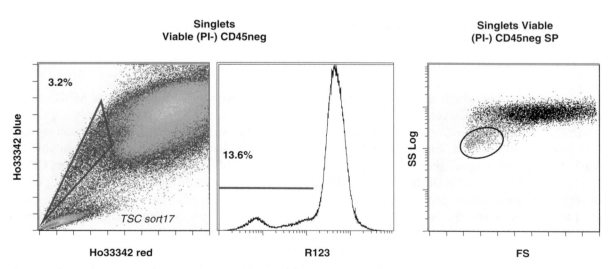

Fig. 5. Light scatter properties of cells co-transporting Hoechst 33342 (Ho) and rhodamine 123 (R123). From *left to right*: The Ho transporting *side population* (3.2%) is visualized within nonhematopoietic tumor cells as Ho dim events with greater blue than red fluorescence intensity. R123 transporting cells comprised 13.6% of nonhematopoietic tumor cells. Cells cotransporting both dyes (color-evented red) represented 0.43% of nonhematopoietic tumor cells; most (68.6%) had low light scatter properties consistent with small resting cells.

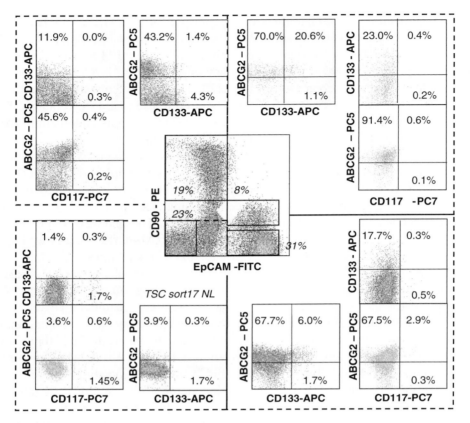

Fig. 6. Expression of ABCG2 and stem/progenitor markers on tumor cells subsetted on the basis of EpCAM and CD90 expression in normal lung tissue. The sample was obtained from grossly normal tissue from a lung lobe resected for NSC lung cancer. The central histogram shows four populations based on the expression of the epithelial differentiation marker EpCAM, and the stem/progenitor marker CD90 within nonhematopoietic normal lung cells. Adjacent to each corner of the central histogram are three additional histograms showing coexpression of CD117, ABCG2, and CD133 within each EpCAM/CD90 subpopulation.

are tumorigenic, but which cells are both tumorigenic and express properties (such as MDR) which render them therapy resistant.

ABCG2 Expression in Untreated NSC Lung Carcinoma and Normal Lung. Lung resection is often first line therapy for NSC lung cancer. Untreated tumor and adjacent normal lung are available for study, facilitating comparison. Figure 6 shows the coexpression of the stem/progenitor markers CD90, CD117, and CD133, the MDR transporter ABCG2, and the epithelial differentiation antigen EpCAM in single cell suspensions prepared from disaggregated normal lung adjacent to the tumor (the same sample as Figs. 4 and 5). Nonhematopoietic single cells with DNA content ≥ 2N were identified according to a gating strategy that will be described in Fig. 8.

Nonhematopoietic cells were classified by expression of EpCAM and CD90. The remaining markers were then analyzed as outcomes on the four nonoverlapping EpCAM vs. CD90 populations. It should be noted that the normal lung preparation results from dissociation of a complex tissue with airway, vascular, and alveolar components, and is subject to artifacts due to selective recovery during tissue digestion. EpCAM and CD90 classifiers reveal several discrete populations (Fig. 6) also present in the tumor (Fig. 7). These include EpCAM-/CD90–, EpCAM^{dim}/CD90^{bright}, EPCAM^{bright}/CD90^{dim},

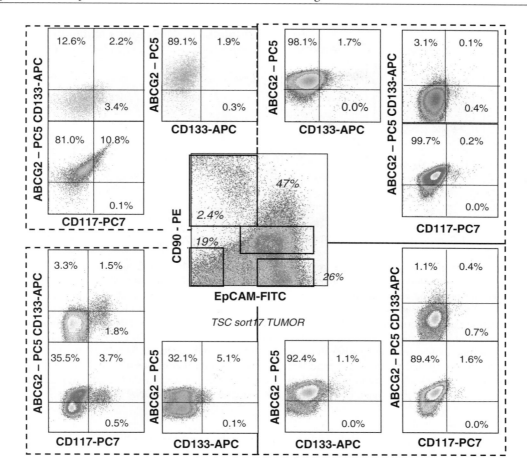

Fig. 7. Expression of ABCG2 and stem/progenitor markers on tumor cells subsetted on the basis of EpCAM and CD90 expression in a previously untreated, newly diagnosed NSC lung cancer. The tumor was obtained from the same resected lobe as the normal tissue shown in Fig. 6. The histogram layout is identical to that of Fig. 6.

and EpCAM^{bright}/CD90– populations (note that EpCAM^{dim} cells were resolved with the FITC conjugate). The EpCAM– (nonepithelial or undifferentiated) CD90– population is ABCG2–/CD133– with a small population of CD117+ cells (2%). The EpCAM^{dim}/CD90^{bright} population (epithelial stem cell candidate) is CD117–/CD133–, and contains a significant subpopulation (46%) of ABCG2+ cells. The EpCAM^{bright}/CD90^{dim} cells (progenitor candidate) are uniformly CD117–/ABCG2+ (92%), and have a subpopulation coexpressing CD133 (23%), a phenotype shared by EpCAM^{bright}/CD90– cells (mature epithelium). These results indicate that ABCG2 is highly expressed in normal airway epithelial cells and suggest that it is activated during the stem stage and amplified at the progenitor stage. CD133 marks a subset of epithelial committed progenitor cells, and CD117 is not normally expressed in the airway epithelium.

In the tumor digest (Fig. 7), the EpCAM^{bright}/CD90^{dim} population predominates (47%), but the other populations highlighted in normal lung are also present. Unlike normal lung, the EpCAM– (nonepithelial or undifferentiated) CD90– population is ABCG2+ (39%), with significant subpopulations of CD133+ (4.8%) and CD117+ (4.2%) cells. The EpCAM^{dim}/CD90^{bright} population (epithelial stem cell candidate) is strongly ABCG2+ (92%) and contains a subpopulation of CD117+ (6%). The EpCAM^{bright}/

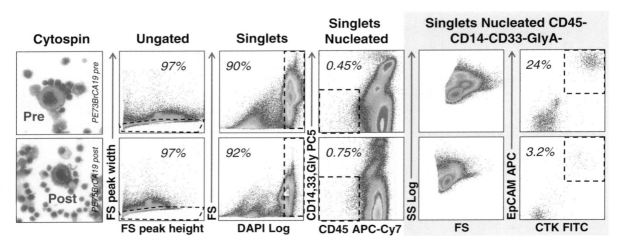

Fig. 8. Gating strategy for analysis of tumor cell survival after therapy. Pleural Effusions were collected from a patient with previously untreated metastatic breast cancer before (*top panels*) and nine weeks after therapy (*bottom panels*) with the antiproliferative nucleotide analog capecitabine. From *left to right*: Cytocentrifuge preparations (Wright Giemsa) shows preferential survival of lymphoid cells; forward light scatter pulse analysis is used to identify singlets (eliminating cell clusters); noncellular debris and apoptotic cells with <2N DNA are eliminated by DAPI staining; CD45− (nonhematopoietic) cells are identified (note relative enrichment of nonhematopoietic cells and loss of CD33+ polymorphonuclear leukocytes after therapy); loss of high light scatter cells reflects the loss of polymorphonuclear leukocytes, activated macrophages, and large tumor cells after therapy, as well as preferential survival of small cells (low light scatter); Cytokeratin positive, EpCAM positive cells are reduced but not eliminated after therapy. Subsequent analyses (Fig. 9) are gated on CD45 negative singlets with ≥ 2N DNA.

CD90^{dim} (progenitor candidate) and EpCAM^{bright}/CD90− cells (mature epithelium) cells are uniformly ABCG2+, and have small subpopulations expressing CD117 (0.5%) or CD133 (3.2%).

Compared with normal lung, the tumor is remarkable for high ABCG2 and moderate CD117 expression among the EpCAM− population, high ABCG2 and CD117 expression among the EpCAM^{dim}/CD90^{bright} population, and overrepresentation of the EpCAM^{bright}/CD90^{dim} population. Another important finding is that MDR expression and MDR constitutive activity (Fig. 4) in the same tumor sample are strikingly discordant, emphasizing that MDR transport is inducible, and the presence of an MDR transporter in the membrane does not indicate that it is constitutively active. These results also support the interpretation that MDR activity or expression by itself can not be used as a surrogate stem/progenitor marker in the lung because it is also present in differentiated tissue. This is not to say that it is absent in stem cells (cancer or otherwise), or to negate its importance in therapy resistance.

Identity of Metastatic Breast Cancer Cells which Survive Therapy: A Case Report. The median survival of breast cancer patients after developing a malignant pleural effusion is 7–8 months *(34)*, with virtually no patients achieving durable remission. The ability to monitor malignant pleural effusion cells before and after therapy can provide a detailed snapshot of the cells that survive therapy. The patient, a 56-year-old female diagnosed with ER− PR− Her2− invasive lobular breast carcinoma presented with a malignant pleural effusion 2 months after initial diagnosis. She was treated with Xeloda® (capecitabine), a prodrug converted to the active thymidine analog 5-fluorouracil by intracellular thymidine phosphorylase. Pleural effusion samples were obtained before and 9 weeks after initiation of treatment. Prior to treatment the effusion consisted chiefly of a mononuclear cell infiltrate, with 0.5% nonhematopoietic cells, 24% of which were cytokeratin and EpCAM positive (Fig. 8, top row). Fifty-nine percent of cytokeratin+ cells had >2N DNA (Fig. 9), indicating a significant proportion of aneuploid or proliferating tumor cells. Among the cytokeratin+ cells, 85% expressed the adhesion molecule CD44, and 12% were positive for the multiple drug resistance transporter ABCG2. CD117

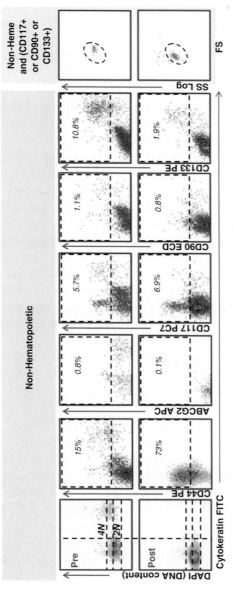

Fig. 9. Survival of CD44+ and CD117+ small cells after therapy. Pleural effusion cells collected before (*top panels*) and after therapy (*bottom panels*) were gated as described in Fig. 8. From *left to right*: DNA content vs. cytokeratin shows the loss of cytokeratin+ cycling cells after therapy. Although CD44+/cytokeratin+ cells are entirely abrogated, 73% of nonhematopoietic cells surviving therapy were CD44+/cytokeratin negative; ABCG2 expression was not prominent in surviving cells; the proportion of CD117+ and CD90+ cells did not change after therapy, but the majority of CD133+ cells were eliminated; surviving cells bearing either CD117, CD90, or CD133 were CD44+ (80%, not shown) and had homogenous low light scatter and 2N DNA content, consistent with small, resting morphology. The *dashed elliptical* region shown in the rightmost panels was set to include 85% of CD45[bright] (lymphoid) cells in the pretreatment sample.

expression was most prominent in cytokeratin negative nonhematopoietic cells, whereas CD90+ cells comprised a small proportion of cytokeratin positive and negative cells, and CD133 was expressed almost exclusively on cytokeratin positive tumor cells. The morphology of cells expressing either CD117, CD90, or CD133, as reflected in light scatter characteristics, was comparable to resting lymphoid cells.

Following therapy, there was a dramatic loss of high light scatter cells (Fig. 8), which included granulocytes, activated macrophages, and large tumor cells. Although the proportion of nonhematopoietic cells nearly doubled, cytokeratin+/EpCAM+ cells declined by almost an order of magnitude (24–3.2%). The majority (97%) of nonhematopoietic cells had 2N DNA (Fig. 9), consistent with abrogation of proliferation, but 27% of the few remaining cytokeratin+ cells had >2N DNA.

The results of this case study illustrate how the most dramatic changes following antimitotic chemotherapy occur in the hematopoietic compartment, with dramatic ablation of the most reactive cells. Among tumor cells, the most mature fraction (EpCAM+/cytokeratin+) was most visibly depleted, including the CD44+ subset. The majority of nonhematopoietic cells remaining after treatment were cytokeratin–/EpCAM–/CD44+, suggesting that CD44 plays an important role in tumor cell survival, but does not unambiguously mark the therapy resistant tumorigenic cell. ABGG2+, CD117+, and CD90+ tumor cells survived in approximately the same proportion as were present before therapy. CD133+ cells were reduced fivefold, but surviving CD133+ cells marked the few surviving cytokeratin+ cells. The light scatter of cells expressing either CD90, CD117, or CD133 (alone or in combination) remained within a lymphoid pattern, indicating small size and low morphologic complexity. Taken together, in the case reported here, mature tumor cells and activated hematopoietic cells comprised the majority of cells eliminated by therapy, whereas stem/progenitor marker bearing cells remained detectable. The fact that such treatment is considered palliative, with a high probability of tumor recurrence, suggests that the tumorigenic, therapy resistant, recurrence-initiating cells are within the population of surviving tumor cells detected here.

Targeting MRD not MDR: Considering the parameters that comprise therapeutic index for antineoplastic therapy, we are struck by the similarities between the protective mechanisms naturally expressed in normal tissue stem cells and those retained or acquired by tumor cell subsets, which are sometimes rare, but in other cases constitute a considerable proportion of the tumor. Targeting tumor cells that achieve therapy resistance through mechanisms that protect normal tissue stem cells has been proposed (such as inhibition of MDR transporters), and tested in phase I clinical trials *(35)*, but has been unsuccessful precisely because it decreases the ED_{50} while failing to improve therapeutic index. It is easy to imagine that many other therapies targeted against shared protective mechanisms (e.g., stem cell niche interactions and detoxifying enzymes) may fail for similar reasons. It is for this reason that we hypothesize that the most fruitful avenue for increasing the true therapeutic index, particularly for metastatic or recurrent cancers, is to study the properties of the cells that constitute minimal residual disease (MRD). Not long ago this would have been a *non sequitur*. Minimal residual disease was inferred from cancer recurrence, but was itself undetectable. Preparative and analytical techniques such as immunomagnetic separation *(36)* and multiparametric flow cytometric cell sorting *(37)* now permit very rare cells to be detected and isolated from the peripheral circulation, or from other accessible metastatic sites. These methods coupled with sensitive and quantitative analytical techniques, such as gene expression array and RT-PCR, in vitro growth assays, and xenotransplantation models, facilitate the systematic study of cells remaining after therapy and comparison to tissue stem cells. It is in this comparison that modalities which drive a therapeutic wedge between MRD and normal tissue stem cells may be discovered.

METHODS

Sample Preparation: Specimens were collected in accordance with a protocol approved by the University of Pittsburgh Internal Review Board. Single cell suspensions were obtained from excised tumors, normal tissue, and metastatic pleural effusions. Tissue was minced and multicellular clumps in tissue and pleural fluid were digested with type I collagenase (4% in RPMI 1640 medium, Sigma Chemicals, St. Louis MO) and disaggregated through 100 mesh stainless steel screens *(38)*. Viable cells were concentrated and separated from erythrocytes and debris on a ficoll/hypaque gradient (Histopaque 1077, Sigma Chemicals).

Staining and Flow Cytometry: To minimize nonspecific binding of fluorochrome-conjugated antibodies pelleted cell suspensions were preincubated for 5 min with neat decomplemented (56°C, 30 min) mouse serum (5 μL) *(39)*. Prior to intracellular cytokeratin staining, cells were stained for surface markers (2 μL each added to the cell pellet, 15–30 min on ice; CD90-biotin (BD, Cat. No. 555594), Streptavidin-ECD (Beckman Coulter, Cat. No. IM3326), ABCG2-APC (R&D Systems, Cat. No. FAB995A), CD117-PC7 (Beckman Coulter, Cat. No. IM3698), CD133-APC (Miltenyi Biotech, Cat. No. 120001241), CD133-PE (Miltenyi Biotech, Cat. No. 130-080-801), HEA-APC (Miltenyi Biotech, Bergisch Gladbach, Germany, Cat. No. 12000420), CD45-APCC7 (BD, Cat. No. 557833)), and fixed with 2% methanol-free formaldehyde. Cells were then permeabilized with 0.1% saponin (Beckman Coulter, Fullerton, CA) in phosphate buffered saline with 0.5% human serum albumin (10 min at room temperature). Permeabilized cells were pelleted by centrifugation at $400 \times g$ for 7 min at room temperature, supernatant was discarded, and cell pellets were incubated with 5 μL of neat mouse serum for 5 min, centrifuged, and decanted. The cell pellet was disaggregated and incubated with 2 μL of anti-pan cytokeratin-FITC (Beckman Coulter, Cat. No. IM2356) for 30 min. Cells pellets were diluted to a cell concentration of 10 million cells/400 μL of staining buffer and DAPI (Sigma Chemicals, St. Louis MO, Cat. D1306) was added to a final concentration of 5 μg/mL.

Eight-color analysis was performed using the 3-laser, 9-color CyAn LX cytometer (Beckman Coulter-Cytomation, Fort Collins, CO). Analysis requiring an ultraviolet laser for the detection of Ho33342 was performed on a 3-laser 8-color Beckman Coulter-Cytomation MoFlo. An effort was made to acquire a total of 5–10 million cells per sample at rates not exceeding 10,000 events/second. The cytometers were calibrated to predetermined photomultiplier target channels prior to each use using SpectrAlign beads (Dako, Cat. No. KO111) and 8-peak Rainbow Calibration Particles (Spherotech, Libertyville, IL, Cat. No. RCP-30-5A). Color compensation matrices were calculated for each staining combination within each experiment using single-stained mouse IgG capture beads (Becton Dickinson, Cat. No. 552843) for each antibody.

Offline compensation and analysis were performed using VenturiOne, an analytical package utilizing scalable parallel processing and designed specifically for multiparameter rare event problems (Applied Cytometry, Dinnington, Sheffield, UK). In all analyses, doublets and clusters were eliminated using forward scatter peak width vs. height as a discriminator. For cell sorting, propidium iodide staining (PI, 10 μg/mL) was used to eliminate nonviable cells. For intracellular staining, DAPI nuclear staining was used to eliminate hypodiploid cells, erythrocytes, and subcellular debris. In most experiments, a hematopoietic lineage cocktail (CD14, CD33, and glycophorin A vs. CD45) was used to eliminate hematopoietic cells.

Simultaneous measurement of the exclusion of Hoechst 33342 and rhodamine 123: Antibody stained suspended tumor cells were incubated simultaneously with Hoechst 33342 (8 μM) plus R123 (0.13 μM) for 90 min at 37°C. Cells were then washed and resuspended in ice cold staining buffer and held at 4°C. Propidium iodide (PI, 10 μg/mL) was added immediately before sample acquisition. All events were gated on PI excluding (live), nonhematopoietic (CD45−) singlets (doublet discrimination based on forward light scatter pulse analysis). In all experiments, a cocktail of MDR inhibitors cyclosporine (5 μM, Novartis) and fumitremorgin (Fumitremorgin C 1 μM, Alexis, Cat. No. ALX-350-127)) was added to a replicate sample at the time of dye addition, as an MDR transporter specificity control.

Immunohistochemical Staining: Immunohistochemistry was performed by using the EnVision™+ Dual Link Kit (Dako). Briefly, 6 μm paraffin sections mounted on glass microscope slides were heated (60°C, 20 min) deparaffinized (3 min washes: xylene × 3, absolute EtOH × 2, 90% EtOH × 1, 75% EtOH × 1, DI H$_2$O × 1) and rinsed twice in wash buffer (Dako). Endogenous Enzyme Block (Dako) was applied for 10 min to quench any endogenous peroxidase. After two washes, the tissue sections were incubated for 60 min in a blocking solution (PBS, 5% goat serum, 0.05% Tween 20) to reduce nonspecific antibody binding. Anti-cytokeratin (1:100 in blocking solution, Dako, cat. No. M0821), anti-CD117 (1:200, Dako, cat. No. A4502), or anti-CD90 (1:50, BD Pharmingen, cat. No. 550402) primary antibodies were layered directly on the sections. N-Universal Negative Control (Dako, cat. No. N1698) was substituted for primary antibody as a negative control. All primary antibodies and controls were incubated for 60 min at room temperature. Tissue sections were washed three times prior to applying horse radish peroxidase-labeled polymer (Dako) for 30 min at room temperature. After two washes in wash buffer, staining was completed by incubating the sections with 3,3′-diaminobenzidine (DAB+) substrate-chromogen for 5–10 min (as determined by microscopic observation). Finally, the sections were washed twice in wash buffer and cell nuclei were stained for 3 min with Hematoxylin (Dako). Sections were washed in DI H$_2$O and sequentially immerged for 1 min in 75% ethanol, 90% ethanol, 100% ethanol and three times in xylene. Slides were mounted in nonaqueous medium (Cytoseal™280, Richard-Allan Scientific) and photographed under brightfield microscopy using a digital camera and software (Spot Insight 2 Meg FW Color Mosaic model 18.2, Diagnostic Instruments, Inc.).

ACKNOWLEDGMENTS

This work was supported by grants BC032981 and BC044784 from the Department of Defense, the Hillman Foundation and the Glimmer of Hope Foundation. Vera Donnenberg is a CDMRP Era of Hope Scholar. The authors thank Ms. Darlene Monlish, Ms. Melanie Pfeifer, Mr. E. Michael Meyer, and Mr. Ludovic Zimmerlin for their expert technical assistance, and Drs. Rodney Landreneau and Shannon Puhalla for providing samples and clinical expertise. We also thank Mr. Peter Nobes and Mr. David Roberts of Applied Cytometry for the opportunity to collaborate on the development of software specifically designed for multiparameter rare event analysis on large datafiles.

REFERENCES

1. Thomas E, Storb R, Clift RA, et al. Bone-marrow transplantation (first of two parts). N Engl J Med 1975;292(16):832–43.
2. Santos GW, Owens AH, Jr. Allogeneic marrow transplants in cyclophosphamide treated mice. Transplant Proc 1969;1(1):44–6.
3. Mathe G, Amiel JL, Schwarzenberg L, Cattan A, Schneider M. Haematopoietic chimera in man after allogenic (homologous) bone-marrow transplantation. (control of the secondary syndrome. Specific tolerance due to the chimerism). Br Med J 1963;2(5373):1633–5.
4. Quastler H. Studies on roentgen death in mice. I. Survival time and dosage. Am J Roentgenol 1945;45:449–56.
5. Mehta J, Powles R, Sirohi B, et al. Impact of cytogenetics on the outcome of autotransplantation for acute myeloid leukemia in first remission: is the benefit of intensive pretransplant therapy limited to patients with good karyotypes? Bone Marrow Transplant 2003;32(2):157–64.
6. Dingli D, Michor F. Successful therapy must eradicate cancer stem cells. Stem Cells 2006;24(12):2603–10.
7. Blazar BR, Orr HT, Arthur DC, Kersey JH, Filipovich AH. Restriction fragment length polymorphisms as markers of engraftment in allogeneic marrow transplantation. Blood 1985;66(6):1436–44.

8. Frei E, 3rd, Elias A, Wheeler C, Richardson P, Hryniuk W. The relationship between high-dose treatment and combination chemotherapy: the concept of summation dose intensity. Clin Cancer Res 1998;4(9):2027–37.

9. Mertens AC. Cause of mortality in 5-year survivors of childhood cancer. Pediatr Blood Cancer 2007;48(7):723–6.

10. Hassett MJ, O'Malley AJ, Pakes JR, Newhouse JP, Earle CC. Frequency and cost of chemotherapy-related serious adverse effects in a population sample of women with breast cancer. J Natl Cancer Inst 2006;98(16):1108–17.

11. Ceelen WP, Morris S, Paraskeva P, Pattyn P. Surgical trauma, minimal residual disease and locoregional cancer recurrence. Cancer Treat Res 2007;134:51–69.

12. Vidal-Vanaclocha F, Mendoza L, Telleria N, et al. Clinical and experimental approaches to the pathophysiology of inter-leukin-18 in cancer progression. Cancer Metastasis Rev 2006;25(3):417–34.

13. Paus R, Cotsarelis G. The biology of hair follicles. N Engl J Med 1999;341(7):491–7.

14. Alonso L, Fuchs E. Stem cells of the skin epithelium. Proc Natl Acad Sci USA 2003;100(Suppl 1):11830–5.

15. Aguirre-Ghiso JA. Models, mechanisms and clinical evidence for cancer dormancy. Nat Rev Cancer 2007;7(11):834–46.

16. Kern SE, Shibata D. The fuzzy math of solid tumor stem cells: a perspective. Cancer Res 2007;67(19):8985–8.

17. Al-Hajj M, Wicha MS, Benito-Hernandez A, Morrison SJ, Clarke MF. Prospective identification of tumorigenic breast cancer cells. Proc Natl Acad Sci USA 2003;100(7):3983–8.

18. Li C, Heidt DG, Dalerba P, et al. Identification of pancreatic cancer stem cells. Cancer Res 2007;67(3):1030–7.

19. O'Brien CA, Pollett A, Gallinger S, Dick JE. A human colon cancer cell capable of initiating tumour growth in immunodeficient mice. Nature 2007;445(7123):106–10.

20. Szotek PP, Pieretti-Vanmarcke R, Masiakos PT, et al. Ovarian cancer side population defines cells with stem cell-like characteristics and Mullerian Inhibiting Substance responsiveness. Proc Natl Acad Sci USA 2006;103(30):11154–9.

21. Singh SK, Clarke ID, Terasaki M, et al. Identification of a cancer stem cell in human brain tumors. Cancer Res 2003;63(18):5821–8.

22. Dirks PB. Cancer: stem cells and brain tumours. Nature 2006;444(7120):687–8.

23. Patrawala L, Calhoun-Davis T, Schneider-Broussard R, Tang DG. Hierarchical organization of prostate cancer cells in xenograft tumors: the CD44+alpha2beta1+ cell population is enriched in tumor-initiating cells. Cancer Res 2007;67(14):6796–805.

24. Donnenberg VS, Luketich JD, Landreneau RJ, DeLoia JA, Basse P, Donnenberg AD. Tumorigenic epithelial stem cells and their normal counterparts. Ernst Schering Found Symp Proc 2006;5:245–63.

25. Giangreco A, Shen H, Reynolds SD, Stripp BR. Molecular phenotype of airway side population cells. Am J Physiol Lung Cell Mol Physiol 2004;286(4):L624–30.

26. Cereghini S, Yaniv M, Cortese R. Hepatocyte dedifferentiation and extinction is accompanied by a block in the synthesis of mRNA coding for the transcription factor HNF1/LFB1. Embo J 1990;9(7):2257–63.

27. Rulifson IC, Karnik SK, Heiser PW, et al. Wnt signaling regulates pancreatic beta cell proliferation. Proc Natl Acad Sci USA 2007;104(15):6247–52.

28. Huntly BJ, Gilliland DG. Cancer biology: summing up cancer stem cells. Nature 2005;435(7046):1169–70.

29. Pierce GB, Speers WC. Tumors as caricatures of the process of tissue renewal: prospects for therapy by directing differentiation. Cancer Res 1988;48(8):1996–2004.

30. Bertoncello I, Williams B. Hematopoietic stem cell characterization by Hoechst 33342 and rhodamine 123 staining. Methods Mol Biol 2004;263:181–200.

31. Rege TA, Hagood JS. Thy-1 as a regulator of cell-cell and cell-matrix interactions in axon regeneration, apoptosis, adhesion, migration, cancer, and fibrosis. Faseb J 2006;20(8):1045–54.

32. Chaudhary PM, Roninson IB. Expression and activity of P-glycoprotein, a multidrug efflux pump, in human hematopoietic stem cells. Cell 1991;66(1):85–94.

33. Zhou S, Zong Y, Lu T, Sorrentino BP. Hematopoietic cells from mice that are deficient in both Bcrp1/Abcg2 and Mdr1a/1b develop normally but are sensitized to mitoxantrone. Biotechniques 2003;35(6):1248–52.

34. Singer TS, Sulkes A, Biran S. Pleural effusion in breast cancer: influence upon clinical course and survival. Chemioterapia 1986;5(1):66–9.

35. Lum BL, Fisher GA, Brophy NA, et al. Clinical trials of modulation of multidrug resistance. Pharmacokinetic and pharmacodynamic considerations. Cancer 1993;72(11 Suppl):3502–14.

36. O'Hara SM, Moreno JG, Zweitzig DR, Gross S, Gomella LG, Terstappen LW. Multigene reverse transcription-PCR profiling of circulating tumor cells in hormone-refractory prostate cancer. Clin Chem 2004;50(5):826–35.

37. Donnenberg AD, Donnenberg VS. Rare-event analysis in flow cytometry. Clin Lab Med 2007;27(3):627–52, viii.

38. Elder E, Whiteside, TL. Processing of Tumors for Vaccine and/or Tumor Infiltrating Lymphocytes. In: Rose N, Conway de, Macario, E, Fahey, JL, Friedman, H, Prnn, GM, eds. Manual of Clinical Laboratory Immunology, 4th Edition: American Society for Microbiology; 1992:817–9.

39. Donnenberg VS, Landreneau RJ, Donnenberg AD. Tumorigenic stem and progenitor cells: implications for the therapeutic index of anti-cancer agents. J Control Release 2007;122(3):385–91.

Index